Rhinology and Endoscopic Skull Base Surgery

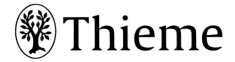

Rhinology and Endoscopic Skull Base Surgery

Series Editors

Professor Emeritus Milind V. Kirtane, M.S. (ENT)
Seth G. S. Medical College & KEM Hospital
P. D. Hinduja National Hospital & Research Centre
Breach Candy Hospital
Prince Ali Khan Hospital
Saifee Hospital
Mumbai, India

Chris E. de Souza, M.S., D.O.R.L., D.N.B., F.A.C.S.
ENT Consultant
Lilavati Hospital
Holy Family Hospital
Holy Spirit Hospital
Tata Memorial Hospital
Mumbai, India

Visiting Assistant Professor
Department of Otoloaryngology
SUNY Brooklyn, New York, USA
Department of Otolaryngology
LSUHSC, Shreveport, Louisiana, USA

Volume Editors

Anand K. Devaiah, M.D., F.A.C.S.
Associate Professor
Department of Otolaryngology - Head and Neck Surgery
Department of Neurological Surgery
Department of Ophthalmology
Boston University School of Medicine
Boston Medical Center, Massachusetts, USA

Bradley F. Marple, M.D., F.A.A.O.A.
Professor and Vice Chair Department of Otolaryngology
University of Texas Southwestern Medical Center
Dallas, Texas, USA

Associate Dean for Graduate Medical Education
University of Texas Southwestern Medical Center
Dallas, Texas, USA

Thieme Medical and Scientific Publishers Private Limited
A-12, Second Floor, Sector - 2
Noida, Uttar Pradesh - 201 301, India
Email: customerservice@thieme.in
www.thieme.com

Thieme
Delhi • Stuttgart • New York

Thieme Medical and Scientific Publishers Private Limited
A-12, Second Floor, Sector - 2
Noida, Uttar Pradesh - 201 301, India

Managing Editor: Sangeeta P.C.
Production Editor: Sangeeta Gaur
National Sales and Marketing Director: Harish Singh Bora
Chief Executive Officer: Ajit Kohli

Rhinology and Endoscopic Skull Base Surgery/[edited by] Anand K. Devaiah and Bradley F. Marple.

Includes bibliographical references and index.

ISBN 978-93-82076-01-8

Devaiah, Anand K. II Marple, Bradley F.

Important note: Medical knowledge is ever changing. As new research and clinical experience broaden our knowledge, changes in treatment and drug therapy may be required. The authors and editors of the material herein have consulted sources believed to be reliable in their efforts to provide information that is complete and in accord with the standards accepted at the time of publication. However, in view of the possibility human error by the authors, editors, or publishers of the work herein or changes in medical knowledge, neither the authors, editors, nor publishers, nor any other party who has been involved in the preparation of this work, warrants that the information contained herein is in every respect accurate or complete, and they are not responsible for any errors or omissions or for the results obtained from use of such information. Readers are encouraged to confirm the information contained herein with other sources. For example, readers are advice to check the product information sheet included in the package of each drug they plan to administer to be certain that the information contained in this publication is accurate and that changes have not been made in the recommended dose or in the contraindications for administration. This recommendation is of particular importance in connection with new or infrequently used drugs. Some of the product names, patents, and registered designs referred to in this book are in fact registered trademarks or proprietary names even though specific reference to this fact is not always made in the text. Therefore, the appearance of a name without designation as proprietary is not to be construed as a representation by the publishers that it is in the public domain.

5 4 3 2 1

ISBN: 978-93-82076-01-8
eISBN: 978-93-82076-07-0

Rhinology and Endoscopic Skull Base Surgery
Published by Thieme Medical and Scientific Publishers Private Limited
A-12, Second Floor, Sector - 2, Noida, Uttar Pradesh - 201 301, India
Email: customerservice@thieme.in
www.thieme.com
Printer: Gopsons Papers Limited, Noida

Foreword

This text comes at a time when important leaps in patient care are occurring in endoscopic skull base surgery and rhinology. These disciplines encompass some of the most exciting areas of research, collaboration, and innovation. While team-based care is in varying states of evolution for areas of medicine, there are not many areas where one sees such a rich and rapid convergence of diverse multidisciplinary care and coordination. Similarly, when viewing endoscopic skull base surgery and rhinology in an integrated way, we strive to create a foundation for learning, discussion, and development. It is our sincere hope that residents, fellows, practitioners, and patients will find this text a necessary reference.

This text represents a truly international effort, with contributors from around the globe. This is most fitting, given that innovation in endoscopic skull base surgery and rhinology is occurring on a worldwide scale, and it is the global community of patients who we strive to help.

The many individuals who have contributed to this text cannot be thanked enough for giving their time and expertise. Indeed, the editors and authors for the entire series of texts are to be congratulated on a world-class comprehensive reference. The series editors, Drs. Kirtane and de Souza, have done an extraordinary job in putting this entire project together.

It is our delight and privilege to present this book to the reader, and hope that it serves you well in your pursuit of knowledge and innovative patient care.

Anand K. Devaiah, M.D., F.A.C.S.
Bradley F. Marple, M.D., F.A.A.O.A.

Acknowledgments

It is impossible to acknowledge everyone I need to acknowledge, but a few individuals bear mention in the context of this text.

My many mentors in training, particularly Drs. Larry Hoover, Doug Girod, and Terry Tsue, gave me opportunities to learn the foundations and facets of endoscopic skull base surgery, open skull base surgery, and rhinology. This happened at a time when many of the concepts, we now take for granted, were still being envisioned by them and others around the globe. My partners in clinical care and research have been wonderful collaborators, both locally and worldwide. This also includes the many exceptional residents who have been part of our program and care team for my patients over the years. Their questions of "how" and "why" have been a great source of intellectual curiosity.

The patients and their families who put their trust in me cannot be thanked enough. It is ultimately because and for them that this text exists. They have been my most important teachers.

No acknowledgment would be complete without recognizing the love and support from my wife, Manju; my boys, Jayanth and Deven; and my parents, Kulachandra and Vani.

Anand K. Devaiah, M.D., F.A.C.S.

Otolaryngology is, and has always been, a close community. Those who train in our profession experience a unique opportunity to not only read about its innovators but also learn directly from them. This way we are all linked by a common professional heritage.

I feel fortunate to have undertaken my otolaryngology training at a time when endoscopic techniques were first introduced in the United States. The inherent challenge of dim light sources, poor hemostasis, lack of equipment, and ill-defined procedures served to stimulate innovation, development, and opportunity. This, in turn, provided the foundation for a paradigm shift that has become contemporary rhinology and endoscopic skull base surgery.

With this in mind, I would like to take this opportunity to acknowledge a few of the many individuals who have not only contributed to my personal growth and development but also meaningfully contributed to the field of Rhinology. Drs. Steve Schaefer and Lanny Close taught me the early techniques of ESS, but more importantly instilled a drive to develop and move those same techniques forward. Role models, such as Drs. Peter Roland, Scott Manning, and Matthew Ryan, taught me the value of critical thinking and the importance of maintaining just a hint of skepticism. Richard Mabry, M.D., deserves special recognition for continually reminding me that as a Rhinologist it is critical to consider the entire patient.

Bradley F. Marple, M.D., F.A.A.O.A.

A Note from Series Editors

Rhinology as a separate scientific discipline has gained credence with the development of endoscope, allowing excellent visualization of structures which was not possible earlier. External approaches to the nasal cavity that had external incisions have now become endoscopic surgeries with no disfiguring external incisions. This has all been possible because of the endoscope, marvelous optics, robotics and navigation systems, and newer generations of CT scans and MRIs. Rhinology is finally coming into its own. Debates still rage. However, as time passes by and patients are closely followed up, it will become clear what paths we need to follow to treat effectively and competently.

Otology as a science has predated that of rhinology. This is evidenced as it was only in 2004 that Dr. Linda Buck and Dr. Richard Axel were awarded the Nobel Prize for their seminal work on olfaction. The Nobel Prize for the physiology of hearing was given almost 45 years ago. The technology and expertise to treat nasal and paranasal problems has evolved very quickly. There are now many centers that treat rhinologic problems and have expanded their applications to include the anterior skull base. This has caused closer cooperation between rhinologists and neurosurgeons. This is an exciting new field. Technology, optics, and dedicated training in this area has led to the development and refining of Rhinology not only as a science but also as an art as well.

The editors and authors of this excellent book are well aware that we are on a continuum. All efforts of this book are directed to smoothing the path of rhinologists by providing current, easy to understand, and up-to-date information to the reader. This book will help prepare the rhinologist well so that when a patient presents in the office with a rhinologic complaint the reader of this book will be better prepared to understand how to go about giving expert treatment. For this we thank the editors and authors of this book.

Milind V. Kirtane, M.S.
Chris E. de Souza, M.S., D.O.R.L., D.N.B., F.A.C.S.

Introduction

Rhinology is one of the most dynamic and exciting subspecialties within Otorhinolaryngology—head and neck surgery. Driving forces have been technological advances in endoscopic instrumentation and image-guided navigation, improved understanding of endoscopic anatomy, parallel advancements in related surgical disciplines, and a spirit of collaboration. There has been a rapid evolution of surgical techniques with expansion to the skull base, orbit, and beyond.

Rapid change brings new challenges. How do rhinologists keep abreast of the latest medical and surgical advances? There is a need to incorporate best practices into decision making and not simply follow the latest fad. The authors in this book are all experts in their respective topics and offer medical and surgical solutions based on a wealth of clinical experience as well as a balanced sense of current practices. Rhinologic surgery does not exist in isolation. The rhinologic surgeon must be mindful of the anatomical and medical foundations of rhinology so that proper decisions are made and nonsurgical alternatives are considered. It follows that good surgical outcomes are dependent on a holistic approach to management and surgical intervention is just one aspect of patient care. Increasingly, care is provided by a multidisciplinary team and the rhinologic surgeon must be conversant with divergent practices and philosophies.

In this volume, Drs. Devaiah and Marple have succeeded in assembling a premier list of international authors who are all thought leaders in rhinology. The content is logically divided into three sections: *Foundations of Rhinology and Endoscopic Skull Base Surgery*, *Rhinology and Paranasal Sinus Surgery*, and *Endoscopic Skull Base Surgery and Related Skull Base Surgery*. These chapters provide a comprehensive snapshot of the current state of the art and offer hints of future directions.

Carl H. Snyderman, M.D., M.B.A.

Contributors

Nithin D. Adappa, M.D.
Division of Rhinology and Skull Base Surgery
Department of Otorhinolaryngology – Head and Neck
Surgery
Hospital of the University of Pennsylvania
Philadelphia, Pennsylvania, USA

Vijay K. Anand, M.D.
Department of Otolaryngology – Head and Neck Surgery
Weill Cornell Medical Center
New York, New York, USA

Ashwin Ananth
Department of Otolaryngology Head and Neck Surgery
University of Kansas School of Medicine
Kansas City, Kansas, USA

Michael S. Benninger, M.D.
Head and Neck Institute
The Cleveland Clinic
Cleveland, Ohio, USA

Department of Surgery
Lerner College of Medicine
Case Western Reserve University
Cleveland, Ohio, USA

Ricardo L. Carrau, M.D., F.A.C.S.
Department of Otolaryngology – Head and Neck Surgery
Skull Base Surgery Program
The Ohio State University Medical Center
Columbus, Ohio, USA

Rakesh K. Chandra, M.D.
Department of Otolaryngology – Head and Neck Surgery
Northwestern University Feinberg School of Medicine
Chicago, Illinois, USA

Philip G. Chen, M.D.
Department of Otolaryngology – Head and Neck Surgery
University of Virginia
Charlottesville, Virginia, USA

Alexander G. Chiu, M.D.
Division of Otolaryngology – Head and Neck Surgery
Department of Surgery
University of Arizona
Tucson, Arizona, USA

Daniel T. T. Chua, M.D.
Comprehensive Oncology Centre
Hong Kong Sanatorium and Hospital
Happy Valley, Hong Kong, China

Noam A. Cohen, M.D., Ph.D.
Department of Otorhinolaryngology – Head and Neck Surgery
Philadelphia Veterans Affairs Medical Center
University of Pennsylvania
Philadelphia, Pennsylvania, USA

Anand K. Devaiah, M.D., F.A.C.S
Department of Otolaryngology - Head and Neck Surgery
Department of Neurological Surgery
Department of Ophthalmology
Boston University School of Medicine
Boston Medical Center
Boston, Massachusetts, USA

Angela M. Donaldson, M.D.
Department of Otolaryngology – Head and Neck Surgery
University of Cincinnati Medical Center
Cincinnati, Ohio, USA

Wolfgang Draf, M.D., Ph.D., F.R.C.S. (Ed)
Department of Ear, Nose and Throat Diseases, Head and
Neck Surgery
International Neuroscience Institute
Hannover, Germany

Ivan H. El-Sayed, M.D., F.A.C.S.
Department of Otolaryngology – Head and Neck Surgery
Center for Minimally Invasive Skull Base Surgery
University California San Francisco
San Francisco, California, USA

Juan C. Fernandez-Miranda, M.D.
Department of Neurological Surgery
University of Pittsburgh School of Medicine
Pittsburgh, Pennsylvania, USA

Elisa N. Flower, M.D.
Division of Neuroradiology
Department of Radiology
Boston Medical Center
Boston University School of Medicine
Boston, Massachusetts, USA

Paul A. Gardner, M.D.
Department of Neurological Surgery
University of Pittsburgh School of Medicine
Pittsburgh, Pennsylvania, USA

Andrew N. Goldberg, M.D., M.S.C.E., F.A.C.S.
Division of Rhinology and Sinus Surgery
Departments of Otolaryngology – Head and Neck Surgery
and Neurological Surgery
University of California, San Francisco
San Francisco, California, USA

Mitchell Ray Gore, M.D., Ph.D.
Greensboro Ear, Nose, and Throat Associates
Greensboro, North Carolina, USA

Satish Govindaraj, M.D., F.A.C.S.
Department of Otolaryngology – Head and Neck Surgery
Icahn School of Medicine at Mount Sinai
New York, New York, USA

Timothy Haffey, M.D.
Department of Otolaryngology
Head and Neck Institute
Cleveland Clinic Foundation
Cleveland, Ohio, USA

Brendan C. Hanna, M.B.B.Ch., Ph.D., F.R.C.S.I.
Department of Otolaryngology – Head and Neck Surgery
The Queen Elizabeth Hospital
Adelaide, South Australia, Australia

Ehab Y. Hanna, M.D., F.A.C.S.
Departments of Head and Neck Surgery and Neurosurgery
MD Anderson Cancer Center
The University of Texas
Houston, Texas, USA

Eric H. Holbrook, M.D.
Department of Otology and Laryngology
Harvard Medical School
Massachusetts Eye and Ear Infirmary
Boston, Massachusetts, USA

F. Christopher Holsinger, M.D., F.A.C.S.
Department of Head and Neck Surgery
Stanford University
Stanford, California, USA

Larry A. Hoover, M.D., F.A.C.S
Department of Otolaryngology – Head and Neck Surgery
The University of Kansas School of Medicine
Kansas City, Kansas, USA

David W. Kennedy, M.D., F.A.C.S., F.R.C.S.I.
Department of Otorhinolaryngology – Head and Neck Surgery
Perelman School of Medicine
University of Pennsylvania
Philadelphia, Pennsylvania, USA

Eleanor Pitz Kiell, M.D.
Department of Otolaryngology
Wake Forest University Baptist Medical Center
Winston Salem, North Carolina, USA

Nataliya Kovalchuk, Ph.D.
Department of Radiation Oncology
Boston Medical Center
Boston, Massachusetts, USA
Harvard School of Medicine
Boston, Massachusetts, USA

Greg A. Krempl, M.D., F.A.C.S.
Department of Otorhinolaryngology
University of Oklahoma Health Sciences Center
Oklahoma City, Oklahoma, USA

John M. Lee, M.D., F.R.C.S.C., M.Sc.
Department of Otolaryngology – Head and Neck Surgery
St. Michael's Hospital
University of Toronto
Toronto, Ontario, Canada

Paul A. Levine, M.D.
Department of Otolaryngology – Head and Neck Surgery
University of Virginia School of Medicine
Charlottesville, Virginia, USA

Larry G. Linson, D.O.
Department of Otolaryngology
Ohio University College of Osteopathic Medicine
Columbus, Ohio, USA

Rodney Lusk, M.D.
ENT Institute
Boys Town National Research Hospital
Omaha, Nebraska, USA

Elizabeth Mahoney Davis, M.D., F.A.C.S., F.A.A.O.A.
Department of Otolaryngology – Head and Neck Surgery
Boston University Medical Center
Boston, Massachusetts, USA

Bradley F. Marple, M.D., F.A.A.O.A.
Department of Otolaryngology – Head and Neck Surgery
University of Texas Southwestern Medical Center
Dallas, Texas, USA
Graduate Medical Education University of Texas
Southwestern Medical Center
Dallas, Texas, USA

Edward D. McCoul, M.D., M.P.H.
Department of Otolaryngology – Head and Neck Surgery
Weill Cornell Medical Center
New York, New York, USA

Colby G. McLaurin, M.D.
Department of Otorhinolaryngology
The University of Oklahoma Health Sciences Center
Oklahoma City, Oklahoma, USA

Ralph Metson, M.D.
Department of Otology and Laryngology
Harvard Medical School
Boston, Massachusetts, USA

James Whit Mims, M.D.
Department of Otolaryngology
Wake Forest University School of Medicine
Winston Salem, North Carolina, USA

Amir Minovi, M.D.
Department of Otorhinolaryngology
St. Elisabeth Hospital
Ruhr University Bochum
Bochum, Germany

Candace A. Mitchell, M.D.
Department of Otolaryngology – Head and Neck Surgery
University of North Carolina School of Medicine
Chapel Hill, North Carolina, USA

Rohini N. Nadgir, M.D.
Department of Radiology
Boston Medical Center
Boston University School of Medicine
Boston, Massachusetts, USA

A. Omer Nawaz, M.S., D.A.B.R.
Department of Radiation Oncology
Boston Medical Center
Boston University School of Medicine
Boston, Massachusetts, USA
Paoli Hospital Cancer Center
Main Line Health Systems
Paoli, Pennsylvania, USA

Bradley A. Otto, M.D.
Department of Otolaryngology – Head and Neck Surgery
The Ohio State University
Columbus, Ohio, USA

Stephen S. Park, M.D.
Division of Facial Plastic Surgery
Department of Otolaryngology – Head and Neck Surgery
University of Virginia Health System
Charlottesville, Virginia, USA

Aaron N. Pearlman, M.D.
Department of Otolaryngology – Head and Neck Surgery
New York Presbyterian Hospital
Weill Cornell Medical College
New York, New York, USA

Michael P. Platt, M.D.
Department of Otolaryngology – Head and Neck Surgery
Boston University School of Medicine
Boston, Massachusetts, USA

Steven D. Pletcher, M.D.
Department of Otolaryngology – Head and Neck Surgery
University of California, San Francisco
San Francisco, California, USA

Rosser Kennedy Powitzky, M.D.
Division of Otolaryngology
Texas A&M Health Sciences Center
Scott & White Health Systems
Temple, Texas, USA

Daniel M. Prevedello, M.D.
Department of Neurosurgery
The Ohio State University
Columbus, Ohio, USA

Alkis J. Psaltis, M.D., Ph.D., F.R.A.C.S.
Division of Rhinology and Skull Base
Department of Otolaryngology – Head and Neck Surgery
Medical University of South Carolina
Charleston, South Carolina, USA

Paul B. Romesser, M.D.
Department of Radiation Oncology
Memorial Sloan-Kettering Cancer Center
New York, New York, USA

Austin S. Rose, M.D.
Division of Pediatric Otolaryngology – Rhinology, Allergy and Sinus Surgery
Department of Otolaryngology – Head and Neck Surgery
University of North Carolina School of Medicine
Chapel Hill, North Carolina, USA

Osamu Sakai, M.D., Ph.D.
Department of Radiology
Boston Medical Center
Boston University School of Medicine
Boston, Massachusetts, USA

Rodney J. Schlosser, M.D.
Ralph H. Johnson VA Medical Center
Charleston, South Carolina, USA
Division of Rhinology
Department of Otolaryngology – Head and Neck Surgery
Medical University of South Carolina
Charleston, South Carolina, USA

Brent A. Senior, M.D., F.A.C.S, F.A.R.S.
Division of Rhinology, Allergy, and Endoscopic Skull Base Surgery
Department of Otolaryngology – Head and Neck Surgery
University of North Carolina
Chapel Hill, North Carolina, USA

David C. Shonka, Jr., M.D.
Department of Otolaryngology – Head and Neck Surgery
University of Virginia School of Medicine
Charlottesville, Virginia, USA

Anthony G. Del Signore, Pharm.D., M.D.
Department of Otolaryngology – Head and Neck Surgery
Mount Sinai School of Medicine
New York, New York, USA

Raj Sindwani, M.D., F.A.C.S., F.R.C.S.(C)
Department of Rhinology, Sinus and Skull Base Surgery
Head and Neck Institute
Cleveland Clinic Foundation
Cleveland, Ohio, USA

Stephanie Shintani Smith, M.D.
Department of Otolaryngology – Head and Neck Surgery
Northwestern University Feinberg School of Medicine
Chicago, Illinois, USA

Carl H. Snyderman, M.D., M.B.A.
Departments of Otolaryngology and Neurological Surgery
University of Pittsburgh School of Medicine
Pittsburgh, Pennsylvania, USA

Zachary M. Soler, M.D., M.Sc.
Department of Otolaryngology – Head and Neck Surgery
Medical University of South Carolina
Charleston, South Carolina, USA

Nicholas C. Sorrel, M.D.
Department of Otorhinolaryngology
University of Texas Medical Center
Houston, Texas, USA

James A. Stankiewicz, M.D.
Department of Head and Neck Surgery
Stritch School of Medicine
Loyola University
Maywood, Illinois, USA

Michael G. Stewart, M.D., M.P.H.
Department of Otolaryngology – Head and Neck Surgery
New York Presbyterian Hospital
Weill Cornell Medical College
New York, New York, USA

Jonathan Y. Ting, M.D.
Department of Otology and Laryngology
Harvard Medical School
Boston, Massachusetts, USA

Minh Tam Truong, M.D.
Department of Radiation Oncology
Boston University School of Medicine
Boston, Massachusetts, USA
Department of Radiation Oncology
Boston Medical Center
Boston, Massachusetts, USA

Craig R. Villari, M.D.
Department of Otolaryngology
Emory University
Atlanta, Georgia, USA

Patrick C. Walz, M.D.
Department of Otolaryngology – Head and Neck Surgery
The Ohio State University Medical Center
Columbus, Ohio, USA

Eric W. Wang, M.D.
Department of Otolaryngology
University of Pittsburgh School of Medicine
The Eye and Ear Institute
Pittsburgh, Pennsylvania, USA

William I. Wei, F.R.C.S., F.R.C.S.E., F.A.C.S. (Hon.)
Department of Surgery
Li Shu Pui ENT Head and Neck Surgery Centre
Hong Kong Sanatorium and Hospital
Happy Valley, Hong Kong, China

Sarah K. Wise, M.D.
Department of Otolaryngology
Emory University
Atlanta, Georgia, USA

Troy D. Woodard, M.D.
Department of Otolaryngology
Cleveland Clinic Foundation
Head and Neck Institute
Cleveland, Ohio, USA

Peter-John Wormald, M.D., F.R.A.C.S., F.C.S. (SA), F.R.C.S. (Ed.), M.B.Ch.B.
Department of Otolaryngology – Head and Neck Surgery
University of Adelaide
Adelaide, South Australia, Australia

Arthur William Wu, M.D.
Division of Endoscopic Sinus and Skull Base Surgery
Department of Otolaryngology – Head and Neck Surgery
Cedars-Sinai Medical Center
Los Angeles, California, USA

Bharat B. Yarlagadda, M.D.
Department of Otolaryngology – Head and Neck Surgery
Boston Medical Center
Boston University School of Medicine
Boston, Massachusetts, USA

Adam M. Zanation, M.D.
Department of Otolaryngology – Head and Neck Surgery
University of North Carolina School of Medicine
University of North Carolina at Chapel Hill
Chapel Hill, North Carolina, USA

Lee A. Zimmer, M.D., Ph.D.
Department of Otolaryngology – Head and Neck Surgery
University of Cincinnati College of Medicine
Cincinnati, Ohio, USA

Table of Contents

SECTION I: Foundations of Rhinology and Endoscopic Skull Base Surgery

1 Embryology of the Nose and Paranasal Sinuses

Michael P. Platt

All surgeons strive for mastery of surgical anatomy that takes its origin in embryological developments. Successful performance of operative procedures is dependent on a keen awareness of the relevant anatomical structures and their relationships within the operative field. Embryology is the basis for understanding anatomy, and thus is of great importance to those who undertake surgical endeavors. Within the nose and paranasal sinuses, surgeons often use embryological principles to obtain successful outcomes or avoid deleterious complications. Additionally, clinical pathology resulting from abnormal embryological development is seen within the sinuses affected with diseases such as choanal atresia, nasal dermoid tumors, and congenital encephaloceles. This chapter provides an overview of sinonasal embryology with clinically relevant applications to head and neck surgeons.

Embryological Development

Nose, Septum, and Nasal Cavity

The nose and nasal cavities develop on the face between the 4th and 10th week of fetal development.[1,2] The facial structures are formed by a fusion of five prominences: a single frontonasal process, paired maxillary prominences, and paired mandibular prominences (**Fig. 1.1**). These prominences develop under the stimulation of neural crest cells that migrate from the dorsal embryo onto the face. It is this neural crest mesenchyme that establishes the structural framework (cartilage and bone) of the nose and sinuses, and directs development of the sinonasal structures. The internal mesenchyme is covered by an ectoderm lining, which provides a mature respiratory mucosal interface that lines the nasal and sinus passages.

The midline frontonasal process gives rise to two nasal placodes inferiorly. Under the stimulus of neural crest cells, the nasal cavity begins as a pit at the center of each placode. The placodes develop into horseshoe-shaped medial and lateral processes, which resemble the nasal alar cartilages. As the two parallel pits in the nasal placode deepen toward the nasopharynx, a primitive choana is formed when the burrowing placodes fuse with the endoderm-lined posterior pharyngeal walls. This junction of endoderm and ectoderm has clinical significance as the bounds of the ectoderm-derived "Schneiderian membrane," from which inverted papillomas arise. An oronasal membrane, which separates these primitive nasal cavities from the oral cavity, ruptures to allow for a temporary continuous oronasal cavity. Later migration of the palatal shelves forms a permanent separation of the oral and nasal cavities with completion of the true choana. Cleft palates are seen as a failure of palatal shelf migration to separate the oral and nasal cavities.[2]

The frontonasal process forms a mesoderm-lined projection that is the basis for the nasal septum. Neural crest mesenchyme migrates posteriorly to form the quadrangular cartilage, vomer, and perpendicular plate of the ethmoid. In the sixth week, growth of the medial nasal processes and maxillary processes contact each other to form the columella, philtrum, and upper lip, whereas the lateral nasal processes invaginate to form the lacrimal duct. By 10 weeks of gestation, the cartilaginous and bony frameworks for the facial, nasal, and septal structures are in place.[1,2]

Nasal Turbinates and Paranasal Sinuses

As the nasal cavity and septum develop, a series of ridges on the lateral nasal wall called turbinals (ethmoturbinals and maxilloturbinals) coalesce into three or four main projections from which the sinus cavities and nasal turbinates develop.[3] The tremendous variation in sinus anatomy, complexity of the ethmoid labyrinth, and limitations in embryological study results in multiple opinions regarding paranasal sinus development with varying numbers of turbinals and turbinal origin of the sinonasal structures.[3–6] Neural crest mesenchyme migration provides a cartilaginous framework that later ossifies into bone of the turbinates and sinus septations. As these projections and invaginations extend from the rudimentary nasal cavity, ectoderm-derived mucosa provides the lining of the natural mucociliary

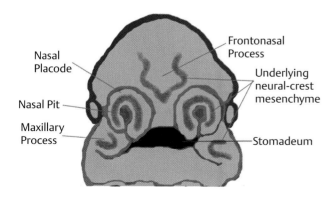

Figure 1.1 The developing human embryo. Neural crest mesenchyme directs development of the facial and sinonasal structures.

Nasal Placode

Nasal Pit

Maxillary Process

Frontonasal Process

Underlying neural-crest mesenchyme

Stomadeum

sinonasal drainage pathways. The outgrowth of sinus cavities from a common nasal cavity establish the pattern of mucociliary clearance that determines how sinus secretions are cleared into the diverticular spaces around the turbinals (inferior, middle, and superior meatii), and coalesce to a single pathway in the nasopharynx.

The first or anterior projection (ethmoturbinal) in the nasal cavity forms the agger nasi cells and the uncinate process. The space between this projection becomes the ethmoid infundibulum, hiatus semilunaris, and frontal recess. The frontal sinus develops as an extension of the first ethmoturbinal in an anterosuperior direction.[3] Pneumatization of the frontal sinus within the frontal bone does not begin until age 2 and is completed during adolescence.

The superior projections (ethmoturbinals) in the nasal cavity form the middle and superior turbinates. A lateral mass of mesenchyme from the superior ethmoturbinal forms the remaining ethmoid air cells adjacent to the superior and middle turbinates. The ethmoid air cells continue to develop through secondary invaginations resulting in a complex network of sinuses that have drainage pathways for the anterior and posterior ethmoid sinuses on either side of the basal lamella.

An inferior projection (maxilloturbinal) forms the inferior turbinate, inferior meatus, and the maxillary sinus. The middle meatus is established as an area between the projections from the anterior and inferior turbinals to drain the maxillary, anterior ethmoid, and frontal sinuses. The inferior aspect of the invagination of the lateral nasal process, forms which the nasolacrimal duct, is located below the inferior maxilloturbinal in the region known as the inferior meatus.

The sphenoid sinus develops from invagination of nasal mucosa in the ethmoid recess into the sphenoid cartilage.[5] A pouch forms within the cartilage, which later ossifies and continues to pneumatize through childhood until around the age of 12 when the sphenoid is fully developed.

The olfactory placode originates from neural ectoderm. These intracranial cells are stimulated by nasal mesenchymal cells to enter the nasal cavity at the area of the cribriform plate and develop into the olfactory mucosa that lines the superior nasal cavity. Olfactory neuroepithelial development failure is commonly seen with congenital anosmia.

Variations of Sinus Development

Anatomical variations that occur during normal sinus embryogenesis have clinical implications in the treatment of sinus disease. The pattern of sinus aeration demonstrates wide variability. Identification of specific embryological variant entities will allow for optimal surgical treatment of sinus disease.

Sinus Aplasia/Hypoplasia

Sinus development and pneumatization can vary greatly among individuals and even between the sides of the same

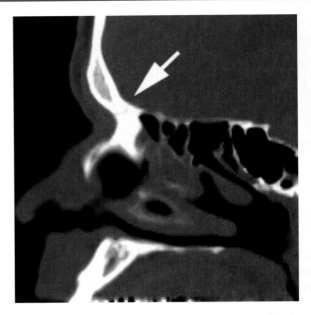

Figure 1.2 Aplasia of the frontal sinus (arrow) is an embryological variant where the frontal sinus fails to develop.

person. Sinus pneumatization can be limited by inflammatory conditions or by other unknown factors. Hypoplasia of the sinuses is often seen in inflammatory sinus diseases, including cystic fibrosis and primary ciliarydyskinesia, where there is active inflammation during the teenage period of sinus development. Osteitis and osteoneogenesis are often seen in the areas of limited pneumatization.

Sinus aplasia or hypoplasia can occur in the frontal, maxillary, or sphenoid sinuses (**Fig. 1.2**). It remains unknown why one or more sinuses do not develop in an otherwise healthy individual. There is no known consequence to having an aplastic or hypoplastic sinus; however, identification of an aplastic or hypoplastic sinus is of extreme importance when planning for surgical entry into the sinuses. Failure to recognize a hypoplastic maxillary sinus can result in orbital entry during uncinectomy or sinus probing. Failure to recognize an aplastic frontal sinus during attempted frontal sinusotomy can result in penetration of the skull base with cerebrospinal fluid (CSF) leak and further intracranial injury.

Ethmoid Sinus

Numerous variations exist within the ethmoid sinuses because of their complex anatomy and higher number of septations. It is important to recognize these anatomical variants when performing sinus surgery, as failure to do so can result in complication or suboptimal outcome.

A posterior ethmoid cell that overlies the sphenoid sinus and has contact with the optic nerve is known as Onodi cell (**Fig. 1.3**). If this variant is not recognized on preoperative imaging and surgical dissection proceeds in the posterolateral ethmoid, injury to the optic nerve may occur. An infraorbital ethmoid cell, known as Haller cell, may narrow the natural maxillary sinus drainage pathway. Aeration of the middle

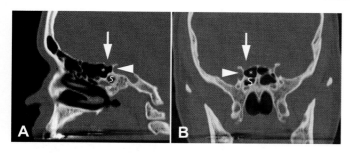

Figure 1.3 An Onodi cell (*), seen on (A) sagittal and (B) coronal computed tomography scans, is an embryological variant in the posterior ethmoid sinus. The optic nerve (arrow) and carotid artery (arrowhead) are found adjacent to the Onodi cell instead of the sphenoid sinus(S).

turbinate, a concha bullosa, can similarly narrow the middle meatus region. A low-lying cribriform plate (Keros type 3) can place the patient at increased risk for CSF leak during surgery. Congenital absence of a portion of the lamina papyracea can result in focal dehiscence of orbital contents. If this entity is not recognized at the time of ethmoidectomy, orbital injury may ensue.

A final anatomical variant seen within the ethmoid sinus is with the location of the anterior ethmoid artery. This artery traverses the skull base between the orbit and the anterior cranial fossa. In a small subset of patients, this artery is surrounded by ethmoid air cells and not within the bone of the skull base. In such a scenario, care must be taken during frontal sinusitis to not transect the artery.

Frontal Sinus

Development of the frontal sinus has several anatomical variants. Massive pneumatization of the frontal sinuses, or pneumosinus frontalis dilitans, is an infrequent variant that can have aesthetic implication. A supraorbital ethmoid cell can extend into the frontal recess and frontal sinus creating a narrow frontal drainage pathway. A frontal cell within the frontal sinus can also present as a mucocele variant described as a frontal bullosa.[7] The interfrontal cell drains to either frontal sinus.[8]

Sphenoid Sinus

Variation of development within the sphenoid sinus can have devastating outcome if not considered during sphenoid surgery. The optic nerve and carotid artery are usually seen at the lateral sphenoid sinus. A dehiscence of the bone overlying the optic or carotid canal can place these structures at risk during sphenoid sinus surgery. Entry to the sphenoid is safely performed through the natural sphenoid ostium, which is opposite the carotid and optic nerves within the sinus. The intersinus septum may insert into the bone overlying the carotid artery. If removal of this bone is needed for the procedure, methods that do not use lateral torquing force (i.e., high-speed drill) are preferred

to prevent carotid injury. Last, a sphenoid sinus with wide lateral pneumatization is often the site of spontaneous sphenoid sinus CSF leak.

Abnormal Embryological Development

Choanal Atresia

Choanal atresia is a potentially life-threatening congenital anomaly.[9] Failure of the choana to canalize during embryological development results in complete nasal airway obstruction. Newborns are obligate nasal breathers for the first 3 months of life. Symptoms of choanal atresia appear at birth, where signs of hypoxia are only seen when a baby is not crying (oral breathing). Unilateral atresia is sometimes identified by the inability to pass a flexible suction catheter through the nasal cavity; however, this obstruction is sometimes not identified until later in life when there is mucopurulent nasal drainage or symptomatic nasal obstruction.

Choanal atresia can be seen in conjunction with CHARGE syndrome (coloboma, heart defects, choanal atresia, retardation of growth and/or development, genitourinary abnormalities, and ear problems) or as an isolated abnormality. Mutation in the *CHD7* gene has been identified in more than half of the patients with CHARGE syndrome.[10] The embryological cause of isolated choanal atresia remains unknown. Several theories regarding choanal atresia revolve around failure of developmental membranes to rupture, abnormal ingrowth from surrounding bony structures (septum and lateral nasal wall), adhesion formation, and misdirection of neural crest cell migration.[9] Obstruction of the nasal cavity in choanal atresia has been seen at sites, which vary in loci and tissue composition (membranous or bone), suggesting that there may be more than one mechanism that leads to the formation of atresia.[9]

Dermoid Cyst

Nasal dermoid cysts are epithelial-lined inclusion cysts that contain dermal features of hair follicles and exocrine glands. These cysts represent abnormal embryological development where a remnant of epithelium become trapped without a drainage pathway.[11] Between the frontal and nasal bones is the fonticulus nasofrontalis, a membrane that allows for a potential space—the prenasal space. During embryogenesis, developing dura passes through a bony opening in the skull, the foramen cecum. The foramen cecum and fonticulus nasofrontalis are normally obliterated by growth of surrounding bone; however, the potential for trapping of abnormal tissue in this prenasal space exists. It is theorized that the epithelial rests maintain attachment to the underlying fibrous tissue and are pulled into the prenasal space.[12] Dermoid cysts can have both skin and dural attachments because of the embryological origin adjacent to these potential spaces. In rare presentations, dermoid cysts are seen at the medial canthal region, possibly representing abnormal development of the lacrimal duct during closure of the lateral nasal process.

Encephalocele and Glioma

The presence of neural tissue in the nose or sinonasal cavity can occur from abnormal embryological development. A nasal glioma contains heterotopic rests of brain tissue with or without rudimentary connection to the brain. Gliomas can be seen within the sinonasal cavity or extranasally as a mass on the nasal dorsum or glabella.

An encephalocele is a herniation of neural tissue that is continuous with the subarachnoid space through a defect in the skull base (**Fig. 1.4**). Encephaloceles are usually intranasal but can also be seen on the external nose. There are multiple theories for the development of encephaloceles and gliomas, which describe abnormal deposition of neural tissue during embryogenesis, failure of tissue separation during neuropore closure, and abnormal neural crest cell migration at the skull base. The size and location of the encephalocele will determine the clinical presentation. External nasal lesions are often seen early, whereas intranasal and sinus encephaloceles may not be recognized until later in life as an incidental finding on imaging. Other possible presenting symptoms of an encephalocele include nasal obstruction, sinusitis from sinus outflow obstruction, or meningitis from spread of nasal flora to the intracranial cavity.

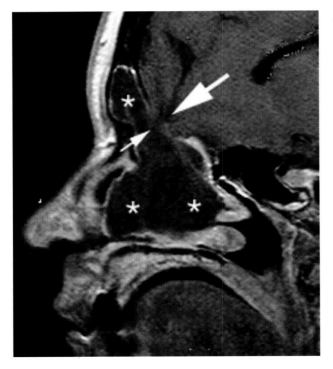

Figure 1.4 An encephalocele (*) can result from embryological failure of the skull base to close (arrows), resulting in herniation of intracranial contents into the sinus cavities.

Rare Congenital Nasal Deformities

Median nasal cleft can be seen as a small midline scar on the nose or as a more significant separation of the nasal cartilages. Lateral nasal clefts result in a defect in the ala or upper lateral cartilage and can vary in severity. Frontonasal syndrome includes nasal clefts in association with hypertelorism and frontal bone defects. The complete congenital absence of a nose (arhinia) or a double nose (polyrhinia) is an extremely rare entity that occurs from embryological defects.

Nasal Lacrimal Anomalies

The nasolacrimal duct forms by infolding of the lateral process of the nasal placode. The involution of ectoderm is completed with detachment from the external facial surface and connection as a cylindrical structure. During this process, any ectoderm cell that becomes trapped within the mesenchymal tube can proliferate to form a lacrimal cyst. These cysts can present with nasolacrimal obstruction causing epiphora or dacryocystitis, or with nasal obstruction from an intranasal mass in the anterior nasal cavity. Newborns with large or bilateral nasolacrimal cysts can demonstrate airway compromise in the postnatal period.

Pyriform Aperture Stenosis

Congenital nasal obstruction can be caused by narrowing of the anterior nasal cavity because of pyriform aperture stenosis.[13] Overgrowth of the nasal process of the maxilla leads to bone narrowing that restricts nasal airflow.

Conclusion

Embryological development of the nose and paranasal sinuses is a complex series of events. Numerous anatomical variations as well as disorders that arise from abnormal embryological development lead to clinically relevant entities that must be recognized by head and neck surgeons. Understanding of the embryological origins and pathways by which the sinuses develop will help surgeons optimize their outcomes and prevent complications.

References

1. Larsen WJ. Human Embryology. New York: Churchill Livingstone; 1993
2. Moore KL. The Developing Human: Clinical Oriented Embryology. Philadelphia: WB Saunders; 1998
3. Stammberger H. Functional endoscopic sinus surgery: the Messerklinger Technique. Philadelphia, PA: BC Decker; 1991
4. Schaffer JP. The Nose, Paranasal Sinuses, Nasolacrimal Passageways and Olfactory Organ in Man: A Genetic, Developmental and Anatomico-Physiological Consideration. Philadelphia, PA: P Blakiston's Sib; 1920
5. Van Alyea OE. Nasal Sinuses: An Anatomical and Clinical Consideration. Baltimore, MD: Williams and Wilkins; 1951

6. Bingham B, Wang RG, Hawke M, Kwok P. The embryonic development of the lateral nasal wall from 8 to 24 weeks. Laryngoscope 1991;101(9):992–997

7. Reh DD, Lewis CM, Metson R. Frontal bullosa: diagnosis and management of a new variant of frontal mucocele. Arch Otolaryngol Head Neck Surg 2010;136(6):625–628

8. Goldsztein H, Pletcher SD, Reh DD, Metson R. The frontal wishbone: anatomic and clinical implications. Am J Rhinol 2007;21(6):725–728

9. Hengerer AS, Brickman TM, Jeyakumar A. Choanal atresia: embryologic analysis and evolution of treatment, a 30-year experience. Laryngoscope 2008;118(5):862–866

10. Vissers LE, van Ravenswaaij CM, Admiraal R, et al. Mutations in a new member of the chromodomain gene family cause CHARGE syndrome. Nat Genet 2004;36(9):955–957

11. Pratt LW. Midline cysts of the nasal dorsum: embryologic origin and treatment. Laryngoscope 1965;75:968–980

12. Luongo RA. Dermoid cyst of the nasal dorsum. Arch Otolaryngol 1933;17:755–765

13. Brown OE, Myer CM III, Manning SC. Congenital nasal pyriform aperture stenosis. Laryngoscope 1989;99(1):86–91

2 Surgical Endoscopic Anatomy of the Nose, Paranasal Sinuses, and Skull Base

Craig R. Villari and Sarah K. Wise

An understanding of the embryological material discussed in Chapter 1 will serve as a solid foundation for understanding the complex relationships between the nasal cavity and paranasal sinuses. Knowledge of these relationships is necessary for evaluating nasal and paranasal sinus pathology and subsequently completing safe and effective endoscopic and open procedures. This chapter explores basic considerations of skull base anatomy, while other chapters emphasize on specific areas and procedures.

Primarily, the nasal cavity and the paranasal sinuses are protected by components of the maxilla and the ethmoid, sphenoid, and frontal bones. The vomer, the lacrimal, and the zygomatic bones also contribute to the overall structure of the nasal and sinus cavities. Given the number of bones involved and the contiguous and vital structures that these bones protect, thorough attention must be paid to all aspects of the nasal cavity and the paranasal sinuses.

Nasal Cavity

The right and left nasal cavities are often considered mirror images of each other; however, precise symmetry between these sides is typically an exception and almost never the rule. The anterior border of the nasal cavity is the nasal vestibule, which contains the transition zone from the external squamous epithelium of skin to the respiratory mucosa that lines the nasal cavity and paranasal sinuses. Medially, the nasal cavity is bordered by the nasal septum, which contains contributions from the maxillary crest and vomer inferiorly, the quadrangular cartilage anteriorly, and the perpendicular plate of the ethmoid bone superiorly. Anterolaterally, the nasal bones, the upper and lower lateral cartilages, and the soft tissue gives shape to the external nasal pyramid. The choana serves as a posterior limit to the nasal cavity and transition into the nasopharynx. The lateral portion of the nasal cavity contains the most complex anatomy and will be covered in depth in subsequent sections within this chapter.

Maxillary Sinus

The maxillary sinus is bordered by the alveolar portion of the maxillary bone anteriorly, the orbital floor superiorly, the zygoma laterally, the pterygopalatine and infratemporal fossae posteriorly, and the lateral nasal wall medially[1] (**Fig. 2.1**). Entry into the maxillary sinus is usually through the solitary natural ostium identified within the posterior

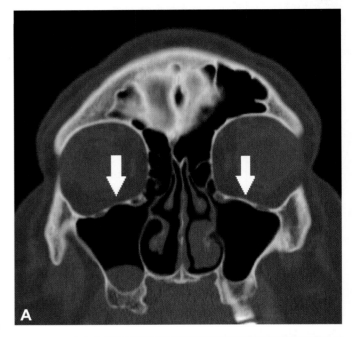

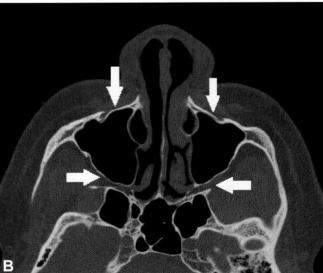

Figure 2.1 Computed tomography scan images in bone window algorithm demonstrating the bony anatomical borders of the maxillary sinuses. (A) Coronal image demonstrating the orbital floor (vertical arrows), zygoma, and lateral nasal wall as the superior, lateral, and medial bony walls of the maxillary sinus, respectively. (B) Axial image demonstrating the maxilla (vertical arrows) and pterygopalatine fossa (horizontal arrows) as the anterior and posterior boundaries of the maxillary sinus, respectively.

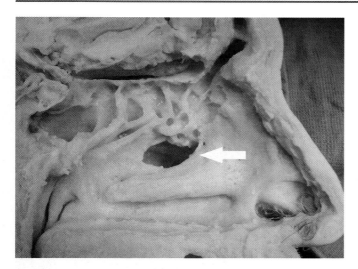

Figure 2.2 Parasagittal image of a gross cadaveric dissection of the lateral nasal wall. The uncinate process has been partially resected, and the maxillary ostium has been widened (arrow).

third of the ethmoid infundibulum[2] (**Figs. 2.2** and **2.3**). However, in up to 23% of patients, accessory ostia may form through the anterior or posterior fontanelles.[2] The fontanelles are located within the lateral nasal wall and are devoid of bone; in certain cases, the overlying mucosa and connective tissue are deficient, resulting in an additional drainage pathway of the sinus.

Two anatomical variants of maxillary sinus are important for an endoscopic surgeon. Usually 15 cm³ in volume, the maxillary sinus can have variable pneumatization, potentially resulting in a hypoplastic sinus. As the maxillary sinus decreases in volume, the orbital contents tend to fill a larger volume of the midface. Small maxillary sinus volumes and relatively large orbital volumes are seen in young children before full aeration of the maxillary sinuses, cystic fibrosis, and silent sinus syndrome of the maxillary sinus (**Fig. 2.4**). Infraorbital ethmoid (Haller) cells must also be considered during endoscopic intervention as they tend to narrow the outflow tract of the maxillary sinus. Although they overwhelmingly originate from the anterior ethmoid sinus, they can emanate from the posterior ethmoid cells in roughly 12% of patients.[3,4] Special preoperative radiographic attention must be paid to identify and properly address these on endoscopic intervention.

Ethmoid Sinus

The ethmoid sinus is not one sinus, but a complex of ethmoid sinus cells with contributions from the middle and superior turbinates. The ethmoid sinus is the only sinus that is not a self-contained singular cell with one clear ostium. Because of the complexity of the ethmoid sinus, stepwise discussion of its key components will help highlight several important relationships.

Uncinate Process

The hook-shaped uncinate process is a curved bony extension from the lateral nasal wall that is often one of the first structures encountered on endoscopic intervention.

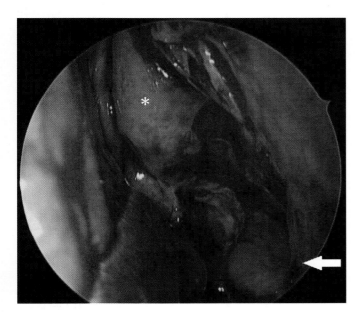

Figure 2.3 Endoscopic image of the left middle meatus and left maxillary sinus ostium, which has been partially enlarged (arrow). The middle turbinate is held medially, and the ethmoid bulla is visualized (*). The uncinate process has been resected.

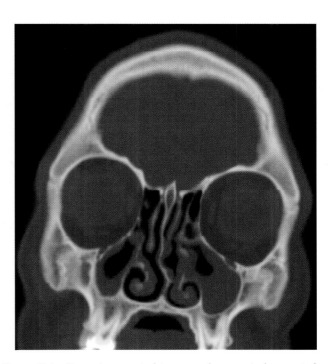

Figure 2.4 Coronal computed tomography scan in bone window algorithm of a patient with cystic fibrosis. Image demonstrates hypoplastic maxillary sinuses bilaterally, with relatively larger orbital volumes compared with the maxillary sinus volumes.

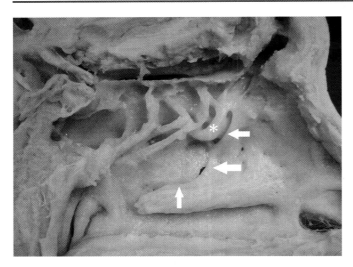

Figure 2.5   Parasagittal image of the lateral nasal wall. The hook-shaped uncinate process is demonstrated by the arrows. Note that the uncinate process has both vertical and horizontal portions (arrows). Also note that the uncinate process partially covers the maxillary sinus ostium and the ethmoid bulla (*).

The uncinate process attaches superiorly to the maxilla near the lacrimal bone and then sweeps inferiorly and posteriorly to a free edge without bony attachment[5] (**Fig. 2.5**). This sweeping curve gives the uncinate process both vertical and horizontal portions.

The superior attachment of the vertical portion of the uncinate process is variable and thus affects the drainage pattern of the frontal sinus.[3,5] The vertical uncinate process most commonly attaches to the lamina papyracea. In this arrangement, drainage of the frontal sinus courses into the middle meatus, medial to the uncinate process. However, if the uncinate process attaches superiorly to the middle turbinate itself or directly to the skull base, frontal sinus drainage will occur lateral to the uncinate process and into the ethmoid infundibulum. Failure to identify this arrangement can lead to an inadequate drainage of the postoperative frontal sinus.

The posterior edge of the uncinate process also forms a boundary of the hiatus semilunaris, a two-dimensional space that serves as an "entrance" to the three-dimensional ethmoid infundibulum. The ethmoid infundibulum is bordered anteromedially by the uncinate process, posteriorly by the ethmoid bulla, and laterally by the lamina papyracea. The ethmoid infundibulum is a noteworthy structure, given that it is a natural drainage pathway for maxillary sinuses and often a drainage pathway for the frontal sinuses.

Ethmoid Bulla

The ethmoid bulla is located in the anterior ethmoid cavity, just posterior to the vertical portion of the uncinate process (**Figs. 2.3** and **2.5**). Approximately 92% of patients have well-pneumatized ethmoid bullae, and this structure continues to be a very consistent landmark for the anterior ethmoid

sinuses during endoscopic intervention.[6] The ethmoid bulla is bordered laterally by the lamina papyracea, posteriorly by the vertical portion of the middle turbinate basal lamella and retrobullar recess, and anteriorly by the ethmoid infundibulum and the vertical uncinate process.

Agger Nasi Cells

The agger nasi cells are the most anterior of the anterior ethmoid sinus cells. Although they may not be present if the cells are not pneumatized, the region rests anterior and inferior to the frontal sinus and the frontal recess. It lies superior to the lateral connection of uncinate process and is positioned between the nasal bones, the lacrimal bones, and the maxilla. The position of the agger nasi region is very important in a thorough dissection of the frontal recess and frontal sinus. Any remnant or residual sinus tissue or septations left behind in the agger nasi region may result in obstruction of the frontal sinus outflow.[7]

Middle Turbinate

The middle turbinate is a deceptively complex structure. It begins in the parasagittal plane anteriorly but then changes orientation to the semicoronal and then to the semiaxial planes as it travels posteriorly (**Figs. 2.6** and **2.7**). The change in orientation is key to understanding the ethmoid sinuses as the middle turbinate serves as both the posterior and the medial boundary to the anterior ethmoid complex.

The free edge of the middle turbinate is in the parasagittal orientation; as we follow the turbinate posteriorly past the ethmoid bulla, the vertical portion of the basal lamella can be

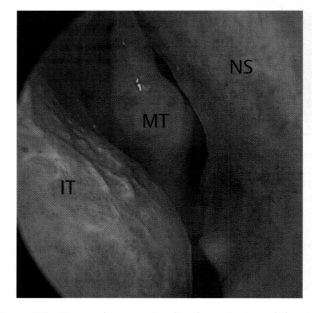

Figure 2.6   Commonly encountered endoscopic view of the right nasal cavity. The nasal septum (NS) and inferior turbinate (IT) are seen in the foreground. The parasagittal portion of the middle turbinate (MT) is seen more posteriorly.

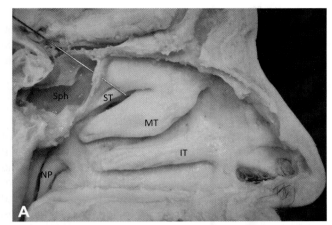

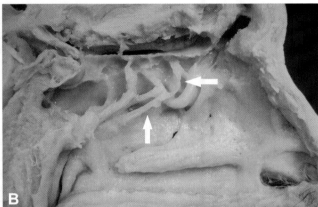

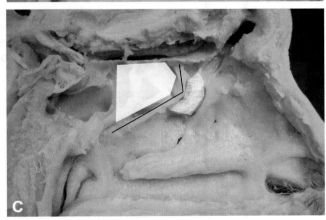

Figure 2.7 Gross cadaveric dissection of the lateral nasal wall. (A) The inferior turbinate (IT), middle turbinate (MT), and superior turbinate (ST) are intact and in their native position. A metal probe is in the natural ostium of the sphenoid sinus (Sph). The nasopharynx (NP) is visualized posteriorly. (B) The parasagittal portions of the MT and ST have been removed. The vertical and horizontal portions of the MT basal lamella can be visualized (arrows). (C) The vertical and horizontal portions of the MT basal lamella are outlined with a black solid line. This separates the anterior ethmoid cavity (light-shaded region) from the posterior ethmoid cavity (solid-shaded region).

turbinate is the horizontal portion of the basal lamella. This posterior attachment can serve as a landmark for locating the sphenopalatine foramen and may be useful in surgical treatment of epistaxis.[1,3]

The middle turbinate can become pneumatized. The location of the pneumatized portion determines the structure's name, but recognizing these structures on preoperative computed tomography can be key to maintaining orientation during surgical dissection.

If the anterior parasagittally oriented portion is pneumatized, it is called a concha bullosa (**Fig. 2.8**). If the vertical portion of the basal lamella is pneumatized, it is called an interlamellar cell.[1,3,6]

Posterior Ethmoid Complex

As stated earlier, the anterior boundary of the posterior ethmoid complex is the vertical portion of the basal lamella. The remainders of its boundaries are the anterior face of the sphenoid sinus posteriorly, the lamina papyracea laterally, the superior turbinate medially, and the skull base superiorly.

A sphenoethmoid, or Onodi, cell is specifically named posterior ethmoid cell. These cells are seen in as many as 30% of patients and are of great clinical importance.[8] The sphenoethmoid cell is actually the hyperpneumatized posterior ethmoid cell that has continued to develop in a superolateral direction with respect to the true sphenoid sinus. In the case of a well-pneumatized sphenoethmoidal cell, one can easily confuse this cell for a sphenoid sinus. It is important to identify sphenoethmoid cells radiographically

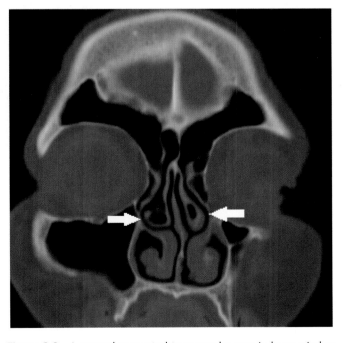

Figure 2.8 A coronal computed tomography scan in bone window algorithm demonstrating bilateral middle turbinate concha bullosae (arrows).

identified, which divides the anterior and posterior ethmoid complexes. Following the turbinate more posteriorly reveals that the basal lamella position changes again to a more semiaxial orientation. This posterior portion of the

before dissecting the sinuses for two reasons. First, failure to recognize them preoperatively can lead to incomplete dissection. Second, structures commonly seen in the walls of the sphenoid sinus (the optic nerve and the carotid artery) may be present along the outer limits of the sphenoethmoid cell (**Fig. 2.9**).

Skull Base

The skull base slopes in a three-dimensional pattern. It is at its most superior position anterolaterally and then slopes inferiorly in medial and posterior directions. The skull base is thickest laterally and posteriorly, and then thins medially and anteriorly to a thickness of only 0.2 mm along the cribriform plate. This makes it a likely site for iatrogenic cerebrospinal fluid (CSF) leak.[9]

The Keros classification system can be used to help identify potential risk of iatrogenic CSF leak with surgery involving the lateral olfactory region. The classification stratifies the height of the olfactory sulcus into three types—Keros type 1 contains an olfactory sulcus depth from 1 to 3 mm, Keros type 2 contains those with a depth from 4 to 7 mm, and Keros type 3 involves those with a depth from 8 to 16 mm. As the Keros type increases, the theoretical risk of entering the olfactory groove from a lateral position (thus causing a CSF leak) increases. Fortunately, it appears that Keros type 1 is the most common presentation at almost 83% of cases.[10]

The anterior ethmoid artery is also incorporated into the ethmoid skull base. It should be identified radiographically before intervention and is usually seen in the same coronal plane as the most anterior visualization of the optic nerve before visualizing the globe. It usually runs along the skull base in an anteromedial direction but can be dehiscent of the skull base, dropping below the actual ethmoid roof anywhere from 1 to 3 mm (**Fig. 2.10**).[9]

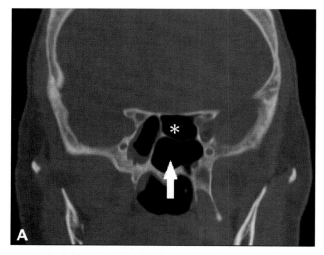

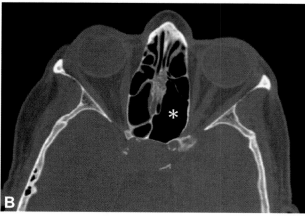

Figure 2.9 Computed tomography scan in bone window algorithm showing (A) coronal and (B) axial views of a left-sided sphenoethmoid (Onodi) cell (*). The true left sphenoid sinus (denoted by an arrow) is located inferior to the large left sphenoethmoid cell on the coronal image. Also note the proximity of the optic nerve canal to the sphenoethmoid cell.

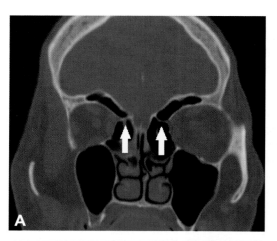

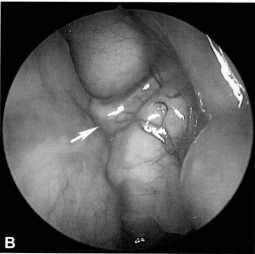

Figure 2.10 (A) Coronal computed tomography scan in bone window algorithm demonstrating bilateral anterior ethmoid arteries present in bony mesenteries below the ethmoid skull base (arrows). (B) Endoscopic photo of the right frontal recess. The anterior ethmoid artery is visible just below the bony skull base, running in a posterolateral-to-anteromedial direction.

Frontal Sinus

The frontal sinus is bordered by the anterior table of the frontal bone anteriorly, the posterior table posteriorly, and their confluence superiorly. Medially, there is a frontal intersinus bony septum (**Fig. 2.11**). The lateral floor of the frontal sinus is the orbital roof.

As discussed in the preceding sections, there is a tremendous interplay between the arrangement of the anterior ethmoid complex and the outflow tract from the frontal sinus. The frontal recess is an area that the endoscopic surgeon should thoroughly understand. It is an hourglass-shaped region through which the frontal sinus contents exit to drain into the nasal cavity.[3] Although there are various potential drainage pathways from the frontal sinus dependent on the superior insertion of the uncinate process, the bony components to the frontal recess itself are relatively constant. The frontal sinus is the superior limit of the frontal recess, whereas the nasal cavity is the inferior limit. The agger nasi cells form the anterior border of the frontal recess, the ethmoid bulla forms the posterior border. The lamina papyracea bounds the frontal recess laterally, and the anterior superior portion of the middle turbinate bounds the frontal recess medially.

There are several additional pneumatized cells that must be considered when discussing the frontal sinus and frontal recess. The frontal intersinus septum can become pneumatized; this frontal intersinus septal cell will drain into either the right or the left frontal sinus. Theoretically, the endoscopic surgeon could enter this intersinus septal cell and convince himself that he has adequately drained the

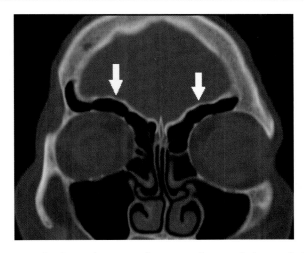

Figure 2.12 Coronal computed tomography scan in bone window algorithm demonstrating bilateral supraorbital ethmoid cells. These cells arch laterally over the orbital roof and their ostia may be mistaken for frontal sinus ostia on endoscopic dissection. However, the supraorbital ethmoid cell ostium will drain posterolaterally to the true frontal sinus ostium.

opposite frontal sinus. The surgeon may also come across supraorbital ethmoid cells—ethmoid cells that, as their name depicts, pneumatize in a superolateral direction over the orbit (**Fig. 2.12**). Both the intersinus septal cell and the supraorbital ethmoid cell may disorient the surgeon if not adequately mapped out on preoperative imaging. When viewed endoscopically, however, the frontal intersinus septal cell ostium will drain medially to the true frontal sinus ostium, and the supraorbital ethmoid cell ostium will drain posterolaterally to the true frontal sinus ostium (**Fig. 2.13**).

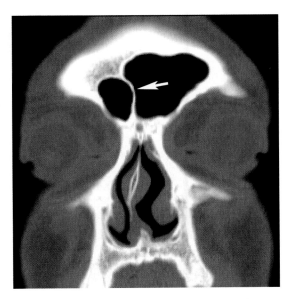

Figure 2.11 Coronal computed tomography scan in bone window algorithm demonstrating the right and left frontal sinuses divided medially by the frontal intersinus septum. As with the nasal cavity and other paranasal sinuses, symmetry between sides is typically the exception rather than the rule. In this image, the right frontal sinus is considerably smaller than the left one.

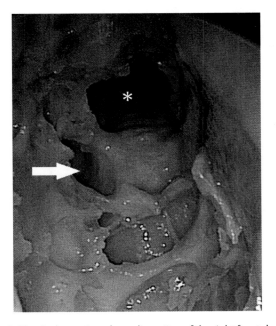

Figure 2.13 Endoscopic cadaver dissection of the right frontal recess. The ostium of the supraorbital ethmoid cell (arrow) is posterolateral to the true frontal sinus ostium (*).

Frontal cells must also be considered for adequate treatment of the frontal sinuses. In certain cases, cells can pneumatize superior to the agger nasi cells and may or may not extend into the frontal sinus proper.[11] A type 1 frontal cell is a single anterior ethmoid cell that pneumatizes above the agger nasi cell but does not extend into the frontal sinus. A type 2 frontal cell is described as multiple "stacked" cells above the agger nasi cell; these may or may not involve the frontal sinus. A type 3 frontal cell is a single, large cell, again superior to the agger nasi cell that extends into the frontal sinus and communicates with the frontal recess. The final frontal cell is the type 4 cell in which the named cell is located entirely within the frontal sinus and attached to the thicker anterior table of the frontal sinus.[12] These frontal cells must be identified preoperatively to develop a thorough surgical plan.

Two additional anatomic entities must also be considered as they may impinge on the frontal sinus outflow tract and be mistaken for the true frontal sinus ostium during endoscopic surgical dissection. The suprabullar recess is an anatomical region that exists when the ethmoid bulla does not extend to the skull base. As its name denotes, it lies superior to the ethmoid bulla but inferior to the skull base. A surgeon could easily convince himself that he has entered the frontal recess when he has only fallen into the suprabullar recess. When the suprabullar space is an open space, it is termed the suprabullar recess; when it is contained, it is termed a suprabullar cell. Next, a frontal bulla cell exists when an ethmoid cell pneumatizes into the frontal recess and along the posterior table of the frontal sinus. The ostium of the frontal bulla cell opens posterior to the true frontal sinus ostium. Noticing this frontal bulla cell on preoperative imaging is important in protecting the skull base and also correctly opening the frontal sinus ostium in endoscopic dissections.

Sphenoid Sinus

The anterior wall of the sphenoid sinus sits at the posterior aspect of the nasal cavity, just superior to the choana. The roof of the sphenoid sinus, the planum sphenoidale, comprises a portion of the posterior skull base. The roof transitions posteriorly to become the common skull base between the sinus and the sella turcica—allowing transphenoidal approach to the pituitary gland. Inferior to the sella rests the thicker bone of the clivus. The floor of the sphenoid sinus and sphenoid rostrum attaches anteriorly to the vomer. Medially, the intersinus septum divides the right and the left sphenoid sinus. The sphenoid intersinus septum is seldom perfectly within the midline sagittal plane, and volume differences between the right and the left sphenoid sinuses are the norm (**Fig. 2.14**).

The natural ostium of the sphenoid sinus sits roughly 1 to 1.5 cm above the superior rim of the choana and is usually located about halfway between the nasal septum and the posterior insertion of the superior turbinate.[13] The

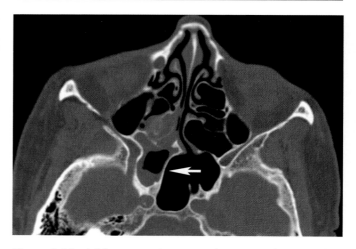

Figure 2.14 Axial computed tomography scan in bone window algorithm demonstrating asymmetric right and left sphenoid sinuses. The sphenoid intersinus septum inserts onto the bony canal of the right internal carotid artery. The right sphenoid sinus is also partially opacified with mucosal disease.

ostium opens into the superior aspect of the sinus and can alternatively be identified using a 30-degree angle from the nasal spine—using this approach, the ostium is roughly 7 cm posterior to the nasal spine (**Fig. 2.7A**).

When working within the sphenoid sinus, one must be cognizant of several vital surrounding structures. As discussed in the preceding sections, the pituitary gland is located posterior and superior to the sphenoid cavity, in a relatively midline position. The optic chiasm is located superior to the pituitary gland, with the optic nerves extending laterally from the chiasm toward the orbital apices. When viewed from the sphenoid cavities, the internal carotid arteries are located lateral to the pituitary gland and clivus. The optic nerves and carotid arteries will often leave impressions in the sphenoid sinus walls and create the opticocarotid recesses. The cavernous sinus lies lateral to the sphenoid sinus and contains cranial nerves III, IV, V_1, V_2, and VI. One more neural structure, the vidian nerve, may also be seen as an impression into the sphenoid sinus, but this is along the inferolateral aspect of the sinus floor.

As discussed previously, the sphenoid intersinus septum rarely inserts perfectly midline along the posterior sinus wall, and studies have demonstrated insertion of the septum onto the bony canals of the optic nerve or internal carotid artery, or near a frankly dehiscent structure[8] (**Fig. 2.14**). Given the potentially disastrous outcomes from injury to one of these structures, understanding the anatomy and spatial arrangement of these abutting structures can make intervention much safer.

Conclusion

The nasal cavity and paranasal sinuses are a complex series of structures. There are almost innumerable combinations of anatomical variants that the surgeon may encounter.

Despite their complexity, the endoscopic surgeon can perform safe, effective intervention by recalling the normal "best case" anatomy and then adapting their approach for each patient with a thorough review of any available preoperative imaging.

References

1. Bolger W. Anatomy of the paranasal sinuses. In: Kennedy D, Bolger W, Zinreich S, eds. Diseases of the Sinuses: Diagnosis and Management. Hamilton, Ontario: B.C. Decker, Inc., 2001:1–11

2. Van Alyea O. The ostium maxillare: anatomic study of its surgical accessibility. Arch Otolaryngol 1936;24:553–569

3. Stammberger HR, Kennedy DW, Bolger W, et al; Anatomic Terminology Group. Paranasal sinuses: anatomic terminology and nomenclature. Ann Otol Rhinol Laryngol Suppl 1995;167(Suppl 167):7–16

4. Kainz J, Braun H, Genser P. Haller's cells: morphologic evaluation and clinico-surgical relevance. Laryngorhinootologie 1993;72(12):599–604

5. Bolger WE, Woodruff WW Jr, Morehead J, Parsons DS. Maxillary sinus hypoplasia: classification and description of associated uncinate process hypoplasia. Otolaryngol Head Neck Surg 1990;103(5, pt 1):759–765

6. Stammberger H. Functional Endoscopic Sinus Surgery: the Messerklinger Technique. Philadelphia, PA: B.C. Decker;1991

7. Kuhn F, Bolger W, Tisdal R. The agger nasi cell in frontal recess obstruction: an anatomic, radiologic, and clinical correlation. Oper Tech Otolaryngol Head Neck Surg 1991;2:226–231

8. Batra PS, Citardi MJ, Gallivan RP, Roh HJ, Lanza DC. Software-enabled CT analysis of optic nerve position and paranasal sinus pneumatization patterns. Otolaryngol Head Neck Surg 2004;131(6):940–945

9. Kainz J, Stammberger H. The roof of the anterior ethmoid: a place of least resistance in the skull base. Am J Rhinol 1989;3:191–199

10. Solares C, Lee W, Batra P, Citardi M. Lateral lamella of the cribiform place. Arch Otolaryngol 2008;134:285–289

11. Van Alyea O. Frontal cells: an anatomic study of these cells with consideration of their clinical significance. Arch Otolaryngol 1941;34:11–23

12. Bent J, Cuilty-Siller C, Kuhn F. The frontal cell as a cause of frontal sinus obstruction. Am J Rhinol 1994;8:185–191

13. Yanagisawa E, Yanagisawa K, Christmas DA. Endoscopic localization of the sphenoid sinus ostium. Ear Nose Throat J 1998;77(2): 88–89

3 Applied Physiology of the Paranasal Sinuses

Nithin D. Adappa and Noam A. Cohen

Although the exact functional contribution of the paranasal sinuses to the respiratory system is not completely understood, it is logical to assume that the sinuses are an extension of the nasal cavity and play a role in cleansing and conditioning the air inspired for ventilation. Thus, from a cellular standpoint, the physiological contribution of the paranasal sinuses involves mucociliary clearance and both innate and adaptive immune defense of the respiratory system. Persistent pathophysiological processes involving the paranasal sinuses result in chronic rhinosinusitis (CRS) that affects more than 35 million Americans annually.[1] This chapter focuses on the paranasal sinuses, primary innate defense system and mucociliary clearance as well as evaluates the current literature on biofilms and the implication of the nitric oxide (NO) on the sinonasal cavity.

Mucociliary Clearance

Mucosa

The paranasal sinus mucosa consists of a superficial layer of epithelium with variable numbers of goblet cells, an acellular basement membrane, a thick lamina propria containing vascular and glandular layers, and periosteum. The sinus epithelium consists predominantly of simple ciliated columnar cells.[2] Both ciliated and nonciliated columnar cells have hundreds of immotile microvilli along their surface, which are tiny hair-like projections of actin filaments 1 to 2 mm in length covered by the cell membrane. The microvilli increase the total surface area of the columnar cells, which likely aids the sinonasal mucosa in mucus production, secretion, and sensation.[3] The goblet cells, interspersed throughout the columnar cells, aid in mucus production via secretory granules that contain mucin, a glycoprotein essential to the viscosity and elasticity of mucus (**Fig. 3.1**).

Beneath the thin basement membrane lies the lamina propria, the layer containing the glands, vasculature, and nerves supplying the sinonasal mucosa. The lamina propria has a superficial glandular layer, a vascular layer, and a deep glandular layer. Sympathetic fibers run through lamina propria, which appear to play a more significant role in mucosal vasoconstriction and decongestion than in regulating nasal secretions.[4]

Sinus Mucus

The epithelium is covered in a mucus blanket that traps cellular debris, pathogens, and particulate matter that

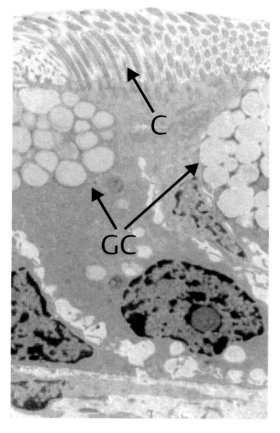

Figure 3.1 Transmission electron micrograph of two goblet cells (GCs) containing secretory granules and overlying cilia (C). The granules will be released between cilia and are an essential component to viscosity and elasticity of the mucus.

precipitates from inspired air. Mucus consists of two layers, namely the *gel phase*, which is a discontinuous outer viscous layer that rides along the tips of extended cilia; and the *sol phase*, which surrounds the shafts of cilia as a continuous inner layer of lower viscosity composed of water and electrolytes (Na^+, K^+, Ca^{2+}, and Cl^-). The sinonasal mucosa produces approximately 600 to 1800 mL of mucus per day.[5]

Mucin proteins are secreted by goblet cells and are an essential component of mucus that gives the gel phase its characteristic rheologic properties of viscosity and elasticity. They are a group of large, thread-like glycoproteins that contain peptide backbones and oligosaccharide side chains. Mucin proteins are secreted in condensed form and undergo hydration to form a gel, facilitating mucociliary clearance by creating a unique fluid structure that can retain trapped debris while maintaining a pliable and easily transportable medium. Mucus contains many proteins that aid in the local immune defense.

Ciliary Structure and Function

Respiratory cilia clear the mucus blanket containing pathogens and debris from both the upper and lower respiratory passages by beating in a coordinated and rhythmic manner. There are approximately 50 to 200 cilia per epithelial cell, each measuring 5 to 7 μm in length and 0.2 to 0.3 μm in diameter (**Fig. 3.2**).[5] Each cilium is composed of a bundle of interconnected microtubules, termed the axoneme, and an overlying membrane that is part of the cell plasma membrane. The axonemes of motile cilia contain two central singlet microtubules surrounded by nine doublet microtubules.

Each cilium movement is defined by a forward power stroke followed by a recovery stroke. During the recovery stroke, the cilium bends 90 degrees and sweeps back to its starting point. The mechanism of ciliary motion depends on a series of adenosine triphosphate–dependent molecular motors that cause the outer doublets of the axoneme to slide relative to each other producing a vectorial force. Although it is well established that cilia beat in a coordinated fashion, referred to as a metachronous wave, the mechanism of coordination is not entirely understood. One theory that explains the coordinated, wave-like motion of cilia is that gap junctions connecting adjacent epithelial cells may allow a directional propagation of intracellular calcium waves driving the microtubule interactions and ultimately the entire metachronous wave.[6] Another possible mechanism relies on the close relationship between the cilia and the hydrodynamic forces surrounding them in their partly liquid environment, where only a relatively small number of coordinated cilia would be necessary to generate a hydrodynamic wave that, in turn, forces the timed coordinating beating of nearby cilia.[7] Once a metachronous wave is established, spontaneous beating can range from approximately 9 to 15 Hz in humans, and the cilia tip reaches a velocity of 600 to 1000 mm/s.

Sinonasal Mucociliary Clearance Patterns

The cilia create coordinated, microscopic wave movements that propel mucus in a direction-oriented fashion. The mucus of the paranasal sinuses is directed toward the nasal cavity, where it then travels to the posterior nasopharynx and is eventually ingested by the immunologically active gastrointestinal tract.

In the maxillary sinus, mucus must flow superomedially, against gravity, from the most inferior portion of the cavity. The anterior ethmoid cells direct their mucus toward their individual ostia, then into the middle meatus, whereas the posterior ethmoid cells direct their mucus toward the superior meatus and eventually into the sphenoethmoidal recess. The sphenoid sinus also drains through its natural ostium into the sphenoethmoidal recess. The mucus flow pattern in the frontal sinus appears to be unique in that it demonstrates both retrograde and anterograde motions. Mucus along the medial portion of the sinus is carried superiorly, away from the frontal ostium, and then laterally along the roof of the sinus. The mucus along the floor and the inferior portions of the anterior and posterior walls is then carried medially toward the frontal ostium, where it then drains into the frontal recess and the ethmoid infundibulum.

Ciliary Dysfunction

Mucociliary clearance is dependent on normal cilia function and mucus composition. Disease states that compromise this essential mode of defense tend to result in impaired clearance of inhaled pathogens and ultimately recurrent sinopulmonary infections. In addition to inherited pathologies, such as primary ciliary dyskinesia and cystic fibrosis, exposure to various environmental pathogens can also alter the normal mucociliary clearance system. Common bacterial pathogens such as *Haemophilus influenzae, Streptococcus pneumoniae, Staphylococcus aureus,* and *Pseudomonas* produce specific toxins to impair ciliary motion and coordination.[7] Viruses responsible for common upper respiratory infections disrupt the microtubule function of ciliated columnar cells and change the viscosity of surrounding mucus. Impairing the local defense system facilitates the infectious pathogens' upper airway colonization. Although CRS is multifactorial, a common pathophysiological sequela is ineffective sinonasal mucociliary clearance, resulting in stasis of sinonasal secretions and subsequent chronic infection and/or persistent inflammation. Two latest topics of great

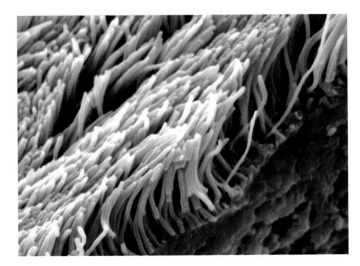

Figure 3.2 Scanning electron micrograph (6400×) of the paranasal sinus epithelium showing numerous cilia. The cilia beat in a coordinated fashion to clear debris.

interest in the otolaryngic community, which ultimately affect mucociliary clearance, are biofilms and paranasal sinus NO levels.

Biofilms

It is presently estimated that at least 65% of all human bacterial infections may involve biofilm formation. Biofilms have also been implicated in several conditions seen in an otolaryngology practice, including otitis media, CRS, chronic tonsillitis, adenoiditis, and device infections.[8] Bacterial biofilms are described as surface-associated communities of microorganisms encased in a protective extracellular matrix. Biofilms are initiated when free-floating, planktonic bacteria anchor to biological or inert surfaces. The attached bacteria multiply and progress from a state of monolayer to a microcolony and then to a critical mass, in which interbacterial crosstalk occurs, triggering a phenomenon known as quorum sensing that leads to the biofilm phenotype. The bacteria respond collectively to express factors that are specific to the biofilm phenotype, which leads to the secretion of an exopolysaccharide matrix. Under the right environmental conditions, free-floating bacteria are released from the biofilms, and the cycle is continued at other surfaces.[9,10]

Bacteria in biofilms are resistant to host defenses because the extracellular matrix that makes up most of the biofilm serves to protect the bacteria against antibodies, immune system phagocytosis, and antibiotics. Increased antibiotic resistance is a trait common to biofilm bacteria. Bacteria in biofilms show 10- to 1000-fold less sensitivity to antibiotics than bacteria growing in culture.[9]

Bacterial biofilms have been implicated in the chronic nature of CRS.[11] Of late, studies have shown that patients with biofilms have more persistence of postoperative symptoms, ongoing mucosal inflammation, and infections.[12,13] It was reported that biofilms existed on the sinus mucosa of patients with CRS both before and after functional endoscopic sinus surgery (FESS), and they contributed to an increased likelihood of unfavorable outcomes in FESS.[12,14,15]

A variety of techniques have been evaluated to manage and treat biofilm. These treatments include surgery, topical antimicrobials, and other adjuvant therapies. Newer treatments are aimed at interfering with the biofilm life cycle and targeting bacterial attachment and quorum-sensing mechanisms.

Paranasal Sinus Nitric Oxide

NO has been implicated in several physiological components, including neurotransmission, bronchodilation,[16] and mucociliary regulation.[17] Strong evidence supports NO production from the paranasal sinuses.[18] There has been some recent concern regarding decreased concentration of NO following endoscopic sinus surgery. Given the studies demon-

strate the implication of NO on mucociliary clearance, and a natural concern of mucociliary clearance in CRS patients, further evaluation is justified. In the rhinologic community, the debate over optimal surgical enlargement of sinuses often centers around NO levels. Proponents of smaller surgical ostia point to decreased disruption of NO levels as a reason. Additionally, a growing body of literature also demonstrates that biofilm formation is increased in the presence of low NO levels.[19,20] Studies have demonstrated that the majority of NO in the airways is generated from the paranasal sinuses, specifically the sinus mucosa. Given the identified bacteriostatic role in *S. aureus* in vitro, in addition to the proximity of the sinuses to the bacterially active nasal and oral cavities, one proposed possibility is host defense.[21]

Phillips et al performed a systematic review of NO and sinonasal disease evaluating all previous publications that demonstrated this correlation with specific criteria including only evaluating those studies that specifically measured gaseous NO concentrations.[18] Although they found a wide range of measurement techniques introducing a large variability in NO results in the respective studies, they did attempt to answer the debate as to the optimal opening of sinus cavities because of potential decreases in NO concentration. They stated that based on present data, no definitive conclusion can be drawn about optimal ostium size. They further report that NO levels, do in fact, seem to be related to ciliary beat frequency,[22] but based on the review, it is unclear whether this is a cause or effect of the underlying disease process.[18]

Although evidence suggests that NO aids in upper airway homeostasis and immunity by modulating blood flow, augmenting mucociliary clearance, and acting as an antiviral and antimicrobial agent, NO may also be toxic under certain conditions. The complicated biological pathways of NO in the upper airways, especially involving the pathogenesis of chronic inflammatory disorders such as CRS and nasal polyposis, demand further investigation. The elucidation of NO's precise role in these inflammatory diseases may allow for earlier and more accurate diagnosis, noninvasive follow-up monitoring, and new therapeutic approaches that will prevent the harmful direct and indirect effects mediated by NO.

Conclusion

Although CRS is a multifactorial disease process, disruption of mucociliary clearance is the common endpoint resulting in the vast majority of symptomatology associated with the disease. Normal function of the sinus mucosa, mucus, and cilia are critical for optimal clearance. Recent investigations on biofilms and NO levels in the paranasal sinuses are two important factors that ultimately affect mucociliary function, and further investigations will aid in future treatment applications.

References

1. Murphy MP, Fishman P, Short SO, Sullivan SD, Yueh B, Weymuller EA Jr. Health care utilization and cost among adults with chronic rhinosinusitis enrolled in a health maintenance organization. Otolaryngol Head Neck Surg 2002;127(5):367–376

2. Wagenmann M, Naclerio RM. Anatomic and physiologic considerations in sinusitis. J Allergy Clin Immunol 1992;90(3, pt 2):419–423

3. Busse WW. Mechanisms and advances in allergic diseases. J Allergy Clin Immunol 2000;105(6, pt 2):S593–S598

4. Naclerio R. Clinical manifestations of the release of histamine and other inflammatory mediators. J Allergy Clin Immunol 1999;103(3, pt 2):S382–S385

5. Lamblin G, Lhermitte M, Klein A, et al. The carbohydrate diversity of human respiratory mucins: a protection of the underlying mucosa? Am Rev Respir Dis 1991;144(3, pt 2):S19–S24

6. Yeh TH, Su MC, Hsu CJ, Chen YH, Lee SY. Epithelial cells of nasal mucosa express functional gap junctions of connexin 43. Acta Otolaryngol 2003;123(2):314–320

7. Gheber L, Priel Z. Synchronization between beating cilia. Biophys J 1989;55(1):183–191

8. Solomon DH, Wobb J, Buttaro BA, Truant A, Soliman AM. Characterization of bacterial biofilms on tracheostomy tubes. Laryngoscope 2009;119(8):1633–1638

9. Davies D. Understanding biofilm resistance to antibacterial agents. Nat Rev Drug Discov 2003;2(2):114–122

10. Richards JJ, Melander C. Controlling bacterial biofilms. Chem Bio Chem 2009;10(14):2287–2294

11. Psaltis AJ, Ha KR, Beule AG, Tan LW, Wormald PJ. Confocal scanning laser microscopy evidence of biofilms in patients with chronic rhinosinusitis. Laryngoscope 2007;117(7):1302–1306

12. Psaltis AJ, Weitzel EK, Ha KR, Wormald PJ. The effect of bacterial biofilms on post-sinus surgical outcomes. Am J Rhinol 2008;22(1):1–6

13. Singhal D, Psaltis AJ, Foreman A, Wormald PJ. The impact of biofilms on outcomes after endoscopic sinus surgery. Am J Rhinol Allergy 2010;24(3):169–174

14. Bendouah Z, Barbeau J, Hamad WA, Desrosiers M. Biofilm formation by *Staphylococcus aureus* and *Pseudomonas aeruginosa* is associated with an unfavorable evolution after surgery for chronic sinusitis and nasal polyposis. Otolaryngol Head Neck Surg 2006;134(6):991–996

15. Prince AA, Steiger JD, Khalid AN, et al. Prevalence of biofilm-forming bacteria in chronic rhinosinusitis. Am J Rhinol 2008;22(3):239–245

16. Belvisi MG, Stretton CD, Yacoub M, Barnes PJ. Nitric oxide is the endogenous neurotransmitter of bronchodilator nerves in humans. Eur J Pharmacol 1992;210(2):221–222

17. Runer T, Cervin A, Lindberg S, Uddman R. Nitric oxide is a regulator of mucociliary activity in the upper respiratory tract. Otolaryngol Head Neck Surg 1998;119(3):278–287

18. Phillips PS, Sacks R, Marcells GN, Cohen NA, Harvey RJ. Nasal nitric oxide and sinonasal disease: a systematic review of published evidence. Otolaryngol Head Neck Surg 2011;144(2):159–169

19. Barraud N, Hassett DJ, Hwang SH, Rice SA, Kjelleberg S, Webb JS. Involvement of nitric oxide in biofilm dispersal of *Pseudomonas aeruginosa*. J Bacteriol 2006;188(21):7344–7353

20. Schlag S, Nerz C, Birkenstock TA, Altenberend F, Götz F. Inhibition of staphylococcal biofilm formation by nitrite. J Bacteriol 2007;189(21):7911–7919

21. Hoehn T, Huebner J, Paboura E, Krause M, Leititis JU. Effect of therapeutic concentrations of nitric oxide on bacterial growth in vitro. Crit Care Med 1998;26(11):1857–1862

22. Lundberg JO, Farkas-Szallasi T, Weitzberg E, et al. High nitric oxide production in human paranasal sinuses. Nat Med 1995;1(4):370–373

4

Imaging of the Paranasal Sinuses and Anterior Skull Base

Rohini N. Nadgir, Elisa N. Flower, Anand K. Devaiah, and Osamu Sakai

Imaging of the nasal cavity, paranasal sinuses, and anterior skull base has become an important component in the evaluation and management of disease in these areas. Infectious, inflammatory, traumatic, and neoplastic disease processes can be delineated with imaging modalities to improve patient care. Although radiographs provide some information and were more heavily relied upon in the past, the improved anatomic detail provided by computed tomography (CT) has made this modality the mainstay of sinonasal imaging. Magnetic resonance imaging (MRI) is typically performed for complex pathologies, when there is a need for better soft tissue delineation or for determining extension of disease outside of the sinonasal cavity. In these cases, CT and MRI are often complementary to each other.

This chapter focuses on the role of imaging in various clinical conditions rather than a complete review of pathologic processes that can be seen in this region. Although the imaging strategy may vary from one patient to another depending on the clinical question, this chapter provides guidance in the radiologic evaluation of suspected sinonasal/anterior skull base disease.

Imaging Techniques

Computed Tomography

CT provides an excellent definition of bone and air-filled spaces, and it is the primary modality for imaging of the sinuses. It is particularly useful in the evaluation of sinus inflammation and nasal polyposis.[1] CT is based on electron density and follows the same principles as that of radiography. Denser structures (such as metal and bone) stop more X-rays and are seen as relatively hyperdense structures, whereas less dense structures (such as air) stop fewer X-rays and are relatively hypodense structures. Presently, most CT examinations are performed with multidetector-row CT (MDCT). This can provide submillimeter slices through regions of interest with much less motion artifact than older generation scanners. In evaluation of the sinonasal cavities, the coronal plane of imaging is most relevant to the endoscopist, and CT data can be acquired in the coronal plane with the patient in the prone position.

At our institution and many others, sinonasal imaging is now performed in the axial plane with the patient in the supine position. High-quality sagittal and coronal-reformatted images can be obtained from the axially acquired thin section "volume data."[2,3] Images are reconstructed with soft tissue and bone algorithms and reviewed in soft tissue and bone window settings, respectively, to fully evaluate the integrity of bony structures and relevant soft tissues. Three-dimensional reconstructions can also be performed based on the axially acquired data.

Magnetic Resonance Imaging

MRI has a much higher soft tissue contrast resolution compared with CT. It is very good at differentiating among various soft tissues and fluids.[4] Depending on the clinical issue, submillimeter slice thickness in any plane can help delineate small structures such as skull base foramina and cranial nerves. MRI relies on the signal generated from excited hydrogen nuclei (protons). Radiofrequency pulses are applied to stimulate a proton, and then the coil captures the signal emitted as the nucleus relaxes. The terms T1 and T2 refer to different types of relaxation of the nuclei.

On MRI, fat on T1-weighted images demonstrates a very high signal, appearing as "white," or hyperintense, on the image. Fluid, such as cerebrospinal fluid (CSF), is dark on T1-weighted images although it is not completely black, whereas cortical bone and air have almost no signal and are seen as "black," or hypointense on T1-weighted images. Administration of intravenous gadolinium-based contrast material shortens the T1 of tissues and results in an increase in the signal or brightness on T1-weighted images.

T2-weighted images demonstrate simple fluids such as CSF as bright or high signal. Cortical bone and air appear dark on T2-weighted images. Fat on fast-spin echo technique T2-weighted image is bright. However, various forms of fat suppression techniques may be used, reducing this tissue's innate T2 hyperintensity.

Gadolinium-based contrast agents are intravenously administered and are typically used in the evaluation of soft tissues. Hypervascular lesions show an increased signal on MRI after intravenous contrast administration; subtle extension of disease into other adjacent compartments (i.e., orbit and brain) and along nerves (i.e., perineural spread) may be appreciable only on postcontrast images. Fat-suppression techniques can be applied after contrast administration to better delineate enhancing lesions into the fat or bone marrow; however, inhomogeneous fat suppression and susceptibility artifacts may cause image "blurring" and make the diagnosis of perineural tumor spread difficult, particularly near bone/air interfaces. Therefore, careful evaluation of precontrast T1-weighted images is essential, and performing postcontrast T1-weighted imaging both with and without fat suppression is ideal.

Positron Emission Tomography

The use of positron emission tomography (PET) in diagnostic imaging of malignancy has grown considerably in the past decade. PET imaging involves intravenous administration of a radiotracer tagged to a commonly occurring substance in the body, a gamma ray detector that senses positron-emitting radiotracers, and computer-based processing that assembles these measured emissions into images. In clinical practice, 2-[fluorine-18]fluoro-2-deoxy-D-glucose is the most commonly used radiotracer, which aggregates in metabolically active processes including most malignancies. Once the radiotracer has had adequate time for tissue uptake (60 to 90 minutes), emissions are measured by the gamma detector during the next 30 to 60 minutes.

In evaluating malignancy, PET examinations provide information for treatment planning and post treatment follow-up. The malignant process being imaged must be "PET-avid," meaning that the neoplasm takes up more radiotracer than surrounding non-neoplastic tissue, so that the neoplasm may be distinguished from non-neoplastic tissue. Given the normal high degree of metabolic activity and glucose uptake in the brain, lesions within the brain and adjacent skull base typically cannot be clearly delineated with PET. Most PET studies are now performed along with CT (PET/CT), and images can be fused together to improve anatomic detail of the disease process.

Imaging Evaluation

It is critical for the radiologist to know the clinical presentation and expected diagnosis to tailor the imaging study, including the choice of modality as well as imaging planes and relevant sequences. Anatomic location of the suspected disease process is critical for the radiologist to protocol the study properly as well as for interpretation. For example, on the basis of the clinical concern, the radiologist must decide whether the imaging should focus on the bony or soft tissue anatomy or both, and whether or not contrast should be used for the imaging study requested. Furthermore, imaging studies can be used for intraoperative navigation.

There are other anatomic and pathologic considerations when deciding on which scans to use for a particular clinical scenario. The CT scan is the workhorse for sinus and skull base pathology. In the event that the information about a neoplastic or vascular process is needed, contrast should be given with this scan. MRI with contrast is most useful when evaluating soft tissue detail, examining for neoplastic invasion, or when other detailed angiographic information is needed. PET, with or without CT, can be useful in neoplastic processes that are PET avid. The most useful and cost-effective role of PET for otolaryngologic diseases is still under study, but shows great promise.

Some general statements about sinus and skull base imaging can be made, despite the variations that exist because of clinical presentation. Sinus inflammatory disease (e.g., polyps) is usually studied appropriately with a noncontrast CT. If skull base lesions or disorders are suspected, an MRI can be useful in delineating soft tissue detail, dural integrity, and intracranial involvement.

Conditions Affecting the Sinonasal Cavity and Anterior Skull Base

Congenital

Although rare, in a pediatric patient with nasal mass, with or without midline craniofacial anomaly, congenital lesions including nasal glioma, dermoid, and cephalocele must be considered.[5] Occasionally, these lesions are identified incidentally in pediatric and adult patients for examinations performed for other reasons. Imaging is essential before biopsy, to exclude the possibility of cephalocele.

Nasal glioma, consisting of ectopic glial tissue arising most commonly at the nasal dorsum or less commonly within the nasal cavity, can maintain attachment to the skull base but does not extend intracranially. Nasal dermoid, consisting in part of fatty tissue, may be associated with a sinus tract extending through foramen cecum and cribriform plate with dural attachment. Cephaloceles, consisting of herniated brain tissue (encephalocele), meninges (meningocele), or both (meningoencephalocele), can be seen extending through frontonasal, nasoethmoidal, and nasoorbital defects (**Fig. 4.1**). In distinguishing these entities from one another, MRI is the preferred imaging modality because of superior soft tissue contrast resolution. For example, MRI can show small amounts of fatty tissue to make the diagnosis of dermoid that can be imperceptible by CT. MRI can also show other intracranial developmental defects that may coexist in the setting of cephalocele. However, CT plays an important role in demonstrating the integrity of the bony anterior skull base, including foramen cecum, crista galli, and cribriform plate for the purposes of surgical planning.[5,6]

Choanal atresia can be diagnosed clinically in the neonatal period, but imaging is necessary to fully evaluate the severity of the atresia. Excellent bony definition provided by CT can help distinguish stenosis from complete atresia and membranous from bony atresias before surgical correction.[7]

In patients with anosmia, high-resolution coronally acquired T2-weighted images can show absence or hypoplasia of the olfactory bulbs at the anterior skull base.[8] Without associated parenchymal gliosis, this finding is most compatible with congenital etiology.

Trauma

The sinuses and nasal cavity are subject to direct traumatic injury. Hemorrhage layering within a sinus, sinuses, and/or nasal cavity in the setting of facial swelling and a

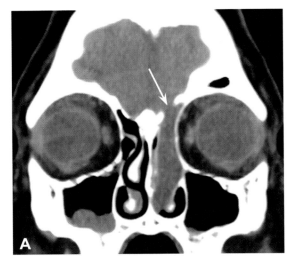
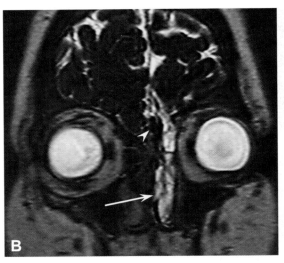

Figure 4.1 Frontoethmoid cephalocele. (A) Coronal unenhanced computed tomography image demonstrates a fluid-attenuation mass in the left nasal cavity associated with a defect in the left ethmoid roof (arrow). (B) High-resolution coronal T2-weighted magnetic resonance image shows predominantly fluid nature of this mass (arrow) and focal dysplastic brain tissue in the frontal sinus (arrowhead). Findings are consistent with meningoencephalocele.

history of recent trauma can be specific for acute fracture injury. Although such injuries can be initially evaluated by radiography, CT can provide a greater anatomic detail in an expedited fashion.[9] Bony discontinuities of the nasolacrimal duct, orbital structures, and skull base may indicate additional unsuspected injuries. Focal hemorrhages in the sinuses, soft tissues of the face, and orbits can be identified on images reconstructed by soft tissue algorithm. Air within or adjacent to the carotid canal can indicate potential for internal carotid artery injury, and an angiographic study should follow to address patency of this vessel.[10,11] Three-dimensional reformations of the facial bones can help in diagnosis and surgical planning (**Fig. 4.2**). MRI does not play an important role in the acute traumatic setting.

Infectious/Inflammatory Disease

When complications from acute sinusitis are suspected, such as orbital, soft tissue/facial, and intracranial extension of infection, imaging is very useful. The presence of air–fluid level within a sinus on imaging can be consistent with acute inflammation in the appropriate clinical setting, but is not very specific.

In patients with recurrent or chronic sinusitis being considered for surgical management, noncontrast CT should be obtained for diagnosis and surgical planning purposes.[2,3] CT can demonstrate the extent of sinus inflammation and can identify anatomic variations or lesions that may be the cause of recurring symptoms.[12] An odontogenic source of sinus inflammation, typically from periodontal disease, is not uncommon. The offending tooth as well as associated sinus inflammation can be identified by CT.[13] Enlarged Haller air cells, antrochoanal polyps, and mucoceles may cause obstruction at critical sites of mucociliary draining, resulting in recurring episodes of sinus inflammation and can also be readily evaluated by CT.[14] Impact of an enlarged Haller air cell on the ostiomeatal unit can be elegantly demonstrated on coronal CT images. The presence of a polypoid lesion

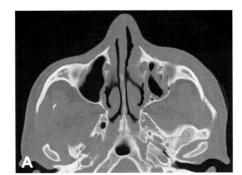
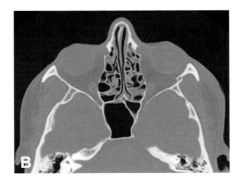
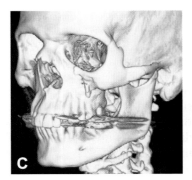

Figure 4.2 Zygomaticomaxillary complex fracture. (A) Axial computed tomography image demonstrates acute fractures of the anterior and posterolateral walls of the left maxillary sinus and depressed fracture. (B) More superiorly, there is a comminuted disruption of the left lateral orbital wall. (C) Three-dimensional volume-rendered image demonstrates the characteristic findings of the zygomaticomaxillary complex fracture. Anterior maxillary wall fracture extends to the orbital rim.

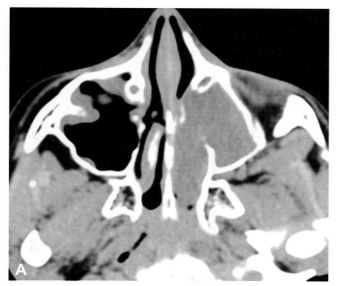 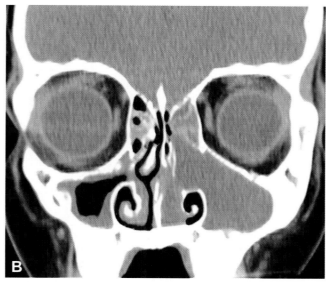

Figure 4.3 Antrochoanal polyp. (A) Axial and (B) coronal unenhanced computed tomography images demonstrate a fluid-attenuation lesion occupying and expanding the left maxillary sinus with extension through the maxillary ostium into the left nasal cavity.

arising from the maxillary sinus extending into the nasal cavity through the ostium with typical watery density and bony remodeling on CT can be specific for antrochoanal polyp[15] (**Fig. 4.3**). Mucoceles, occurring as a result of chronic inflammation or earlier trauma, result in sinus expansion, typically within the frontal sinus although all sinuses can be affected, and contain complex proteinaceous components. CT can show bony remodeling by the mucocele with bone thinning and/or frank dehiscence. Both CT and MRI can show the complex cystic nature of these lesions and identify extension outside of the sinus into the adjacent nasal cavity, orbit, and brain with associated mass effect on these structures[16] (**Fig. 4.4**).

In patients with chronic sinus inflammation, thickening and sclerosis of paranasal sinus walls can be seen. Occasionally, linear or chunky calcifications may be present within the involved sinus(es). This should not be confused with the expansion of hematopoietic marrow within facial bones seen in patients with the chronic anemia of thalassemia or sickle cell disease.[17] In the chronically inflamed sinus, contents may be hyperdense on CT. This is related to inspissated debris, fungal superinfection, or allergic reaction associated with fungal infection that may be otherwise clinically unsuspected (**Fig. 4.5**). On MRI, this same fungal material results in signal dropout or "blackness" within the sinus on T1- and T2-weighted images from iron and manganese deposits. This results in the appearance of a "clear" sinus, although in reality the sinus is opacified. For this reason, fungal sinusitis can be difficult to identify on MRI. Therefore, CT should be the first-line modality when sinus disease is suspected. Extensive hyperdense material within sinuses on CT should raise concern for allergic fungal sinusitis.[1,18,19]

Imaging is often performed in the setting of complicated sinus infection. Extension of sinus inflammation into the adjacent orbit, brain, and bone itself can be identified on

CT and MRI.[19,20] In younger patients, direct extension along vascular channels typically from the ethmoid sinus into the medial orbit is not uncommon. Both CT and MRI with contrast can demonstrate the presence of inflammatory tissue in the orbit with or without an organized fluid collection (**Fig. 4.6**); CT would be the preferred modality in these cases as it is typically more readily available at most institutions and images are more quickly acquired. MRI with contrast better evaluates intracranial manifestations of disease extension including empyema, meningitis, and encephalitis.[21] Abnormal meningeal and parenchymal enhancement may be seen in these cases. Both CT venogram and MRI of the skull base with contrast can demonstrate associated cavernous sinus thrombosis as a filling defect within an enlarged cavernous sinus. Given the small caliber of the venous component within the cavernous sinuses, patency may be difficult to confirm on MR venograms performed using typical phase-contrast technique. Cavernous sinus patency can be more reliably assessed on contrast-enhanced MR venography and in comparison of pre and postcontrast images through this region.[22] Optic neuritis as a result of sinus infection has been reported[23] and can be demonstrated on MRI with increased T2 signal, increased caliber, and abnormal enhancement within the affected optic nerve and sheath complex. Inflammation with or without abscess formation may cross the bone into the overlying extracranial soft tissues and can be identified on CT or MRI with contrast. Pott's puffy tumor is frontal bone osteomyelitis with extracranial subperiosteal abscess secondary to frontal sinusitis, which presents as a fluctuant mass. An organized abscess can be identified as a discrete fluid density or signal region on CT and MRI, respectively, with peripheral rim enhancement. However, MRI can also identify intracranial extension of infection including small extra-axial abscesses, meningeal enhancement, and

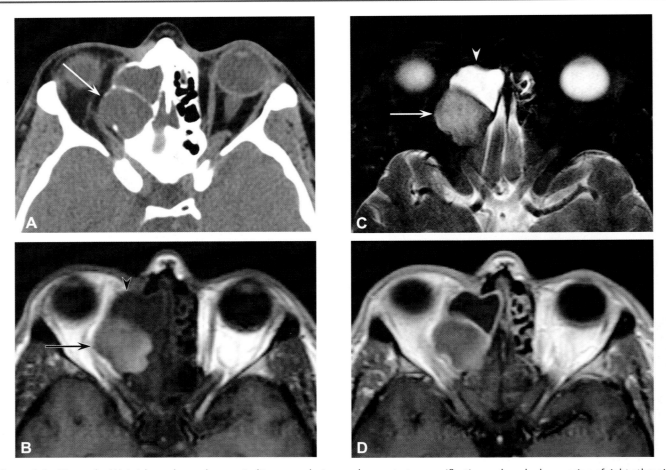

Figure 4.4   Mucocele. (A) Axial unenhanced computed tomography image demonstrates opacification and marked expansion of right ethmoid air cells with bony remodeling of the overlying lamina papyracea (arrow). (B) Axial T1-weighted and (C) T2-weighted magnetic resonance images demonstrate that the more posterior expanded ethmoid air cell contains proteinaceous material with T1 hyperintensity and T2 hypointensity (arrows), whereas the more anterior air cell contains serous fluid with simple fluid signal (arrowheads). (D) Axial postcontrast T1-weighted image shows no solid-enhancing component, confirming fluid nature of the lesion.

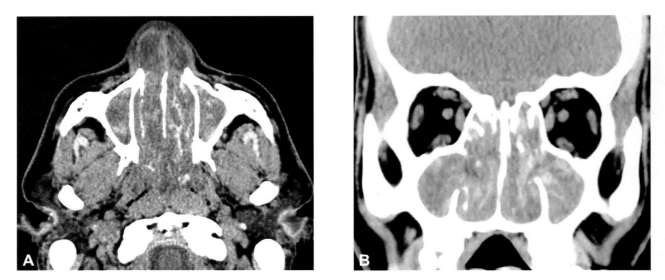

Figure 4.5   Nasal polyposis with allergic fungal sinusitis. (A) Axial computed tomography (CT) image demonstrates ovoid expansile fluid-attenuation masses within the anterior nasal cavity bilaterally consistent with nasal polyps. (B) Coronal unenhanced CT image shows a total opacification of the ethmoid sinuses, maxillary sinuses, and nasal cavity bilaterally with areas of high density secondary to fungal infection. Note expansile nature of this process with lateral bowing of the lamina papyracea.

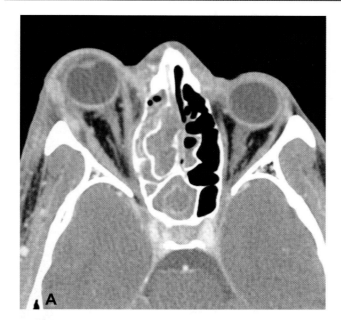

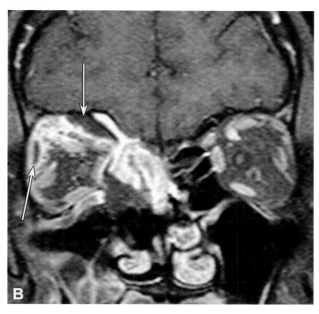

Figure 4.6 Orbital abscess due to ethmoid sinusitis. (A) Axial postcontrast computed tomography image demonstrates right proptosis associated with right-sided ethmoid and sphenoid sinus opacification. Note increased density in the extraconal fat within the right orbit. (B) Coronal postcontrast T1-weighted magnetic resonance image shows that parts of the inflammatory tissue in the superior and lateral orbit are fluid in nature, indicating abscess formation (arrows).

parenchymal signal changes that can be imperceptible on CT; therefore, MRI is indicated in this clinical setting.[24]

There are numerous inflammatory/granulomatous disease processes that can affect the sinonasal regions and anterior skull base, including but not limited to granulomatosis with polyangiitis (formerly Wegener granulomatosis), sarcoidosis, tuberculosis, and less commonly syphilis. Although there are no findings specific to these conditions, the combination of mucosal thickening, mucosal ulceration,

and bony destruction should raise concern for inflammatory process, best seen on CT. In aggressive cases, direct orbital, skull base, and intracranial extension of inflammatory tissue can be seen. CT can define the extent of bony erosion (**Fig. 4.7A**). MRI can show soft tissue involvement of the skull base, orbit, face, and brain (**Fig. 4.7B** and **C**). Although CT can appreciate soft tissue extension, dural enhancement is best seen on MRI; however, direct meningeal involvement and reactive meningeal enhancement are difficult to

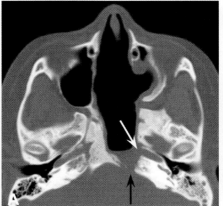
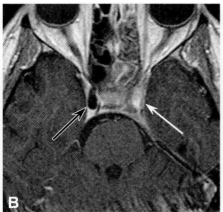
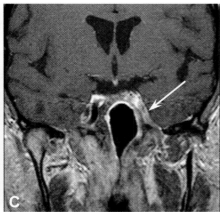

Figure 4.7 Granulomatous polyangiitis (formerly Wegener granulomatosis). (A) Axial computed tomography image demonstrates destruction of the nasal septum, anterior and posterior walls of the sphenoid sinus, and left aspect of the clivus (black arrow). The carotid canal is also focally destroyed medially (white arrow). Medial wall of the left maxillary sinus and turbinates have been surgically resected. Hyperostosis of the remaining sphenoid sinus and left maxillary sinus walls indicates chronic inflammation. (B) Axial postcontrast T1-weighted magnetic resonance (MR) image shows asymmetric enhancing soft tissue within the cavernous sinus on the left (white arrow), accounting for the patient's presenting symptom of left-sided sixth nerve palsy. Note the absence of the internal carotid artery flow void on the left compared with normal appearance on the right (black arrow). (C) Coronal postcontrast T1-weighted MR image shows asymmetric enhancement of the left Meckel cave (white arrow) with extension along V3 through the foramen ovale.

distinguish on imaging. Nasal septal perforation is not uncommonly seen in the setting of inflammatory sinusitis, although it may also be a post-traumatic, iatrogenic, or drug-related phenomenon. Lymphoma may also result in septal perforation.[18,25]

Benign Tumors and Tumor-Like Conditions

Polypoid lesions within the nasal cavity are easily appreciated on clinical examination. Sinus CT can be performed to evaluate the extent of these lesions and to assess for aggressive features that may indicate malignancy or malignant transformation.[26] Nasal polyps are not uncommon and typically arise from the lateral nasal wall.[27] In patients with sinonasal polyposis, polypoid masses can be seen involving nasal cavity and paranasal sinuses, with near-total opacification, expansion, and even bony erosion in severe cases. Polyps usually demonstrate fluid characteristics on CT and MRI but mixed density chronic inflammatory contents can also be seen on CT because of chronic inflammation from trapped fluid within the nasal cavity and sinuses (**Fig. 4.5**). In particular, allergic fungal sinusitis occurring in atopic patients may accompany sinonasal polyposis and can be suspected on imaging when mixed-attenuation contents of multiple sinuses or pansinus opacification are seen.

Inverted papillomas often arise from the lateral wall of the nasal cavity and extend into the maxillary sinus through the ostium. They are typically heterogeneous in density with expansile osseous change and often with calcification. Bony destructive change raises concern for concomitant malignancy or malignant transformation. On MRI, inverted papillomas may demonstrate the classic cerebriform pattern on T2- and postcontrast T1-weighted images.[28]

Juvenile angiofibroma is a benign, but locally aggressive, highly vascular lesion, often noted to extend into the nasal cavity at the time of clinical presentation. Extension of the lesion via the pterygopalatine fossa into the infratemporal fossa, brain, and orbit can be seen in more advanced cases. On CT, expansion of the pterygopalatine fossa and anterior displacement of the posterolateral wall of the maxillary sinus is often seen (**Fig. 4.8A**). On MRI, these lesions will show prominent "flow voids" or serpiginous dark signal within vessels on T1- and T2-weighted images. These lesions enhance on postcontrast imaging because of their highly vascular nature (**Fig. 4.8B** and **C**). These lesions should be embolized before surgical resection, to avoid significant intraoperative blood loss.[29,30]

Benign bony lesions in the sinonasal cavity can be incidentally identified on imaging performed for other reasons. Osteomas are commonly seen within the paranasal sinuses, most often in the frontal and ethmoid sinuses, and are usually asymptomatic, although multiple osteomas may be associated with Gardner syndrome. On CT, they appear as rounded, usually homogeneously dense masses, similar to the density of cortical bone. When large, they can obstruct mucociliary drainage and may require resection.[31]

Fibrous dysplasia can result in a marked expansile change within multiple facial bones. In advanced cases, proptosis, facial asymmetries, and functional obstruction of the paranasal sinus and nasal cavity drainage may result. The characteristic "ground glass" appearance of involved bony structures can be elegantly demonstrated on CT, although occasionally lytic and sclerotic areas may be seen (**Fig. 4.9**). On MRI, involved marrow will be abnormally dark on T1- and T2-weighted images, with variable degrees of enhancement after contrast administration.[32,33]

Meningioma is the most common benign intracranial tumor, and the olfactory groove is a common site of origin. When large, extracranial extension can be seen at the anterior skull base. On MRI, the tumor itself is similar in intensity to brain on T1- and T2-weighted images, and enhances homogeneously, often with a "dural tail" of enhancement.[34] On CT, hyperostosis, or "blistering," can be seen at the anterior

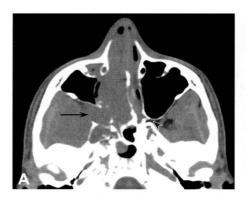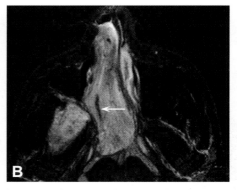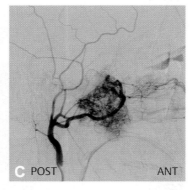

Figure 4.8 Juvenile angiofibroma. (A) Unenhanced computed tomography image demonstrates soft tissue density lesion in the right nasal cavity and pterygopalatine fossa (PPF) (arrow), widening the right PPF and displacing the posterolateral wall of the maxillary sinus anteriorly. Note the normal-sized left PPF with preserved fat attenuation (arrowhead). (B) Axial T2-weighted magnetic resonance image demonstrates an intermediate to hyperintense lesion within the nasopharynx and nasal cavity with extension laterally via the PPF into the retroantral fat and masticator space on the right. Focal curvilinear hypointensity (arrow) is compatible with flow void indicating hypervascular nature of this lesion. (C) External carotid angiogram, lateral projection, demonstrates a tumor blush and markedly enlarged internal maxillary artery feeding the lesion.

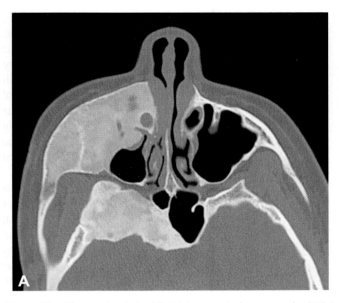
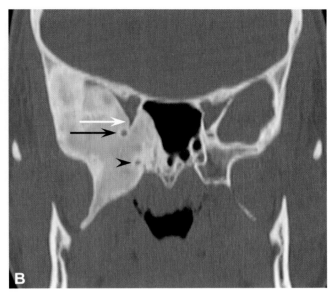

Figure 4.9 Fibrous dysplasia. (A) Axial computed tomography (CT) image demonstrates the classic "ground glass" density and expansion of the affected bone, involving the right zygoma, maxilla, and sphenoid bone. (B) Coronal CT image shows the lesion surrounding the foramen rotundum (black arrow) with narrowing of the vidian canal (arrowhead) and infraorbital fissure (white arrow).

skull base and may reflect reactive change from the tumor or may represent direct bone involvement by the tumor.

Malignant Tumors

CT and MRI typically fulfill complementary roles in the work-up of sinonasal malignancies. The use of PET or PET/CT in this setting is under investigation, with some early studies suggesting value in identifying nodal and distant metastases.[35] Although it is often difficult to provide the precise histopathologic identification of the process based on imaging alone, the extent of tumor involvement within bone, adjacent soft tissue compartments, skull base foramina, and lymph nodes can be evaluated by imaging. This can help in diagnostic and treatment planning.

Squamous cell carcinoma (SCC) is the most common malignancy to affect the paranasal sinuses and nasal cavity.[36] The maxillary sinus is most commonly affected. Patients may not present until the tumor is advanced, with the development of sinonasal obstruction from growth of the tumor. On CT, unilateral sinus opacification with associated aggressive bony erosion and destruction can be seen (**Fig. 4.10A**). Soft tissue tumor changes can also be seen extending beyond the primary site of involvement into

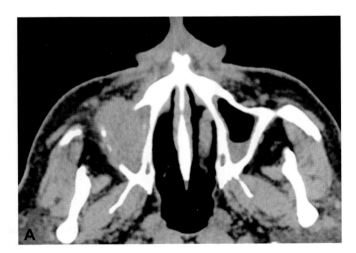
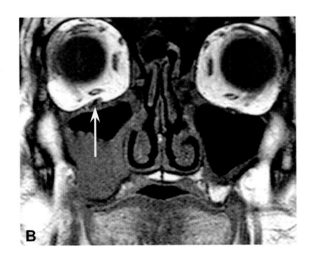

Figure 4.10 Squamous cell carcinoma. (A) Axial computed tomography image demonstrates a soft tissue mass centered in the right maxillary sinus that erodes through the anterior and posterolateral walls of the maxillary sinus. There is invasion into the anterior buccal space and retroantral fat. (B) Coronal T1-weighted magnetic resonance image shows tumor in the right maxillary sinus and enlargement of the infraorbital nerve, indicating perineural tumor spread (arrow).

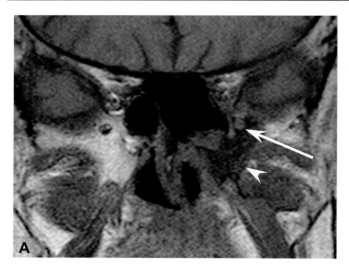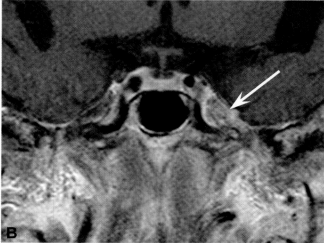

Figure 4.11 Perineural tumor spread in recurrent maxillary squamous cell carcinoma. (A) Coronal T1-weighted magnetic resonance images show abnormal dark marrow signal within the left sphenoid bone (arrowhead) because of direct tumor extension from the maxilla (not pictured). There is enlargement of the V2 in the left foramen rotundum (white arrow), indicating perineural tumor spread. (B) Coronal postcontrast T1-weighted image shows abnormal enhancement and expansion of the left Meckel cave (arrow).

adjacent sinuses, nasal cavity, buccal fat, facial tissues, and orbits. Bony destruction of the anterior skull base and orbital walls can be easily identified on CT, and the degree of soft tissue involvement both intracranially and intraorbitally can be assessed better on MRI[37] (**Fig. 4.10B**). It may be difficult to differentiate tumor from secondary inflammatory change within affected and adjacent sinuses on unenhanced CT. Therefore, postcontrast images on CT and MRI are critical to make the distinction. In general, SCC appears darker than inflammatory tissue on T2-weighted images, and it enhances less avidly than inflammatory tissue after contrast administration.[38]

Perineural tumor spread should be assessed on imaging, including involvement of the infraorbital groove and pterygopalatine fossa and associated conduits for spread into the palate, nasal cavity, infratemporal fossa, brain, and orbit. On CT, involvement can be suspected on the basis of enlargement of the skull base foramina/canals, permeative bony change extending up to the margin of the foramina, or loss of expected normal fatty attenuation within the foramina. On MRI, perineural tumor extension can be suspected with loss of fatty signal and abnormal enhancement within or near the skull base foramina or canals (**Fig. 4.11**). Furthermore, denervation injury can be identified on MRI. Early denervation shows an abnormal increased signal on T2-weighted or short T1 inversion recovery images and enhancement within muscle groups whereas chronic denervation shows fatty atrophy within these muscle groups.[39, 40]

Although distinguishing tumor types on imaging is difficult, certain imaging characteristics can help narrow the differential diagnosis. On imaging, lymphoma may appear similarly to SCC; however, lymphoma is often homogeneous in density or signal without necrosis and with relative T2 hypointensity (**Fig. 4.12**). Lymphoma more often extends

across bony structures with a relatively preserved bony architecture, whereas SCC tends to show bony compartment destruction.[41] Salivary gland malignancies arising from minor salivary glands within the nasal mucosa are much less common than SCC and lymphoma, but they tend to demonstrate perineural tumor spread at the time of diagnosis.[42]

Soft tissue tumors centered at the anterior skull base may arise from the superior nasal cavity or intracranial compartment. Patients typically present with nasal congestion and anosmia because of tumor involvement of the nasal cavity and olfactory epithelium at the cribriform plate, respectively. SCC arising from the superior nasal cavity is the most common malignancy in this region and can be seen with bony destruction of the anterior skull base on CT and intracranial involvement on CT and MRI.[43] Dural enhancement is best identified on MRI and can indicate reactive change; thickened dural enhancement with nodularity is a strong indicator of direct dural involvement with tumor. On CT and MRI, sinonasal undifferentiated carcinoma is difficult to distinguish from SCC or neuroendocrine tumors. These tumors can demonstrate metabolic activity on PET (**Fig. 4.13**). Esthesioneuroblastoma arising from olfactory epithelium can also present in this location. This lesion is also difficult to distinguish from other tumors in this location; however, the diagnosis can be suspected when peritumoral cysts (cysts along the intracranial margins of the tumor) are identified on postcontrast CT or MR images[44] (**Fig. 4.14**).

CT can demonstrate tumor matrix in malignancies arising from the bone marrow itself. Osteosarcoma in facial bones may arise de novo or may be secondary to earlier radiotherapy.[45] These arise from the alveolar ridge of the maxilla or body of the mandible and show marked aggressive bone destruction and sclerotic components.

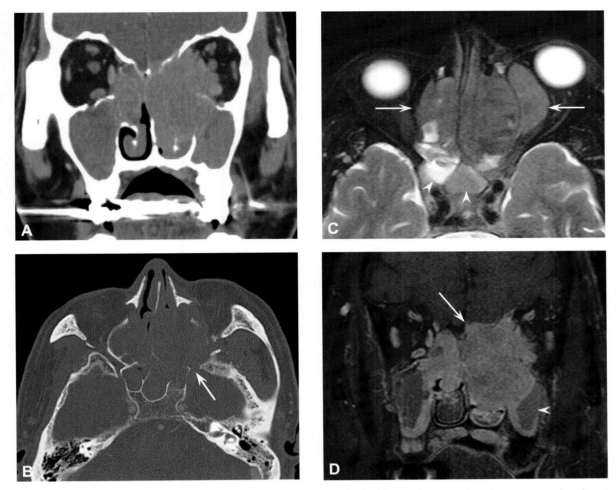

Figure 4.12 Lymphoma. (A) Coronal contrast-enhanced computed tomography (CT) image demonstrates a homogeneously enhancing lesion within the bilateral ethmoid and maxillary sinuses and nasal cavity extending into both orbits and the left anterior skull base. (B) Axial bone window CT image shows widening of the left foramen rotundum (arrow) indicating perineural tumor extension. (C) Axial T2-weighted magnetic resonance (MR) image shows a typical homogeneous T2-intermediate signal lesion, suggestive of high cellularity, involving ethmoid sinus and medial orbits bilaterally (arrows). Note relatively hyperintense fluid in the sphenoid sinus because of obstructed sinus outflow (arrowheads). (D) Coronal postcontrast fat-suppressed T1-weighted image shows a homogeneously enhancing lesion invading both orbits and anterior skull base with intracranial extension along the dura (arrow). The margins of the lesion are more clearly distinguishable from the sinus opacification because of outflow obstruction (arrowhead) on postcontrast MRI compared with CT.

Chondrosarcomas may arise on the maxillary sinus wall, nasal septum, or undersurface of the sphenoid bone and may be associated with Maffucci syndrome. Although slow growing, these lesions are aggressive and destructive as well. CT can show characteristic cartilaginous matrix.[46]

In all cases of suspected malignancy, associated adenopathy can be identified as enlargement and/or necrosis of lymph nodes as the best indicators on CT and MRI of tumor involvement.

Postsurgical Appearances and Complications

Imaging may be difficult to interpret in the postoperative period. The variety of surgical techniques and materials used for skull base reconstruction is reflected in the wide range of CT and MRI appearances of the postoperative bed.[47] Dural-based extra-axial hematomas at the surgical bed can be difficult to distinguish on imaging from dural graft material. Smooth linear dural enhancement is often seen underlying the bone flap and can persist for decades after surgery. Postoperative pneumocephalus is an expected finding following surgery, and the volume of air should decrease over time. The appearance of the bone flap is variable; marrow can demonstrate focal lucencies over time with resorption and irregularity along its margins. PET imaging can be difficult to interpret in the immediate postoperative period, as the response for healing and inflammation will be PET avid. It is generally avoided for a minimum of 6 weeks post-therapy, and is often postponed until 3 months post-treatment.

Imaging can be used in evaluating postsurgical sequelae.[48] CSF leaks can be identified using CT cisternography (CT images obtained after intrathecal administration of iodinated

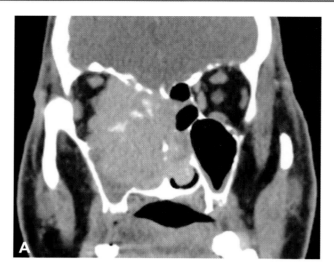
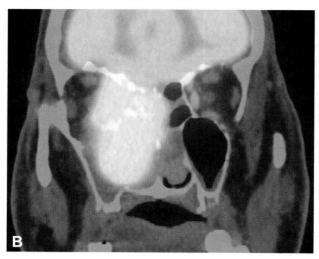

Figure 4.13 Sinonasal undifferentiated carcinoma. (A) Coronal computed tomography (CT) image shows aggressive soft tissue mass centered in the right nasal cavity with extension into the ethmoid air cells, maxillary sinus, and orbit on the right. (B) Coronal-fused positron emission tomography CT image shows hypermetabolic nature of this lesion. Note that intracranial involvement is difficult to assess because of normal high 2-[fluorine-18]fluoro-2-deoxy-D-glucose avidity of the brain tissue.

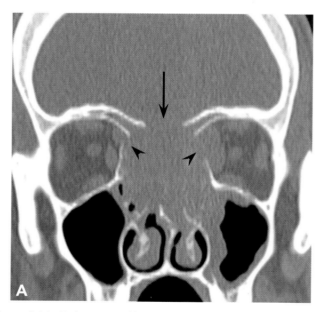
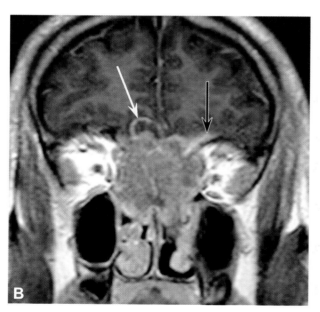

Figure 4.14 Esthesioneuroblastoma. (A) Coronal computed tomography image in bone window shows cortical discontinuity at the anterior skull base (arrow) and medial orbital walls bilaterally (arrowheads) because of intracranial and intraorbital tumor extension, respectively. (B) Coronal postcontrast T1-weighted magnetic resonance image shows heterogeneously enhancing expansile lesion centered at the superior nasal cavity/anterior skull base. There is an extension laterally into ethmoid sinuses and medial orbits bilaterally and superiorly into the cranial cavity with dural-based enhancement along the left anterior skull base (black arrow). Peritumoral cyst along the superior margin of the tumor (white arrow) is often seen associated with esthesioneuroblastoma.

contrast material) or high-resolution T2-weighted MRI through the skull base; the same techniques can be used to identify other post-traumatic or spontaneous CSF leaks. In the setting of postsurgical infection, imaging may be performed to evaluate for intracranial extension and presence of drainable collections. The bone flap is susceptible to osteomyelitis and may show areas of lysis. Frontal lobe retraction injuries may occur during surgery, and this will show as focal areas of hemorrhage within the inferior frontal and anterior frontal lobe regions. On CT, the parenchymal hemorrhages will be hyperdense with surrounding low density relative to normal brain, indicating blood products surrounded by vasogenic edema. Depending on the age of the hemorrhage, variable signal can be seen on T1- and T2-weighted MR images. Other less common complications that may be seen include tension pneumocephalus, with air collection causing mass effect on the underlying brain. Herniation of brain and/or meninges (meningoencephalocele) is best seen on coronal

MR images, and it may occur if the skull base reconstruction is not adequate. Tumor recurrence rates vary with pathology. However, any new soft tissue nodularities in the surgical bed, better seen on postcontrast MRI, can raise suspicion for recurrence of tumor.

Summary

Imaging of the nasal cavity, paranasal sinuses, and anterior skull base has become an integral component in the evaluation of various sinonasal/anterior skull base conditions. The anatomic detail provided by CT has made this modality the mainstay of sinonasal imaging. MRI is typically performed for more complex pathologies, when there is a concern for contiguous extension of disease outside of the sinonasal cavity into the face, brain, and orbit. In these cases, CT and MRI are often complementary to each other. The role of PET and PET/CT is under investigation.

References

1. Mafee MF, Tran BH, Chapa AR. Imaging of rhinosinusitis and its complications: plain film, CT, and MRI. Clin Rev Allergy Immunol 2006;30(3):165–186

2. Hoang JK, Eastwood JD, Tebbit CL, Glastonbury CM. Multiplanar sinus CT: a systematic approach to imaging before functional endoscopic sinus surgery. AJR Am J Roentgenol 2010;194(6):W527–W536

3. Zinreich SJ, Kennedy DW, Rosenbaum AE, Gayler BW, Kumar AJ, Stammberger H. Paranasal sinuses: CT imaging requirements for endoscopic surgery. Radiology 1987;163(3):769–775

4. Lloyd GA. Diagnostic imaging of the nose and paranasal sinuses. J Laryngol Otol 1989;103(5):453–460

5. Hedlund G. Congenital frontonasal masses: developmental anatomy, malformations, and MR imaging. Pediatr Radiol 2006;36(7):647–662, quiz 726–727

6. Barkovich AJ, Vandermarck P, Edwards MS, Cogen PH. Congenital nasal masses: CT and MR imaging features in 16 cases. AJNR Am J Neuroradiol 1991;12(1):105–116

7. Thomas BP, Strother MK, Donnelly EF, Worrell JA. CT virtual endoscopy in the evaluation of large airway disease: Review. AJR Am J Roentgenol 2009; 192(3, Suppl)S20–S30, quiz S31–S33

8. Qu Q, Liu J, Ni D, et al. Diagnosis and clinical characteristics of congenital anosmia: case series report. J Otolaryngol Head Neck Surg 2010;39(6):723–731

9. Avery LL, Susarla SM, Novelline RA. Multidetector and three-dimensional CT evaluation of the patient with maxillofacial injury. Radiol Clin North Am 2011;49(1):183–203

10. Feiz-Erfan I, Horn EM, Theodore N, et al. Incidence and pattern of direct blunt neurovascular injury associated with trauma to the skull base. J Neurosurg 2007;107(2):364–369

11. Uyeda JW, Anderson SW, Sakai O, Soto JA. CT angiography in trauma. Radiol Clin North Am 2010;48(2):423–438, ix–x

12. Laine FJ, Smoker WR. The ostiomeatal unit and endoscopic surgery: anatomy, variations, and imaging findings in inflammatory diseases. AJR Am J Roentgenol 1992;159(4):849–857

13. Longhini AB, Branstetter BF, Ferguson BJ. Unrecognized odontogenic maxillary sinusitis: a cause of endoscopic sinus surgery failure. Am J Rhinol Allergy 2010;24(4):296–300

14. Kantarci M, Karasen RM, Alper F, Onbas O, Okur A, Karaman A. Remarkable anatomic variations in paranasal sinus regon and their clinical importance. Eur J Radiol 2004;50(3):296–302

15. Sakai O, Flower E. Antrochoanal polyp. In: Sakai O, ed. Head and Neck Imaging Cases. New York, NY: McGraw Hill; 2011:232–234

16. Rao VM, Sharma D, Madan A. Imaging of frontal sinus disease: concepts, interpretation, and technology. Otolaryngol Clin North Am 2001;34(1):23–39

17. Saito N, Nadgir RN, Flower EN, Sakai O. Clinical and radiologic manifestations of sickle cell disease in the head and neck. Radiographics 2010;30(4):1021–1034

18. Branstetter BF IV, Weissman JL. Role of MR and CT in the paranasal sinuses. Otolaryngol Clin North Am 2005;38(6):1279–1299, x

19. Lund VJ, Lloyd G, Savy L, Howard D. Fungal rhinosinusitis. J Laryngol Otol 2000;114(1):76–80

20. Curtin HD, Rabinov JD. Extension to the orbit from paraorbital disease. The sinuses. Radiol Clin North Am 1998;36(6):1201–1213, xi

21. Hoxworth JM, Glastonbury CM. Orbital and intracranial complications of acute sinusitis. Neuroimaging Clin N Am 2010;20(4):511–526

22. Leach JL, Fortuna RB, Jones BV, Gaskill-Shipley MF. Imaging of cerebral venous thrombosis: current techniques, spectrum of findings, and diagnostic pitfalls. Radiographics. 2006;26 (Suppl 1):S19–S41

23. Ergene E, Rupp FW Jr, Qualls CR, Ford CC. Acute optic neuritis: association with paranasal sinus inflammatory changes on magnetic resonance imaging. J Neuroimaging 2000;10(4):209–215

24. Blumfield E, Misra M. Pott's puffy tumor, intracranial, and orbital complications as the initial presentation of sinusitis in healthy adolescents, a case series. Emerg Radiol 2011;18(3):203–210

25. Lanier B, Kai G, Marple B, Wall GM. Pathophysiology and progression of nasal septal perforation. Ann Allergy Asthma Immunol 2007;99(6):473–479, quiz 480–481, 521

26. Eggesbø HB. Radiological imaging of inflammatory lesions in the nasal cavity and paranasal sinuses. Eur Radiol 2006;16(4):872–888

27. Larsen PL, Tos M. Origin of nasal polyps: an endoscopic autopsy study. Laryngoscope 2004;114(4):710–719

28. Ojiri H, Ujita M, Tada S, Fukuda K. Potentially distinctive features of sinonasal inverted papilloma on MR imaging. AJR Am J Roentgenol 2000;175(2):465–468

29. Paris J, Guelfucci B, Moulin G, Zanaret M, Triglia JM. Diagnosis and treatment of juvenile nasopharyngeal angiofibroma. Eur Arch Otorhinolaryngol 2001;258(3):120–124

30. Romani R, Tuominen H, Hernesniemi J. Reducing intraoperative bleeding of juvenile nasopharyngeal angiofibroma. World Neurosurg 2010;74(4-5):497–500

31. Ledderose GJ, Betz CS, Stelter K, Leunig A. Surgical management of osteomas of the frontal recess and sinus: extending the limits of the endoscopic approach. Eur Arch Otorhinolaryngol 2011;268(4):525–532

32. Lisle DA, Monsour PA, Maskiell CD. Imaging of craniofacial fibrous dysplasia. J Med Imaging Radiat Oncol 2008;52(4):325–332

33. Abdelkarim A, Green R, Startzell J, Preece J. Craniofacial polyostotic fibrous dysplasia: a case report and review of the literature. Oral Surg Oral Med Oral Pathol Oral Radiol Endod 2008;106(1):e49–e55

34. Sheporaitis LA, Osborn AG, Smirniotopoulos JG, Clunie DA, Howieson J, D'Agostino AN. Intracranial meningioma. AJNR Am J Neuroradiol 1992;13(1):29–37

35. Lamarre ED, Batra PS, Lorenz RR, et al. Role of positron emission tomography in management of sinonasal neoplasms – a single institution's experience. Am J Otolaryngol 2012;33(3):289–295

36. Daele JJ, Vander Poorten V, Rombaux P, Hamoir M. Cancer of the nasal vestibule, nasal cavity and paranasal sinuses. B-ENT 2005;(Suppl 1):87–94, quiz 95–96

37. Hermans R, De Vuysere S, Marchal G. Squamous cell carcinoma of the sinonasal cavities. Semin Ultrasound CT MR 1999;20(3):150–161

38. Loevner LA, Sonners AI. Imaging of neoplasms of the paranasal sinuses. Magn Reson Imaging Clin N Am 2002;10(3):467–493

39. Caldemeyer KS, Mathews VP, Righi PD, Smith RR. Imaging features and clinical significance of perineural spread or extension of head and neck tumors. Radiographics 1998;18(1):97–110, quiz 147

40. Ginsberg LE. MR imaging of perineural tumor spread. Magn Reson Imaging Clin N Am 2002;10(3):511–525, vi

41. Yasumoto M, Taura S, Shibuya H, Honda M. Primary malignant lymphoma of the maxillary sinus: CT and MRI. Neuroradiology 2000;42(4):285–289

42. Alleyne CH, Bakay RA, Costigan D, Thomas B, Joseph GJ. Intracranial adenoid cystic carcinoma: case report and review of the literature. Surg Neurol 1996;45(3):265–271

43. Boo H, Hogg JP. Nasal cavity neoplasms: a pictorial review. Curr Probl Diagn Radiol 2010;39(2):54–61

44. Som PM, Lidov M, Brandwein M, Catalano P, Biller HF. Sinonasal esthesioneuroblastoma with intracranial extension: marginal tumor cysts as a diagnostic MR finding. AJNR Am J Neuroradiol 1994;15(7):1259–1262

45. Lee YY, Van Tassel P, Nauert C, Raymond AK, Edeiken J. Craniofacial osteosarcomas: plain film, CT, and MR findings in 46 cases. AJR Am J Roentgenol 1988;150(6):1397–1402

46. Lee YY, Van Tassel P. Craniofacial chondrosarcomas: imaging findings in 15 untreated cases. AJNR Am J Neuroradiol 1989;10(1):165–170

47. Sinclair AG, Scoffings DJ. Imaging of the post-operative cranium. Radiographics 2010;30(2):461–482

48. Deschler DG, Gutin PH, Mamelak AN, McDermott MW, Kaplan MJ. Complications of anterior skull base surgery. Skull Base Surg 1996;6(2):113–118

SECTION II: Rhinology and Paranasal Sinus Surgery

5 Rhinosinusitis

Stephanie Shintani Smith and Rakesh K. Chandra

Rhinosinusitis (RS) is a group of disorders characterized by symptomatic inflammation of the nose and paranasal sinuses. These disorders affect approximately 15% of the Western population, have substantial effects on the quality of life, and impose a great financial burden to society. Therefore, an appropriate and cost-effective treatment of RS is critical.

There are dramatically different forms of RS. To foster effective treatment and research, several major expert panels have convened to put forth standardized definitions and management guidelines for RS, such as the Rhinosinusitis Task Force,[1] European Position Paper on Rhinosinusitis and Nasal Polyps (EP³OS),[2] the Joint Task Force of Practice Parameters,[3] and Clinical Practice Guideline: Adult Sinusitis (CPG:AS).[4] For simplicity, this chapter will use the guidelines defined in the CPG:AS and/or EP³OS. Note that fungal RS, including fungus ball, allergic fungal rhinosinusitis (AFRS), acute invasive fungal sinusitis, and chronic fungal RS will be discussed in subsequent chapters.

Rhinosinusitis: Definition, Diagnosis, and Classification

By definition, RS must involve both (1) inflammation of the paranasal sinuses and nasal cavity and (2) related signs/symptoms. If both criteria are not met, the diagnosis is not RS. The term *rhinosinusitis* is preferred over the term *sinusitis*, though they are often used interchangeably. RS describes the concomitant inflammation of the contiguous nasal and sinus mucosa, as sinus mucosa is rarely clinically inflamed in the absence of nasal inflammation.

The signs and symptoms of RS generally include purulent nasal drainage, nasal obstruction, and facial pain, pressure, or fullness. It has been debated whether physical examination and history are sufficient to establish the diagnosis of RS, without endoscopy and/or radiographic evidence. Particularly with chronic rhinosinusitis (CRS), when management decisions include costly options of prolonged medical therapy and surgery, objective evidence of the condition is favorable. Key diagnostic criteria will be discussed later in the chapter.

Classification by Duration of Symptoms

RS definitions are generally classified on the basis of symptom duration. RS is defined as "acute" (ARS) (less than 4 weeks), "subacute" (4 to 12 weeks), or "chronic" (CRS) (more than 12 weeks).[1] Another category of RS, called "recurrent ARS," refers to three to four episodes of ARS occurring within 1 year with complete interval resolution of symptoms.[3,4] Different

expert panels use slight variations in these durations and definitions. Typically, ARS denotes symptoms lasting less than 4 weeks, but some definitions use 12 weeks as the cutoff; for example, the most recent EP³OS guidelines define ARS as symptom duration of less than 12 weeks.[2] Subacute RS is an additional subcategory used by some systems, and refer to intermediate RS symptom duration as noted above. While CRS typically refers to RS symptoms lasting longer than 12 weeks, some definitions have used 8 weeks as the threshold.

Classification of Chronic Rhinosinusitis by Phenotypical Subtype: Presence or Absence of Polyps

CRS is also classified by phenotypical subtype, with the presence or absence of polyps. Chronic rhinosinusitis with nasal polyposis (CRSwNP) is characterized by nasal polyps (**Fig. 5.1**) and eosinophilic inflammation initiated and sustained by interleukin (IL)-5 and eotaxin. Chronic rhinosinusitis without nasal polyposis (CRSsNP) is characterized by the absence of polyps and neutrophilic inflammation. AFRS is characterized by eosinophilic mucin and noninvasive fungal elements.

Classification by Severity of Symptoms

An additional level of subclassification, based on the severity of symptoms, allows for tailored management strategies of

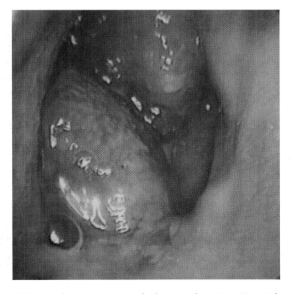

Figure 5.1 Endoscopic view of chronic rhinosinusitis with nasal polyposis, right nasal cavity.

RS. The EP³OS guidelines classify severity based on a visual analog scale that has been statistically validated for use in RS. On this scale, patients rate their symptoms from 0 ("not troublesome") to 10 ("worst thinkable troublesome"). Scores from 0 to 3 are considered mild, 4 to 7 moderate, and 8 to 10 severe.[2]

Staging

Multiple staging systems exist to stratify severity of CRS based on symptoms, endoscopic findings, computed tomography (CT) scan findings, or a combination thereof. The variety of systems likely reflects the failure of any single system to accurately stratify patients. For most of the staging systems, the criteria are too complex for routine clinical use.

The Lund-McKay system is based solely on CT findings and is the most widely used system. Each individual sinus (frontal, maxillary, anterior ethmoid, posterior ethmoid, and sphenoid) is scored as follows: 0 = clear, 1 = partial opacification, and 2 = total opacification. The ostiomeatal complex is unique because it is scored in a binary manner as follows: 0 = clear and 2 = occluded.[5]

Acute Rhinosinusitis

Pathophysiology and Microbiology

In ARS, an inflammatory reaction to a viral upper respiratory tract infection characterizes most cases. Odontogenic sources also account for a minority of cases of maxillary sinusitis (**Fig. 5.2**). The pathophysiology of ARS involves interplay between a predisposing condition (e.g., allergic rhinitis, septal deformity, immune deficiency, and environmental factors), infection, and consequent inflammatory response in the sinonasal mucosa. The inflammatory response involves edema, fluid extravasation, and mucus production. The inflammatory cascade involves T-helper type 1 cytokine polarization associated with tumor necrosis factor-β and interferon-γ. Proinflammatory cytokines such as IL-1β, IL-6, and IL-8 are potent chemoattractive agents for neutrophils.[6]

Mucosal inflammation may lead to obstruction of normal sinus outflow tracts. This obstruction impedes normal ventilation and drainage leading to a lower partial pressure of oxygen, decreased ciliary clearance, and stasis of secretions. A secondary bacterial infection may develop. However, more than 90% of the time ARS is viral. Rhinovirus, coronavirus, influenza, respiratory syncytial virus, and parainfluenza virus are the common instigators.[6,7]

The common bacteria in adult acute bacterial rhinosinusitis (ABRS) are *Streptococcus pneumoniae* (20 to 45%), *Haemophilus influenzae* (20 to 35%), *Moraxella catarrhalis* (2 to 10%), other streptococci (0 to 10%), and *Staphylococcus aureus* (0 to 10%).[7] *S. aureus* was considered a contaminant in the past, but meta-analysis suggests that

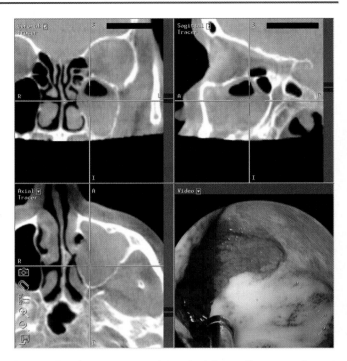

Figure 5.2 Rhinosinusitis involving the left maxillary sinus, from an odontogenic source. This patient developed symptoms of rhinosinusitis, refractory to medical management, following dental implantation.

it is a true pathogen in approximately 10% of ABRS cases in adults.[8] Anaerobes may also be implicated.

Widespread use of vaccination has resulted in changes in the bacteriology of ABRS. However, there is no strong evidence of a change in the incidence of ABRS after widespread use of conjugate pneumococcal vaccination. The l.f. type B vaccine reduced the incidence of invasive disease and likely played a role in ABRS. However, as the vaccination strains became less prevalent, other serotypes emerged as potential causes of invasive disease.[9]

Diagnosis

ARS has been historically diagnosed on the basis of clinical history. However, some expert guidelines recommend special assessments to confirm the diagnoses. Other guidelines provide two sets of recommendations: one for primary care providers and another for otolaryngologists. The CPG:AS and EP³OS diagnostic criteria for ARS are listed in **Table 5.1**.

Most otolaryngologists believe that nasal endoscopy is helpful to assess the middle meatus and sphenoethmoidal recess for purulence (**Fig. 5.3**), which should be cultured in severe disease. CT is the preferred imaging option in cases of severe disease, immunocompromised states, or suspected complications. Plain radiography is neither cost-effective nor useful.

A critical step for the clinician is to differentiate ARS into ABRS and viral rhinosinusitis (VRS). This is clinically challenging and the distinction is made by duration of symptoms. VRS is suspected when symptoms last less than

Table 5.1 Diagnostic Criteria for Acute Rhinosinusitis

Summary of CPG:AS Guidelines	Summary of EP³OS Guidelines
Up to 4 wk of purulent nasal drainage accompanied by nasal obstruction, facial pain-pressure-fullness, or both • Purulent nasal discharge may be reported or observed on physical examination • Nasal obstruction may be reported as nasal obstruction, congestion, blockage, or stuffiness, or observed on physical examination	Up to 12 wk of two or more symptoms, one of which should be either nasal obstruction or discharge (anterior/posterior nasal drip): • ± Facial pain/pressure • ± Reduction or loss of smell[a] • Endoscopic signs of polyps and/or mucopurulent discharge and/or edema/mucosal obstruction • CT mucosal changes

Sources: Fokkens W, Lund V, Mullol J. European position paper on rhinosinusitis and nasal polyps 2007. *Rhinol Suppl* 2007;20:99.
Rosenfeld RM, Andes D, Bhattacharyya N, et al. Clinical practice guideline: adult sinusitis. *Otolaryngol Head Neck Surg* 2007;137(Suppl 3):S7.
[a]For general practice and/or epidemiologic studies, the definition is based on symptomatology without ENT examination or radiology.
CPG:AS, Clinical Practice Guideline: Adult Sinusitis; EP³OS, European Position Paper on Rhinosinusitis and Nasal Polyps; wk, week(s); CT, computed tomography.

10 days. ABRS is suspected when symptoms last more than 10 days or worsens after initial improvement.[4]

Treatment

The goals of treatment of ARS are to alleviate or minimize symptoms, reduce inflammation, eradicate pathogens, and promote sinus drainage. The fundamental difficulty in treating ARS is determining which cases warrant antibiotics. Though only an estimated 1 to 2% of ARS has a bacterial etiology, survey data show overuse of antibiotics for 80 to 90% of ARS.[10]

Therefore, initial treatment is determined by the severity and duration of symptoms. The majority of ARS cases resolve spontaneously within 2 weeks, so it is reasonable to initially implement "watchful waiting" in mild ARS with symptomatic therapy including analgesics, antipyretics, decongestants, nasal irrigation, and steam inhalation.[11] In moderate ARS, an intranasal steroid (INS) is added. In

severe cases, both antibiotics and topical steroids should be added.[2] Further intervention is required in cases that do not respond to this treatment. Treatment recommendations are summarized in **Table 5.2**.

INSs inhibit transcription of proinflammatory mediators upregulated during the inflammatory response. They reduce mucosal inflammation, edema, and nasal congestion. INSs can also help in cases of comorbid allergic rhinitis. Treatment with INSs has proven to be safe and well tolerated, with limited systemic absorption.

In patients with severe symptoms, or when symptoms worsen or persist, antibiotic therapy should be added to INSs. Antibiotic choice depends on local bacterial resistance patterns, effectiveness, and safety. In the United States, the first-line therapy is amoxicillin. Trimethoprim-sulfamethoxazole or macrolide are alternatives for patients

Table 5.2 Suggested Treatment for Acute Rhinosinusitis

Severity	Recommended Therapy (Level of Evidence)
Mild ARS	Symptomatic treatment
Moderate ARS	Symptomatic treatment Add intranasal corticosteroid (Ib) after 5 d Add antibiotic after 5–14 d (Ia) If no response after 14 d, reconsider diagnosis and perform endoscopy
Severe ARS	Intranasal corticosteroids Antibiotics Oral corticosteroids (to reduce pain in severe disease) If no improvement in 48 h, consider nasal endoscopy, culture, and CT Consider intravenous antibiotics, imaging, and surgery
Comorbid allergic rhinitis	Add oral antihistamine

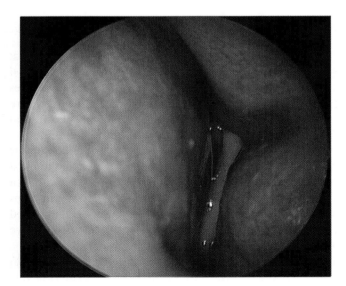

Figure 5.3 Purulence in the middle meatus, in acute bacterial rhinosinusitis.

ARS, acute rhinosinusitis; d, day(s); h, hour(s); CT, computed tomography.

allergic to amoxicillin. If there is an increased likelihood of bacterial resistance, amoxicillin/clavulanate or a fluoroquinolone is recommended. The duration of treatment remains debatable, as studies comparing 5 days of treatment with 10 days have not shown significant differences.[12]

Chronic Rhinosinusitis

Pathophysiology and Microbiology

CRS is characterized by chronic inflammation of the sinonasal mucosa, cytokine release, and tissue remodeling. It is a heterogeneous condition in which host factors, environmental factors, allergic factors, viruses, bacteria or fungi, biofilms, and superantigens variably contribute. Furthermore, growing evidence indicates that CRSwNP and CRSsNP are two separate entities with specific inflammatory pathways and cytokine profiles.

Structural and anatomic factors may contribute to CRS, and these must be examined in light of other factors. Obstruction may be caused by multiple anatomic variants, including septal deviation, concha bullosa, paradoxic middle turbinates, and scarring from previous trauma. Patency of the pathways through which the sinuses drain is crucial for adequate mucociliary function, sinus ventilation and drainage. Ostial obstruction may lead to fluid stagnation, creating a moist, hypoxemic environment ideal for pathogens.

Some patients with CRS are physiologically predisposed to chronic paranasal sinus inflammation. The association between allergic rhinitis and RS has been well established. In patients with CRS, the incidence of allergy has been found to be higher than that in the general population. Airway hyperactivity, with or without aspirin hypersensitivity, and with or without nasal polyps, is a well-known risk factor associated with CRS. However, other factors such as immunodeficiency, ciliary dysfunction (e.g., Kartagener syndrome), cystic fibrosis, autoimmune disease, and granulomatous disorders (e.g., Wegener granulomatosis and sarcoidosis) can also contribute. Smoking is also a risk factor for RS and is associated with poorer outcomes after surgery.[13]

The role of microorganisms in CRS is controversial because bacteria and fungi can both infect or simply colonize the sinuses. Thus, CRS has recently been recognized primarily as an inflammatory, rather than infectious, disorder. Whether they be normal flora or cause for infection, the organisms cultured in CRS include *S. pneumoniae, H. influenzae, M. catarrhalis, S. aureus, Pseudomonas aeruginosa,* and other anaerobes. These organisms are typically prone to be resistant to commonly prescribed antibiotics.

Recent studies suggest that bacterial superantigens may directly activate the inflammatory cascade. For example, staphylococcal enterotoxin may activate T cells, bypassing the normal antigen-presenting mechanism of T-cell activation. Bacterial colonization with enterotoxin-producing *S. aureus* is found with an increased prevalence in patients with nasal polyps. In contrast, patients with CRS without polyps do not have an increased prevalence of enterotoxin-specific immunoglobulin E antibodies.[14]

Bacterial biofilms have also been suggested as possible contributors to CRS. A biofilm is a complex polysaccharide matrix synthesized by bacteria, which serves as a protective microenvironment for bacterial colonies. Such biofilms may explain the persistent crusting and symptoms despite antibiotic treatment in CRS.[15]

Local osteitis of the underlying bone also plays a role in CRS, and it can be found in 36 to 53% of patients with CRS, using both radiographic and pathologic criteria, respectively. It is thought to elaborate CRS by inducing persistent inflammatory changes in the mucosa.[16]

The role of fungus in CRS has been debated since the first publication by Ponikau et al in 1999,[17] which proposed that ubiquitous fungi cause intense eosinophilic infiltration essentially in all cases of CRS. This theory has been widely discussed, but a universal role of fungus in CRS is not universally accepted. Rather, a separate entity of allergic fungal sinusitis remains widely accepted.

Diagnostic Special Considerations

CRS must be differentiated from other conditions that mimic symptoms including sinonasal mass, atypical facial pain, migraine headache, allergic/nonallergic rhinitis, and fungal RS. It is also important to address comorbid conditions in CRS, such as cystic fibrosis, allergic rhinitis, and anatomic variation. Guidelines for CRS diagnosis are presented in **Table 5.3**.

To confirm a diagnosis of CRS and also to uncover other important diagnoses, diagnostic evaluation such as CT and/or nasal endoscopy should be performed.[2,12] Nasal endoscopy can be performed in the clinic, and may show purulent mucus, edema of the middle meatus and ethmoids, and the presence of nasal polyp to support a diagnosis of CRS. Sinus CT scan without intravenous contrast is recommended to evaluate the evidence for mucosal inflammation, anatomic obstruction, and masses. Furthermore, CT scan is important for preoperative planning if surgery is pursued. Although subjective symptom-based criteria allow both primary care providers and specialists to diagnose CRS, many physicians recognize the diagnostic usefulness of CT as an objective criterion. Recent studies have shown that a wide range (40 to 65%) of patients with symptoms of CRS actually have the disease when measured against the gold standard CT scan.[18–20]

Allergy and/or immunologic studies should be performed for patients who fail to improve or who have symptoms of both allergy and CRS. Allergy skin testing is the study of choice to determine immunoglobulin E-mediated sensitivity. Radioallergosorbent testing is an alternative to skin testing. For patients who fail aggressive medical and surgical treatment, immunologic and HIV testing should also be considered.[12]

Table 5.3 Diagnostic Criteria for Chronic Rhinosinusitis

Summary of CPG:AS Guidelines	Summary of EP³OS Guidelines

More than 12 wk of two or more of the following signs and symptoms:
• Mucopurulent drainage (anterior, posterior, or both)
• Nasal obstruction (congestion)
• Facial pain-pressure-fullness
• Decreased sense of smell and inflammation is documented by one or more of the following findings:
   • Purulent mucus or edema in the middle meatus or ethmoid region
   • Polyps in nasal cavity or the middle meatus
   • Radiographic images showing inflammation of the paranasal sinuses
	More than 12 wk of two or more symptoms:
	• One of which should be either nasal blockage/obstruction/congestion, or nasal discharge (anterior/posterior nasal drip), ± facial pain/pressure, ± reduction or loss of smell, and
	• Anterior rhinoscopy or endoscopic signs of polyps and/or endoscopic signs of mucopurulent discharge primarily from middle meatus, and/or edema/mucosal obstruction primarily in middle meatus
	Optional:
	• CT for otolaryngologists (not for primary care)

Sources: Fokkens W, Lund V, Mullol J. European position paper on rhinosinusitis and nasal polyps 2007. *Rhinol Suppl* 2007(20):101.
Rosenfeld RM, Andes D, Bhattacharyya N, et al. Clinical practice guideline: adult sinusitis. *Otolaryngol Head Neck Surg* 2007;137(Suppl 3):S18.
CPG:AS, Clinical Practice Guideline: Adult Sinusitis; w, week(s); EP³OS, European Position Paper on Rhinosinusitis and Nasal Polyps; CT, computed tomography.

Treatment

The treatment of CRS is complex because of its variable etiologies and difficulty in distinguishing them clinically. Treatment varies significantly across geographic regions and across physician specialties, indicating the need for a widely accepted evidence-based treatment protocol.[21] Nevertheless, the mainstays of CRS treatment include antibiotics, steroid therapy, and nasal saline irrigations. Additional therapies that may be useful include concomitant allergy treatment with antihistamines, leukotriene inhibitors, decongestants, and antifungal agents.

CRS should be treated according to its three major subtypes: CRSsNP, CRSwNP, and AFRS. The recommendations are listed in **Table 5.4**. The role of antibiotics in CRS is controversial, though widely accepted for acute exacerbations.

Antibiotic selection should be guided by culture when possible via transantral puncture or middle meatus culture using a small wire brush. Antibiograms should be consulted to match the cultured organisms. If empiric treatment is necessary, broad-spectrum antibiotics should cover *S. aureus*, Gram-negative bacilli, and anaerobes. Though there is a lack of randomized controlled trials that reveals an optimal duration, the commonly recommended duration of antibiotic treatment is a prolonged course of 4 to 12 weeks.

Topical antibiotics, such as mupirocin suspended in saline, has been reportedly effective. Parenteral antibiotic treatment is typically reserved for severe or complicated infections. Topical INSs are routinely used in CRS for a localized anti-inflammatory effect. The typical form is an intranasal spray. Drops are also available. Oral steroids may be used for exacerbations of CRSwNP and CRSsNP. Oral

Table 5.4 Treatment Recommendations for Chronic Rhinosinusitis

CRS without Nasal Polyposis	CRS with Nasal Polyposis
Mild • INS • Nasal lavage • If failure after 3 mo, treat as moderate/severe and consider CT and surgery **Moderate/severe** • INS • Nasal lavage • Long-term macrolide therapy • Culture **Cases that improve** • INS • Nasal lavage • ±Long-term macrolide therapy **Cases that fail** • Consider CT and surgery	**Mild** • INS for 3 mo • If beneficial, continue and review every 6 mo • If no improvement, add oral steroids • If still no improvement, consider CT and surgery • If improved after 1 mo, switch to topical steroid drops, review after 3 mo **Moderate** • INS for 3 mo • If beneficial, continue and review every 6 mo • If no improvement after 3 mo, add a short course of oral steroids, consider CT and surgery **Severe** • Short course of oral steroids plus INS for 1 mo • If beneficial, INS only, review after 3 mo • If no improvement, perform CT and consider surgery

Source: Fokkens W, Lund V, Mullol J. European position paper on rhinosinusitis and nasal polyps 2007. *Rhinol Suppl* 2007;20:1–136.
CRS, chronic rhinosinusitis; mo, month(s); INS, intranasal steroid; CT, computed tomography.

steroids are also commonly given in the preoperative period. Nasal irrigations with isotonic or hypertonic saline are beneficial in terms of alleviation of symptoms, endoscopic findings, and quality of life in patients with CRS.

Surgery is considered in cases that do not respond to medical management and in cases showing any complication. The extent of surgery depends on the extent of sinuses involved and transition areas. The details of surgery are discussed later in this text.

Complications

Complications of sinusitis occur when inflammation or infection extend outside the paranasal sinuses and nasal cavity (e.g., neurologic, ophthalmologic, or soft tissue involvement). CT scans of the sinuses and CT of the orbits and/or brain (with contrast) should be obtained when complications are suspected.

Because the paper thin and often dehiscent lamina papyracea is the barrier between the orbit and ethmoid sinuses, direct extension of infection to the orbit is the most common complication of acute sinusitis. Additionally, thrombophlebitis can occur via the valveless ophthalmic venous system that communicates with the ethmoid veins. The course of untreated orbital infection typically progresses according to the Chandler classification: periorbital (preseptal) cellulitis, orbital cellulitis, subperiosteal abscess, orbital abscess, and cavernous sinus thrombosis. Physical examination and imaging differentiate between these complications.

Periorbital cellulitis and orbital cellulitis require intravenous antibiotics. In adults, subperiosteal abscesses require surgical decompression and drainage of the infected sinus. In children, some small subperiosteal abscesses without evidence of vision loss or decreased extraocular movement may respond to intravenous antibiotics. Orbital abscesses require surgical decompression and drainage of the offending sinus.

Septic emboli may flow posteriorly through the ophthalmic venous system causing infection, inflammation, and cavernous sinus thrombosis. Signs/symptoms include picket fence spiking fevers, toxemia, chemosis, sluggish pupillary response, ophthalmoplegia, and blindness. CT/magnetic resonance imaging may show intraluminal enhancement. The Tobey-Ayer or Queckenstedt test may show that external compression of the jugular vein on the unobstructed side increases cerebrospinal fluid pressure. Intravenous antibiotic treatment should be instituted immediately, and, if indicated, the involved sinuses should be surgically drained. The role of anticoagulation to prevent further thrombus formation and systemic steroid therapy is controversial.

Meningitis usually occurs by extension of infection from the sinuses. Diagnosis may be suggested by headache, lethargy, nuchal rigidity, fever, Kernig sign, Brudzinski sign, seizures, and photophobia; diagnosis is established by lumbar puncture. Treatment of meningitis requires intravenous antibiotics and surgical drainage of the involved sinus.

An epidural abscess may occur by direct extension of infection, typically from the frontal sinus. Signs/symptoms include headache, low-grade to spiking fever, and mental status changes. Further direct extension or hematogenous seeding may lead to subdural empyema and brain abscess, causing more neurologic sequelae. Treatment requires surgical drainage of the abscess and treatment of the involved sinus with wide exposure of dura.

Other complications of RS include Pott puffy tumor (osteomyelitis or subperiosteal abscess of the frontal bone caused by invasion through the diploic vein), osteitis, superior orbital fissure syndrome, orbital apex syndrome, and sinocutaneous fistula. These can require evacuation or decompression of the disease, antibiotics, and other interventions to reverse these adverse sequelae of RS.

Conclusion

RS represents a diverse spectrum of disease with a significant burden on human health. The pathophysiology and management of this disease continues to evolve. Successful management can require both medical and surgical intervention. The risk of complications from disease warrants careful evaluation and management.

References

1. Lanza DC, Kennedy DW. Adult rhinosinusitis defined. Otolaryngol Head Neck Surg 1997;117(3, pt 2):S1–S7
2. Fokkens W, Lund V, Mullol J; European Position Paper on Rhinosinusitis and Nasal Polyps group. European position paper on rhinosinusitis and nasal polyps 2007. Rhinol Suppl 2007;20: 1–136
3. Slavin RG, Spector SL, Bernstein IL, et al; American Academy of Allergy, Asthma and Immunology; American College of Allergy, Asthma and Immunology; Joint Council of Allergy, Asthma and Immunology. The diagnosis and management of sinusitis: a practice parameter update. J Allergy Clin Immunol 2005;116(6, Suppl):S13–S47
4. Rosenfeld RM, Andes D, Bhattacharyya N, et al. Clinical practice guideline: adult sinusitis. Otolaryngol Head Neck Surg 2007;137(3, Suppl):S1–S31
5. Lund VJ, Kennedy DW; The Staging and Therapy Group. Quantification for staging sinusitis. Ann Otol Rhinol Laryngol Suppl 1995;167:17–21
6. Eloy P, Poirrier AL, De Dorlodot C, Van Zele T, Watelet JB, Bertrand B. Actual concepts in rhinosinusitis: a review of clinical presentations, inflammatory pathways, cytokine profiles, remodeling, and management. Curr Allergy Asthma Rep 2011;11(2):146–162
7. Anon JB, Jacobs MR, Poole MD, et al; Sinus And Allergy Health Partnership. Antimicrobial treatment guidelines for acute bacterial rhinosinusitis. Otolaryngol Head Neck Surg 2004;130(1, Suppl):1–45
8. Payne SC, Benninger MS. *Staphylococcus aureus* is a major pathogen in acute bacterial rhinosinusitis: a meta-analysis. Clin Infect Dis 2007;45(10):e121–e127
9. Benninger MS, Manz R. The impact of vaccination on rhinosinusitis and otitis media. Curr Allergy Asthma Rep 2010;10(6):411–418

10. Meltzer EO, Hamilos DL. Rhinosinusitis diagnosis and management for the clinician: a synopsis of recent consensus guidelines. Mayo Clin Proc 2011;86(5):427–443

11. Marple BF, Brunton S, Ferguson BJ. Acute bacterial rhinosinusitis: a review of U.S. treatment guidelines. Otolaryngol Head Neck Surg 2006;135(3):341–348

12. Pearlman AN, Conley DB. Review of current guidelines related to the diagnosis and treatment of rhinosinusitis. Curr Opin Otolaryngol Head Neck Surg 2008;16(3):226–230

13. Briggs RD, Wright ST, Cordes S, Calhoun KH. Smoking in chronic rhinosinusitis: a predictor of poor long-term outcome after endoscopic sinus surgery. Laryngoscope 2004;114(1):126–128

14. Van Zele T, Gevaert P, Watelet JB, et al. *Staphylococcus aureus* colonization and IgE antibody formation to enterotoxins is increased in nasal polyposis. J Allergy Clin Immunol 2004;114(4):981–983

15. Harvey RJ, Lund VJ. Biofilms and chronic rhinosinusitis: systematic review of evidence, current concepts and directions for research. Rhinology 2007;45(1):3–13

16. Lee JT, Kennedy DW, Palmer JN, Feldman M, Chiu AG. The incidence of concurrent osteitis in patients with chronic rhinosinusitis: a clinicopathological study. Am J Rhinol 2006;20(3):278–282

17. Ponikau JU, Sherris DA, Kern EB, et al. The diagnosis and incidence of allergic fungal sinusitis. Mayo Clin Proc 1999;74(9):877–884

18. Bhattacharyya N, Lee LN. Evaluating the diagnosis of chronic rhinosinusitis based on clinical guidelines and endoscopy. Otolaryngol Head Neck Surg 2010;143(1):147–151

19. Stankiewicz JA, Chow JM. A diagnostic dilemma for chronic rhinosinusitis: definition accuracy and validity. Am J Rhinol 2002;16(4):199–202

20. Hwang PH, Irwin SB, Griest SE, Caro JE, Nesbit GM. Radiologic correlates of symptom-based diagnostic criteria for chronic rhinosinusitis. Otolaryngol Head Neck Surg 2003;128(4):489–496

21. Lee LN, Bhattacharyya N. Regional and specialty variations in the treatment of chronic rhinosinusitis. Laryngoscope 2011;121(5):1092–1097

6 Evidence-Based Medicine in the Diagnosis and Treatment of Chronic Rhinosinusitis

Michael S. Benninger and Troy D. Woodard

Chronic rhinosinusitis (CRS) is a complex disorder that has many potential etiologies and associated disorders. There are few, if any, predictable etiologies. The spectrum of disease can vary dramatically from individual to individual and the responsiveness to treatment is often unpredictable. As a result, there are multiple potential diagnostic approaches and many differing treatment options that may be used in isolation or in combination. The literature related to CRS is growing rapidly in an effort to add some clarity to this problem and to improve treatment. Unfortunately, much of the CRS literature is poorly controlled and there is little level A or level B evidence. This chapter will attempt to identify the highest quality of the reported evidence to establish the most predictable principles of evidence-based management of CRS. The evidence is then broken down into four grades from A (best evidence) to D (worst evidence) and then subcategorized into eight levels of evidence (1a, 1b, 2a, 2b, 3a, 3b, 4, and 5).[1] Where possible, the highest evidence in the different areas will be discussed. This chapter will focus on the treatment of CRS because the scope of this chapter does not allow for an evaluation of the evidence as it relates to diagnosis.

Definitions

To evaluate the quality of the evidence, it is important to rely on a well-defined statement. Until 2003, CRS was not clearly defined and the general term *sinusitis* was commonly used. In 1997, a general categorization of rhinosinusitis was applied to these disorders because it was clear that both the nose and sinuses are involved.[2] A task force under the direction of the Sinus and Allergy Health Partnership and supported by the American Rhinologic Society, the American Academy of Otolaryngic Allergy, and the American Academy of Otolaryngology-Head and Neck Surgery used the literature to create universally acceptable definitions for rhinosinusitis and CRS.[3]

The task force proposed that because it has become clear that inflammation is the major universal finding in all patients with rhinosinusitis, newer definitions have been developed to describe rhinosinusitis. The newer definitions are as follows: *Rhinosinusitis* is a group of disorders characterized by inflammation of the mucosa of the nose and paranasal sinuses. *Chronic rhinosinusitis* is rhinosinusitis of at least 12 consecutive weeks' duration. Therefore, *CRS* is a group of disorders characterized by inflammation of the mucosa of the nose and paranasal sinuses of at least 12 consecutive weeks' duration.[3] This definition was supported by a large multispecialty group of otolaryngologists and allergists representing six national societies[4] and was used to identify articles from the literature to include in this review.

Antibiotics and Antifungals

There are several reviews that suggest the roles of antimicrobials and antifungals in the management of CRS. A thorough review in 2005 by the European Academy of Allergology and Clinical Immunology (EAACI), along with the European Rhinologic Society, examined the literature in relationship to the treatment of CRS and nasal polyps.[5] They graded the evidence from A (strong evidence) to D (no evidence). They also tried to determine the relevance of the evidence. Although there was good evidence of the effectiveness of antibiotics for the treatment of acute bacterial rhinosinusitis (ABRS), the overall evidence for antimicrobial treatment of CRS was poor.[5] The evidence for oral antibiotics used for less than 2 weeks was graded at level 3 (case–control trials) but with a recommendation of C with no relevance. For a long-term treatment with antibiotics, the data were also rated a recommendation C but with some relevance. There was poor evidence to support either short-term or long-term antibiotic treatment for nasal polyps.[5]

A Cochrane Collaboration review in 2001 also looked at the evidence for antibiotics in comparison with placebo in the treatment of CRS without polyps.[6] A thorough review of the literature identified only one study where antibiotics were compared with placebo in CRS without polyps. Their findings state that "There is limited evidence from one small study to support the use of systemic antibiotics for the curative treatment of chronic rhinosinusitis in adults."[6] This recommendation also suggested that the risk of bias supporting the results in this one study was high. Their final recommendations were that further good quality trials, with large sample sizes, are needed to evaluate the use of antibiotics in CRS.[6] Finally, Clinical Practice Guidelines published in 2007 by the American Academy of Otolaryngology-Head and Neck Surgery recommend antibiotics for the treatment of ABRS and suggest a benefit of nasal irrigations in CRS; however, no mention is made regarding the antimicrobial treatment in CRS.[7]

One application of antibiotics may be for the reduction of inflammation associated with CRS by low-dose, long-term macrolide therapy. A review in 2009 suggests that "low-dose, long-duration macrolide therapy is a viable option for patients refractory to standard medical or surgical therapy," although the authors admit that this is based on limited evidence and that even in the best circumstances, the control of symptoms would be expected to be modest and not fully controlled.[8] "Daily clarithromycin (250 mg), azithromycin (250 mg), or roxithromycin (150 mg) should be continued for at least 12 weeks to achieve measurable results."[8]

There has been a substantial interest in the role of nasal antibiotic irrigations or nebulized antibiotics for the treatment of CRS.[9] In addition, there has been recent recognition of the potential roles of biofilms and superantigens that are produced by bacteria and may play a role in the etiology, propagation, or potentially resisting therapy.[3,4] In such cases, antibiotic irrigants or nebulization may be of benefit. Despite this interest, controlled studies have been poorly performed or were not randomized. In addition, given that there is some evidence to support the use of nasal irrigations independently, it is hard to isolate the effects of antibiotics in comparison with irrigations alone. Although anecdotal cases of good responsiveness are seen in clinical practice there is little evidence to support the use of antibiotic irrigations in CRS with or without polyps.

The effectiveness of oral antibiotics in the treatment of CRS either with or without polyps is poor. Oral antibiotics may be considered in patients who develop an acute purulent exacerbation of CRS. Whether or not antibiotic irrigations have an effect under these circumstances is not known, although controlling infection or even colonization of methicillin-resistant *Staphylococcus aureus* by mupirocin irrigations would seem reasonable.

There has been a substantial interest in the role of fungus in the development of inflammation in CRS.[10,11] One of the problems with assessing the role of fungus is that there are numerous ways in which fungus can be relevant in rhinosinusitis: acute fungal infections, allergic fungal rhinosinusitis (AFS), and chronic nonimmunoglobulin E-mediated inflammation. Overall there is a sense that "the current evidence supports the notion that AFS is part of a spectrum of severe CRS with polyps,"[12] but that an immunologic response to fungus is not universally associated with rhinosinusitis.[11] Furthermore, although there is some evidence that anti-inflammatory therapy may be an effective treatment in patients who may have fungal-mediated CRS, there is very little good evidence that either systemic or topical antifungal therapy has any role in the treatment of CRS either with or without polyps. The EAACI report suggests that there were no data supporting the role of systemic antifungals and that the level of recommendation for topical antifungals is a D.[5] A systematic review of the literature, published in 2011, does not support the use of topical amphotericin B for the treatment of CRS.[13]

Saline Irrigations

Saline irrigations are frequently used to treat patients with sinonasal symptoms. Initially there was only anecdotal evidence and saline irrigations were regarded as a homeopathic therapy to be adjunctively used with other medical therapy for chronic sinusitis. However, during the past decade there has been increasing evidence that saline irrigations are not only inexpensive and well tolerated but also have a valuable role in improving sinonasal health and quality of life in patients with CRS.

Saline solution can be administered to the nasal cavity by a variety of devices including bottle, spray, or nebulizer. There is no standard recipe for making saline solution. While some solutions are isotonic, others have hypertonic and buffered concentrations. Personal preference typically determines the concentration used; however, many practitioners prefer hypertonic saline solution as it has been associated with increased mucociliary clearance. A study by Talbot et al demonstrated an increased mucociliary clearance of saccharin after using buffered hypertonic saline irrigations in healthy volunteers.[14] Interestingly, another study by Ural et al demonstrated decreased mucociliary transit times with hypertonic saline irrigations in patients with chronic sinusitis. In contrast, patients with allergic rhinitis and acute sinusitis had improved mucociliary clearance with isotonic saline irrigations.[15]

Several studies demonstrate benefits from using hypertonic and isotonic saline irrigations. Rabago et al[16] conducted a 6-month randomized control trial testing the efficacy of daily hypertonic saline irrigations in patients with sinusitis. Subjective outcomes were measured with the Medical Outcomes Survey Short Form-12, the Rhinosinusitis Disability Index, and a Single-Item Sinus-Symptom Severity Assessment. Not only did the experimental subjects report an overall improvement of sinus-related quality of life, but they also reported fewer 2-week periods with sinus-related symptoms ($p < 0.05$), less use of antibiotics ($p < 0.05$), and less use of nasal spray ($p = 0.06$).[16] In the subsequent study, which was an uncontrolled 12-month follow-up study, there was still a sustained improvement in the quality of life in patients using hypertonic saline nasal irrigations for sinonasal symptoms.[17] In contrast, the usage of isotonic saline irrigations was demonstrated in a study by Bachmann et al.[18] This randomized controlled double-blind trial compared the effectiveness of endonasal irrigations with isotonic EMS salt (balneotherapeutic water) solution to that of isotonic sodium chloride solution in the treatment of adult patients with CRS. Subjective complaints, endonasal endoscopy, and radiography results revealed a significant improvement in both groups ($p = 0.0001$). In comparison, the two groups were not significantly different in outcome.[18]

The benefit of hypertonic saline solution has been demonstrated in the pediatric population as well. Shoseyov et al performed a randomized double-blind study to compare the effect of nasal wash with hypertonic saline versus isotonic saline on pediatric patients with CRS.[19] All patients were evaluated by two clinical scores (cough and nasal secretions/postnasal drip) and by a radiology score at the beginning of the study and after 4 weeks. The hypertonic saline group had significantly improved symptom scores in all areas. However, the isotonic saline group showed a significant improvement only in the postnasal drip score.

A 2007 Cochrane review evaluated the effectiveness and safety of topical saline in the management of chronic sinusitis.[20] Eight trials met the search criteria. Three studies compared saline irrigations with no treatment, one study compared saline irrigations with placebo, one study compared it as an adjunct with an intranasal steroid, and another compared it against an intranasal steroid spray. The latter two studies compared hypertonic saline solution with isotonic saline solution. Based on the review, there was evidence that saline irrigation is beneficial in the treatment of symptoms related to CRS when used alone and as an adjunct. There was no difference between hypertonic and isotonic saline solutions. Although intranasal steroids were more effective than saline, there was no superiority when saline was compared with reflexology "placebo."

Intranasal and Systemic Corticosteroids

Intranasal corticosteroids (INSs) are commonly used for the treatment of patients with CRS with or without polyps. There is good basic evidence that INSs can reduce the immune response and decrease inflammation. They have been shown to improve nasal symptoms, inspiratory flow rates and mucociliary clearance in comparison with placebo, and also to decrease eosinophils and cytokines, both of which are important mediators of inflammation in CRS, in nasal tissues.[21] There is, however, no good evidence of the roles of INSs in reducing symptoms or improving inflammation in patients with CRS without polyps. There have, however, been well-done prospective trials that do show that INSs can reduce the size of polyps, improve airflow, and reduce symptoms in patients with CRS with polyps.[22,23] A Cochrane report has reviewed the literature for the role of INSs in the treatment of patients with cystic fibrosis with nasal polyps, and they have concluded that although there is a reduction in nasal polyps there is no good demonstrable evidence of improvement in nasal symptom scores.[24]

Similar to INS therapy, systemic steroids are widely used for controlling symptoms, decreasing inflammation, and reducing the size of polyps in CRS. They appear to be particularly valuable in patients who have associated allergy or asthma, and they are commonly used to reduce the size of nasal polyps with good, if not temporary, results. The data related to the role of systemic steroids in patients with CRS without polyps are not as robust. A systematic evidence-based review found no randomized controlled trials of oral steroid use in CRS without polyps and articles supporting

this use are based largely on evidence-based medicine levels 4 and 5 studies.[25]

Endoscopic Sinus Surgery

As mentioned earlier, CRS has many etiologies including a variety of host, acquired, and environmental factors that result in an increase in the inflammatory response.[5] Because of the multifactorial nature of this illness, there is no one therapy that works for every patient. Medical management is the primary therapy for chronic sinusitis. While some people respond well to medical management, others do not and require surgery. Surgery has a vital role in the treatment schema of chronic sinusitis and is performed more than 2,00,000 times a year.[26] Traditional open approaches have now given way to more modern endoscopic techniques.

Despite endoscopic sinus surgery (ESS) being the gold standard for treating sinusitis unresponsive to medical therapy, there is very little level 1a evidence that demonstrates its effectiveness in treatment. In a 2009 Cochrane review on functional endoscopic sinus surgery (FESS), the authors evaluated studies that compared FESS versus medical treatment, FESS versus conventional sinus surgery, FESS plus medical therapy versus medical treatment, and FESS plus medical treatment versus conventional sinus surgery. They were able to identify only three qualifying studies that were suitable for inclusion in the review.[27] One study was an unpublished randomized control trial comparing endoscopic middle meatal antrostomy with conventional inferior meatal antrostomy in 33 patients. The median follow-up time was 12 months. This study found no significant difference in symptom scores between the two groups.[27] Another study by Hartog et al compared patients with chronic maxillary sinusitis.[27,28] FESS with sinus irrigation and medical treatment was compared with sinus irrigation and medical treatment only. While there was a significant reduction in the purulent discharge and hyposmia in the surgical group, there was no significant difference in the overall cure rates at 12 months. The study by Ragab et al compared FESS with medical treatment in comparison with medical treatment alone in 90 patients with CRS.[29] Subjective and objective outcomes were significantly improved in both the medical and surgical treatment groups. There were no significant differences between the groups except for an improvement in total nasal volume during acoustic rhinometry after surgery in CRS patients without polyps. Because there was no much difference between the two groups, the authors concluded that medical therapy should be initially attempted with surgery reserved for cases refractory to medical therapy.[29]

Despite the lack of many randomized control trials, there is substantial observational evidence demonstrating improvements in symptoms and quality of life after ESS.[30–37] In a systematic review evaluating the evidence supporting ESS in the management of adult CRS by Smith et al, the authors found an overwhelming majority of level 4 evidence with a few level 2 studies demonstrating that ESS is effective in improving symptoms and quality of life in adults with CRS.[38] According to Smith et al, there were approximately 32 retrospective studies and 11 prospective studies that demonstrated symptom improvement after FESS. The lack of higher level studies may be because of several factors. First, it is difficult to standardize surgeries, especially in multicenter trials. Second, randomization may pose ethical concerns and it is difficult to blind patients to a surgical procedure.[38,39]

In contrast to primary ESS, revision ESS has been shown to be successful in 50 to 90% of the cases.[40] McMains et al demonstrated improvements in both objective and subjective measures in patients who failed maximal medical therapy and earlier FESS for CRS.[41] They did note that patients with nasal polyps were more apt to fail previous surgery than patients with other comorbid conditions. In addition, Smith et al demonstrated that patients with primary ESS were twice as likely to improve after surgery compared with patients having revision ESS.[42]

Since its inception in the 1980s, ESS has flourished to become the standard of surgical care for medically resistant rhinosinusitis. Although hundreds of publications discuss the usage and effectiveness of this surgical modality, there is still a paucity of levels 1 and 2 evidence supporting ESS. As a result, there needs to be the development of higher level prospective studies with comparison groups to cause the pendulum to shift to a more evidence-based approach.

Balloon Sinus Dilation

Balloon sinus catheterization is a newly designed procedure that has gained much popularity during the past few years. Introduced in 2005, the balloon catheter technology uses a minimally invasive technique that has been previously applied in other areas such as cardiac angioplasty and urology. Balloon sinuplasty was the first developed and most studied system that employs a guide wire, which is endoscopically passed through the obstructed ostium and into the sinus under fluoroscopic guidance or transillumination. Subsequently, an uninflated balloon catheter is threaded over the guide wire and into the sinus. Once position across the ostium is confirmed, the balloon is inflated. The balloon is then deflated and the complex is removed, leaving a dilated ostium.

Compared with traditional ESS, this technique is less invasive and results in less bleeding.[43] It has been associated with less mucosal trauma or stripping that may be found with conventional ESS and under certain circumstances can be performed under local anesthesia.[43] These characteristics make balloon sinuplasty an attractive option in treating select patients whose overall medical status is too poor to subject them to the risks associated with conventional ESS.

Despite these positive attributes, there have not been any randomized controlled trials comparing endoscopic balloon sinus dilation with endoscopic, conventional, and/or medical therapy for chronic sinusitis. Several studies demonstrate that balloon sinuplasty is a safe and feasible method of dilating obstructed sinus ostia in select patients with CRS.[43–45] In a multicenter nonrandomized trial, involving 115 patients, the efficacy, safety, and initial outcomes at 24 weeks postoperation were measured.[44] At 24 weeks postprocedure, 80.5% of the previously dilated ostia were patent, 1.6% were not patent, and the patency of 17.9% of the ostia could not be determined. This trial also reported a significant improvement in patient's sinonasal outcome test 20 (SNOT-20) scores and demonstrated no serious adverse events associated with sinus balloon catheterization. Conclusions from this trial were that balloon sinus catheterization is a safe and effective tool in dilating the sinus ostia for a durable time period.[44] Subsequent 1- and 2-year follow-up studies on the same cohort of patients have demonstrated long-term efficacy of balloon dilation and sustainability of low SNOT-20 scores.[46,47] Even though this series of studies provide long-term insight into balloon sinuplasty, this study is a single-armed, uncontrolled, and observational study. Therefore, its interpretation and applicability to chronic sinusitis patients is limited.

To date, there is only one comparative study that compares balloon sinus dilation to ESS. Friedman et al conducted a retrospective review of a cohort of patients who had recurrent acute sinusitis or CRS.[48] Patient symptoms and satisfaction using the SNOT-20 questionnaire, postoperative narcotic use, and costs were compared after 3-month follow-up. Both patient groups had significant improvements in SNOT-20 scores. However, patient satisfaction was higher and postoperative narcotics usage was less in patients who had endoscopic balloon dilation. While the cost for primary procedures was similar, the cost for revision surgery using endoscopic balloon dilation was considerably less.[48]

Similar to the aforementioned technique, other new technologies use an inflatable balloon to dilate the sinus ostia. However, these systems differ in the manner in which the tool is operated. While one system uses a transantral sinus balloon dilation method, the other uses a "one size fits all sinuses" balloon dilation kit that has a single flexible balloon that can be used to dilate the maxillary, sphenoid, and frontal sinuses. The transantral balloon dilation of the ethmoid infundibulum was substantiated when Stankiewicz et al reported a significant reduction in SNOT 20 scores at 1-year posttransantral dilation of the ethmoid infundibulum.[49] A 2011 Cochrane review summarized the literature related to balloon dilation of sinus openings with the authors concluding, "At present there is no convincing evidence supporting the use of endoscopic balloon sinus ostial dilation compared to conventional surgical modalities in the management of CRS refractory to medical treatment. With the escalating use of balloon sinuplasty, there is an urgent need for more randomised controlled trials to determine its efficacy over conventional surgical treatment modalities."[50]

Despite the definite advantages, balloon sinus catheterization is not a panacea and must be used in proper settings. Its versatile nature gives it the potential to have a broad and favorable impact within the management of chronic sinusitis. However, there are several areas of concern that can only be addressed by conducting prospective controlled studies that compare balloon sinus catheterization with standard of care chronic sinusitis treatment paradigms.

Conclusion

CRS is a complex disease with multiple interrelating potential etiologies and therefore multiple evaluations and treatment options. Perhaps because of these multiple interrelated factors, it has been difficult to design and implement studies with high levels of evidence to support any specific recommendations. The literature is largely filled with levels 3 to 5 studies and there is a great paucity of levels 1 or 2 information. Treatment at this time will in many cases be empiric, trial and error, and specifically designed for the individual patient.

References

1. Stewart MG, Neely JG, Paniello RC, Fraley PL, Karni RJ, Nussenbaum B. A practical guide to understanding outcomes research. Otolaryngol Head Neck Surg 2007;137(5):700–706
2. Lanza DC, Kennedy DW. Adult rhinosinusitis defined. Otolaryngol Head Neck Surg 1997;117(3, pt 2):S1–S7
3. Benninger MS, Ferguson BJ, Hadley JA, et al. Adult chronic rhinosinusitis: definitions, diagnosis, epidemiology, and pathophysiology. Otolaryngol Head Neck Surg 2003;129(Suppl 3):S1–S32
4. Meltzer EO, Hamilos DL, Hadley JA, et al; American Academy of Allergy, Asthma and Immunology (AAAAI); American Academy of Otolaryngic Allergy (AAOA); American Academy of Otolaryngology--Head and Neck Surgery (AAO-HNS); American College of Allergy, Asthma and Immunology (ACAAI); American Rhinologic Society (ARS). Rhinosinusitis: establishing definitions for clinical research and patient care. J Allergy Clin Immunol 2004;114(Suppl 6):155–212
5. Fokkens W, Lund V, Bachert C, et al; EAACI. EAACI position paper on rhinosinusitis and nasal polyps executive summary. Allergy 2005;60(5):583–601
6. Piromchai P, Thanaviratananich S, Laopaiboon M. Systemic antibiotics for chronic rhinosinusitis without nasal polyps in adults. Cochrane Database Syst Rev 2011;(5):CD008233
7. Rosenfeld RM. Clinical practice guideline on adult sinusitis. Otolaryngol Head Neck Surg 2007;137(3):365–377
8. Soler ZM, Smith TL. What is the role of long-term macrolide therapy in the treatment of recalcitrant chronic rhinosinusitis? Laryngoscope 2009;119(11):2083–2084
9. Vaughan WC, Carvalho G. Use of nebulized antibiotics for acute infections in chronic sinusitis. Otolaryngol Head Neck Surg 2002;127(6):558–568
10. Ponikau JU, Sherris DA, Kern EB, et al. The diagnosis and incidence of allergic fungal sinusitis. Mayo Clin Proc 1999;74(9):877–884
11. Orlandi RR, Marple BF, Georgelas A, Durtschi D, Barr L. Immunologic response to fungus is not universally associated with rhinosinusitis. Otolaryngol Head Neck Surg 2009;141(6):750–756, e1–e2
12. Pant H, Schembri MA, Wormald PJ, Macardle PJ. IgE-mediated fungal allergy in allergic fungal sinusitis. Laryngoscope 2009;119(6):1046–1052
13. Isaacs S, Fakhri S, Luong A, Citardi MJ. A meta-analysis of topical amphotericin B for the treatment of chronic rhinosinusitis. Int Forum Allergy Rhinol 2011;1(4):250–254
14. Talbot AR, Herr TM, Parsons DS. Mucociliary clearance and buffered hypertonic saline solution. Laryngoscope 1997;107(4):500–503
15. Ural A, Oktemer TK, Kizil Y, Ileri F, Uslu S. Impact of isotonic and hypertonic saline solutions on mucociliary activity in various nasal pathologies: clinical study. J Laryngol Otol 2009;123(5):517–521
16. Rabago D, Zgierska A, Mundt M, Barrett B, Bobula J, Maberry R. Efficacy of daily hypertonic saline nasal irrigation among patients with sinusitis: a randomized controlled trial. J Fam Pract 2002;51(12):1049–1055
17. Rabago D, Pasic T, Zgierska A, Mundt M, Barrett B, Maberry R. The efficacy of hypertonic saline nasal irrigation for chronic sinonasal symptoms. Otolaryngol Head Neck Surg 2005;133(1):3–8
18. Bachmann G, Hommel G, Michel O. Effect of irrigation of the nose with isotonic salt solution on adult patients with chronic paranasal sinus disease. Eur Arch Otorhinolaryngol 2000;257(10):537–541
19. Shoseyov D, Bibi H, Shai P, Shoseyov N, Shazberg G, Hurvitz H. Treatment with hypertonic saline versus normal saline nasal wash of pediatric chronic sinusitis. J Allergy Clin Immunol 1998;101(5):602–605
20. Harvey R, Hannan SA, Badia L, Scadding G. Nasal saline irrigations for the symptoms of chronic rhinosinusitis. Cochrane Database Syst Rev 2007;(3):CD006394
21. Marple BF, Stankiewicz JA, Baroody FM, et al; American Academy of Otolaryngic Allergy Working Group on Chronic Rhinosinusitis. Diagnosis and management of chronic rhinosinusitis in adults. Postgrad Med 2009;121(6):121–139
22. Ruhno J, Andersson B, Denburg J, et al. A double-blind comparison of intranasal budesonide with placebo for nasal polyposis. J Allergy Clin Immunol 1990;86(6, pt 1):946–953
23. Jankowski R, Schrewelius C, Bonfils P, et al. Efficacy and tolerability of budesonide aqueous nasal spray treatment in patients with nasal polyps. Arch Otolaryngol Head Neck Surg 2001;127(4):447–452
24. Beer H, Southern KW, Swift AC. Topical nasal steroids for treating nasal polyposis in people with cystic fibrosis. Cochrane Database Syst Rev 2011;(5):CD008253
25. Lal D, Hwang PH. Oral corticosteroid therapy in chronic rhinosinusitis without polyposis: a systematic review. Int Forum Allergy Rhinol 2011;1(2):136–143
26. Osguthorpe JD. Surgical outcomes in rhinosinusitis: what we know. Otolaryngol Head Neck Surg 1999;120(4):451–453
27. Khalil HS, Nunez DA. Functional endoscopic sinus surgery for chronic rhinosinusitis. Cochrane Database Syst Rev 2006;(3):CD004458
28. Hartog B, van Benthem PP, Prins LC, Hordijk GJ. Efficacy of sinus irrigation versus sinus irrigation followed by functional endoscopic sinus surgery. Ann Otol Rhinol Laryngol 1997;106(9):759–766
29. Ragab SM, Lund VJ, Scadding G. Evaluation of the medical and surgical treatment of chronic rhinosinusitis: a prospective, randomised, controlled trial. Laryngoscope 2004;114(5):923–930
30. Soler ZM, Smith TL. Quality of life outcomes after functional endoscopic sinus surgery. Otolaryngol Clin North Am 2010;43(3):605–612
31. Chester AC, Antisdel JL, Sindwani RS. Symptom-specific outcomes of endoscopic sinus surgery: a systematic review. Otolaryngol Head Neck Surg 2009;140(5):633–639
32. Ling FT, Kountakis SE. Rhinosinusitis Task Force symptoms versus the Sinonasal Outcomes Test in patients evaluated for chronic rhinosinusitis. Am J Rhinol 2007;21(4):495–498
33. Chester AC, Sindwani R, Smith TL, Bhattacharyya N. Fatigue improvement following endoscopic sinus surgery: a systematic review and meta-analysis. Laryngoscope 2008;118(4):730–739

34. Lund VJ, MacKay IS. Outcome assessment of endoscopic sinus surgery. J R Soc Med 1994;87(2):70–72

35. Senior BA, Kennedy DW, Tanabodee J, Kroger H, Hassab M, Lanza D. Long-term results of functional endoscopic sinus surgery. Laryngoscope 1998;108(2):151–157

36. Soler ZM, Mace J, Smith TL. Symptom-based presentation of chronic rhinosinusitis and symptom-specific outcomes after endoscopic sinus surgery. Am J Rhinol 2008;22(3):297–301

37. Benninger MS, Khalid AN, Benninger RM, Smith TL. Surgery for chronic rhinosinusitis may improve sleep and sexual function. Laryngoscope 2010;120(8):1696–1700

38. Smith TL, Batra PS, Seiden AM, Hannley M. Evidence supporting endoscopic sinus surgery in the management of adult chronic rhinosinusitis: a systematic review. Am J Rhinol 2005;19(6):537–543

39. Lund VJ. Evidence-based surgery in chronic rhinosinusitis. Acta Otolaryngol 2001;121(1):5–9

40. Moses RL, Cornetta A, Atkins JP Jr, Roth M, Rosen MR, Keane WM. Revision endoscopic sinus surgery: the Thomas Jefferson University experience. Ear Nose Throat J 1998;77(3):190–202, 193–195, 199–202

41. McMains KC, Kountakis SE. Revision functional endoscopic sinus surgery: objective and subjective surgical outcomes. Am J Rhinol 2005;19(4):344–347

42. Smith TL, Litvack JR, Hwang PH, et al. Determinants of outcomes of sinus surgery: a multi-institutional prospective cohort study. Otolaryngol Head Neck Surg 2010;142(1):55–63

43. Brown CL, Bolger WE. Safety and feasibility of balloon catheter dilation of paranasal sinus ostia: a preliminary investigation. Ann Otol Rhinol Laryngol 2006;115(4):293–299, discussion 300–301

44. Bolger WE, Brown CL, Church CA, et al. Safety and outcomes of balloon catheter sinusotomy: a multicenter 24-week analysis in 115 patients. Otolaryngol Head Neck Surg 2007;137(1):10–20

45. Vaughan WC. Review of balloon sinuplasty. Curr Opin Otolaryngol Head Neck Surg 2008;16(1):2–9

46. Kuhn FA, Church CA, Goldberg AN, et al. Balloon catheter sinusotomy: one-year follow-up–outcomes and role in functional endoscopic sinus surgery. Otolaryngol Head Neck Surg 2008;139(3)(Suppl 3):S27–S37

47. Weiss RL, Church CA, Kuhn FA, Levine HL, Sillers MJ, Vaughan WC. Long-term outcome analysis of balloon catheter sinusotomy: two-year follow-up. Otolaryngol Head Neck Surg 2008;139(3)(Suppl 3):S38–S46

48. Friedman M, Schalch P, Lin HC, Mazloom N, Neidich M, Joseph NJ. Functional endoscopic dilatation of the sinuses: patient satisfaction, postoperative pain, and cost. Am J Rhinol 2008;22(2):204–209

49. Stankiewicz J, Truitt T, Atkins JJ Jr. One-year results: transantral balloon dilation of the ethmoid infundibulum. Ear Nose Throat J 2010;89(2):72–77

50. Ahmed J, Pal S, Hopkins C, Jayaraj S. Functional endoscopic balloon dilation of sinus ostia for chronic rhinosinusitis (Review). Cochrane Collab 2011;7:1–16

7 Fungal Diseases of the Paranasal Sinuses

Anand K. Devaiah and Bradley F. Marple

Fungal involvement in sinus disease has a wide variety of manifestations. It has been implicated in sinus disease, from acute infection to chronic disease and invasive disease. There have been debates on direct pathogenic role of fungus versus host response to the fungus. Whether fungus has any role in sinus disease—that it may simply be ubiquitous and seen as a colonizing organism—has been debated for several disease subsets. This chapter will explore different areas of fungus involvement in sinus disease. There have been several methods of classification based on the pathology and epidemiology,[1-3] but the disease can be divided into the following categories: noninvasive fungal rhinosinusitis (allergic fungal rhinosinusitis [AFRS] and mycetoma) and invasive fungal rhinosinusitis (acute invasive, chronic invasive, and granulomatous).

Noninvasive Fungal Rhinosinusitis

Allergic Fungal Rhinosinusitis

AFRS is the most common form of fungal rhinosinusitis. It is characterized by dark, thick, inspissated mucus filling the paranasal sinuses. This allergic or eosinophilic mucin is thick and very tenacious, which can be difficult to extract from the sinuses. On microscopic examination, it has onion-skin layers of necrotic and degranulating eosinophils in the background, few fungal hyphae, and small hexagonal lysophospholipase crystals (also known as Charcot-Leyden crystals).[4-6] The most common organisms isolated are dematiaceous fungi such as bipolaris and curvularia.[7,8]

The disease classically manifests as unilateral disease. Patients exhibit slow, progressive nasal congestion, postnasal drainage, nasal obstruction, and anosmia. The thick, mucinous debris is commonly found in the nasal discharge. If the fungal element of this disease is not recognized, a patient may have disease refractory to conventional treatments and even have multiple surgeries in an effort to clear the disease process. Patients may have proptosis or telecanthus at presentation.[9-12] Diagnostic computed tomography (CT) scans may suggest the diagnosis by demonstrating opacification of multiple sinuses with areas of central hyperattenuation from mucin, mucoceles, and remodeling of the paranasal sinuses including lamina papyracea. Magnetic resonance imaging (MRI) may also demonstrate similar sinus findings on T1 and T2 imaging, particularly elevated peripheral signal from mucosal inflammation and central signal attenuation from mucin.

Patients are typically young, atopic, and immunocompetent.[8,10] The pathogenesis of the disease has been assumed to be fungal hypersensitivity culminating in Gell and Coombs types 1 and 3 reactions to fungal allergens, similar to *Aspergillus* bronchopulmonary disease.[13] Given the association with allergy and with elevated immunoglobulin (Ig) G and IgE levels to fungal antigens, this appears to be a valid hypothesis for one part of the pathogenic mechanism.[9,13-15] Although other investigators have suggested different diagnostic criteria, Bent and Kuhn[16] published criteria that have remained the most reliable in establishing the diagnosis. Their criteria include establishing the following: type 1 hypersensitivity by history, skin tests, or in vitro testing; characteristic CT scan findings as illustrated above; demonstration of nasal polyposis; confirming eosinophilic mucus; finding positive fungal stains in specimens from sinus surgery; and the absence of fungal invasion into sinus tissue. It is believed that the key to successful long-term management of this disease will hinge on developing more effective classification and disease characterization, given the overlap with other forms of chronic rhinosinusitis.

AFRS is treated through a combination of medical and surgical methods. Surgery is employed to open and evacuate the paranasal sinuses, particularly if there is evidence of extensive remodeling and risk of orbital or intracranial complication. Extensive resection of mucosa is not necessary, but re-establishing drainage pathways is essential. Different medical treatments have been used, each with varying success and each carries merit in their use. Immunotherapy, leukotriene inhibitors, systemic steroids, topical nasal steroids, macrolides, and antifungals may be used in management.[10,17-20] Amphotericin B lavage has been advocated in the treatment of rhinosinusitis, targeting fungal etiology, but the data are inconclusive in showing an acceptable risk:benefit ratio.[21] However, this and other antifungal irrigations may fail because of the inability to properly penetrate the mucinous sinus debris. Despite this inability interventions are chosen, AFRS still has a high risk of recurrence.[22] Successful treatment results in a reversal of any sinus and orbit remodeling (i.e., proptosis and volume reduction), as well as resolution of mucin production.

The production of mucin with the presence of fungus is a diagnostic hallmark and helps guide treatment. However, there are variations of the disease that do not have fungal elements identified in the mucin, yet they respond to AFRS treatments. Ferguson[23] proposed eosinophilic mucin rhinosinusitis (EMRS) to describe this variant. Subsequently, Ponikau et al[24] reported that fungi was ubiquitous in sinus disease and could be identified using more sensitive testing in chronic rhinosinusitis patients. They postulated that the chronic rhinosinusitis disease may be a cell-mediated hypersensitive response to fungi. These and other reports point to conflicting evidence in the literature; some of the findings have been replicated by other observers, whereas others have not. Additional studies have supported the hypothesis that IgE- and IgG-dependent mechanisms lead to a fungal antigen hypersensitivity response in patients with AFRS and EMRS.[25,26] These incompletely understood mechanisms are presumptively responsible for the production of eosinophilic mucin seen in AFRS and EMRS. Regardless, the exact relationship of fungus in rhinosinusitis continues to be an area of debate (and is further discussed in another chapter), but in AFRS the diagnostic and treatment findings directed toward fungus appear to have utility as well as suggestion of underlying mechanisms. The differences seen in diagnostic and clinical performance of patients likely represent variability in disease pathogenesis as well as the need to identify other key factors to better tailor diagnosis and treatment algorithms.

Mycetoma

This is a form of noninvasive rhinosinusitis that is most often caused by *Aspergillus* species.[27] It has been well characterized as a separate entity given the noninvasive nature of the disease. It has been described classically in the immunocompetent patients. Other reports indicate that they can occur in immunocompromised patients and may also involve Mucorales order organisms.[28] It should be noted that in an immunocompromised patient in particular, diagnosis of mycetoma versus invasive fungal rhinosinusitis should be very carefully considered, as the treatments and the overall prognosis are significantly different.

The presentation of mycetoma should be suspected under certain conditions. There is typically a paucity of sinus involvement, and a singular sinus can be involved. The sinuses typically involved are the maxillary (most common) and sphenoid sinuses. The mycetoma grows in the sinus, exerting mass effect. CT is especially useful in supporting the diagnosis, whereas MRI may be useful in some patients where soft tissue delineation may be needed. The classic appearance on CT shows intrasinus inspissation with hyperattenuated areas suggestive of calcification (**Fig. 7.1**). Sinus remodeling and hyperostosis can be seen as well. On MRI, one sees low signal intensity on T1- and T2-weighted imaging, which can sometimes make diagnosis difficult if used as the sole modality. In general, CT is more useful in supporting the diagnosis.

The diagnosis of mycetoma is made through physical examination and surgical intervention to remove the material within the sinus. No signs of invasion should be seen in the sinus or surrounding tissues. The typical "peanut

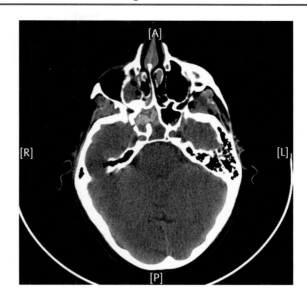

Figure 7.1 A noncontrast computed tomography scan of a right sphenoid mycetoma. Note the increased signal associated with the fungal lesion (arrow).

butter" appearance of the mycetoma is seen when opening the involved area. Opening the sinus and removal of all the debris is the mainstay of the treatment. Medical therapy is generally not needed, as surgical evacuation is generally adequate to eradicate the disease.

Invasive Fungal Rhinosinusitis

On the other end of the spectrum is invasive fungal rhinosinusitis. This disease represents a life-threatening disorder. Fungi invade sinus mucosa, vasculature bone, and adjacent structures such as the eye and brain. There are several methods of classification, and controversy exists about how to best distinguish the forms of the disease. It can be subdivided into three forms: acute invasive, chronic invasive, and granulomatous. Several organisms have been shown to be causative for the different forms. Most often, the causative organisms for these diseases are the Ascomycota phylum, *Aspergillus* species, or those within the Mucorales order (phylum Zygomycetes), specifically *Mucor*, *Rhizomucor*, and *Rhizopus*. Other agents have been described and include *Candida* species, *Dermatiaceous* species, *Fusarium* species, and *Pseudoallescheria* species.[29] Different species may coexist in the same patient's disease as well.

Patients at risk are immunocompromised in some fashion, with the exception of the chronic granulomatous form, which is seen almost exclusively in immunocompetent individuals. Common immunodeficiency-associated risk factors include diabetes (with or without ketoacidosis), acquired immunodeficiency syndrome (AIDS), hematologic malignancies with leukopenia (either absolute or functionally), leukopenia for other reasons (e.g., leukopenia induced for bone marrow transplant), and

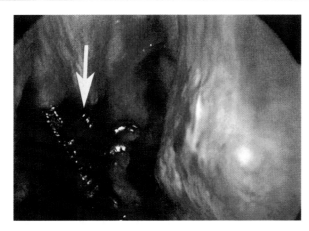

Figure 7.2 Endoscopic view of a patient's nasal cavity with invasive fungal rhinosinusitis, resulting from neutropenia associated with leukemia. This is a view of the left nasal cavity through a surgical defect from the initial debridement, looking through the septum to the posterior nasal cavity. The crusting seen (arrow) is an area of involvement proven by biopsy. This also illustrates the importance of repeat examinations and debridement to ensure the disease is controlled.

immunomodulation for solid organ transplantation. Other factors include iron overload with or without a need for deferoxamine therapy and protein malnutrition.

Patients who are immunocompromised and present with signs of rhinosinusitis should be examined with nasal endoscopy for signs of invasive fungal rhinosinusitis. Sloughing, crusting, necrosis, or hypovascular areas should raise the suspicion for invasive fungal sinusitis (**Fig. 7.2**). Mucorales pathogens may present early on as necrotic-appearing tissue when examined endoscopically, along with having elements of microvascular invasion. Although *Aspergillus* also presents with necrotic tissue changes, it may also present with pale, hypovascular tissue presumably because of early predilection for microvasculature. Patients may also report epistaxis, infection of the facial soft tissues, periorbital edema, proptosis, decreased vision, mental status change, or seizure. The granulomatous form often presents with mass effect and can mimic malignancy. Biopsy of involved tissue and adjacent normal-appearing tissue is the most reliable method of making the diagnosis.

Histologically, one sees invasion of the sinus mucosa, blood vessels, bone, or adjacent structures by fungal elements. This is best seen on silver stain, but it may also be seen on hematoxylin and eosin. In the granulomatous form, there is a granulomatous reaction and dense fibrosis[30] and typically less vascular invasion. On microscopic examination, the organisms have differentiating characteristics. *Aspergillus* has thin hyphae with numerous septations. The hyphae branch at acute (45-degree) angles. Pathogenic *Mucor* species exhibit broad hyphae with few to no septations and have a 90-degree angle branching.

CT and MRI can be helpful as adjunctive studies, but do not supplant microscopic examination of tissue. In a

study that looks at MRI and CT for acute invasive fungal rhinosinusitis, Groppo et al[31] found MRI was more sensitive than CT (average 86% vs. 63%). Positive predictive value was higher (94% for MRI and 91% for CT), but average negative predictive value was lower (86% for MRI and 56% for CT). MRI was better for detecting extra sinus involvement (e.g., orbital involvement). Hence, having CT and MRI is useful to help support the diagnosis, identify extra sinus involvement, and help surgical planning, but physical examination and surgical findings during debridement should be the primary determinant of surgical extent.

Mortality depends on several factors. The form of the disease, extent of involvement, use of combination surgical with medical therapy, and patient immune function are important factors. The chronic and granulomatous forms have lower mortality than acute invasive disease. Mortality for acute invasive disease has been quoted as ranging from 18 to 80% from different sources. Mortality is higher when accompanied by poor immune function, specifically low absolute neutrophil count (ANC). In one study, having an ANC < 500/mm^3 for more than 10 days carried a greater risk of developing invasive fungal rhinosinusitis.[32] Having a low ANC is also associated with a higher disease mortality. Other factors that increase mortality include intracranial involvement, with some sources indicating 70% mortality. Being unable to control underlying comorbidities also carries higher mortality. The combination of surgery and antifungals has reduced mortality overall, with one literature analysis quoting overall survival in acute invasive zygomycosis at 70% when surgery and antifungals are used.[33]

Acute Invasive Fungal Rhinosinusitis

The acute form is typically present for less than 4 weeks and progresses rapidly, as the name implies. The infection will progress quickly over a very short time, which can manifest even over hours. Therefore, this should be considered an emergency, and patients with the acute invasive form should be treated rapidly, shortly after discovering the presence of the disease as long as they are able to undergo treatment. Even over a period of a few hours, the effects can be devastating. Tissue involvement can spread quickly from the sinuses into adjacent tissues (**Fig. 7.3**). The invasive and disseminated form of the disease is most commonly caused by *Aspergillus fumigatus*. In severe disseminated disease, this typically involves the pulmonary system and central nervous system and is seen in severe immunocompromised states with neutropenia. Disease in patients with diabetes is often because of *Mucor*.

Treatment is both surgical and medical. The surgical debridement should continue ideally until clear margins on frozen section are obtained. This may result in radical excisions of tissue including removal of the orbital contents, overlying soft tissues of the face, and some involved intracranial tissues. Endoscopic management of disease can be employed if the disease is amenable to this method and

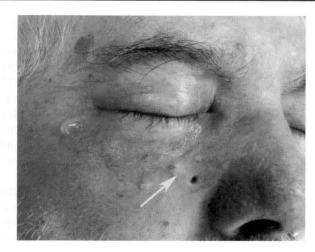

Figure 7.3 Invasive fungal rhinosinusitis involving the soft tissues. Figure shows a patient with involvement of the right melolabial area (arrow) and right eyelid. In this case, these areas exhibited subtle erythema and edema and were confirmed as involved with invasive fungus spread from the paranasal sinuses.

the surgeon is comfortable with endoscopic techniques. Follow-up examinations and repeat debridements in the operating room are recommended; one needs to ensure that further progression of the disease is halted, as progression can continue despite adequate initial debridement and initiation of antifungal therapy. Daily examinations and periodic surgical debridements are recommended until there is no sign of necrotic tissue.

Medical therapy should be initiated as soon as possible and takes two forms: antifungal therapy and therapy directed against the underlying immunocompromise. There are several regimens that can be considered,[29,34] and asking assistance from an infectious disease specialist is essential. Antifungal therapy is generally directed against the causative organism. If the agent has not been identified, amphotericin or similar broad-spectrum antifungal medicine should be administered initially. For *Aspergillus*, *Fusarium*, and *Pseudoallescheria*, voriconazole or other agents active against these pathogens are considered. *Candida* can be treated with fluconazole in non-neutropenic patients; for neutropenic patients, using agents such as amphotericin or voriconazole should be considered. Taking the necessary steps to correct any underlying immune suppression, if possible, is also important in the treatment of this disease. Aggressive treatment of contributing conditions, such as diabetes, should be undertaken.

Chronic Invasive Fungal Rhinosinusitis

This is a disease that has slow progression and has been present and showing invasive features for 3 months. Hence, it has a relatively low grade of invasion. It is more often seen in those with diabetes, chronic steroid use, and AIDS. *A. fumigatus* is the pathogen associated with this form of the disease. It is not uncommon to see orbital apex syndrome

(ophthalmoplegia, visual loss, and hypesthesia of the upper face) in this disease.

Treatment modalities are generally the same as that for acute invasive rhinosinusitis. However, the less aggressive nature of the disease will often allow for being more sparing of sensitive structures, such as the eye and brain, if possible. The disease can still progress or become more opportunistic, so proper follow-up and treatment directed at controlling the disease and comorbidities is important.

Granulomatous Fungal Rhinosinusitis

This disease results in a granulomatous reaction and mass effect with invasion of the surrounding tissue. This is a slowly progressing disease, with a time course that measures over months. It commonly involves the orbit at some point in the disease process, leading to proptosis or other visual problems. Other sites of involvement can include any of the paranasal sinuses, the face, and nose. *Aspergillus flavus* is the causative organism in this disease. It is more typically seen in India, Pakistan, Saudi Arabia, and Sudan. Treatment for this disease is surgical and medical, similar to what is typically employed in chronic invasive rhinosinusitis.

Summary

Fungal rhinosinusitis takes on noninvasive and invasive forms. The treatment for these diseases continues to evolve and can involve both surgical and medical options. Recognition of the differences between these forms and their subtypes is essential for patients, given the great differences in the clinical pictures and outcomes.

References

1. Ryan MR, Marple BF. Allergic fungal sinusitis: diagnosis and management. Curr Opin Otolaryngol Head Neck Surg 2007; 15: 18–22
2. Saravanan K, Panda NK, Chakrabarti A, Das A, Bapuraj RJ. Allergic fungal rhinosinusitis: an attempt to resolve the diagnostic dilemma. Arch Otolaryngol Head Neck Surg 2006;132(2):173–178
3. Chakrabarti A, Denning DW, Ferguson BJ, et al. Fungal rhinosinusitis: a categorization and definitional schema addressing current controversies. Laryngoscope 2009;119(9):1809–1818
4. Katzenstein AL, Sale SR, Greenberger PA. Allergic Aspergillus sinusitis: a newly recognized form of sinusitis. J Allergy Clin Immunol 1983;72(1):89–93
5. Safirstein BH. Allergic bronchopulmonary aspergillosis with obstruction of the upper respiratory tract. Chest 1976;70(6):788–790
6. Miller JW, Johnston A, Lamb D. Allergic aspergillosis of the maxillary sinuses. Thorax 1981;36:710
7. Manning SC, Schaefer SD, Close LG, Vuitch F. Culture-positive allergic fungal sinusitis. Arch Otolaryngol Head Neck Surg 1991;117(2):174–178
8. Ence BK, Gourley DS, Jorgensen NL, et al. Allergic fungal sinusitis. Am J Rhinol 1990;4:169–178
9. Marple BF. Allergic fungal rhinosinusitis: current theories and management strategies. Laryngoscope 2001;111(6):1006–1019

10. Schubert MS, Goetz DW. Evaluation and treatment of allergic fungal sinusitis. II. Treatment and follow-up. J Allergy Clin Immunol 1998; 102(3):395–402

11. McClay JE, Marple B, Kapadia L, et al. Clinical presentation of allergic fungal sinusitis in children. Laryngoscope 2002;112(3):565–569

12. Manning SC, Vuitch F, Weinberg AG, Brown OE. Allergic aspergillosis: a newly recognized form of sinusitis in the pediatric population. Laryngoscope 1989;99(7, pt 1):681–685

13. Schubert MS. Allergic fungal sinusitis: pathogenesis and management strategies. Drugs 2004;64(4):363–374

14. Manning SC, Holman M. Further evidence for allergic pathophysiology in allergic fungal sinusitis. Laryngoscope 1998; 108(10):1485–1496

15. Stewart AE, Hunsaker DH. Fungus-specific IgG and IgE in allergic fungal rhinosinusitis. Otolaryngol Head Neck Surg 2002;127(4):324–332

16. Bent JP III, Kuhn FA. Diagnosis of allergic fungal sinusitis. Otolaryngol Head Neck Surg 1994;111(5):580–588

17. Kuhn FA, Javer AR. Allergic fungal sinusitis: a four-year follow-up. Am J Rhinol 2000;14(3):149–156

18. Folker RJ, Marple BF, Mabry RL, Mabry CS. Treatment of allergic fungal sinusitis: a comparison trial of postoperative immunotherapy with specific fungal antigens. Laryngoscope 1998;108(11, pt 1): 1623–1627

19. Bent JP III, Kuhn FA. Antifungal activity against allergic fungal sinusitis organisms. Laryngoscope 1996;106(11):1331–1334

20. Rains BM III, Mineck CW. Treatment of allergic fungal sinusitis with high-dose itraconazole. Am J Rhinol 2003;17(1):1–8

21. Orlandi RR, Marple BF. The role of fungus in chronic rhinosinusitis. Otolaryngol Clin North Am 2010;43(3):531–537, viii

22. Kupferberg SB, Bent JP III, Kuhn FA. Prognosis for allergic fungal sinusitis. Otolaryngol Head Neck Surg 1997;117(1):35–41

23. Ferguson BJ. Eosinophilic mucin rhinosinusitis: a distinct clinico-pathological entity. Laryngoscope 2000;110(5, pt 1):799–813

24. Ponikau JU, Sherris DA, Kern EB, et al. The diagnosis and incidence of allergic fungal sinusitis. Mayo Clin Proc 1999;74(9):877–884

25. Pant H, Kette FE, Smith WB, Wormald PJ, Macardle PJ. Fungal-specific humoral response in eosinophilic mucus chronic rhinosinusitis. Laryngoscope 2005;115(4):601–606

26. Collins M, Nair S, Smith W, Kette F, Gillis D, Wormald PJ. Role of local immunoglobulin E production in the pathophysiology of noninvasive fungal sinusitis. Laryngoscope 2004;114(7):1242–1246

27. Ferreiro JA, Carlson BA, Cody DT III. Paranasal sinus fungus balls. Head Neck 1997;19(6):481–486

28. Robey AB, O'Brien EK, Richardson BE, Baker JJ, Poage DP, Leopold DA. The changing face of paranasal sinus fungus balls. Ann Otol Rhinol Laryngol 2009;118(7):500–505

29. Johnson MD, Gleeson TD. Invasive Fungal Sinusitis. In: Hospenthal DR, ed. http://infections.consultantlive.com/display/article/1145625/1526057#. Published February 2010. Accessed June 23, 2012

30. Das A, Bal A, Chakrabarti A, Panda N, Joshi K. Spectrum of fungal rhinosinusitis; histopathologist's perspective. Histopathology 2009;54(7):854–859

31. Groppo ER, El-Sayed IH, Aiken AH, Glastonbury CM. Computed tomography and magnetic resonance imaging characteristics of acute invasive fungal sinusitis. Arch Otolaryngol Head Neck Surg 2011;137(10):1005–1010

32. Chen CY, Sheng WH, Cheng A, et al. Invasive fungal sinusitis in patients with hematological malignancy: 15 years experience in a single university hospital in Taiwan. BMC Infect Dis 2011;11:250

33. Roden MM, Zaoutis TE, Buchanan WL, et al. Epidemiology and outcome of zygomycosis: a review of 929 reported cases. Clin Infect Dis 2005;41(5):634–653

34. Walsh TJ, Anaissie EJ, Denning DW, et al; Infectious Diseases Society of America. Treatment of aspergillosis: clinical practice guidelines of the Infectious Diseases Society of America. Clin Infect Dis 2008;46(3):327–360

8 Evaluation and Treatment of Olfactory Disorders

Arthur William Wu and Eric H. Holbrook

Often overlooked in comparison to our other senses, the sense of smell is still an important way by which we experience the world around us. As in other animals, smell at its basic level tells us whether a substance or environment is good or bad, safe or dangerous. It can act as a warning system detecting smoke from a fire or the stench of spoiled food. Smell also imparts flavor to food, and by doing so, changes a necessity of daily survival into a matter of enjoyment. It greatly affects our quality of life and can trigger some of our deepest memories; it triggers emotion with the smell of a holiday dinner or of a spouse's cologne or perfume. The quality and intensity of this perception depend on the anatomic state of the nasal epithelium and the status of the peripheral and central nervous systems. Dysfunction at any one of the many steps along the olfactory pathway can disable a patient's sense of smell and greatly affect his or her quality of life.

Anatomy and Physiology

The relevant anatomy and physiology of olfaction explain how an odor is carried into the nose and eventually is perceived by the brain as a distinct smell. Before an odorant can activate a receptor it must first reach the olfactory cleft. The pathway of odorant exposure to the nasal cavity is usually thought to occur through an anterior pathway via the nares and anterior nasal cavity. It has become clear, however, that a retronasal stimulation of the olfactory epithelium is also important and probably plays a role in flavor appreciation during eating.[1] This secondary pathway is important in cases of anterior nasal obstruction from polyp disease, in which odor identification appears to be more effective through a retronasal route.[2]

As the odorant molecule traverses the narrow passageway of the nasal cavity, it must first cross from the air phase to the mucus phase to gain access to the olfactory receptors. The odorant molecules must be not only soluble in the mucus but also free enough within the mucus to interact with receptors on the olfactory epithilium.[3] Changes in the character of the mucus can influence the diffusion time required for odorant molecules to reach the receptor sites.[4]

The olfactory epithelium corresponds to an area in the superior recess of the right and left nasal cavities, between the septum and middle/superior turbinates, and below the cribriform plate, termed the olfactory cleft. The epithelium is a continuous sheet at birth but develops irregular borders and is progressively replaced with respiratory epithelium in patches thereafter.[5] This respiratory metaplasia is thought to increase in size even in normal-functioning adults. The area of olfactory epithelium in adults generally includes the surface of the superior turbinates and occasionally the anterior extent of the middle turbinates, covering an area of roughly 1 to 2 cm^2.[6,7]

The olfactory mucosa is a pseudostratified columnar neuroepithelium. In the deepest layer are the basal cells, which are the putative stem cells that give rise to all components of the epithelium. In all primates and mammals the olfactory neurons are continually being replaced by the dividing basal cells. The combined presence of immature olfactory neurons with mature neurons and mitotic cells in the basal layer of the olfactory epithelium in human autopsy specimens strongly supports the presence of regenerating olfactory neurons in humans.[7] It is this unique ability of the olfactory mucosa to renew itself that enables the possibility of full recovery after injury to the epithelium. In fact, intensive research studying the multipotency of these basal cells is ongoing. The cells have been shown to harbor the ability to become neuronal, as well as nonneuronal, cells outside of the olfactory system.[8] Microvillar-capped sustentacular cells occupy the most apical layer of the epithelium. Beneath the basement membrane, serous Bowman glands send ducts through the epithelium to the surface. The olfactory neurons occupy the region superficial to the basal cells, with more mature cell bodies residing apically. They are bipolar in shape with dendrites terminating in knobs with immotile cilia at the surface of the mucosa. These cilia contain the olfactory receptors providing increased surface area for sampling the odorants introduced into the nasal cavity. The olfactory axons exit through the basal lamina and converge with other axons into nerve bundles, termed fila olfactoria (cranial nerve I), that travel through the lamina propria and eventually traverse the cribriform plate to contact the olfactory bulb. The axons are surrounded by special olfactory ensheathing cells that are unique because they share characteristics that are common with both Schwann cells and central glial cells. Because of the unique regenerative properties of this neuroepithelium, there has been interest in the role of the ensheathing cells in this process and its possible therapeutic potential for repair of peripheral nerve injury. These same axons make first-order synapses in the glomeruli of the olfactory bulb. Further signal transduction proceeds along the olfactory tract to higher processing centers of the olfactory cortex at the base of the frontal lobes and medial aspect of the temporal lobes. From the olfactory cortex, information is sent to the insular cortex in the thalamus where olfactory and taste information is integrated.[9]

The gene family responsible for olfactory receptors is the largest within the human genome, coding for close to 700 different transmembrane G-protein receptor types, although a large proportion of these are nonfunctional pseudogenes.[10] Each olfactory neuron expresses one single receptor type. In rodents, olfactory neurons with the same receptor type converge on an average of two glomeruli per bulb, creating the beginning of a specialized odorant map. It is clear that one odorant does not activate one receptor type but many receptor types are activated to various degrees. Therefore, by stimulating a combination of different receptor types, a pattern of glomerular activation occurs. In this way, the system can encode an almost limitless number of different odorants.

Evaluation

History

The most important element in the evaluation of a patient with an olfactory disorder is obtaining the history. A detailed history will provide a diagnosis in the vast majority of cases. The physician should first assess what type of olfactory disorder the patient is describing. Quantitative disorders are deficiencies of detection. *Hyposmia* is the decreased ability to detect odors, and *anosmia* is an inability to detect odors. Patients with qualitative disorders may have difficulty identifying an odor (*parosmia*) or they may perceive odors when none are present (*phantosmia*).

Although there are many proposed etiologies of olfactory disorders, the most common are because of upper respiratory infections (URIs), head trauma, and rhinosinusitis; therefore, significant time should be directed toward identifying these causes in the history.[11-15] Given the large contributions of smell to flavor, it is not unusual for patients to describe a loss of taste as the presenting complaint. By confirming that the patient can detect salty, sweet, sour, or bitter tastes, one may then focus specifically on olfaction. This also gives the clinician an opportunity to educate patients on the differences between smell, taste, and flavor. Patients should be asked about the severity of the smell loss and how it affects their everyday life. Descriptions of hazardous events including the inability to detect cooking fires, natural gas leaks, or spoiled food are often relayed by the patient and it presents an opportunity to counsel the patient on the risks of smell loss.

Timing of the onset of the disorder can be very helpful. Sudden onset of smell loss is usually related to an URI or trauma, whereas gradual smell loss is usually associated with causes such as aging, neurodegenerative disease, and long-term chronic rhinosinusitis (CRS). Fluctuation in the ability to smell is associated frequently with CRS and polyps. Having no memory of the ability to smell implies a congenital smell loss. In this case, further questions relating

to a delay in sexual maturity and family history of the same should be asked to check for Kallmann syndrome and an endocrine referral should be considered if the patient is prepubescent.[16]

Physicians should inquire about the presence of URI symptoms, head trauma (regardless of severity), acute or chronic exposure to chemicals, changes in medications, and use of over-the-counter medications. Inquiry should be made into the use of topical nasal zinc preparations. These medications, designed to prevent or shorten URIs, have been implicated in causing sudden smell loss.[17,18] Patients who have reported this phenomenon describe the smell loss occurring immediately or within hours of the use of the medication, coinciding with a burning sensation in the nasal cavity when the medication was applied. It may be difficult to prove a causal relationship between zinc sprays and olfactory loss, as most patients take this medication for URI, which itself is a leading cause of olfactory disorders.

When inquiring about other symptoms and medical problems, nasal obstruction, drainage, facial pressure/pain, ear complaints, and fatigue suggest CRS and/or allergic rhinitis. Unilateral symptoms of obstruction and epistaxis raise concerns for a nasal mass. Patients should be queried regarding memory loss, confusion, and cognitive dysfunction that may suggest a neurodegenerative disorder such as Alzheimer disease or Parkinson disease. Olfactory loss is an early symptom in Alzheimer disease, and diminished olfactory ability on testing may be an important early signal for further development of this disorder.[19] Vision changes, headaches, and sensory or motor changes should prompt a work-up for intracranial mass or central nervous system abnormality. Medical and surgical history should be reviewed to uncover possible sources such as nasal trauma, previous nasal surgery, stroke, and thyroid disorders.

Patients with parosmia or phantosmia should be asked for a history of migraines or seizure disorder in addition to questions regarding rhinosinusitis. Patients with phantosmia thought to be related to abnormal olfactory signal processing will often confirm a unilateral presentation to the distorted smell when asked. They often experience relief after periods of sleep and may notice a decrease during episodes of crying or bending over. The abnormal odor is described usually as having a rotten, moldy, swampy, or burning quality, and is often associated with a decreased sense of smell on the side of the distortion.[20] This information can help distinguish a causal relationship with a disorder of the olfactory nerves from more central disorders.

Physical Examination

In addition to a routine otolaryngologic examination, cranial nerve function should be assessed to rule out any localizing intracranial lesion, and special attention should be given to the examination of the nose. We recommend that rhinoscopy, nasal endoscopy, and administration of local anesthetic or decongestant sprays be delayed until

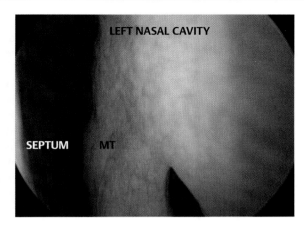

Figure 8.1 A normal olfactory cleft can be seen superiorly between the middle turbinate (MT) and the septum during endoscopy of the left nasal cavity.

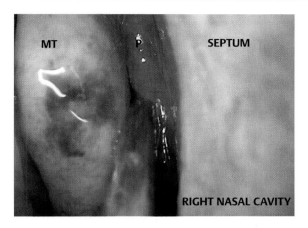

Figure 8.2 A large polyp (P) is obstructing the olfactory cleft between the middle turbinate (MT) and the septum in the right nasal cavity.

olfactory testing has been performed to avoid potential confounding effects. Anterior rhinoscopy alone has been shown to fail in the diagnosis of a conductive/obstructive olfactory loss in 51% of cases compared with 9% of cases with the use of nasal endoscopy.[12] For this reason, nasal endoscopy should be performed in all patients presenting with smell disorders to look for evidence of CRS, nasal polyposis, allergic rhinitis, or a nasal mass. Close attention should be given to the olfactory cleft, noting mucosal edema, thickened mucus, or other subtle signs of CRS (**Figs. 8.1** and **8.2**). In patients presenting with smell loss after nasal or sinus surgery, endoscopic inspection of the olfactory cleft looking for evidence of scarring or recurrent disease is useful in directing further management. In cases of patients complaining of phantosmia, unilateral occlusion of the nostril will usually result in temporary relief of symptoms if the disorder is related to airflow on the blocked side. This will also help localize the problem to the right or left side. In addition, unilateral topical nasal application of 4% cocaine solution with the body in a supine position and the head extended will anesthetize the olfactory neurons and provide relief of phantosmia if it is related to a disorder of olfactory signal transduction. This procedure will not help with more centrally related causes.[20]

Olfactory Testing

An integral component of the evaluation of a patient with smell disorder is olfactory testing. The two most common types of clinical tests for olfaction are threshold detection testing and identification testing. In threshold detection testing, the ability to detect odors is assessed through forced choice testing of gradually increased concentrations of an odorant, such as butyl alcohol, presented along with a blank sample.[11] The concentration at which the odor is detected consistently and correctly against the blank is the threshold of detection and is compared with a normal average. The drawbacks of this testing are its length and

need for a knowledgeable test administrator. Tests of identification involve presentation of a battery of different stimuli to the individual and asking the patient to choose the correct smell from the list of possibilities. The Sniffin' Sticks test uses odorant-impregnated, felt-tipped pens to test detection threshold, identification, and discrimination.[21-23] A composite score is again derived and compared with normative data. The test can be reused and is easy to perform, but it requires time commitment from a test administrator. The most widely used olfactory test in the United States is the University of Pennsylvania Smell Identification Test, commercially marketed as the Smell Identification Test (Sensonics, Haddon Heights, New Jersey). This is a self-administered forced-choice smell identification test using microencapsulated beads to present an odor in a scratch-and-sniff manner. Forty items are presented and patients must select the identity of the odor from four multiple choice answers. Results are compared with normal data stratified among age and sex. The test categorizes the patient as normal, hyposmic, anosmic, or possibly malingering. The test has a good reproducibility and correlates well with threshold tests.[24]

Imaging

The history and physical examination should dictate the need for further imaging. Patients with a clear history of causation such as URI-related anosmia and a collaborating normal physical examination need no further radiographic work-up.[25] In the setting of an identifiable cause based on history and the absence of abnormal findings on complete examination, magnetic resonance imaging (MRI) is not indicated as part of the evaluation.[26] In patients with atypical history, no clear identifiable cause, or with neurological findings, an MRI should be obtained to rule out an intracranial mass. In cases of congenital anosmia presenting in pediatric patients before the onset of puberty, an MRI can be useful in identifying the absence of olfactory bulbs found in association with Kallmann syndrome, although genetic studies have become a more definitive form of testing for this disorder. Patients with olfactory disorders related to CRS should undergo computed tomography (CT) scanning of the sinuses to evaluate the extent of disease. CT scans may also be used to evaluate for isolated obstruction of the olfactory clefts.[27]

Management

Sensorineural Causes

A main source of frustration for physicians presented with a patient complaining of smell disorders is in the management of these disorders. Although knowledge regarding the causes of sensorineural olfactory loss is improving, the ability to reverse olfactory dysfunction in the more common causes, such as upper respiratory tract infections and traumatic head injury, remains poor. Various nutritional supplements and medical therapies have been tried, including topical and systemic steroids, but controlled studies have been lacking. Blomqvist et al looked at patients with a decreased sense of smell including those resulting from an URI and CRS with polyps (not significant enough for surgery) placed on oral steroids with simultaneous fluticasone spray for 10 days. A surprising 83% showed improvement in olfactory testing with the oral steroids, including those with URI as a cause. Those who improved with oral steroids were given either fluticasone or a placebo. All subjects were found to maintain the improved sense of smell, suggesting a lack of benefit from nasal steroid sprays.[28] Similar results were found in a separate study looking at the use of oral prednisolone or topical mometasone in patients with idiopathic, sinonasal-related, or URI-related loss.[29] Although mometasone did not significantly improve symptoms, improvement of olfactory function occurred in all categories of patients after oral prednisolone. As short courses of oral steroids are relatively safe and inexpensive, steroid therapy may be worth trying electively for most patients presenting with sensorineural smell loss. In a study on the use of theophylline in patients with hyposmia, the authors reported improvements in smell with the use of this medication.[30] However, it is important to note that the patients with severe smell loss had only modest improvements.

Conductive Causes

The most common conductive cause of olfactory loss is CRS with or without polyps. These patients usually recount a history of fluctuating smell loss with episodes of anosmia associated with an increase in nasal obstruction and drainage. Endoscopic sinus surgery has been shown to provide significant improvements in the sense of smell of affected patients.[31,32] However, it has become increasingly clear that CRS and polyposis are not pure conductive causes of smell loss. Management with nasal and oral steroids as well as sur-

gery can improve olfactory function by removing obstructing polyps or edema, but over years there can be a decline in function often leading to complete anosmia refractory to oral steroids. There is evidence based on biopsy studies that a direct effect of inflammation from CRS on the olfactory epithelium contributes to this type of olfactory loss.[33,34] A tapering dose of oral steroids can provide information on whether smell loss in patients with CRS has progressed to a more permanent loss. With a better understanding of the mechanisms and inflammatory mediators of CRS, we may become more efficient in the prevention or even the treatment of this form of olfactory dysfunction.

Phantosmia/Parosmia

The typical course of phantosmia or parosmia is that symptoms lessen over time to tolerable levels. However, in the patients where symptoms are still very bothersome, intervention may be necessary. In patients with phantosmia related to nasal airflow, nasal saline drops may be administered in the head down position to temporarily occlude the olfactory cleft or nasal decongestants may be purposefully used to produce rhinitis medicamentosa in the offending side. In patients in whom symptoms are so severe that they cause weight loss or severe depression, surgical intervention to endoscopically denude or chemically destroy the olfactory epithelium may provide relief.[20] Careful work-up of these patients is critical to rule out central causes such as migraine disorder, epilepsy, or functional disorders before surgical interventions are considered.[35]

Conclusion

Our understanding of the mechanisms of olfaction and olfactory disorders is growing, but much is still unknown. Outcomes for patients with obstructive causes are more promising than idiopathic, traumatic, or post-viral losses. Steroid therapy may reduce edema or polyps, but surgery may ultimately be necessary in some cases when mechanical obstruction is not relieved medically. Unfortunately, effective medical treatments for a large portion of patients presenting with olfactory loss do not exist. Further basic science and clinical research is needed to provide novel therapeutic options that may help those suffering from this sensory loss.

References

1. Small DM, Gerber JC, Mak YE, Hummel T. Differential neural responses evoked by orthonasal versus retronasal odorant perception in humans. Neuron 2005;47(4):593–605
2. Landis BN, Giger R, Ricchetti A, et al. Retronasal olfactory function in nasal polyposis. Laryngoscope 2003;113(11):1993–1997
3. Laffort P, Patte F, Etcheto M. Olfactory coding on the basis of physicochemical properties. Ann N Y Acad Sci 1974;237(0):193–208
4. Getchell TV, Margolis FL, Getchell ML. Perireceptor and receptor events in vertebrate olfaction. Prog Neurobiol 1984;23(4):317–345

5. Nakashima T, Kimmelman CP, Snow JB Jr. Structure of human fetal and adult olfactory neuroepithelium. Arch Otolaryngol 1984; 110(10):641–646

6. Leopold DA, Hummel T, Schwob JE, Hong SC, Knecht M, Kobal G. Anterior distribution of human olfactory epithelium. Laryngoscope 2000;110(3, pt 1):417–421

7. Holbrook EH, Wu E, Curry WT, Lin DT, Schwob JE. Immunohistochemical characterization of human olfactory tissue. Laryngoscope 2011;121(8):1687–1701

8. Murrell W, Féron F, Wetzig A, et al. Multipotent stem cells from adult olfactory mucosa. Dev Dyn 2005;233(2):496–515

9. Shipley MT, Ennis M. Functional organization of olfactory system. J Neurobiol 1996;30(1):123–176

10. Reed RR. After the holy grail: establishing a molecular basis for mammalian olfaction. Cell 2004;116(2):329–336

11. Cain WS, Gent JF, Goodspeed RB, Leonard G. Evaluation of olfactory dysfunction in the Connecticut Chemosensory Clinical Research Center. Laryngoscope 1988;98(1):83–88

12. Seiden AM, Duncan HJ. The diagnosis of a conductive olfactory loss. Laryngoscope 2001;111(1):9–14

13. Miwa T, Furukawa M, Tsukatani T, Costanzo RM, DiNardo LJ, Reiter ER. Impact of olfactory impairment on quality of life and disability. Arch Otolaryngol Head Neck Surg 2001;127(5):497–503

14. Temmel AF, Quint C, Schickinger-Fischer B, Klimek L, Stoller E, Hummel T. Characteristics of olfactory disorders in relation to major causes of olfactory loss. Arch Otolaryngol Head Neck Surg 2002;128(6):635–641

15. Reden J, Maroldt H, Fritz A, Zahnert T, Hummel T. A study on the prognostic significance of qualitative olfactory dysfunction. Eur Arch Otorhinolaryngol 2007;264(2):139–144

16. Murphy C, Doty RL, Duncan HJ. Clinical disorders of olfaction. In: Doty RL, ed. Handbook of Olfaction and Gustation. 2nd ed. New York, NY: Marcel Dekker, Inc.; 2003:461–478

17. Jafek BW, Linschoten MR, Murrow BW. Anosmia after intranasal zinc gluconate use. Am J Rhinol 2004;18(3):137–141

18. Alexander TH, Davidson TM. Intranasal zinc and anosmia: the zinc-induced anosmia syndrome. Laryngoscope 2006;116(2):217–220

19. Nordin S, Monsch AU, Murphy C. Unawareness of smell loss in normal aging and Alzheimer's disease: discrepancy between self-reported and diagnosed smell sensitivity. J Gerontol B Psychol Sci Soc Sci 1995;50(4):187–192

20. Leopold DA, Loehrl TA, Schwob JE. Long-term follow-up of surgically treated phantosmia. Arch Otolaryngol Head Neck Surg 2002;128(6):642–647

21. Kobal G, Hummel T, Sekinger B, Barz S, Roscher S, Wolf S. "Sniffin' sticks": screening of olfactory performance. Rhinology 1996; 34(4):222–226

22. Hummel T, Sekinger B, Wolf SR, Pauli E, Kobal G. 'Sniffin' sticks': olfactory performance assessed by the combined testing of odor identification, odor discrimination and olfactory threshold. Chem Senses 1997;22(1):39–52

23. Hummel T, Konnerth CG, Rosenheim K, Kobal G. Screening of olfactory function with a four-minute odor identification test: reliability, normative data, and investigations in patients with olfactory loss. Ann Otol Rhinol Laryngol 2001;110(10):976–981

24. Doty RL, Shaman P, Kimmelman CP, Dann MS. University of Pennsylvania Smell Identification Test: a rapid quantitative olfactory function test for the clinic. Laryngoscope 1984;94(2, pt 1): 176–178

25. Sugiura M, Aiba T, Mori J, Nakai Y. An epidemiological study of postviral olfactory disorder. Acta Otolaryngol Suppl 1998;538: 191–196

26. Konstantinidis I, Haehner A, Frasnelli J, et al. Post-infectious olfactory dysfunction exhibits a seasonal pattern. Rhinology 2006;44(2):135–139

27. Biacabe B, Faulcon P, Amanou L, Bonfils P. Olfactory cleft disease: an analysis of 13 cases. Otolaryngol Head Neck Surg 2004;130(2): 202–208

28. Blomqvist EH, Lundblad L, Bergstedt H, Stjärne P. Placebo-controlled, randomized, double-blind study evaluating the efficacy of fluticasone propionate nasal spray for the treatment of patients with hyposmia/anosmia. Acta Otolaryngol 2003;123(7):862–868

29. Heilmann S, Huettenbrink KB, Hummel T. Local and systemic administration of corticosteroids in the treatment of olfactory loss. Am J Rhinol 2004;18(1):29–33

30. Henkin RI, Velicu I, Schmidt L. An open-label controlled trial of theophylline for treatment of patients with hyposmia. Am J Med Sci 2009;337(6):396–406

31. Ling FT, Kountakis SE. Important clinical symptoms in patients undergoing functional endoscopic sinus surgery for chronic rhinosinusitis. Laryngoscope 2007;117(6):1090–1093

32. Litvack JR, Mace J, Smith TL. Does olfactory function improve after endoscopic sinus surgery? Otolaryngol Head Neck Surg 2009;140(3):312–319

33. Kern RC. Chronic sinusitis and anosmia: pathologic changes in the olfactory mucosa. Laryngoscope 2000;110(7):1071–1077

34. Kern RC, Conley DB, Haines GK III, Robinson AM. Pathology of the olfactory mucosa: implications for the treatment of olfactory dysfunction. Laryngoscope 2004;114(2):279–285

35. Stein DJ, Le Roux L, Bouwer C, Van Heerden B. Is olfactory reference syndrome an obsessive-compulsive spectrum disorder?: two cases and a discussion. J Neuropsychiatry Clin Neurosci 1998;10(1): 96–99

9   Allergy and Chronic Rhinosinusitis

Elizabeth Mahoney Davis

Traditional perspectives on the pathophysiology of chronic rhinosinusitis (CRS) focus on a cycle of anatomic obstruction, osteomeatal occlusion, stasis of mucosal secretions, and bacterial infection. Recognizing that this paradigm may be overly simplistic, applying only to a segment of patients with CRS, our understanding of the pathogenesis of CRS has evolved in recent years to focus on other chronic inflammatory processes. Although a specific cause effect correlation between allergy and CRS is not established, epidemiologic data do support a relationship between allergic rhinitis and rhinosinusitis.[1,2] Further, there has been increasing support for the concept of the "unified airway," a model of respiratory disease that connects inflammatory disease in the upper and lower airways and regards the entire respiratory tract, from the sinonasal mucosa to the lungs, as an integrated system influenced by both local and systemic inflammatory mediators.[3] Krouse et al allege that upper airway inflammatory diseases, such as allergic rhinitis and sinusitis, and lower airway inflammatory disease, such as asthma, often coexist, and physicians should approach these diseases as a spectrum of inflammatory disorders. Studies have shown that interventions directed at one airway disease process often prove beneficial to other airspace inflammatory processes. For example, studies have demonstrated an improvement in asthma control with treatment of allergic rhinitis. Based on this same reasoning, improved control of allergic rhinitis in the patient suffering from CRS may be an important component of the overall treatment strategy.

Mechanisms

Allergic rhinitis is characterized by an immunoglobulin (Ig) E-mediated, type 1 hypersensitivity reaction. When this type 1 hypersensitivity reaction occurs in response to an inhaled antigen, mast cells degranulate and release preformed mediators including histamine, tryptase, and cytokines including interleukin (IL)-5. These cytokines then act as chemoattractants and stimulate migration of other inflammatory mediators including neutrophils, eosinophils, T lymphocytes, and macrophages.[4] This migration of additional mediators is associated with the late-phase allergic response, occurring hours after initial antigen exposure; this late-phase response is believed to correlate with the more chronic nature of inflammatory disease, as is seen in CRS.

A critical player in this late-phase allergic response is the eosinophil that releases additional tissue-damaging mediators including peroxidases and major basic protein. Eosinophilia is considered central to the allergic response

and is a common feature in other airway inflammatory disorders including asthma and many subsets of CRS. In fact, tissue samples of sinus mucosa of adults with CRS have shown high levels of both IL-5 and eosinophils.[5] High levels of IL-5 and eosinophils are also seen in the polypoid tissue in patients with chronic rhinosinusitis with nasal polyposis (CRSwNP). Although nasal polyposis (NP) is not always associated with atopy, the predominance of IL-5 and eosinophils in polypoid tissue argue for a relationship with mast cell pathophysiology. Many therapies for CRS are now directed at these chronic inflammatory pathways, and allergic disease is regarded as an inflammatory factor that should be considered in the evaluation and management of the patient with CRS.

Allergy Diagnostics

Patient history and physical examination lie at the core of allergy diagnosis. In fact, the vast majority of patients with allergic rhinitis do not require confirmatory diagnostic testing. If a patient is poorly controlled with medical therapy, if a patient desires to implement environmental controls, and/or if a firm diagnosis of allergy will influence treatment including consideration of immunotherapy, then allergy diagnostic testing is reasonable. Options for allergy testing can be classified as either in vivo or ex vivo. The gold standard for allergy testing is in vivo challenge. Typically reserved for experimental situations, select antigens can be administered to the bronchial, nasal, or conjunctival tissues and clinical manifestations are observed.

A more accessible and similarly reliable tissue to test is the skin. The skin harbors tissue mast cells. When these cells are sensitized to a particular antigen, they will degranulate, and the skin will develop a wheal and flare reaction (**Fig. 9.1**). Such skin tests can be administered via either epicutaneous prick tests or intradermal tests.[6] It is important to highlight the fact that any in vivo challenge carries a risk of severe, life-threatening allergic reaction and such testing should be performed in a clinical setting prepared to manage anaphylaxis. An alternative to skin testing is the in vitro testing modality of allergen-specific serum IgE testing. All in vitro testing modalities are premised on measurement and quantification of antigen-specific IgE in the patient's serum. In vitro testing has been shown to correlate well with skin testing and offers a safety advantage with no risk of anaphylaxis. An in-depth discussion regarding the selection and application of allergy testing techniques is beyond the scope of this chapter.

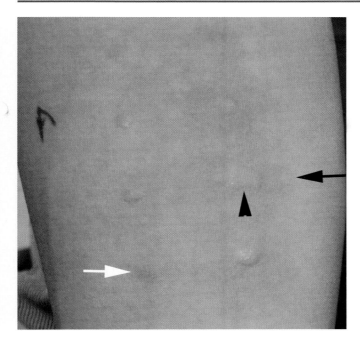

Figure 9.1 Skin prick testing. Figure shows typical skin responses to prick testing. The white arrow shows a negative prick test. The black arrowhead shows the whealing response associated with a positive skin test. The black arrow shows the erythema (flare) associated with skin testing.

Allergy Treatment

There are three broad categories of allergy treatment: environmental control, pharmacotherapy, and immunotherapy.

Environmental Control

The first arm of allergy treatment involves environmental control. Avoidance of allergic triggers is, in theory, the most effective treatment for allergy, yet the least practical. As many inhalant triggers are quite ubiquitous, environmental control focuses on reduction of the exposure recognizing that complete avoidance may not be possible. Patient education is important in implementing appropriate avoidance measures. Verbal counseling with the provision of printed materials with specific control regimens for antigens such as animal dander, dust mites, molds, and pollens is helpful. Despite a patient's best efforts, complete antigen avoidance is difficult to execute and additional allergy therapeutics are often necessary.

Pharmacotherapy

The second arm of allergy treatment involves pharmacotherapy. Several classes of pharmacotherapeutic agents exist and can be classified into two main categories: symptom controllers and immune modulators. Those directed at symptom control typically block "downstream" allergic mediators. These include antihistamines, decongestants, mucolytics,

mast cell stabilizers, and anticholinergics. Separate from the agents directed at symptom control, those pharmacotherapeutics directed at immune modulation are more involved "upstream" and participate in downregulation of the allergic cascade. Many of the medications used for allergic rhinitis that fall in the immune-modulatory category are also used in the treatment of CRS and deserve special consideration, both for the treatment of allergic rhinitis and for their role in the treatment of CRS.

Corticosteroids

A mainstay of treatment in the management of inflammatory disease including CRS, corticosteroids work by downregulating inflammatory cytokines including IL-5, modulating T-helper cell type 2 (TH2) expression, and blocking chemotaxis of inflammatory mediators. Topical corticosteroid sprays are considered a first-line medication in the management of allergic rhinitis and offer the obvious advantage of avoiding the long-term side effects associated with systemic corticosteroid use. Treatment with nasal corticosteroid sprays has been shown to be efficacious in patients with CRSwNP.[7] Interestingly, data to support the use of topical corticosteroid for the treatment of CRS without nasal polyps are scarce. In fact, a recent meta-analysis by Kalish et al failed to show a statistically significant benefit to patients with CRS who were treated with intranasal steroids.[8]

Although oral corticosteroids have enjoyed a long clinical track record in the use of CRS, particularly in the subset of patients with NP, it should be emphasized that oral steroids carry a risk of potential complications. Systemic corticosteroids carry a risk of adrenal suppression, osteoporosis, and gastric ulcers, and their long-term use should be minimized.

Antileukotrienes

Leukotrienes are produced from arachidonic acid via the lipoxygenase pathway and are then stored in mast cells. When mast cell degranulation occurs, leukotrienes are released and act as inflammatory mediators. Leukotriene modifiers including montelukast, zafirlukast, and zileuton have been shown to reduce both peripheral blood eosinophil counts and tissue eosinophilia in asthmatics. The same effect is believed to occur in CRS patients.[9] Leukotriene inhibitors have been shown to be effective in the treatment of CRS in open-label studies, particularly in patients with NP and asthma. In fact, in a small prospective study, a statistically significant benefit for montelukast treatment in patients with NP was observed both via symptom scores and polyp eosinophil counts.[10] Unfortunately, evidence to support the efficacy of leukotriene modifiers in patients with isolated CRS is lacking, but this class of medications may be seen as helpful adjuncts in modulation of the inflammatory cascade, particularly in CRS patients with comorbid asthma or allergic rhinitis.[11]

Immunomodulators

As increasing attention has focused on the inter related inflammatory processes characterizing asthma, allergic rhinitis, and CRS, interest in more focused immune modulation has likewise grown. Mepolizumab, an IL-5 monoclonal antibody, has been shown to significantly reduce asthma exacerbations in patients with sputum eosinophilia.[12,13] Although not studied in the context of CRS, this may bear a promise for certain subsets of CRS patients. Omalizumab, a monoclonal anti-IgE agent, has been noted to be effective in treating allergic asthma and allergic rhinitis.[14] Omalizumab currently has limited indications and is restricted to use in persons older than 12 years of age with moderate to severe asthma, who have a positive skin test or in vitro reactivity to a perennial aeroallergen, and who have failed therapy with inhaled corticosteroids. Further research on immunomodulators is necessary, but the potential for more targeted therapies for allergic rhinitis and CRS seems promising.

Immunotherapy

The third arm of allergy treatment is immunotherapy. Immunotherapy involves the delivery of controlled, escalating amounts of antigen such that the allergic response is downregulated and tolerance is achieved. Immunotherapy is typically reserved for patients in whom avoidance and basic pharmacotherapeutic measures have been inadequate, as well as in patients with more severe and prolonged symptoms who are capable of complying with an extended duration of therapy. Objective evidence of IgE-mediated allergic disease must be documented in the form of either in vitro or skin testing, and the results should plausibly correlate with the patient's symptoms. Immunotherapy is attractive to many patients as it is the only treatment that truly offers the potential to alter the natural course of allergy.

Subcutaneous Immunotherapy

Traditional subcutaneous immunotherapy (SCIT) was first introduced in 1911 when Noon successfully treated hay fever patients with pollen injections.[15] Since then, safe protocols for allergy immunotherapy have been fine-tuned. Most simply, escalating doses of antigen are injected on a regular schedule (often weekly) until a maintenance dose is achieved, and then maintenance injections are continued for a period of 3 to 5 years. Immunotherapy modulates immunoglobulin and lymphocyte responses; specifically, an increase in antigen-specific IgG4 and a decrease in antigen-specific IgE is seen, and a transition from a Th2-cytokine milieu to a Th1-cytokine predominant milieu occurs.[16]

This shift away from a Th2-dominant inflammatory process may have therapeutic benefits for other systemic inflammatory processes, including the possibility of benefit for patients with CRS. Numerous studies have demonstrated the efficacy of immunotherapy for both seasonal and perennial allergens.[17,18] Immunotherapy has also been shown to be beneficial for patients with allergic rhinitis and asthma.[18] It seems theoretically reasonable that the downregulation of both local and systemic inflammation induced by allergen immunotherapy would benefit patients with CRS, although only limited data support a role for immunotherapy in atopic patients with CRS.[19]

Immunotherapy is not without side effects and risks. Patients may have local reactions such as itching or swelling at the site of injection. Systemic side effects include urticaria, angioedema, and anaphylactic shock. The incidence of serious systemic reaction with conventional SCIT is reported to occur among fewer than 2% of injections.[16] Although traditional subcutaneous immunotherapy enjoys a long track record with demonstrated safety and efficacy, there are barriers to successful treatment. Patient compliance and convenience are issues because of the weekly nature of the injections and required duration of therapy. Additionally, some patients are fearful of needles. Finally, there are some patients in whom immunotherapy is relatively contraindicated such as patients with brittle asthma or who are taking β-blocking medications. For these reasons, efforts have been made to develop alternative routes of administering immunotherapy.

Sublingual Immunotherapy

Over the past two decades there has been a mounting interest in sublingual immunotherapy (SLIT). SLIT is similar in principle to SCIT but involves an alternate delivery route; antigen is held under the tongue for an interval and then either swallowed or spit. In 1998, the World Health Organization endorsed SLIT as an acceptable means of immunotherapy.[20] The Allergic Rhinitis and its Impact on Asthma guidelines have also supported SLIT as a viable modality of immunotherapy in adults and children.[18] SLIT is better tolerated than SCIT and appears to have a similar efficacy.[21] A clear advantage of SLIT is that the safety profile allows patients the option to administer the treatment at home, which often results in improved patient convenience and compliance. More robust research about dosing protocols remains necessary, as escalation and maintenance schedules are reported variably in the literature. At the current time, there is no Food and Drug Administration–approved SLIT allergen product available in the United States, yet large numbers of U.S. physicians do offer this as an off-label treatment to their patients. Off-label use of various medications is practiced widely across all specialties of medicine, and it is prudent for individual physicians to review the SLIT literature and make a judgment about the appropriateness of SLIT for their individual patients.

Aspirin Desensitization

A small subset of CRSwNP is classified as having aspirin-exacerbated respiratory disease (AERD), frequently termed Samter triad or aspirin triad. The triad criteria include NP, asthma, and aspirin sensitivity. As highlighted earlier, sinus tissue histology from this subset of CRS patients is significant for high-grade eosinophilia. Part of the common pathophysiology for the disease triad is an excess level of cysteinyl leukotrienes. Interestingly, aspirin desensitization has been shown to downregulate cysL1-receptor expression; therefore, for the aspirin triad subset of CRS patients, aspirin desensitization may be a treatment option. More specifically, aspirin desensitization is best considered for patients who have AERD and rhinosinusitis refractory to traditional therapy including inhaled or oral corticosteroids and leukotriene modifiers. After initial desensitization, the maintenance of aspirin desensitization requires aspirin doses given twice daily. The daily dosing is very important, as subsequent desensitization is recommended if aspirin is missed for more than 48 hours.[22] Although application of this treatment is limited to the subset of CRS patients with AERD, its efficacy has been supported by objective measures, which show a reduction in the incidence of revision sinus surgery as well as the number of sinus infections per year in patients who receive this treatment.[23,24]

Conclusion

The "unified airway" concept of respiratory disease argues for the interrelated nature of airway diseases including asthma, allergic rhinitis, and chronic sinusitis. This model asserts that treatment of one inflammatory process in the airway may have the added benefit of influencing other inflammatory airway processes. Although there is no well-established causal relationship between allergic rhinitis and CRS, consideration of allergic disease as a comorbid condition in patients with CRS is important and it is plausible that reduction of an individual's overall inflammatory load with appropriately selected allergy therapy may be helpful in the management of CRS.

References

1. Gelincik A, Büyüköztürk S, Aslan I, et al. Allergic vs nonallergic rhinitis: which is more predisposing to chronic rhinosinusitis? Ann Allergy Asthma Immunol 2008;101(1):18–22
2. Gutman M, Torres A, Keen KJ, Houser SM. Prevalence of allergy in patients with chronic rhinosinusitis. Otolaryngol Head Neck Surg 2004;130(5):545–552
3. Krouse JH, Brown RW, Fineman SM, et al. Asthma and the unified airway. Otolaryngol Head Neck Surg 2007;136(5 Suppl):S75–S106
4. Ahmad N, Zacharek MA. Allergic rhinitis and rhinosinusitis. Otolaryngol Clin North Am 2008;41(2):267–281, v
5. Eliashar R, Levi-Schaffer F. The role of the eosinophil in nasal diseases. Curr Opin Otolaryngol Head Neck Surg 2005;13(3):171–175
6. Franzese C. Diagnosis of inhalant allergies: patient history and testing. Otolaryngol Clin North Am 2011;44(3):611–623, viii
7. Joe SA, Thambi R, Huang J. A systematic review of the use of intranasal steroids in the treatment of chronic rhinosinusitis. Otolaryngol Head Neck Surg 2008;139(3):340–347
8. Kalish LH, Arendts G, Sacks R, Craig JC. Topical steroids in chronic rhinosinusitis without polyps: a systematic review and meta-analysis. Otolaryngol Head Neck Surg 2009;141(6):674–683
9. Pizzichini E, Leff JA, Reiss TF, et al. Montelukast reduces airway eosinophilic inflammation in asthma: a randomized, controlled trial. Eur Respir J 1999;14(1):12–18
10. Kieff DA, Busaba NY. Efficacy of montelukast in the treatment of nasal polyposis. Ann Otol Rhinol Laryngol 2005;114(12):941–945
11. Brozek JL, Bousquet J, Baena-Cagnani CE, et al; Global Allergy and Asthma European Network; Grading of Recommendations Assessment, Development and Evaluation Working Group. Allergic Rhinitis and its Impact on Asthma (ARIA) guidelines: 2010 revision. J Allergy Clin Immunol 2010;126(3):466–476
12. Haldar P, Brightling CE, Hargadon B, et al. Mepolizumab and exacerbations of refractory eosinophilic asthma. N Engl J Med 2009;360(10):973–984
13. Nair P, Pizzichini MM, Kjarsgaard M, et al. Mepolizumab for prednisone-dependent asthma with sputum eosinophilia. N Engl J Med 2009;360(10):985–993
14. Vignola AM, Humbert M, Bousquet J, et al. Efficacy and tolerability of anti-immunoglobulin E therapy with omalizumab in patients with concomitant allergic asthma and persistent allergic rhinitis: SOLAR. Allergy 2004;59(7):709–717
15. Noon LCB. Prophylactic inoculation against hay fever. Lancet 1911;10:1572–1573
16. Koshkareva YA, Krouse JH. Immunotherapy—traditional. Otolaryngol Clin North Am 2011;44(3):741–752, x
17. Calderon MA, Alves B, Jacobson M, Hurwitz B, Sheikh A, Durham S. Allergen injection immunotherapy for seasonal allergic rhinitis. Cochrane Database Syst Rev 2007;(1):CD001936
18. Bousquet J, Khaltaev N, Cruz AA, et al; World Health Organization; GA(2)LEN; AllerGen. Allergic Rhinitis and its Impact on Asthma (ARIA) 2008 update (in collaboration with the World Health Organization, GA(2)LEN and AllerGen). Allergy 2008;63(Suppl 86):8–160
19. Rosenfeld RM, Andes D, Bhattacharyya N, et al. Clinical practice guideline: adult sinusitis. Otolaryngol Head Neck Surg 2007;137(3 Suppl):S1–S31
20. Bousquet J, Lockey R, Malling HJ, et al. Allergen immunotherapy: therapeutic vaccines for allergic diseases. World Health Organization. American Academy of Allergy, Asthma and Immunology. Ann Allergy Asthma Immunol 1998;81(5, pt 1):401–405
21. Canonica GW, Bousquet J, Casale T, et al. Sub-lingual immunotherapy: World Allergy Organization Position Paper 2009. Allergy 2009;64(Suppl 91):1–59
22. Macy E, Bernstein JA, Castells MC, et al; Aspirin Desensitization Joint Task Force. Aspirin challenge and desensitization for aspirin-exacerbated respiratory disease: a practice paper. Ann Allergy Asthma Immunol 2007;98(2):172–174
23. McMains KC, Kountakis SE. Medical and surgical considerations in patients with Samter's triad. Am J Rhinol 2006;20(6):573–576
24. Berges-Gimeno MP, Simon RA, Stevenson DD. Long-term treatment with aspirin desensitization in asthmatic patients with aspirin-exacerbated respiratory disease. J Allergy Clin Immunol 2003;111(1):180–186

10 Functional Rhinoplasty: Principles and Techniques

Philip G. Chen and Stephen S. Park

Nose plays the central role in respiration, olfaction, humidification of inspired air, and filtration. However, the importance of these factors on quality of life is frequently overlooked until these functions are compromised.[1] Nasal obstruction is a problem frequently encountered by otolaryngologists. The etiologies are legion, yet the nasal valve is an important site of obstruction. Understanding the anatomy and physiology of the nasal valve is critical in evaluation, treatment, and planning for functional rhinoplasty.

Anatomy

The nasal valve was first described over 100 years ago by Mink, referring to the narrow section of the nasal cavity at the border of the upper lateral cartilage (ULC) and lower lateral cartilage (LLC).[2] Since then, the definition has evolved to divide the valve into internal and external components. The internal valve consists of the lateral nasal soft tissue and is bordered by the ULC, nasal septum, and head of the inferior turbinate. The internal valve angle is 10 to 15 degrees in the leptorrhine (European) nose and wider in the platyrrhine (Asian and African) nose,[3] with an average cross-sectional area of 55 to 83 mm^2.[3-5] The external valve represents the alar vestibule and is defined by the nasal sill, alar rim, medial crus, and nasal spine. The external valve has little in the way of structure and is comprised mostly of fibroareolar tissue. A third and critically important, yet ironically less frequently discussed, site of the nasal sidewall is the *intervalve* area. This area has no rigid support except for occasional sesamoid cartilage, and is located at the inferolateral aspect of the lateral crura of the LLC. The corresponding superficial landmark is the supra-alar crease, and a deep supra-alar crease implies that the intervalve is the epicenter of collapse. Pathology there can be due to recurvature of the lateral crus, a paradoxically concave lateral crus, or simply a weak and collapsing soft tissue.

Understanding the nasal valve is crucial because it is the narrowest and flow limiting segment of airway, which accounts for approximately half of the total nasal resistance. Obstruction at the valve can be static or dynamic, and can also be affected by the nasal muscles. Cole and Roithmann described the nasal dilators (nasalis anterior and nasalis posterior) and compressors (procerus, levator labii, superioris alaeque nasi, nasalis, and depressor septi).[5]

Additionally, external changes in nasal shape can impact function. For example, ptosis of the nasal tip is frequently seen in the aging population and can alter the intranasal space and create valve narrowing. Further, tip ptosis is not infrequently seen after primary rhinoplasty when tip support mechanisms are compromised. For this reason, the rhinoplasty surgeon must be mindful when destabilizing these structures. There are major and minor support mechanisms for the nasal tip, although the degree of contribution of each definite structure varies among individuals. The major tip support mechanisms include the inherent strength of the LLC, the attachment of the medial crura of the LLC to the caudal septum (pods), and the attachment of the ULC to the LLC (scroll). The cartilaginous septum can also be considered a major support mechanism because it functions to support much of the lower two-thirds of the nose. Minor tip support mechanisms include attachments of the alar cartilage to the skin, interdomal ligament, and nasal spine.

Physics of Resistance and Airflow

Small decreases in diameter of the nasal passage result in large increases in resistance and therefore nasal obstruction. Resistance to flow is inversely proportional to the radius raised to the fourth power (Poiseuille law). Further, airflow velocity increases when the diameter/cross-sectional area decreases. The higher velocity results in amplified turbulence and resistance, which leads to increasing obstruction in a self-propagating cycle. As per the Bernoulli principle pressure decreases with the increase in rate of flow. Applying this principle to nasal airflow explains the lower pressure at the nasal walls exacerbating collapse. To counteract Bernoulli principle the lateral nasal wall needs to be rigid enough to withstand inward forces, though some degree of collapse is expected at high rates of flow.

Etiology

The differential diagnosis for nasal obstruction is extensive, and the diagnoses and treatments are beyond the scope of this chapter. Clearly, one must rule out masses (polyp, encephalocele, tumor, etc.). Additional possibilities include rhinitis, granulomatous disease, empty nose/paradoxical obstruction, scar bands, and foreign body. When faced with nasal anatomic abnormalities, many otolaryngologists first consider the septum as the site of pathology. While septoplasty is a widely performed procedure, its role in nasal obstruction has been challenged. Constantian and

Clardy[6] evaluated patients before and after surgery with rhinomanometry. They found that septal surgery alone did not show any improvement in mean nasal airflow, while both internal and external valve reconstruction improved flow significantly. Obviously, the exact etiology and degree of improvement varies with each patient.

Some nasal valve obstruction results from etiologies such as trauma, Mohs surgery, facial paralysis, and commonly, iatrogenic collapse after rhinoplasty.[7–10] A reduction rhinoplasty, whether to the dorsum or tip, is a common culprit of creating iatrogenic valve collapse and nasal obstruction. Postrhinoplasty obstruction can be manifest as tip ptosis, destabilization of the vestibule, narrowing of the bony piriform or open roof, or destabilized ULC after dorsal reduction. Middle vault collapse and tip ptosis can also occur from disease processes that compromise the bony framework and produce a subsequent saddle nose deformity. Wegener granulomatosis, septal hematomas with necrosis, and iatrogenic causes can all result in saddle nose deformities.

Anatomic Considerations in Rhinoplasty

Anatomic variation in nasal anatomy is a comprehensive topic that can fill an entire textbook. However, it bears mentioning briefly variants in anatomy that predispose patients to functional obstruction in addition to pitfalls that can occur after rhinoplasty.

Dorsal hump reduction in patients with short nasal bones is challenging, especially when osteotomies are also performed. These patients typically also have long ULCs that lack the same support as nasal bones. Dorsal hump reduction weakens the support between the ULC and dorsal septum. The destabilized ULCs fall into the middle vault with associated contracture of the nasal mucosa and soft tissue envelope, which together obstructs the nasal passage and yields a poor cosmetic appearance. Further, the internal valve is narrowed because the cut edge of the dorsal septum lacks the natural cartilaginous widening present in the native dorsum. In addition to a constricted nasal passage, patients may suffer with cosmetic defects such as the "inverted-V deformity" or the related "hour glass deformity." Osteotomies with medicalization of the bone, by their very nature, narrow the internal nasal valve.

When malformations of the LLC are present, tip-narrowing procedures, such as dome-binding sutures, can create nasal obstruction. Intrinsic weakness of the lateral crura of the LLCs or vertically oriented LLCs each results in weak nasal sidewalls. The poor structure is unable to withstand the negative inspiratory pressure and leads to dynamic collapse of the nasal sidewall and/or external valve (**Fig. 10.1**). Additionally, certain tip procedures cause LLC buckling at the intermediate crura leading to unsightly bossae. Any maneuver, such as additional resection (former complete strip operation), which further compromises

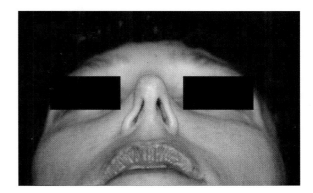

Figure 10.1 Base view demonstrating severe external valve collapse with inspiration. The obstruction is greater on the right, but still severe on the left.

the cartilage must be avoided. The LLCs can also have a paradoxical curvature with the concavity facing intra-nasally and creating a static obstruction. Tip maneuvers frequently medialize the lateral crura and must be considered at the time of surgery.

Although not an anatomic issue per se, the surgeon must be cautious when making intercartilaginous incisions during rhinoplasty. The intercartilaginous cuts can destabilize the scroll area. When they are made too close to the nostril margin, scarring of the external valve occurs, and the destabilized junction of the ULCs and LLCs cannot withstand the forces of contracture. Further blunting at the internal valve angle aggravates obstruction.

Tension nose is a naturally occurring deformity resulting from overgrowth of the quadrangular septal cartilage. This leads to an appearance of a "big nose," with a high nasal dorsum and an anterior septal angle that sits cephalad to the tip-defining point.[11] This combination stretches nasal skin and soft tissue, resulting in alar flattening and a very narrow static internal valve.

A deviated septum is one of the most common causes of nasal obstruction. The caudal septum is more easily addressed with standard septoplasty approaches. However, a more challenging situation is present when the septum is deviated at the dorsal aspect that creates a static narrowing at the internal valve.

Evaluation

As is the rule in functional rhinoplasty, identifying not only the location of obstruction but also the anatomic etiology is the key. A thorough history will uncover previous surgery and trauma. History additionally helps delineate reversibility, seasonal differences, laterality, pain, and epistaxis. It is also important to inquire about impact on daily life.

A physical examination and careful palpation are paramount to identifying the epicenter of pathology. It must be performed both at rest and with inspiration, to distinguish between static and dynamic collapse, respectively. On anterior view of the nose, the examiner pays particular

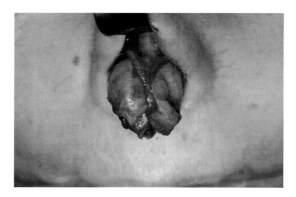

Figure 10.2 Intraoperative view of paradoxical curvature of the lateral crura of the left lower lateral cartilage. Note that the malformation leads to a resting position which impedes airflow.

attention to a narrow middle third, deep supra-alar crease, and deviation of the nasal bones at rest. Inspiration exposes sidewall collapse or a pinched valve. The profile view is helpful to evaluate for saddle nose and tip ptosis. Finally, the base view is helpful in determining the patency of the nasal lobule at rest and with inspiration and paradoxical lateral crura of the LLC (**Fig. 10.2**). Additional information is gained by a modified Cottle maneuver, which can help pinpoint the location of collapse. This is performed by placing the stick of a cotton swab or a cerumen loop at the site of collapse (**Fig. 10.3A** and **B**). The patient inspires and reports subjective improvement in airflow. The examiner also listens for changes in turbulence with inspiration.

Anterior rhinoscopy provides a clear assessment of the septum and nasal mucosa but one must remain cognizant of the blades of the speculum because they stent the nasal sidewall. For example, the nasal speculum is notorious for masking obstruction caused by weakness or recurvature of the LLC. If one is concerned for a mass, then endoscopy is helpful, although not needed in all patients. Facial nerve weakness must be documented because its presence will compromise the function of the nasal dilators and results in nasal obstruction.

Additional studies are rarely needed. Acoustic rhinometry and rhinomanometry have been used to determine airflow,[10,12,13] but findings are poorly correlated with patients' subjective reporting; it has primarily been used as a research tool. Similarly, use of computed tomography has been suggested to study nasal structure and anomalies (bone and cartilage at valve, alar and lateral cartilages, nasal tip, valve angle), especially after previous rhinoplasty. This of course is a static evaluation and may not be clinically relevant in most patients.

Management

Nonsurgical management of valve obstruction is limited. External nasal dilators are effective in some patients with minor collapse.[14] These adhesive strips are placed over the nasal dorsum, and like a flaring suture, widen the lateral

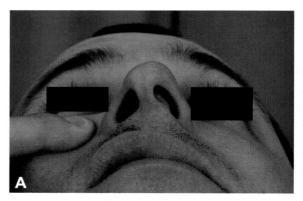

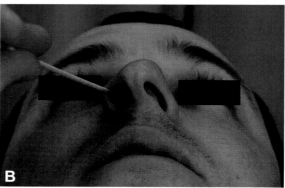

Figure 10.3 Base view of the nose in a patient with intervalve collapse. (A) Lateral distraction of the cheek skin leads to improved airflow, but epicenter of collapse is not identified. (B) Cottle maneuver performed with cotton tipped applicator resulting in significant improvement in nasal airflow at the site of collapse.

nasal wall and valve angle with additional support to prevent collapse. While they can be effective, the adhesive irritates thin nasal skin and allergic reactivity is possible. Vestibular cones (nose cones) have additional theoretical utility in selective patients, although there is a paucity of literature on efficacy. These cone-shaped stents are slipped into the vestibule, which both opens the external valve and provides support to avoid collapse. There are various manufacturers of similar products, but these tend to be a night-time remedy because most individuals prefer not to wear these visible devices in public.

Before proceeding with functional rhinoplasty, other anatomic abnormalities should be addressed. Septal deviation is often a co-contributor and correction is performed concomitantly with a nasal valve repair.

The only definitive option in most cases of nasal valve obstruction is functional rhinoplasty. Patient and surgical selection, however, are not "one-size-fits-all." First, while many surgical options exist, determining the proper rhinoplasty technique is critical based on the site of obstruction. Further, patients have different lifestyles and expectations. For instance, an avid fitness enthusiast with minor obstruction at rest but dynamic collapse on deep inspiration may benefit significantly from surgery. In contrast, a more sedentary patient with the same obstruction may not be as satisfied postoperatively by the seemingly small improvement in breathing.

Alar Batten Grafts

The batten graft is used when there is a collapse at the nasal sidewall, which may be the external or *intervalve* area.[15] This is primarily a static procedure to reinforce the nasal sidewall and prevent collapse during respiration. It is not intended to apply a major change to the resting anatomy nor does it address middle vault narrowing. Both endonasal and open approaches are possible, but the external approach is employed more often because multiple grafts and sutures are frequently used simultaneously. Artificial materials for grafting remain somewhat controversial. Septal or conchal cartilage is readily available without causing much additional morbidity. The conchal cartilage is especially well-suited because of the intrinsic curvature that best supports the sidewall with ample strength to prevent valve collapse.

To place these grafts, the soft tissue envelope of the nose is opened in the standard fashion for external rhinoplasty. A precise pocket must be made, which corresponds exactly to the area of maximal collapse. Most often the epicenter of collapse is at the *intervalve* area, immediately under the supra-alar crease (**Fig. 10.4**). Scissors begin at the lateral most aspect of the lateral crus and dissect in the nasal soft tissue *laterally* and *inferiorly*. The pocket must extend laterally enough to rest on the bony piriform aperture. Care must be taken to stay within the soft tissue envelope, but close to the mucosa. One must resist the tendancy to dissect in a superior direction, which might place the graft over the nasal bones. Pocket size should approximate the graft in order to minimize migration. It is suture secured in place with a rapid absorbing suture, placed through-and-through into the nasal mucosa. This suture pulls the mucosa up to the convex graft and supports this region of the lateral nasal wall. Occasionally, the graft can also be secured to the lateral crus directly in small stitches.

Spreader Grafts and Flaring Suture

Spreader grafts are used to widen the internal valve by lateralizing the ULC and increasing the cross-sectional area.[9,16] The valve angle is minimally affected. These grafts are useful in patients with short nasal bones and long ULCs who are at risk for middle vault collapse. The external approach allows for precise graft positioning and easy suture placement from the dorsal access. Both endonasal and endoscopic approaches can be used effectively.[17] Autologous cartilage grafting is the gold standard, usually septal cartilage and on occasion ear or rib. Alloplasts have been described but are at increased risk for complication. We use septal cartilage when available, but materials such as high-density porous polyethylene are other options.

Cut the cartilage strips into 2 to 3 mm thick pieces, the same length as the ULC. Separate the medial aspects of the ULCs from the dorsal septum, taking care not to violate nasal mucosa as this can introduce contamination and synechiae at the internal valve. Place the strips of the cartilage vertically and parallel to the nasal dorsum between the septum and ULC (**Fig. 10.5A**). A suture is passed through the ULC, dorsal aspect of the graft, and septum to secure the grafts.

Note that this widens the nose on anterior view, and patients should be made aware of this beforehand.[7]

Flaring Sutures

Flaring sutures are used as an adjunct to improve the internal valve—most commonly with spreader grafts.[9,18] Unlike grafts that widen the middle third of the nose, flaring sutures increase the valve angle. Thus, the grafts and sutures act synergistically to dilate the cross-sectional area and decrease resistance at the internal valve.

When placing the flaring suture, it is important to place the suture at the caudal and lateral aspect of the ULC. A permanent monofilament suture is placed in a horizontal mattress fashion. It is tightened over the dorsum, using the nasal dorsum as fulcrum to encourage the ULC to flare outward (**Figs. 10.5A** and **B**). If the suture is placed too lateral, the ULC will buckle inward rather than flare. There is an optimal position for maximal effect. In our practice, this technique has produced lasting results with high patient satisfaction.[18] Other groups have similarly reported the effectiveness of spreader grafts in decreasing the internal valve collapse.[6]

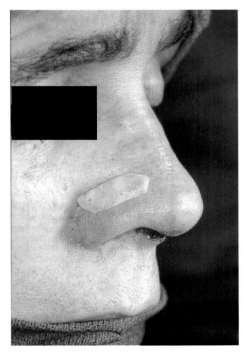

Figure 10.4 Shows the nonanatomic positioning of conchal cartilage used as alar batten grafts. Note that the tip of the graft must be placed laterally and inferiorly onto the piriform aperture.

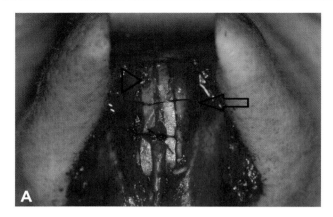

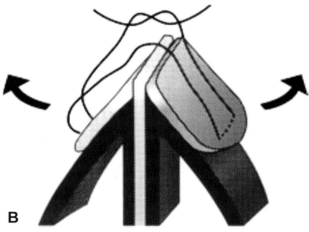

Figure 10.5 (A) Intraoperative photo via external rhinoplasty approach for correction of internal valve collapse with spreader grafts (arrowhead) and a flaring suture (arrow). (B) Schematic diagram representing flaring suture placement. The nasal dorsum is used as a fulcrum to flare open the upper lateral cartilages. The site of the suture placement is important to prevent buckling of the cartilage. *Printed with permission from*: Schlosser RJ, Park SS. Functional nasal surgery. *Otolaryngol Clin North Am* 1999;32:44.

Butterfly Graft

The efficacy of the adhesive external nasal dilator has been studied by measuring the cross-sectional area at the nasal valve with acoustic rhinometry.[14] A significant difference was reported when the device was compared with placebo. Similarly, the butterfly graft is ideal for middle vault reconstruction when the dorsal septum and ULCs are lacking in strength and integrity. It functions as a "permanent" external nasal dilator. The graft can also be used in mild cases of saddle nose deformity with internal valve collapse.

The butterfly graft is placed as an onlay over the supratip and dorsum, which is sutured to the ULCs laterally and lifts them.[19,20] Conchal cartilage is placed at the junction of the ULCs and LLCs and sewn to the underlying cartilage. The natural curvature of the cartilage helps flare the ULC and LLC to open the nasal valve. Patients should be aware that the graft will lead to supratip fullness and even may be palpable in patients with thin nasal tip skin.

Surgery for Lower Lateral Cartilage

Patients with lateral wall collapse, because of a concave lateral crura, recurvature, or intrinsic weakness, may benefit from lateral crura strut grafts. This graft is placed between the vestibular mucosa and lateral crural cartilage, which provides structure and rigidity. Additionally, a batten graft can be sutured to the LLC to lateralize the crura. When paradoxical concavity is present, the vestibular mucosa can be carefully dissected off the cartilage, allowing one to flip the cartilage such that the concavity faces inward. The cartilage is carefully sutured together to re-establish a firm foundation. Batten grafts may be needed in addition to this "flip-flop" technique. Tip grafts can lend additional support to the joint area. On occasion, the intrinsic deformity is of such magnitude that it is best to simply resect the entire crus and replace it with a large batten graft. A lateral crural flaring suture can also be used to flare this region. It is placed in a similar fashion as the ULC flaring suture.

Tip ptosis can also create obstruction at the valve level by distorting intranasal anatomy. Traditional tip rotation maneuvers can be very effective in these circumstances, such as a columellar strut. On occasion, the ptosis is caused by excessive weight of the skin and soft tissue rather than weakening of tip support. Skin at the supratip can be directly excised, followed by a "tip-lifting" stitch. A 4–0 clear nylon suture is well-suited for this maneuver by placing a simple stitch through the domes of the LLCs and suspending it superiorly to the dorsal septum/anterior septal angle. Only a very small advancement is warranted because this powerful maneuver will quickly distort the nose.

Dorsal Reconstruction

A more complicated situation presents when tip ptosis is secondary to dorsal collapse impacting the middle third of the nasal vault and internal valve.[21] In these cases, it is critical to reestablish the structural support normally provided by the L-strut of the septum. Here, the primary goal is reconstruction of a patent nasal passage. Dorsal augmentation, on the other hand, is a secondary cosmetic benefit. With reconstruction, it is not only important that the dorsal skin be brought out, but also that the internal lining is enlarged. Expected contracture of the skin and mucosa requires a stable graft to be used. Autografts, radiated homografts, and alloplastic materials have all been utilized for dorsal reconstruction. Rib grafts (osseocartilaginous vs. cartilaginous) are particularly well-suited for this purpose because of strength, availability, low infection rate, and low extrusion rate. Additional use of a columellar strut graft is beneficial in providing tip projection and support when the soft tissue envelope has scarred and constricted.

Differences exist for harvesting rib but the 7th rib is large and straight and the floating 11th rib is useful because of its solid bone stock.[22,23] Specifically, the external route is used and the ULCs are separated from the dorsal septum to allow subsequent resuspension to the dorsal graft. A subperiosteal pocket is created over the nasal bones. The cartilage is shaped to support the saddled nasal dorsum, which typically requires tapering at the cephalic and caudal ends. The undersurface of the graft is burred with a drill to ensure that the graft sits snuggly on the nasal dorsum. The ULCs are then secured to the lateral edges of the graft, thus supporting the internal nasal valves and camouflaging the lateral borders of the graft.

To create the columellar strut, a pocket is made between the medial crura of the LLCs onto the nasal spine. A thin rectangular piece of cartilage is sutured between the medial crura to improve tip projection.

Conclusion

There are many structural causes for nasal obstruction, and the septum is just one of many areas that must be evaluated on physical examination. In fact, one study found that the septum was deviated toward the clinically obstructed side in 51% of patients, and patients' subjective complaints were only congruous with objective findings approximately half of the time.[6] Identification of the epicenter of collapse on examination is therefore truly paramount. In general, we have had good success by combining spreader grafts with flaring sutures in patients with narrow internal valves. Alar batten grafts are effective when placed in a nonanatomic position within the intervalve area. There are often multiple foci of obstruction and it is critical to stratify them and address each separately (**Fig. 10.6**). The improvement and impact in quality of life makes this field most rewarding.

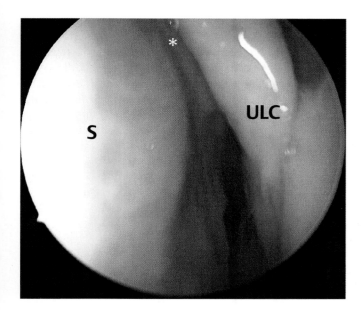

Figure 10.6 Endoscopic view of left nasal cavity showing the presence of a leftward deviated septum (S) with concomitant internal valve collapse in a patient who reported previous septoplasty many years ago. The upper lateral cartilage (ULC) can be clearly identified, which further decreases a narrow valve angle (*).

References

1. Rhee JS, Poetker DM, Smith TL, Bustillo A, Burzynski M, Davis RE. Nasal valve surgery improves disease-specific quality of life. Laryngoscope 2005;115(3):437–440
2. Mink PJ. Le Le nez comme voie respiratory. Belgium: Presse Otolaryngol; 1903;481–496
3. Kasperbauer JL, Kern EB. Nasal valve physiology. Implications in nasal surgery. Otolaryngol Clin North Am 1987;20(4):699–719
4. Haight JS, Cole P. The site and function of the nasal valve. Laryngoscope 1983;93(1):49–55
5. Cole P, Roithmann R. The nasal valve and current technology. Am J Rhinol 1996;10:23–31
6. Constantian MB, Clardy RB. The relative importance of septal and nasal valvular surgery in correcting airway obstruction in primary and secondary rhinoplasty. Plast Reconstr Surg 1996;98(1):38–54, discussion 55–58
7. Khosh MM, Jen A, Honrado C, Pearlman SJ. Nasal valve reconstruction: experience in 53 consecutive patients. Arch Facial Plast Surg 2004;6(3):167–171
8. Elwany S, Thabet H. Obstruction of the nasal valve. J Laryngol Otol 1996;110(3):221–224
9. Schlosser RJ, Park SS. Surgery for the dysfunctional nasal valve. Cadaveric analysis and clinical outcomes. Arch Facial Plast Surg 1999;1(2):105–110
10. Grymer LF. Reduction rhinoplasty and nasal patency: change in the cross-sectional area of the nose evaluated by acoustic rhinometry. Laryngoscope 1995;105(4 Pt 1):429–431
11. Kantas IV, Papadakis CE, Balatsouras DG, et al. Functional tension nose as a cause of nasal airway obstruction. Auris Nasus Larynx 2007;34(3):313–317
12. Roithmann R, Cole P, Chapnik J, Barreto SM, Szalai JP, Zamel N. Acoustic rhinometry, rhinomanometry, and the sensation of nasal patency: a correlative study. J Otolaryngol 1994;23(6):454–458
13. Paniello RC. Nasal valve suspension. An effective treatment for nasal valve collapse. Arch Otolaryngol Head Neck Surg 1996;122(12):1342–1346
14. Griffin JW, Hunter G, Ferguson D, Sillers MJ. Physiologic effects of an external nasal dilator. Laryngoscope 1997;107(9):1235–1238
15. Toriumi DM, Josen J, Weinberger M, Tardy ME Jr. Use of alar batten grafts for correction of nasal valve collapse. Arch Otolaryngol Head Neck Surg 1997;123(8):802–808
16. Sheen JH. Spreader graft: a method of reconstructing the roof of the middle nasal vault following rhinoplasty. Plast Reconstr Surg 1984;73(2):230–239
17. Huang C, Manarey CR, Anand VK. Endoscopic placement of spreader grafts in the nasal valve. Otolaryngol Head Neck Surg 2006;134(6):1001–1005
18. Park SS. The flaring suture to augment the repair of the dysfunctional nasal valve. Plast Reconstr Surg 1998;101(4):1120–1122
19. Clark JM, Cook TA. The 'butterfly' graft in functional secondary rhinoplasty. Laryngoscope 2002;112(11):1917–1925
20. Friedman O, Cook TA. Conchal cartilage butterfly graft in primary functional rhinoplasty. Laryngoscope 2009;119(2):255–262
21. Sykes JM, Tapias V, Kim JE. Management of the nasal dorsum. Facial Plast Surg 2011;27(2):192–202
22. Gentile P, Cervelli V. Nasal dorsum reconstruction with 11th rib cartilage and auricular cartilage grafts. Ann Plast Surg 2009;62(1):63–66
23. Christophel JJ, Hilger PA. Osseocartilaginous rib graft rhinoplasty: a stable, predictable technique for major dorsal reconstruction. Arch Facial Plast Surg 2011;13(2):78–83

11 Rhinogenic Headache

Eleanor Pitz Kiell and James Whit Mims

"Sinus headache" is a term familiar to the general public, the general practitioner, otolaryngologists, and neurologists alike. In the past few decades, however, the clinicians who treat these patients as a referral population have differentiated between headaches with sinonasal symptoms and sinus disorders that include pain as a symptom. Additionally, there may be other relationships such as nasal inflammation that "triggers" an acute exacerbation of a chronic headache condition. Disentangling the sinonasal component from headaches remains clinically challenging.

In 2004, the International Headache Society (IHS) published its guidelines for diagnostic criteria for recognized headache syndromes. Within the guidelines, there is a "headache secondary to rhinosinusitis," which requires a diagnosis of acute sinusitis to meet the criteria.[1] The IHS does not currently accept that chronic sinusitis can be the cause of a headache syndrome. More commonly, the symptoms of a patient with "sinus headaches" will meet the diagnostic criteria associated with one of several other primary headache disorders. Discordantly, most current guidelines for chronic sinusitis recognize facial pain and pressure as a symptom.[2-5] Additionally, some have advocated that anatomic abnormalities might lead to headache even in the absence of infection or inflammation.[6] Surgical intervention in the absence of inflammation remains controversial.

Current research and expert opinion allow us to differentiate most "sinus headaches" into one of the five major categories: (1) acute sinusitis, (2) chronic sinusitis, (3) primary headache disorders including migraines and cluster headaches, (4) trigeminal neuralgia, or (5) anatomic contact point headaches (which are controversial).

Historical Perspective

In the 1940s, Wolff demonstrated that mechanical and chemical stimulation within the nasal cavity led to resultant cephalgia in several healthy volunteers.[7] Despite this knowledge, little research had been undertaken to further describe the relationship between headache and sinonasal abnormalities. With the advent of nasal endoscopes and computed tomography (CT), the ability to evaluate anatomy and pathology within the sinonasal tract has dramatically advanced. Before these modalities, clinicians reasonably presumed sinonasal pathology as the impetus for headaches. However, studies using endoscopy and sinus CT scans revealed a more complicated relationship between headaches and sinonasal pathology.

The IHS released their consensus classification of headaches in 2004. This classification system describes headache syndromes and diagnostic criteria. Headaches with sinus symptoms are restricted to acute rhinosinusitis, migraines with cranial autonomic symptoms, and cluster headaches. Headaches caused by anatomic aberrancies and chronic rhinosinusitis are not an accepted cause of primary headaches by the IHS.

"Sinus Headache": A Misnomer

"Sinus headache" is a common ailment among the general public; however, sinusitis is likely a rare cause of recurrent headaches. Physicians frequently treating sinonasal complaints have recognized that a significant portion of "sinus" headache sufferers have symptoms more consistent with a diagnosis of headache disorder and lack endoscopic and radiographic evidence of sinusitis. As evidenced by the Sinus, Allergy, & Migraine Study by Eross et al, only 3% of patients who believe they suffer from "sinus headache" actually suffer headache secondary to rhinosinusitis. This diagnosis was made based on the IHS criteria following a detailed headache history and complete general and neurological examination by a neurologist. In select cases with high suspicion, investigators utilized brain and sinus imaging.[8]

Several independent studies have found that 58 to 80% of patients who were diagnosed with "sinus headache" meet criteria for migraine.[8-10] Reasons cited for this confusion included pain located over the sinuses, triggered by weather changes, or associated with rhinorrhea. Eross et al in their study had suggested the diagnosis of sinusitis in 78% of these patients.[8] Schreiber et al studied nearly 3000 patients and found a similar over diagnosis of sinus headache which they also attributed to overlapping symptoms. They concluded that there is a lack of recognition that sinonasal symptoms are typical of migraine.[10] With nearly 30 million Americans who suffer from migraines,[11] otolaryngologists should be familiar with the differential diagnosis of headaches in evaluating sinus pain.

Differential Diagnosis of "Sinus Headaches"

Acute Rhinosinusitis

In a patient with new onset headache associated with nasal symptoms, clinicians should consider a sinus infection. The symptoms are particularly suggestive if the patient reports a combination of bilateral, dull, pressure-like, and periorbital facial pain.[12] According to the American Academy of Otolaryngology-Head and Neck Surgery, a diagnosis of acute bacterial rhinosinusitis (ABRS) first requires it to be distinguished from viral rhinosinusitis. Recommendations for making this distinction include that ABRS be diagnosed when (1) symptoms or signs of acute rhinosinusitis are present 10 days or more beyond the onset of upper respiratory tract infection symptoms, or (2) symptoms or signs of acute rhinosinusitis worsen within 10 days after an initial improvement (double worsening). There is no indication for the use of sinus imaging in an uncomplicated ABRS.[5] These represent updated recommendations from a previous system utilizing major and minor criteria for diagnosis based on symptoms. For this constellation of symptoms to be defined as *acute* rhinosinusitis, symptoms must be present for less than 4 weeks. In the patient suffering from headache and who also meets diagnostic criteria for acute rhinosinusitis, the two must be temporally related to attribute the headache symptom to an underlying inflammatory/infectious pathology. The IHS specified this relationship in their consensus statement with a headache caused by rhinosinusitis as the following: (1) frontal headache accompanied by pain in one or more regions of the face, ears, or teeth and fulfilling criteria (3) and (4); (2) clinical, nasal endoscopic, CT scan and/or magnetic resonance imaging (MRI), and/or laboratory evidence of acute or acute-on-chronic rhinosinusitis; (3) headache and facial pain develop simultaneously with onset or acute exacerbation of rhinosinusitis; (4) headache and/or facial pain resolves within 7 days after remission or successful treatment of acute or acute-on-chronic rhinosinusitis.[1] These criteria are summarized in **Table 11.1**.

Treatment of headache in the patient suffering from acute rhinosinusitis, should be directed at underlying cause. Antibiotics are the mainstay of treatment for ABRS. Symptomatic treatment with decongestants, and topical or oral corticosteroids,[2] along with nonsteroidal anti-inflammatory agents are additional recommended options.

Chronic Rhinosinusitis

The IHS maintains that chronic sinusitis is "not validated as a cause of headache or facial pain unless relapsing into an acute stage." The exception to this instance is an acute exacerbation of chronic rhinosinusitis (CRS). This may be characterized by increased nasal mucus or purulence of nasal mucus, worsening congestion and hyposmia, and even systemic symptoms of malaise, fatigue, and occasionally fever. These exacerbations might require systemic corticosteroid therapy in addition to antibiotic therapy (ideally, culture-directed antibiotic therapy).[13]

However, recent otolaryngology, asthma, and allergy consensus guidelines for the diagnosis of chronic rhinosinusitis frequently include facial pain or pressure along with hyposmia, duration greater than 8 to 12 weeks, and objective findings on CT scan or endoscopy.[2–5] The importance of facial pain as a key sign of chronic rhinosinusitis has been called into question. One study examined 75

Table 11.1 Diagnosing Headache Secondary to Acute Rhinosinusitis

Symptoms That Must Be Present for Diagnosis of Acute Rhinosinusitis	
Pressure or Pain in the Face or Teeth	
Discharge from the anterior or posterior nasal cavity that is purulent in nature	
Obstruction of the nasal cavity	
Viral	**Bacterial**
• Signs or symptoms present for less than 10 days • Not worsening or double worsening	• Signs or symptoms present for more than 10 days after the onset of URI symptoms OR • Signs or symptoms improve initially, then worsen within 10 days

Criteria for Diagnosis of Secondary Headache due to Acute Rhinosinusitis
A. Frontal headache in addition to pain in another region of the face, ears or teeth AND fulfilling criteria C and D
B. Clinical, nasal endoscopic, radiographic imaging (CT or MRI), and/or laboratory findings that demonstrate acute or acute-on-chronic rhinosinusitis
C. Headache or facial pain develop coincidentally with onset or acute exacerbation of rhinosinusitis
D. Headache or facial pain resolve within 7 days after successful treatment of acute or acute-on-chronic rhinosinusitis

Printed with permission from: Headache Classification Subcommittee of the International Headache Society. The International Classification of Headache Disorders: 2nd edition. *Cephalalgia*. 2004;24 (Suppl 1):9-160 and Rosenfeld RM, Andes D, Bhattacharyya N, et al. Clinical practice guideline: adult sinusitis. *Otolaryngol Head Neck Surg* 2007;137:S1–31.

d, day(s); URI, upper respiratory tract infection; CT, computed tomography; MRI, magnetic resonance imaging

patients who had persistent facial pain following endoscopic sinus surgery, of these, only half had CT or endoscopic findings consistent with sinus disease at presentation.[14] Another study demonstrated poor correlation between facial pain localization and the affected paranasal sinus by CT scan. Mudgil et al showed no significant difference in the number of points of facial pain regardless of CT findings and that the most frequently cited location of pain was the right temporal area while the most affected sinus was the maxillary sinus.[15]

While facial pain does not seem to be sensitive or specific in CRS, some patients with CRS do report facial pain. For example, authors reviewing chronic sphenoiditis reported headache lasting 4 to 30 months.[16] Chronic rhinosinusitis guidelines continue to include the presence of facial pain or pressure in the diagnostic criteria for chronic rhinosinusitis but emphasize the necessity to correlate with objective findings.

Primary Headache Disorders

The IHS system identifies two primary headache disorders where sinonasal symptoms are included in the diagnostic criteria: migraine and cluster headaches. Criteria for tension headaches do not include sinus symptoms (**Table 11.2**).

Migraine

Migraine is underdiagnosed in the United States. A population-based study in 1999 suggested that only 48% of patients meeting IHS criteria for migraine reported a physician diagnosis.[17] Another study found 66% of those reporting "sinus headache" improved with sumatriptan, a migraine-specific medication.[18] They stated the response rate was similar to other migraine populations. These results suggest that otolaryngologists need to be familiar with the diagnostic criteria for the two most common migraines, typical migraines with and without aura. Symptoms of nausea, vomiting, visual changes, photophobia, and phonophobia should trigger concern that the patient is more likely to be experiencing migraine. Approximately

Table 11.2   Headache Disorders as Described by the International Headache Society

Headache	Typical Symptoms
Migraine	
• Migraine without aura	• More than five attacks lasting 4–72 h • Unilateral • Pulsating quality • Moderate to severe pain severity • Photophobia/phonophobia • Nausea/vomiting
• Migraine with aura	• As above, with migraine aura
Tension-type headache	
• Infrequent episodic tension-type headache	• More than 10 episodes of < 1 d/mo of headache lasting 30 min to 7 d • Bilateral • Pressing/tightening quality • Mild to moderate pain severity • Not aggravated by routine activity
• Frequent episodic tension-type headache	• As above, with > 15 episodes on > 1 but < 15 d/mo in 3 mo
• Chronic tension-type headache	• As above, except > 15 d/mo on average for > 3 mo
Cluster headache and other trigeminal autonomic cephalgias	

• Cluster headache	• At least five attacks with:
	  • Severe or very severe pain
	  • Orbital, supraorbital, or temporal pain
	  • Lasts 15–180 min if untreated
	  • With at least one of the following:
	    – Ipsilateral conjunctival injection and/or lacrimation, nasal congestion and/or rhinorrhea, eyelid edema, forehead and facial sweating, miosis and/or ptosis, or a sense of restlessness

• Paroxysmal hemicranias	• As above with less frequency, and completely preventable by therapeutic doses of indomethacin
• SUNCT	• More than 20 attacks • Unilateral orbital, supraorbital, or temporal pain • Stabbing or pulsating pain • Lasts 5–240 s • Pain accompanied by ipsilateral conjunctival injection and lacrimation • Occur 3–200/d

Printed with permission from: Headache Classification Subcommittee of the International Headache Society. The International Classification of Headache Disorders: 2nd edition. *Cephalalgia*. 2004;24 (Suppl 1):9-160.

h, hour(s); d, day(s); mo, month(s); min, minute(s); SUNCT, short-lasting unilateral neuralgiform headache attacks with conjunctival injection and tearing; s, second(s).

75% of patients who are diagnosed with migraine also experience significant cranial autonomic symptoms. These cranial autonomic symptoms may prove to be distracters when trying to differentiate appropriate diagnosis. The most commonly cited cranial autonomic symptoms include nasal congestion (56%) followed by eyelid edema (37%). Less than a quarter of patients experience rhinorrhea, conjunctival injection, lacrimation, and ptosis.[12] These symptoms are consistent with current findings that associate migraines with cranial vasodilatation followed by release of pain-mediating neuropeptides, such as substance P.[19]

Migraine-specific pharmacotherapy is available and efficacious. In the acute setting, triptans are first-line therapy for moderate or severe migraine. Triptans are a class of selective serotonin 1B/1D receptor agonists that are believed to work by cranial vasoconstriction, peripheral trigeminal inhibition, and prevention of central sensitization.[20,21] Side effects commonly include flushing, bad taste in the mouth, nausea/vomiting, dizziness, nasal irritation, and throat pain. More seriously, hypertensive crisis, stroke, and seizure have been associated with use of triptans. A variety of agents are used for migraine prophylaxis including β blockers, calcium channel blockers, antidepressants, and divalproex sodium. Referral to a headache specialist is often useful to help with medication selection, management of stress, avoidance of triggers, decreasing caffeine, sleep counseling, and eliminating nonsteroidal anti-inflammatory drug rebound.

Cluster Headache

Cluster headache pain is the most severe of the primary headache syndromes. It is characterized by periodic attacks of unilateral pain with associated cranial autonomic symptoms. According to the IHS, patients must experience at least five attacks of severe or very severe unilateral orbital, supraorbital, or temporal pain lasting 15 to 180 minutes if left untreated. It must also be associated with at least one ipsilateral cranial autonomic symptom from the following: conjunctival injection and/or lacrimation, nasal congestion and/or rhinorrhea, eyelid edema, forehead and facial sweating, and miosis and/or ptosis. These symptoms must occur at least once every other day and up to eight times per day.[1] Patients typically pace during an acute attack, whereas migraine sufferers find a secluded place to rest.

Treatment of an acute cluster headache can be challenging as the nature of the pain evolves so quickly. First-line therapy for acute cluster headache is high-flow inhaled oxygen at a standard rate of 7 to 10 L/min. Several studies have shown promising results for the efficacy of high-flow inhaled oxygen at 14 to 15 L/min and hyperbaric oxygen therapy in patients who do not respond to conventional oxygen treatment.[22–24] Pharmacotherapy of choice is subcutaneously injected sumatriptan. It has been well-studied and has a rapid rate of onset with headache severity reduction within 15 minutes of injection. It is safe and effective when used at its regular dose of 6 mg/injection up to twice daily for total daily dose of 12 mg/d. Sumatriptan is contraindicated in patients with coronary artery disease or cerebrovascular disease. Patients who are unable to tolerate triptans may benefit from topically applied lidocaine, ergot derivatives, somatostatin, or octreotide.[25]

Prophylactic therapy for cluster headaches is divided into maintenance prophylaxis and transitional prophylaxis. Maintenance prophylactics are used constantly, while transitional prophylactics are used adjunctively as abortive therapy, during or for short periods, to reduce frequency of attacks. Verapamil is the first-line maintenance prophylactic agent followed by lithium as a second-line agent. Corticosteroids are the mainstay for transitional prophylaxis. More invasive therapies may be beneficial for those resistant or not tolerant of medical management. These include peripheral nerve and sphenopalatine ganglion blocks and stimulation, hypothalamic stimulation and ablative surgical techniques (which are falling out of favor).[25]

More serious causes of headaches or facial pain, such as brain tumors, sinus tumors, invasive fungal sinusitis, or elevated intracranial pressure, need to be considered and appropriately excluded.

Trigeminal Neuralgia

Pain in a facial distribution is often mistaken for "sinus headache." The International Association for the Study of Pain defines trigeminal neuralgia as recurrent episodes of sudden, usually unilateral, severe, brief, stabbing, pain in the distribution of one or more branches of the trigeminal nerve.[26] As the sensory distribution of the trigeminal nerve includes the maxillary and frontal sinuses, it is understandable how trigeminal neuralgia might be confused with sinus pathology. The IHS makes a distinction between classic trigeminal neuralgia (CTN) and symptomatic trigeminal neuralgia (STN). CTN is diagnosed when there is no identifiable etiology for the pain other than possible vascular compression of the trigeminal nerve. There must also be absence of any clinically apparent neurologic deficit. STN results when there is an identifiable anatomic abnormality other than vascular compression such as tumor, multiple sclerosis plaques, or abnormalities in the skull base.[1]

In a patient with pain in the trigeminal distribution, it is important to take a careful history and physical examination, especially a neurologic examination including cranial nerve reflexes. In the absence of identifiable neurologic deficits, an MRI scan will reveal a structural abnormality in approximately 15% of the patients.[27]

Medical treatment is the mainstay for trigeminal neuralgia. First-line therapies are the antiepileptic medications carbamazepine and possibly oxcarbazepine for CTN. One of the hallmarks of CTN is that patients tend to initially respond to carbamazepine. Baclofen, lamotrigine, and pimozide may also be effective for controlling pain in trigeminal neuralgia. There are ongoing trials using lamotrigine, gabapentin, misoprostol, or topiramate in the treatment of multiple sclerosis-plaque associated STN; there are no definitive therapies for trigeminal neuralgia in these patients.[27]

In addition to medical therapies, there are several different procedures that have been proposed in the treatment of trigeminal neuralgia; these are categorized based on the target of the therapy. Peripheral techniques tend to have minimal benefit in terms of pain reduction, with relapse within 1 year but are also relatively low risk. More invasive techniques target the Gasserian ganglion including radiofrequency ablation, ethanol ablation, and gamma knife. Microvascular decompression of the trigeminal nerve may also be utilized. With each of these, up to 90% of patients experience immediate relief and approximately 50% of patients continue to have relief at 3 years.[27] The potential side effects of these procedures include numbness in the distribution of the cranial nerve V, aseptic meningitis, cerebral spinal fluid leak, or corneal numbness leading to keratitis.

Contact Point Headaches

Although IHS does not endorse anatomic abnormalities as a valid etiology of headache, some patients report facial or sinus pain in the absence of acute sinusitis, chronic sinusitis, chronic headache, or neuralgia criteria. It has been theorized that contact points within the nose or sinuses can cause facial pain, but the evidence is mixed and this remains controversial. In patients who do not respond to migraine or neuralgia medication and who do not exhibit evidence of acute inflammation, theories of anatomic causes have arisen from perceived patient need.

Anatomy and Physiology

Contact points are defined as mucosal surfaces that remain adjacent following decongestion by topical medication. These contact points exist in the absence of inflammation and infection. Most commonly, a sharp nasal spur contacts a turbinate. It has also been suggested that a pneumatized middle turbinate, named a concha bullosa, may cause mucosal surface contact between turbinate and septum. The contact between these surfaces was theorized to be irritating because of the high concentration of the neuropeptide, substance P, in the trigeminally derived sensory nerve endings within the nasal mucosa.[28] This hypothesis suggests that the cephalgia derived from rhinologic contact points may be because of the hyperesthesia within the distribution of the trigeminal nerve. A small study disputed this hypothesis by directly testing the presence of facial pain in subjects following the application of pressure, substance P, and adrenaline to their nasal mucosa. They found that none of the subjects experienced facial pain.[29] Casting further doubt on "contact points," Abu-Bakra and Jones also showed an equal occurrence of contact points in individuals with and without headache.[30]

More recent studies suggest that contact points may act as a trigger in those with a headache syndrome, but is not independently the etiology of the pain. Abu-Samra et al studied a total of 42 patients with chronic daily headache, radiographic evidence of nasal contact points and unsatisfactory response to maximal medical therapy. They found that 83% of patients were satisfied following surgery to separate the radiographic contact points. They posit that the contact point irritation serves as a trigger for the activation of a more typical migraine, tension-type, or cluster headaches by potentiating central nervous system hyperresponsiveness.[31] They theorize that stimulation of nasal mucosal receptors cause the release of substance P, both centrally and peripherally. Substance P and calcitonin gene-related peptide are well-recognized mediators in nociceptor pathways within the central nervous system.[29] As with all headache triggers (i.e., nasal contact points, atmospheric pressure changes, and certain foods), there are people who experience these same events without the resultant headache. This is illustrated in **Fig. 11.1**, from a patient who did report improvement in her headaches after septoplasty.

The diagnosis of intranasal "contact points" entails a careful physical examination, nasal endoscopy, and possibly a CT scan. An additional test using local anesthetic in an awake patient who is acutely experiencing headache has been reported. A small amount of local anesthetic (i.e., lidocaine and tetracaine) is applied to the area of contact under direct visualization by the examiner. Should the patient experience more than 50% decrease in pain severity, the test is positive.[32] This test is controversial as there has not been a demonstrable link between test positivity and clinical improvement following sinus surgery.[33]

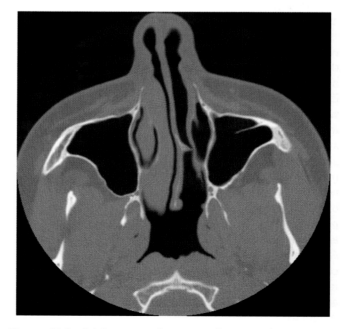

Figure 11.1 Axial computed tomography scan demonstrating mucosal contact points between a septal spur and left middle turbinate.

In 1988, Stammberger et al[6] described an endoscopic approach to sinus disease and headache. This article recommended locating the contact point with CT scans and rigid endoscopy and then also recommended planned modification of the nasal or sinus anatomy. For those with middle turbinate-septum contact, anterior ethmoidectomy was recommended. With superior turbinate-septum contact, the posterior ethmoids are also opened, requiring the removal of the basal lamella. The result of this maneuver may weaken the support maintaining contact between the middle turbinate and septum. Another approach that has been used is to fracture the turbinates along their entire length to displace it away from the septum. This is particularly useful for the inferior turbinate–septum contact point. Many of these patients underwent septoplasty. While Stammberger reported improvement in headache following surgery for contact point headaches, Abu-Bakra and Jones showed no difference.[30] Given the mixed evidence regarding outcomes for these patients after surgery, it remains controversial to suggest surgery for those who suffer from debilitating headaches who have failed maximal medical therapy.

Some patients with recurrent headache or facial pain improve after septoplasty, especially if there is a significant sharp septal spur distorting the turbinate. However, the results are inconsistent and alleviation of facial pain is unreliable as the sole indication for surgery. Endoscopic sinus surgery in the absence of inflammation is not supported in recent guidelines, as outlined by Rosenfeld et al in 2007.[5]

Conclusion

Headache as a presenting symptom for an otolaryngologist can be a confusing and frustrating problem. A thorough history and physical examination is recommended because "sinus headache" is a nonspecific symptom. Most patients with "sinus headache" should be considered for acute rhinosinusitis, a primary headache syndrome (such as migraine or cluster headache), or trigeminal neuralgia. Examination findings and symptom duration consistent with acute bacterial sinusitis (i.e., purulent discharge, inflamed, boggy mucosa, and facial tenderness) warrant antibiotic therapy. Those without ABRS should be asked about inciting events associated with migraines including inciting events, photophobia, phonophobia, nausea, or vomiting. Frequency, distribution, character, and duration of symptoms are helpful in classifying headaches. Educating patients about cranial autonomic symptoms associated with primary headache disorders is frequently necessary. As headache syndromes can have atypical presentations, consulting a headache specialist or mediation trials can be useful. More serious causes including brain or sinus tumors are important to diagnose. Treatment of intranasal contact points as a trigger in those prone to headaches remains controversial. For physicians who see patients complaining of rhinogenic headaches, working knowledge of acute and chronic sinusitis, primary headache disorders, and

trigeminal neuralgia will help guide most patients toward appropriate treatment.

References

1. International Headache Society. The International Classification of Headache Disorders. 2nd ed. Cephalalgia 2004;24 (Suppl 1):9–160
2. Fokkens W, Lund V, Mullol J; European Position Paper on Rhinosinusitis and Nasal Polyps group. European position paper on rhinosinusitis and nasal polyps 2007. Rhinol Suppl 2007;(20):1–136
3. Meltzer EO, Hamilos DL, Hadley JA, et al; American Academy of Allergy, Asthma and Immunology; American Academy of Otolaryngic Allergy; American Academy of Otolaryngology-Head and Neck Surgery; American College of Allergy, Asthma and Immunology; American Rhinologic Society. Rhinosinusitis: Establishing definitions for clinical research and patient care. Otolaryngol Head Neck Surg 2004;131(6, Suppl):S1–S62
4. Slavin RG, Spector SL, Bernstein IL, et al; American Academy of Allergy, Asthma and Immunology; American College of Allergy, Asthma and Immunology; Joint Council of Allergy, Asthma and Immunology. The diagnosis and management of sinusitis: a practice parameter update. J Allergy Clin Immunol 2005;116(6, Suppl):S13–S47
5. Rosenfeld RM, Andes D, Bhattacharyya N, et al. Clinical practice guideline: adult sinusitis. Otolaryngol Head Neck Surg 2007;137(3, Suppl):S1–S31
6. Stammberger H, Wolf G. Headaches and sinus disease: the endoscopic approach. Ann Otol Rhinol Laryngol Suppl 1988;134:3–23
7. Wolff HG. The Nasal, Paranasal, and Aural Structures as Sources of Headache and Other Pain. New York: Oxford University Press; 1948
8. Eross E, Dodick D, Eross M. The Sinus, Allergy and Migraine Study (SAMS). Headache 2007;47(2):213–224
9. Perry BF, Login IS, Kountakis SE. Nonrhinologic headache in a tertiary rhinology practice. Otolaryngol Head Neck Surg 2004;130(4):449–452
10. Schreiber CP, Hutchinson S, Webster CJ, Ames M, Richardson MS, Powers C. Prevalence of migraine in patients with a history of self-reported or physician-diagnosed "sinus" headache. Arch Intern Med 2004;164(16):1769–1772
11. Lipton RB, Stewart WF, Diamond S, Diamond ML, Reed M. Prevalence and burden of migraine in the United States: data from the American Migraine Study II. Headache 2001;41(7):646–657
12. Levine HL, Setzen M, Cady RK, et al. An otolaryngology, neurology, allergy, and primary care consensus on diagnosis and treatment of sinus headache. Otolaryngol Head Neck Surg 2006;134(3):516–523
13. Paul WF, Bruce HH, Lund VJ, et al. Cummings Otolaryngology-Head and Neck Surgery. 5th ed. Philadelphia, PA: Mosby Elsevier; 2010
14. Jones NS, Cooney TR. Facial pain and sinonasal surgery. Rhinology 2003;41(4):193–200
15. Mudgil SP, Wise SW, Hopper KD, Kasales CJ, Mauger D, Fornadley JA. Correlation between presumed sinusitis-induced pain and paranasal sinus computed tomographic findings. Ann Allergy Asthma Immunol 2002;88(2):223–226
16. Gilony D, Talmi YP, Bedrin L, Ben-Shosan Y, Kronenberg J. The clinical behavior of isolated sphenoid sinusitis. Otolaryngol Head Neck Surg 2007;136(4):610–615
17. Lipton RB, Diamond S, Reed M, Diamond ML, Stewart WF. Migraine diagnosis and treatment: results from the American Migraine Study II. Headache 2001;41(7):638–645
18. Cady RK, Schreiber CP. Sinus headache or migraine? Considerations in making a differential diagnosis. Neurology 2002; 58(9, Suppl 6):S10–S14

19. Moskowitz MA. Defining a pathway to discovery from bench to bedside: the trigeminovascular system and sensitization. Headache 2008;48(5):688–690

20. Burstein R, Jakubowski M. Analgesic triptan action in an animal model of intracranial pain: a race against the development of central sensitization. Ann Neurol 2004;55(1):27–36

21. Goadsby PJ. The pharmacology of headache. Prog Neurobiol 2000;62(5):509–525

22. Cohen AS, Burns B, Goadsby PJ. High-flow oxygen for treatment of cluster headache: a randomized trial. JAMA 2009;302(22): 2451–2457

23. Weiss LD, Ramasastry SS, Eidelman BH. Treatment of a cluster headache patient in a hyperbaric chamber. Headache 1989; 29(2): 109–110

24. Di Sabato F, Fusco BM, Pelaia P, Giacovazzo M. Hyperbaric oxygen therapy in cluster headache. Pain 1993;52(2):243–245

25. Ashkenazi A, Schwedt T. Cluster headache—acute and prophylactic therapy. Headache 2011;51(2):272–286

26. Merksey H, Bogduk N. Classification of Chronic Pain: Descriptions of Chronic Pain Syndromes and Definitions of Pain Terms. Seattle: IASP Press; 1994

27. Gronseth G, Cruccu G, Alksne J, et al. Practice parameter: the diagnostic evaluation and treatment of trigeminal neuralgia (an evidence-based review): report of the Quality Standards Subcommittee of the American Academy of Neurology and the European Federation of Neurological Societies. Neurology 2008;71(15):1183–1190

28. Clerico DM. Sinus headaches reconsidered: referred cephalgia of rhinologic origin masquerading as refractory primary headaches. Headache 1995;35(4):185–192

29. Abu-Bakra M, Jones NS. Does stimulation of nasal mucosa cause referred pain to the face? Clin Otolaryngol Allied Sci 2001;26(5):430–432

30. Abu-Bakra M, Jones NS. Prevalence of nasal mucosal contact points in patients with facial pain compared with patients without facial pain. J Laryngol Otol 2001;115(8):629–632

31. Abu-Samra M, Gawad OA, Agha M. The outcomes for nasal contact point surgeries in patients with unsatisfactory response to chronic daily headache medications. Eur Arch Otorhinolaryngol 2011;268(9):1299–1304

32. Mohebbi A, Memari F, Mohebbi S. Endonasal endoscopic management of contact point headache and diagnostic criteria. Headache 2010;50(2):242–248

33. Mariotti LJ, Setliff RC III, Ghaderi M, Voth S. Patient history and CT findings in predicting surgical outcomes for patients with rhinogenic headache. Ear Nose Throat J 2009;88(5):926–929

12 Powered Instrumentation in Endoscopic Sinus Surgery

Timothy Haffey and Raj Sindwani

Throughout history, technological innovations have both facilitated and advanced the practice of endoscopic sinus surgery (ESS). The development of the Hopkins rod provided a high-clarity view of sinonasal anatomy and facilitated the first attempts at endoscopic surgery of the sinuses.[1] With the introduction of the Hopkins rod, one of the surgeon's hands was occupied at all times holding the scope, which means the surgeon needed to change instruments frequently with the remaining hand. This proved cumbersome at times, and predictably led to the development of multifunctional tools that would streamline surgery. This ushered in the era of powered instrumentation for ESS.

As the field of rhinology advanced, surgeons were able to safely venture beyond the confines of the nose and paranasal sinuses to the orbit, skull base, and even into the intracranial cavity. As surgeons push the envelope of endoscopic surgery, they encounter new obstacles, such as the need to safely remove thick bone. New surgical obstacles often become the impetus for technological innovations. In this chapter, we have chosen to focus on technologies that we believe have had, or will have, the greatest impact on the field of ESS: the microdebrider, suction–irrigation drill, radiofrequency ablation, and ultrasonic aspirator.[2-4] This chapter will succinctly outline the basic science of each of these technologies and summarize the available literature on indications for use, safety, and efficacy. We hope to highlight any controversies in the literature, and provide a critical review of the technologies that will allow the reader to determine what role, if any, these technologies may have in the scope of their practice.

Microdebrider

Defined as an electrically powered, cylindrical shaver that uses continuous suction for tissue removal,[5] the microdebrider was first described in the medical literature by the House group as an instrument to morselize acoustic neuromas.[4] It also became a popular tool among orthopedic surgeons as it was used in arthroscopic surgery. Setliff, Goode, and Parsons all published articles describing the use of the microdebrider in ESS for the first time in 1996.[6-8] Since its initial foray into rhinology, there have been many articles published on the use of microdebrider in ESS. The ability of the microdebrider to continuously suction blood away from the surgical field while removing tissue and thin bone have made it the most popular powered instrument used by modern rhinologists. For this reason, many herald the microdebrider as one of the most significant technological advances in the field of rhinology.[5]

Basic Science and Current Technology

There are several companies that manufacture microdebriders for ESS including Olympus-Gyrus (Gyrus, Bartlett, Tennessee, United States), Medtronic-Xomed (Medtronic, Jacksonville, Florida, United States) and Stryker (Stryker Corporation, Kalamazoo, Michigan, United States). Each company offers a product with unique design differences, but all microdebriders consist of a hollow shaft with a rotating, or oscillating, blade within the inner cannula. Continuous suction applied to the inner cannula draws soft tissue and bone chips into the blade. The tissue is cleaved by the oscillation of the blade and suctioned away from the operative field toward the suction canister, where it may be captured in a filter. Importantly, studies have shown that the tissue within the filter is histologically preserved for pathological examination.[5] Some models have a serrated edge on the blade, which allows for better gripping of soft tissue and more aggressive tissue take down. In contrast, straight edges are considered less traumatic and more sparing of adjacent mucosal tissues. Blades can be set to continuously rotate (forward or backward) or oscillate (back and forth across the aperture). For soft tissue removal, the oscillation mode is used at slower speeds of 3000 to 5000 revolutions per minute (RPM) allowing the blade to stay open longer, and more soft tissue to be drawn into the aperture before it is cut. There are also specialized solid burr-like tips available for the microdebrider that allow a drilling action. These tips are beneficial when the surgeon encounters bone that is thicker than the conventional microdebrider blade is able to handle. When used as a drill, however, the rotation settings are much slower for microdebriders than a conventional high-speed drill (15,000 RPM maximum vs. 80,000 to 100,000 RPM, respectively) and thus microdebriders are not as effective at removing thick bone expeditiously (**Fig. 12.1**).

Microdebrider blades come in a variety of angles and offer rotating ports (**Fig. 12.2**). This allows improved access to some hard-to-reach areas of the sinonasal tract. One example is the lateral recesses of the maxillary and sphenoid sinuses, another is the frontal recess. One drawback of using a curved blade is that there are increased rates of obstruction of the inner cannula with debris compared to that with straight cannulas.[5] A recent study performed by Boone

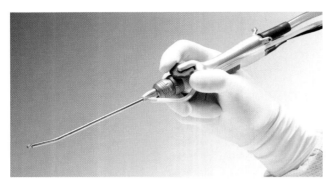

Figure 12.1 Medtronic Straightshot M4 microdebrider and 4-mm × 15-cm anterior skull base burr with a 15-degree bend.

Image courtesy: Medtronic, Jacksonville, Florida, United States.

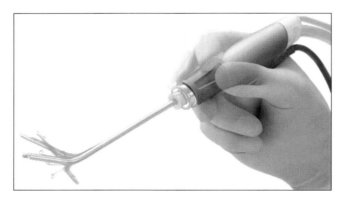

Figure 12.2 Medtronic Straightshot microdebrider with a 30-degree, rotatable blade.

Image courtesy: Medtronic, Jacksonville, Florida, United States.

et al[9] compared a brand new prototype (4.3-mm Medtronic Quadcut blade; Medtronic) with their standard model (4.0-mm Medtronic Tricut blade; Medtronic) to evaluate the issue with clogging. They created a surgical model representing polyp disease (raw oysters) and AFS (minced beef cat food), and found decreased rates of clogging with the prototype in the AFS model. Neither model clogged from the debris in the nasal polyp model.[9]

Recent advances include the ability of navigation systems to track the tips of microdebrider blades. This is most easily accomplished using optical-based systems that can track any rigid instrument or any blade, but a few select blades can now also be tracked using electromagnetic-based platforms as well. Some companies make specialty microdebrider blades with a specific task in mind. For instance, the inferior turbinate blade is a small-diameter blade (2.0 and 2.9 mm sizes) used to perform submucous resection of the vascular erectile tissue of the turbinate while preserving the overlying mucosa. Some models have a beveled guard on the tip of the blade, which can be used to penetrate into the substance of the turbinate and raise the soft tissue away from the turbinate bone, eliminating the need for another instrument change during the procedure. By sparing the surface respiratory epithelium, less crusting and synechiae

formation occur following operation than that when cautery or surface-damaging techniques are employed for turbinate reduction. The incidence of osteitis of the concha, an uncommon complication of turbinate surgery, is also lower when this technology is used.[10]

Instrument Advantages and Evidence

Microdebriders are routinely used by many otolaryngologists as they are thought to spare adjacent mucosa, provide improved precision over standard (nonpowered) instruments, remove tissue more quickly, and provide better visualization as blood is continuously cleared. Despite these anecdotal opinions, however, there are few evidence-based studies actually supporting these contentions.[6–8,11]

Sauer et al conducted a prospective, double-blinded, randomized control trial comparing maxillary antrostomy and ethmoidectomy performed using a microdebrider with those performed with standard instruments. Each patient had the procedure performed bilaterally with one side serving as the internal control. They noted an improvement in symptom and endoscopic scores at 3 weeks in the microdebrider group, but no other differences were noted.[12] It should be mentioned that operating room times and blood loss were not reported in this study.

The ability to simultaneously suction blood away from the surgical field is especially advantageous during ESS for nasal polyps that can bleed considerably during removal. Significant bleeding intraoperatively can increase the risk of complications. Despite the proliferation of microdebriders and their effectiveness at continuously clearing blood from the field, one significant drawback to current platforms is that they do not actually decrease bleeding in any way. The most recent innovation in microdebrider technology now permits the added ability to control bleeding while retaining the shaving and suctioning capabilities of this class of instrument. The PK Diego (Gyrus ACMI-ENT Division, Bartlett, Tennessee, United States) has the ability to provide hemostasis by delivering bipolar energy to the end of its blade. The blade is surrounded by layers of insulation that sandwich inner and outer electrodes (**Fig. 12.3A**). The instrument can be set to low (10 watts [W]), medium (20 W),

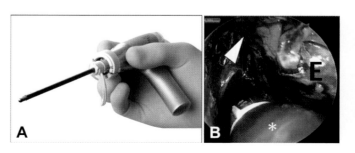

Figure 12.3 (A) PK Diego bipolar-equipped microdebrider with straight blade. (B) Intraoperative view of PK Diego (*) being used to resect an encephalocele (E) along the skull base (arrowhead).

Images courtesy: Gyrus, Bartlett, Tennessee, United States.

or high (40 W) power. One drawback to the current model is that it has a fairly small zone of bipolar cautery, which is located at the distal aspect of the blade, perpendicular to the suction aperture.

A controlled study of 80 patients undergoing surgery for chronic rhinosinusitis with polyps found that the use of the bipolar-equipped PK Diego was associated with significantly less blood loss and shorter operative times compared with surgery performed using a conventional microdebrider.[13] The fact that the PK Diego functions using bipolar instead of monopolar energy is also noteworthy, as this limits the transmission of heat to adjacent intraorbital and intracranial structures. The application of this instrument is also well suited for submucous inferior turbinate reduction where bleeding from the turbinate interior as well as from the entry site can be readily controlled. It can also be beneficial in the endonasal removal of vascularized tissues (e.g., adenoids or tumors) and lesions involving the skull base (**Fig. 12.3B**).

Limitations

Future advances in this technology will likely focus on improving the ability to provide hemostasis during tissue removal, improved torque generation for enhanced drilling capacity, continued improvements in ergonomics, and improving suction flow to decrease clogging (especially in curved blades).

Like any other instrument, microdebriders have certain limitations that must be recognized if these tools are to be used effectively and safely.[4,5] Microdebriders are heavier than conventional instruments and are electrically powered. This means that the tactile feedback during surgery is markedly diminished with microdebriders. This, in addition to the powered nature of these instruments and their use in close proximity to critical structures, has raised concerns about the safety of microdebriders in ESS. Bhatti et al described two cases of ocular injury, one resulting in restrictive ophthalmoplegia and the other in transection of the medial rectus.[14] In both cases, it was argued that the strong suction of the microdebrider allowed orbital fat, or even extraocular muscles, to be pulled through a relatively small defect in the lamina papyracea and into the blade. Berenholz et al described a case of subarachnoid hemorrhage after functional ESS using the microdebrider that was thought to be caused by the strength of suction.[15] Although major complications from ESS are rare, complications that do occur related to microdebrider use may progress more quickly because of the powered nature and suction of this device.[4,5] Finally, microdebriders carry the cost of the system and ongoing costs of disposable components.

Endoscopic Drills

Endoscopic drills are used much less frequently than microdebriders due to the fact that the microdebrider is able

to handle both the soft tissue and the thin bony partitions encountered with most routine endoscopic sinus surgeries. Procedures requiring the removal of thick bone beyond the capacity of the microdebrider led to the development of a variety of drills and burrs. One major advantage of drills over traditional techniques for bone removal is that the drill requires relatively small amount of force to be applied by the operator, permitting expeditious, yet controlled bone removal.[11] This is especially important in rhinologic surgery due to the proximity of crucial structures that must be preserved.

Basic Science and Current Technology

Endoscopic drills have a few key differences that specialize them for use in rhinologic surgery, and separate them from their otologic counterparts. The drills themselves have been designed with a slimmer profile to permit simultaneous use with an endoscope in a narrow surgical field, and to facilitate movement through the nostrils (**Fig. 12.4**). There is a protective sheath along the shaft of the drill burr to protect against collateral friction damage to adjacent tissues (including soft tissues of the nostril). Some also have a sheath to protect the posterior aspect of the burr offering further protection to adjacent structures. Continuous suction/irrigation has also been designed into handpieces to decrease the number of instruments the endoscopic surgeon must manipulate at one time. Suction and irrigation features aim to not only improve visibility, but also function to cool the drill burr and drill–tissue interface in an attempt to limit heat transmission. Other modifications aimed at addressing some of the unique ergonomic and length concerns for endonasal drilling include longer sheaths, extended drill attachments for the skull base, telescoping drill bits, and angulated handpieces. The use of suction–irrigation and some of these other endonasal modifications add to the

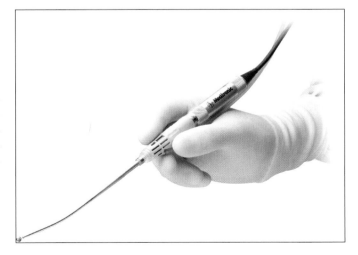

Figure 12.4 EHS Stylus endoscopic drill and round fluted 4 mm × 13 cm transnasal skull base burr with a 15-degree bend.
Image courtesy: Medtronic, Jacksonville, Florida, United States.

caliber of the instrument however, and thus come at the expense of visibility in an already narrow surgical field. There is still opportunity to make great strides in the arena of endoscopic drills.

One fact common to all drills is that the number of flutes on the burr determines how aggressively the drill will take down bone. A burr with few deep flutes will cut very aggressively, resulting in the rapid take down of bone. However, this does come at the expense of fine control. Speed of rotation will also affect how fast bone is drilled away. Something that may be counter-intuitive to the novice user is that faster rotational speeds actually improve control, as there is less chance for chatter or tear out. When more control is needed, diamond burrs are also available, which are generally much less aggressive then fluted (cutting) burrs and are good for smoothing bone edges. Diamond burrs are also used in situations where bone needs to be thinned close to important structures, and controlled movements removing small amounts of bone are needed such as along the skull base and orbital apex.

Instrument Advantages and Evidence

While the drill is not typically needed during standard ESS, there have been numerous articles published outlining how its use has allowed surgery to extend beyond the sinonasal cavities. In 2004, Jho and Ha published a three-part series on the use of endoscopic drils to access the midline anterior fossa skull base, cavernous sinus, clivus, and posterior fossa.[16–18] Endoscopic drills have also been used routinely in the controlled removal of bone from virtually all aspects of the sphenoid sinus: for access to the sella, exposure of the clivus or posterior cranial fossa, or to decompress the optic nerve.

Perhaps the most common contemporary application of endoscopic drilling is in surgery of the frontal sinus. After conservative measures aimed at widening the frontal recess fail, more aggressive techniques targeting the frontal sinus ostium and the floor of the sinus can be pursued.[19] The high-speed drill is very effective at resecting the floor and frontal beak region, and may be used to create a large common aperture draining both frontal sinuses via the endoscopic modified Lothrop procedure (also known as the Draf III or bilateral frontal drillout procedure).[11] This technique has been described by Draf[20] and others in the literature,[21,22] and involves resection of both frontal sinus floors and interfrontal sinus septum through a superior septectomy.

Drills have also had a significant impact on the endoscopic surgery of the orbit and lacrimal system. Endoscopic orbital techniques offer the advantages of enhancing visualization while providing a direct route to the posterior orbit and apex. This has the added benefit that facial incisions and scars are avoided. Performing a successful endoscopic dacryocystorhinostomy (E-DCR) for nasolacrimal duct obstruction requires the creation of a generous bony rhinostomy through, in part, the thick ascending process of the maxilla.

This involves thick bone removal beginning in the region of the maxillary line and proceeding anteriorly. Although many techniques for bone removal have been described including the use of a mallet and osteotome, microdebriders, and lasers,[23–26] many surgeons prefer the finesse and precision best afforded by a high-speed drill. Removal of thick bone during orbital decompression (particularly the lateral and inferior walls) and optic nerve decompressions has also been described in the literature as being augmented by the use of an endoscopic drill.[11]

Limitations

As technological advancements continue, creating a slimmer profile of the endoscopic drill while maintaining the continuous suction–irrigation functions and the quality of the drilling will need to be pursued. The goal is to develop the most ergonomic, superior functioning, endoscopic drill that minimally obstructs the narrow operative field, characteristic of endoscopic rhinologic surgery.

Radiofrequency Ablation

Radiofrequency ablation (coblation) is a technology patented by ArthroCare (Austin, Texas , United States) in 1997, initially intended for use in cartilage ablation during arthroscopy. It was approved in 2000 by the U.S. Food and Drug Administration for use in otolaryngology.[11]

Basic Science and Current Technology

Coblation uses radiofrequency waves to energize electrolytes within a conductive medium (typically saline). This theoretically creates a plasma field, which disrupts molecular bonds within the surrounding tissues at relatively low temperatures (40 to 70°C as compared to over 400°C with monopolar electrocautery). As some studies suggest that a plasma field is unlikely to be created outside a vacuum, Zinder theorized that the decreased thermal damage during coblation has more to do with vaporization of the saline solution than creation of a plasma field.[27] Regardless of the mechanism of action, there is significantly less penetration of thermal energy into the surrounding tissue with the use of this technology, which is advantageous when thermal spread to important structures is not wanted.

The current radiofrequency ablation systems available are the Coblation unit developed by ArthroCare and the Somnus system developed by Somnus Medical Technologies, now with Olympus-Gyrus (Gyrus ACMI-ENT Division, Bartlett, Tennessee, United States) (**Fig. 12.5**).

Advantages and Evidence

The most common use of coblation technology in otolaryngology is for tonsillectomy, where some studies have suggested less postoperative pain and a faster recovery.[28]

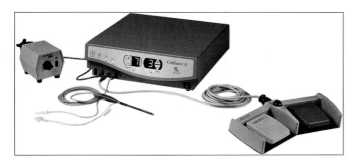

Figure 12.5 Coblator II complete unit and handpiece. *Image courtesy*: ArthroCare ENT, Austin, Texas, United States.

Coblation technology was initially adapted for use in rhinologic surgery for inferior turbinate reduction.[4] The coblator is used to submucosally ablate the erectile tissue of the turbinate providing immediate volume reduction, as well as delayed volume reduction through scarring down as part of the healing process. In 2002, Bäck et al showed significant subjective improvement in nasal obstruction, sneezing, crusting, and nasal discharge using a visual analogue scale after coblation-mediated inferior turbinate reduction.[29]

Recently, other rhinologic applications of this technology have surfaced. A study by Eloy et al compared blood loss with operative time in patients undergoing coblator-assisted polypectomy with those undergoing a microdebrider-assisted polypectomy. There were no differences in disease severity between the groups. The estimated blood loss was 307 mL in the coblation group compared with 627 mL in the microdebrider cohort. The average length of surgery was also shorter in the coblation group. A subgroup analysis revealed that the difference in blood loss was only significant, however, in revision cases.[30] Smith et al also published an article describing the use of the coblation system for the endoscopic resection of encephaloceles. They found a decreased operative time when this technique was compared to traditional bipolar cautery for resection, with no statistical increase in complications noted.[31] Coblation has also been described for use in transnasal tumor resection, where its hemostatic ability could provide ongoing bleeding control during removal of potentially well-vascularized soft tissue.[4]

Limitations

A major limitation to the use of currently available coblation technology to ESS is its inability to address the bony partitions encountered in the ethmoid labyrinth or other areas of the sinonasal tract and skull base. Also, to date there have been no studies examining the extent of heat generation or transmission to adjacent structures during prolonged use of this instrument, as would be necessary for tumor or polyp removal. The theory behind the technology is that radiofrequency ablation of the tissue is supposed to decrease thermal spread. This has yet to be definitively proven in sinus surgery. Other limitations include a relative

paucity of literature documenting clear advantages, associated expense, as well as a limited surgeon experience in the use of this technology for transnasal endoscopic procedures. It should be noted that radiofrequency ablation technology has only recently been introduced to the field of rhinologic surgery, which explains the paucity of data regarding this technology in the literature.

Ultrasonic Aspirators

The sinonasal cavity is bordered by relatively thick bone, with thin bony partitions dividing it into compartments. All surgeries on the sinuses or extending beyond the confines of the sinonasal tract therefore require the controlled take down of varying amounts of bone. Due to the close proximity of important soft tissue structures, it is crucial to take down bone with as little impact on the surrounding soft tissue as possible. A promising recent technological advancement in powered instrumentation impacting ESS has been the bone-cutting ultrasonic aspirator.

Basic Science and Current Technology

Ultrasonic aspirators operate on the converse piezoelectric effect, whereby application of an electric charge to certain crystals creates a reversible mechanical deformation (direct piezoelectric effect refers to electricity being generated by mechanical stress on the crystals). The piezoelectric effect was first described by Pierre and Jacques Curie in the late 19th century. The technology was first described within the medical field in its use for phacoemulsification of the lens during cataract surgery by ophthalmologists. Advances in the field now allow aspirators to expeditiously remove bone while still being respectful of nearby soft tissues.[4,11]

The ultrasonic aspirators currently available are the CUSA NXT by Integra (Integra LifeSciences Corporation, Plainsboro, New Jersey, United States) and the Sonopet Omni Surgical System by Stryker (**Fig. 12.6**). Both models rely on the same general principles of physics. There is a stack of piezoelectric discs, or tubular piezoelectric crystal, within the handpiece that expands and contracts when alternating current is applied causing vibration. This high-frequency vibration breaks down hydrogen bonds in tissue proteins, resulting in their denaturation. The actual cutting of tissue is secondary to cavitation, which is the formation, expansion, and subsequent implosion of small vapor bubbles within the tissue, caused by the ultrasonic waves. The resulting emulsified tissue is then removed by continuous irrigation and suction. The technology was designed such that the frequency of vibration can be adjusted and thus optimized for either bone or soft tissue removal. The ultrasonic aspirator reportedly generates less heat than conventional drills. Power can be adjusted on the ultrasonic aspirator, with greater power resulting in increased amplitude of tip stroke and more aggressive take down of bone or soft tissue.[4,11]

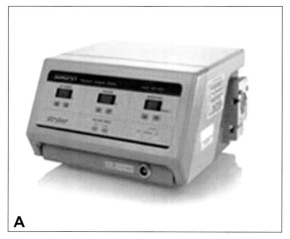

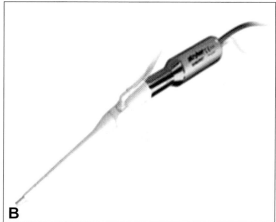

Figure 12.6   Sonopet Omni base unit (A) and handpiece (B).

Image courtesy: Stryker Corporation, Kalamazoo, Michigan, United States.

Instrument Advantages and Evidence

A novel aspect of this new technology and one of its most advantageous features is the programmable selectivity it provides. The endoscopic use of these instruments was first described in otolaryngology literature by Antisdel et al,[32] who reported their experience using an ultrasonic aspirator for the creation of the bony rhinostomy in E-DCR surgery. The authors noted that inadvertent, or even purposeful, contact with the back of the vibrating tip of the aspirator with a mucosa-lined structure such as the nasal septum or middle turbinate, did not cause any identifiable injury.

Unlike most conventional-powered instrumentation, the tip vibrates rather than spinning. The lack of a spinning burr also reduces the risk of skipping or chatter associated with a conventional drill, providing more control. Collateral damage to adjacent structures at risk in the setting of a spinning burr or microdebrider blade is also minimized. It also means that an extra guard to protect the back of the tip from bumping into surrounding structures is not needed. This fact is beneficial, decreasing any further obstruction of the surgical field by the instrument itself, which is important in endoscopic surgery. The use of bone-cutting ultrasonic

aspirators has been described in a variety of neurosurgical procedures, and they have been praised for their ability to minimize damage to soft tissue structures (e.g., vasculature and dura) while removing thick bone in confined spaces. This includes transsphenoidal approaches to fibrous or bony pituitary lesions.[11]

The otolaryngology community also seems to have taken notice of the potential utility of this technology. Greywoode et al described the use of the ultrasonic aspirator for removal of the bony portion of the inferior turbinate, leaving the soft tissues of the inferior turbinate intact.[33] In 2008, Pagella et al reported the successful removal of a frontoethmoid osteoma transnasally using an ultrasonic aspirator.[34] The ability of this technology to selectively remove bone while being respectful of nearby mucosa and soft tissue holds considerable promise for endoscopic transnasal procedures. It is the authors' opinions that the use of the surgical ultrasonic aspirator will likely increase as endoscopic sinus and neurorhinologic techniques continue to expand.

Limitations

This technology, while novel and cutting edge, does not have significant literature supporting rhinologic applications in which it may be advantageous or even preferable. While it theoretically carries benefits over other powered instruments related to its tissue selectivity, the impact of this on actual outcomes has not yet been demonstrated. Another drawback is that the cost of the unit itself is substantial and its use carries the ongoing costs of disposables. Further, this instrument does remove bone more slowly than a high-speed drill and importantly data on heat generation at the tip during bone emulsification are presently lacking.

Conclusion

The adoption of the microdebrider into the field of otolaryngology in the 1990s set off a cascade of development of new innovative powered instrumentation for ESS. As a result, the modern rhinologist has a wide variety of fascinating and evolving tools at their disposal. Recent innovations in powered instrumentation highlighted in this chapter included the microdebrider, endoscopic drill, radiofrequency ablation, and ultrasonic aspirators. The primary drawback of powered instrumentation continues to be the higher costs associated with their utilization, which usually includes both capital expenditures for the system and ongoing costs for disposable parts.

The main advantage of all of these instruments is their ability to accomplish multiple functions with one tool that, importantly, can be operated by the endoscopic surgeon with one hand. The effective utilization of any powered instrument requires an intimate understanding of its capabilities and limitations, and no instrument replaces the need for a thorough understanding of surgical anatomy, expertise, and experience.

References

1. Kennedy DW. Functional endoscopic sinus surgery. Technique. Arch Otolaryngol 1985;111(10):643–649
2. Costa DJ, Sindwani R. Advances in surgical navigation. Otolaryngol Clin North Am 2009;42(5):799–811, ix
3. Batra PS, Ryan MW, Sindwani R, Marple BF. Balloon catheter technology in rhinology: reviewing the evidence. Laryngoscope 2011;121(1):226–232
4. Sindwani R, Manz R. Tehnological innovations in tissue removal during rhinologic surgery. Am J Rhinol Allergy 2012; 26(1):65-69
5. Bruggers S, Sindwani R. Innovations in microdebrider technology and design. Otolaryngol Clin North Am 2009;42(5):781–787, viii
6. Setliff RC III. The hummer: a remedy for apprehension in functional endoscopic sinus surgery. Otolaryngol Clin North Am 1996;29(1):95–104
7. Goode RL. Power microdebrider for functional endoscopic sinus surgery. Otolaryngol Head Neck Surg 1996;114(4):676–677
8. Parsons DS. Rhinologic uses of powered instrumentation in children beyond sinus surgery. Otolaryngol Clin North Am 1996;29(1):105–114
9. Boone JL, Feldt BA, McMains KC, Weitzel EK. Improved function of prototype 4.3-mm Medtronic Quadcut microdebrider blade over standard 4.0-mm Medtronic Tricut microdebrider blade. Int Forum Allergy Rhinol 2011;1(3):198–200
10. Citardi MJ, Batra PS. Image-guided sinus surgery: current concepts and technology. Otolaryngol Clin North Am 2005;38(3):439–452, vi
11. Bruggers S, Sindwani R. Evolving trends in powered endoscopic sinus surgery. Otolaryngol Clin North Am 2009;42(5):789–798, viii
12. Sauer M, Lemmens W, Vauterin T, Jorissen M. Comparing the microdebrider and standard instruments in endoscopic sinus surgery: a double-blind randomised study. B-ENT 2007;3(1):1–7
13. Kumar NS, Sindwani R. Bipolar microdebrider may reduce intraoperative blood loss and operating time during nasal polyp surgery. Ear Nose Throat J 2012;91(8):336–344
14. Bhatti MT, Giannoni CM, Raynor E, Monshizadeh R, Levine LM. Ocular motility complications after endoscopic sinus surgery with powered cutting instruments. Otolaryngol Head Neck Surg 2001;125(5):501–509
15. Berenholz L, Kessler A, Sarfaty S, Segal S. Subarachnoid hemorrhage: a complication of endoscopic sinus surgery using powered instrumentation. Otolaryngol Head Neck Surg 1999;121(5):665–667
16. Jho HD, Ha HG. Endoscopic endonasal skull base surgery: Part 1—The midline anterior fossa skull base. Minim Invasive Neurosurg 2004;47(1):1–8
17. Jho HD, Ha HG. Endoscopic endonasal skull base surgery: Part 2—The cavernous sinus. Minim Invasive Neurosurg 2004;47(1):9–15
18. Jho HD, Ha HG. Endoscopic endonasal skull base surgery: Part 3—The clivus and posterior fossa. Minim Invasive Neurosurg 2004;47(1):16–23
19. Metson R, Sindwani R. Frontal sinusitis: endoscopic approaches. Otolaryngol Clin North Am 2004;37:411–422
20. Draf W. Endonasal micro-endoscopic frontal sinus surgery: the Fulda concept. Oper Tech Otolaryngol Head Neck Surg 1991;2(4):234–240
21. Gross WE, Gross CW, Becker D, Moore D, Phillips D. Modified transnasal endoscopic Lothrop procedure as an alternative to frontal sinus obliteration. Otolaryngol Head Neck Surg 1995;113(4):427–434
22. Close LG, Lee NK, Leach JL, Manning SC. Endoscopic resection of the intranasal frontal sinus floor. Ann Otol Rhinol Laryngol 1994;103(12):952–958
23. Cokkeser Y, Evereklioglu C, Tercan M, Hepsen IF. Hammer-chisel technique in endoscopic dacryocystorhinostomy. Ann Otol Rhinol Laryngol 2003;112(5):444–449
24. Yoon SW, Yoon YS, Lee SH. Clinical results of endoscopic dacryocystorhinostomy using a microdebrider. Korean J Ophthalmol 2006;20(1):1–6
25. Maini S, Raghava N, Youngs R, et al. Endoscopic endonasal laser versus endonasal surgical dacryocystorhinostomy for epiphora due to nasolacrimal duct obstruction: prospective, randomised, controlled trial. J Laryngol Otol 2007;121(12):1170–1176
26. Woog JJ, Sindwani R. Endoscopic dacryocystorhinostomy and conjunctivodacryocystorhinostomy. Otolaryngol Clin North Am 2006;39(5):1001–1017, vii
27. Zinder DJ. Common myths about electrosurgery. Otolaryngol Head Neck Surg 2000;123(4):450–455
28. Magdy EA, Elwany S, el-Daly AS, Abdel-Hadi M, Morshedy MA. Coblation tonsillectomy: a prospective, double-blind, randomised, clinical and histopathological comparison with dissection-ligation, monopolar electrocautery and laser tonsillectomies. J Laryngol Otol 2008;122(3):282–290
29. Bäck LJ, Hytönen ML, Malmberg HO, Ylikoski JS. Submucosal bipolar radiofrequency thermal ablation of inferior turbinates: a long-term follow-up with subjective and objective assessment. Laryngoscope 2002;112(10):1806–1812
30. Eloy JA, Walker TJ, Casiano RR, Ruiz JW. Effect of coblation polypectomy on estimated blood loss in endoscopic sinus surgery. Am J Rhinol Allergy 2009;23(5):535–539
31. Smith N, Riley KO, Woodworth BA. Endoscopic Coblator™-assisted management of encephaloceles. Laryngoscope 2010;120(12):2535–2539
32. Antisdel JL, Kadze MS, Sindwani R. Application of ultrasonic aspirators to endoscopic dacryocystorhinostomy. Otolaryngol Head Neck Surg 2008;139(4):586–588
33. Greywoode JD, Van Abel K, Pribitkin EA. Ultrasonic bone aspirator turbinoplasty: a novel approach for management of inferior turbinate hypertrophy. Laryngoscope 2010;120(Suppl 4):S239
34. Pagella F, Giourgos G, Matti E, Colombo A, Carena P. Removal of a fronto-ethmoidal osteoma using the sonopet omni ultrasonic bone curette: first impressions. Laryngoscope 2008;118(2):307–309

13 Advances in Surgical Navigation

Lee A. Zimmer, Larry G. Linson, and Angela M. Donaldson

Intraoperative image guidance has gained widespread acceptance across many surgical disciplines. These systems allow viewing patient's anatomy from images acquired before surgery. Computed tomography (CT) and magnetic resonance imaging (MRI), as well as combined imaging techniques have been used for acquiring these images. Although several intraoperative systems exist, feedback is essentially provided to the surgeon in a similar manner. The goal of this chapter is to provide a brief history of image-guided systems and discuss the practical use of image guidance in rhinology and skull base surgery.

Image-Guided Surgery Systems

History

While the use of image-guidance technology has gained significant acceptance in the past two decades, the concept of image-guided surgery in the field of neurosurgery began in the 1940s. Stereotactic devices were developed to help drain intracranial abscesses and destroy focal areas of the cerebrum causing abnormal motor activity and pain. Guidance devices relied on framed stereotaxy using plain radiography, fluoroscopy, and anatomic landmarks. With advancements in imaging technology, CT was introduced and it quickly became the image modality of choice for framed stereotaxy procedures. Bergström and Greitz developed a head fixation that was placed during preoperative CT imaging and then used intraoperatively to visualize the trajectory of instrument advancement during a procedure.[1] Some limitations did exist with this system including unreliable assessment of the depth of instruments and limited surgical access because of the sheer size of the headset.

The next step in the evolution of image-guided technology was the elimination of the rigid frame from the headset. Instead of the cumbersome headset used with framed stereotaxy procedures, frameless procedures relied on multiple fiducial markers secured to the patient's head. These markers were worn by the patient during preoperative imaging and remained in place until surgery. Use of early frameless navigational systems was limited due to poor accuracy. Improvement in accuracy was due to various calibration techniques including mobile joint arms with attached probes, acoustic digitizers, and optical encoded systems.

Current Systems

Various computer-aided systems exist for intraoperative imaging. Each system functions by gathering and interpreting either electromechanical, electromagnetic, ultrasound, or optical data. The objectives of computer-aided surgery are to avoid wide-open surgery (the funnel principle) and attempt more minimally invasive procedures (the tunnel principle).[2] Common indications for computer-aided systems in rhinology and endoscopic skull base surgery are discussed later in the chapter.

Image-guided tracking systems finally evolved into the two main calibration types available today: optical (infrared) and electromagnetic (radiofrequency). The most common optical image-guided tracking systems used today include StealthStation (Medtronic, Minneapolis, Minnesota), VectorVision (BrainLab Inc., Feldkirchen, Germany), and Stryker iNtellect Navigation System (Stryker, Portage, Michigan) (**Fig. 13.1A** to **C**). Optical systems use infrared light-emitting diode (LED) technology. These systems have

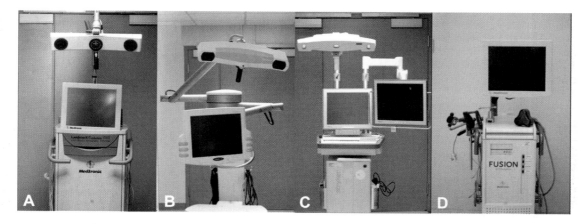

Figure 13.1 Current optical image-guided workstations. (A) StealthStation; (B) VectorVision; (C) Stryker iNtellect Navigation; and (D) Fusion Navigation.

an articulating arm with infrared cameras attached to the main body of the system. Electromagnetic-based systems such as InstaTrak (GE Medical, Waukesha, Wisconsin) and Fusion Navigation System (Medtronic, Minneapolis, Minnesota) have the tracking device attached to the surgical instruments and do not require LEDs (**Fig. 13.1D**).

Image-guidance systems embody four basic units: CT/MRI or combined images viewed in the axial, coronal, and sagittal planes; a workstation to process data from the images; a mechanism to register data from the images to the patient using a headset or fiducial markers secured to the patient; and a mechanism to calibrate instruments so that while they are advanced into the surgical field, movements are visualized. Although slight variations have been reported in the literature, accuracy can reliably be obtained to within 2 mm with all systems.

Optical Systems

The patient is placed in a supine position with the head closest to the image-guided system (IGS) and video monitor. Images are then loaded onto the image-guidance workstation. A headset is placed and secured with a band on the patient's forehead at the level of the brow for sinus surgery (**Fig. 13.2A**). Alternative headsets may be placed anywhere on the head for open procedures via percutaneous

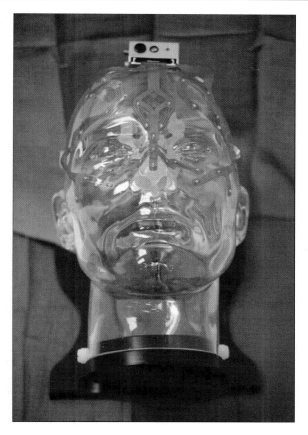

Figure 13.3 Image of the Stryker iNtellect Navigation System with skin surface registration mask and receiver.

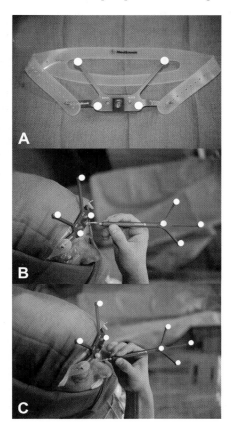

Figure 13.2 (A) Head receiver and strap for the StealthStation; (B) demonstration of registration probe placement in the divot; and (C) demonstration of active skin surface registration.

fixation. Calibration is completed using the system-provided software and placing the tip of the image-guidance probe in a divot on the headset while the foot pedal is depressed (**Fig. 13.2B**). Registration is completed by touching the tip of the straight probe to surface fiducials. Alternatives to fiducial registration are available, including surface (**Fig. 13.2C**), anatomical site, face mask (**Fig. 13.3**), and laser-emitting surface registration.

Typically, fiducial markers are placed at a minimum of three sites plus the nasal dorsum at the level of the medial canthi, the nasal tip, the columella, and the lateral orbital wall at the level of the lateral canthi during imaging.[3] Registration errors may be due to fiducials that have shifted position or become dislodged, the deformation of soft tissues during imaging, and the time between imaging and registration.[4] Designs using face masks and laser surface registration overcome limitations in fiducial-based registration as nothing needs to be placed on the patient during image acquisition.

Once registered, the procedure may begin. Multiple instruments are available for guidance depending on the desired site of surgery and the image is visualized (**Figs. 13.4** and **13.5**). Indeed, several systems allow the attachment of a tracking device to almost any instrument allowing a wide array of options for the surgeon. However, the attachment of tracking devices may change the reach and degree of rotation of the instrumentation.

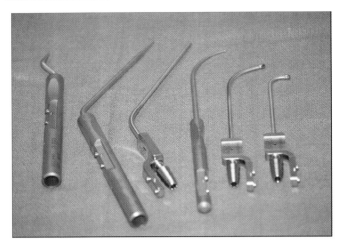

Figure 13.4 Image displaying an array of instrument probes from the Fusion Navigation System.

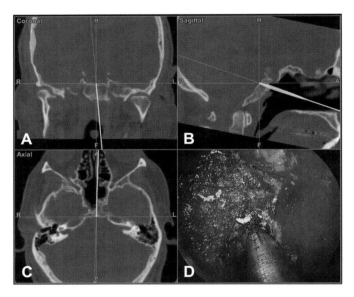

Figure 13.5 Active display image from an endonasal cranial base course using the Stryker iNtellect Navigation System. (A) Coronal computed tomography (CT) images; (B) sagittal CT images; (C) axial CT images; and (D) video display.

As with any technology, limitations exist. Optical-based systems require a clear line of site between the cameras and the LEDs on the instrument. Often this requires a fine "dance" between the camera connected to the endoscope and the selected guidance instrumentation. Furthermore, maintaining a clear line of site between the camera and LED limits the useable space in the operating room for nursing staff and operating room technicians.

Electromagnetic System

Electromagnetic systems require the patient to wear a radiofrequency transmitter on their forehead at the time of imaging and during surgery, and in a single position on the head. The patient is placed in a supine position with the head closest to the IGS and video monitor. The image dataset is then loaded onto the workstation and the headset is placed on the patient. This system uses automatic registration where the headset contains the fiducial markers needed to correspond with the image dataset. Instruments are calibrated in a divot on the headset. The instrument tip is seen as a crosshair on the uploaded images.

A study comparing the EasyGuide (Philips, Eindhoven, The Netherlands), VectorVision, and InstaTrak computer-assisted systems was performed to compare these systems. It revealed that the EasyGuide and VectorVision had differing nearest marker functions (a measurement used to compare accuracy) in the laboratory than in the operating room. Both tested more accurate in the laboratory than they did in the clinic. Possible sources of error included lost fiducial markers, movement of fiducial markers, and soft tissue shifts.[5] InstaTrak, however, tested with similar precision in the laboratory and clinic settings. Possible reasons for lack of error with InstaTrak are the lack of fiducial markers. The headset compensates for a patient's head movement and provides registration of images automatically without having to use fiducial markers as reference points. In this study, the authors concluded that InstaTrak, in using electromagnetic computer-assisted surgery, was the best for paranasal sinus surgeries. VectorVision, with its optical navigation computer-assisted surgery, was more useful for surgery involving the skull base. Another study found that StealthStation's optical computer-assisted surgery system is beneficial for treatment of trauma or lateral and anterior skull base tumors.[6]

The advantage of the electromagnetic systems is ease of registration and can easily be reregistered if accuracy wanes during a procedure. There are some disadvantages in the electromagnetic system, which are not inherent in the optical systems. The presence of metallic objects in the operating room may lead to interference with these IGSs, therefore, instruments, tables, and anesthesia equipment need to be placed far enough away from the operative field to prevent signal disturbances. However, the authors of this chapter have not experienced difficulty with interference while using the electromagnetic system.

Rhinology

Indications

Patient selection for the use of image-guided sinus surgery is surgeon-dependent. The American Academy of Otolaryngology-Head and Neck Surgery has established a policy regarding the use of IGSs that "endorses the intraoperative use of computer aided surgery in appropriately select cases to assist the surgeon in providing localization of anatomic structures."[7] These included revision sinus surgery, distorted sinus anatomy from congenital, postoperative or traumatic causes, extensive sinonasal polyposis, and pathology of the frontal, posterior ethmoid, and sphenoid sinus. Unfortunately, this is a rather vague statement relying on levels 4 (retrospective review) and 5 (expert opinion) evidence in the literature. It provides little guidance for surgical planning and less guidance for earlier authorization through insurers.

Metson and Gray proposed a grouping system to determine the need for image-guided systems in three different clinical scenarios.[8] In group one, patients with localized sinus disease and well-defined anatomical landmarks do not require image guidance. Group two includes patients with more advanced disease or revision surgery with limited landmarks, in which image guidance was not necessary but may be beneficial. Image guidance is recommended for patients in group three, as these patients have disease processes encroaching upon or involving the anterior skull base, pterygomaxillary fossa, infratemporal fossa, or extensive polypoid disease.

Outcomes

Outcomes research in the area of image-guided sinus surgery is both limited and inconclusive at this point. In a physician's survey, 85% of surgeons felts that computer-assisted sinus surgery was associated with increased surgeon confidence. Tabaee et al published the first comparative study looking at the quality of life after endoscopic sinus surgery performed with and without image guidance.[9] Identical SNOT-20 scores were seen between the two cohorts. Additionally, the study found no statistical significance in incidence of complications or need for revision surgery.

Studies indicate that increased operative time is the biggest complaint of image-guided systems.[10] These studies have reported a learning curve for operating room setup and use that starts with an increase of 15 to 30 minutes, but eventually decreases to 5 to 10 minutes. Sindwani and Metson analyzed 33 patients who had either undergone osteoplastic frontal sinus obliteration using image guidance or obliteration via traditional techniques.[11] Image guidance decreased the number of complications during osteoplastic frontal sinus obliteration from 3 to 0. Although the numbers are small, statistical significance was obtained, suggesting that image guidance increased the safety of this complex procedure.

The question as to when it is appropriate to use image-guided systems will probably never be answered with level 1 evidence. An analysis of safety is difficult as the frequency of severe morbidity such as cerebrospinal fluid (CSF) rhinorrhea and orbital injury from sinus surgery is low (< 1%). To appropriately power such a randomized study with significance would require anywhere between 3000 and 30,000 patients. Certainly a task beyond the means of most, if not all, major academic centers. Due to this obstacle, some authors have concluded that guidance based on levels 4 and 5 evidence as provided by the Academy of Otolaryngology statement is sufficient, and to withhold IGS in a randomized study would be unethical.[12]

Endoscopic Skull Base Surgery

History

Skull base surgery developed from the merger of craniofacial and neurosurgery. Open skull base surgery advanced quickly in the 1970s as techniques for surgical exposure and skull base reconstruction using pedicled and free tissue flaps were consistently used. For 40 years, pituitary tumors were removed through a sublabial approach with fluoroscopic guidance. In the 1950s and 1960s, fluoroscopic imaging allowed for the identification of microsurgical instruments in the sphenoid sinus and sella for pituitary surgery. In the 1980s, endoscopic sinus surgery was introduced in the United States and since that time, improvements in endoscopic telescopes and camera systems have allowed sinus surgery to be visualized over video monitoring systems.[13] Transnasal endoscopic pituitary surgery was introduced in the 1990s in Europe and the United States.[14,15] Technological advancements over time have enabled surgeons to increase the success of skull base surgery so much that what was once an inoperable tumor on the skull base can now be removed endoscopically with lower complications, shorter hospital stays, and a lower morbidity rate.[16] To this end, indications for endoscopic approaches to the anterior skull base are broadening every year.

CT imaging was being used intraoperatively as early as the 1980s in neurosurgical procedures. Repeat scans of the operating field were taken intraoperatively to confirm probe tip positions, which was very impractical. It also resulted in excessive amounts of radiation to the patient. This method of image acquisition intraoperatively was abandoned for neurosurgical purposes. Instead, an imaging sequence was taken before surgery and placed on a "CT-dependent frame" for navigation purposes during surgery. However, this still presented complications because the frame of reference in neurosurgery was most often soft tissue, which often became an unreliable source after initiating surgery. In the early 2000s, CT-IGSs were exclusively used for identification of the complex bone anatomy of the skull base during endoscopic, endonasal skull base surgery. As a new approach, few sources of literature were available to study the anatomy, leaving innovative centers to rely on cadaveric dissections before exploring new corridors via the endoscopic approach and IGS was invaluable.

Advancements in understanding of endoscopic anterior skull base surgery anatomy and the refinement of IGS software allowing CT-based guided surgery coupled with MRI (fused) has led to improved accuracy and further delineation of the boundaries between brain, bone, tumor, and vasculature.[17] The MRI offers better soft tissue detail, while the CT offers more distinct bony detail. When coupled together, this technique has been beneficial in situations where anatomy has been altered, such as disease progression, pneumatization anomalies, fibro-osseous lesions, or other bony lesions. Additionally, fused CT/MRI or CT/magnetic resonance venography imaging is strongly encouraged in revision cases or any intracranial lesion where there is a possible distortion of the circle of Willis or the internal carotid arteries.

Indications and Outcomes

The American Academy of Otolaryngology recommends the use of IGSs during endonasal endoscopic cranial base surgery for benign and malignant neoplasms, CSF rhinorrhea, and other skull base defects. IGS is also recommended for any disease involving the skull base, orbit, optic nerve, or carotid artery. Currently, the need for IGS during skull base surgery is antedotal, as there is no data in the literature evaluating the need or improved outcomes with this technology.

Summary

Image-guided sinus surgery has evolved into a valuable adjunct for rhinologic and skull base conditions. The use of optical or electromagnetic navigational systems promises to increase surgeons' confidence and the ability to identify critical structures in distorted surgical fields. Studies quantifying the need for IGS are limited, though levels 4 and 5 evidence strongly suggest the use of this technology in select cases. Further comparative studies with and without image guidance would be helpful to answer two important questions. Does image guidance improve the safety of functional endoscopic sinus surgery and endonasal skull base surgery? Does image guidance improve the quality of the surgery performed and improve long-term benefits? Unfortunately, it may neither be practical nor ethical to perform such studies.

References

1. Bergström M, Greitz T. Stereotaxic computed tomography. AJR Am J Roentgenol 1976;127(1):167–170
2. Caversaccio M, Langlotz F, Nolte L-P, Häusler R. Impact of a self-developed planning and self-constructed navigation system on skull base surgery: 10 years experience. Acta Otolaryngol 2007;127(4):403–407
3. Metson RB, Cosenza MJ, Cunningham MJ, Randolph GW. Physician experience with an optical image guidance system for sinus surgery. Laryngoscope 2000;110(6):972–976
4. Snyderman CH, Zimmer LA, Kassam A. Sources of registration error with image guidance systems during endoscopic anterior cranial base surgery. Otolaryngol Head Neck Surg 2004;131(3):145–149
5. Ecke U, Luebben B, Maurer J, Boor S, Mann WJ. Comparison of different computer-aided surgery systems in skull base surgery. Skull Base 2003;13(1):43–50
6. Wiltfang J, Rupprecht S, Ganslandt O, et al. Intraoperative image-guided surgery of the lateral and anterior skull base in patients with tumors or trauma. Skull Base 2003;13(1):21–29
7. American Academy of Otolaryngology-Head and Neck Surgery. Policy on Intraoperative use of Computer Aided Surgery. AAO-HNS Official Website, Policy Statement, 2002. Available at: http://www.entlink.net/practice/rules/imaging-guiding.cfm
8. Metson R, Gray ST. Image-guided sinus surgery: practical considerations. Otolaryngol Clin North Am 2005;38(3):527–534
9. Tabaee A, Hsu AK, Shrime MG, Rickert S, Close LG. Quality of life and complications following image-guided endoscopic sinus surgery. Otolaryngol Head Neck Surg 2006;135(1):76–80
10. Reardon EJ. The impact of image-guidance systems on sinus surgery. Otolaryngol Clin North Am 2005;38(3):515–525
11. Sindwani R, Metson R. Impact of image guidance on complications during osteoplastic frontal sinus surgery. Otolaryngol Head Neck Surg 2004;131(3):150–155
12. Smith TL, Stewart MG, Orlandi RR, Setzen M, Lanza DC. Indications for image-guided sinus surgery: the current evidence. Am J Rhinol 2007;21(1):80–83
13. Kennedy DW. Functional endoscopic sinus surgery. Technique. Arch Otolaryngol 1985;111(10):643–649
14. Jankowski R, Auque J, Simon C, Marchal JC, Hepner H, Wayoff M. Endoscopic pituitary tumor surgery. Laryngoscope 1992;102(2):198–202
15. Carrau RL, Jho HD, Ko Y. Transnasal-transsphenoidal endoscopic surgery of the pituitary gland. Laryngoscope 1996;106(7):914–918
16. Stamm AM. Transnasal endoscopy-assisted skull base surgery. Ann Otol Rhinol Laryngol Suppl 2006;196:45–53
17. Chisholm EJ, Mendoza N, Nourei R, Grant WE. Fused CT and angiography image guided surgery for endoscopic skull base procedures: how we do it. Clin Otolaryngol 2008;33(6):625–628

14 Surgery of the Inferior Turbinates and Septum: Principles and Techniques

Rosser Kennedy Powitzky, Colby G. McLaurin, and Greg A. Krempl

Septal surgery is one of the most common procedures performed by a rhinologist. Septal abnormalities and turbinate hypertrophy can often prohibit the introduction of endoscopic instruments, and limit good visualization during surgical management of sinus and skull base pathology. Septal surgery is also often required to achieve other important objectives: maximizing nasal tip and dorsal stability, establishing an adequate and long-lasting airway for the patient, and removing any sinus outflow obstructions. While conventional closed septoplasty is a standard surgical approach for many otolaryngologists, conservative and endoscopic techniques are becoming more prominent. This chapter reviews techniques for both approaches as well as turbinate reduction, which commonly accompanies septal deviation surgery.

Anatomy

The nasal septum is the vertical midline structure that extends posteriorly from the columella and divides the nose into roughly symmetric halves. It consists of bone, cartilage, and soft tissue (**Fig. 14.1**). The bony components include the perpendicular plate of the ethmoid bone (PPE), the vomer, the perpendicular plate of the palatine bone, and the palatine extension of the maxilla.[1] The latter two components together are commonly known as the maxillary crest. The cartilaginous septum sits anterior to the vomer and PPE, and is roughly diamond-shaped or quadrangular. A sphenoid extension of cartilage extends between the vomer and PPE up toward the rostrum. The septal cartilage has dense fibrous attachments to the nasal bones and PPE superiorly, the vomer posteroinferiorly, and the palatine process and nasal spine of the maxilla bone caudally. The bony and cartilaginous septal floor is anatomically stabilized in a groove of the maxillary crest.

The inferior turbinates are paired structures consisting of bone and soft tissue that run the length of the inferior meatus from the pyriform aperture anteriorly often to the choana posteriorly. The inferior turbinate bone is a thin, curved bone that articulates with the maxilla at the lateral nasal wall. The nasal septum and inferior turbinates are covered with pseudostratified ciliated (respiratory) epithelium with numerous mucous-producing goblet cells. Beneath the epithelium is the lamina propria, which is rich with seromucinous glands and cavernous vascular tissue with large venous sinusoids. The septal blood flow is supplied by branches from the ethmoidal, sphenopalatine, greater palatine, and labial arteries. Innervation of the septum is from all three divisions of the trigeminal nerve. Knowledge of each branch is important for proper injection of local anesthetics and vasoconstrictors before surgery.[1]

Preoperative Patient Evaluation

Nasal airway obstruction remains the most common indication for surgery of the nasal septum and turbinates. Turbinate and rarely septal mucosal abnormalities can result in turbulent nonlamellar nasal airflow and the subjective sensation of nasal obstruction. Mucosa blood flow cycles can be altered by an inflammatory or infectious process. This can cause inflammatory cell infiltration of the lamina propria, reactive engorgement of the venous sinusoids, and subepithelial edema. Examples of such processes include infectious rhinosinusitis and allergic rhinitis. Secondary changes to the lymphatic and venous drainage, and to the connective tissue within the lamina propria after prolonged inflammation, lead to more permanent hypertrophy of these structures. This renders more resistance to topical decongestants and anti-inflammatory medications such as steroids.

Nasal airflow and/or sinus outflow tracts can also be disrupted by anatomic abnormalities such as septal deviation, spur, fracture, or dislocation from the maxillary crest. These may be caused by former nasal trauma, previous surgery, or congenital factors. When nasal airway obstruction persists despite maximal medical management, such as nasal steroids and topical antihistamines, surgical treatment is indicated.[2,3] Septoplasty may also be indicated for a deviated septum if the patient has epistaxis, intolerance to continuous positive airway pressure (CPAP) treatment, osteomeatal complex obstruction, or access obstruction for sinonasal procedures unrelated to the septum.

A proper history and physical examination with nasal fiberoptic evaluation is used to rule out other potential causes of nasal obstruction that may need to be addressed.[2]

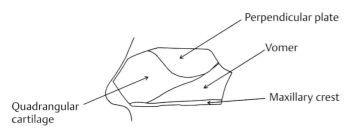

Quadrangular cartilage · Perpendicular plate · Vomer · Maxillary crest

Figure 14.1 Nasal septal anatomy.

Allergic rhinitis, rhinitis medicamentosum, polyps, neoplasms, concha bullosa, adenoid hypertrophy, choanal and pyriform stenosis, severe nasal dorsal deformity, lateral nasal wall collapse, and poor tip support should be properly diagnosed and managed. A history of obstructive sleep apnea (OSA) and CPAP intolerance should prompt a thorough evaluation of the entire upper airway. The region of septal deflection should also be noted during the examination as this will guide proper surgical planning and technique. A more caudal deviation may prompt a traditional closed approach to the septum, for example, while an isolated more posterior deviation or spur may be better addressed endoscopically.[4,5] Septal surgery can be complicated by congenital or traumatic pathology, former attempts at septoplasty or septectomy, preexisting septal perforation, or other obstructing intranasal pathology such as polyps. Complex cases should prompt an open and honest discussion with the patient concerning the higher risk for complications and reasonable expectations.

Although not always necessary, CT imaging may be useful to provide detailed anatomy of the septum and further evaluate concurrent sinonasal disease, such as chronic rhinosinusitis, concha bullosa, congenital narrowing of the pyriform or choana, nasal polyposis, or a neoplastic process. Patients should also be informed preoperatively about what to expect after surgery and the common and most severe complications that can occur.

Surgical Technique

Septoplasty

Traditional Closed Headlight Approach

Septoplasty can be performed with appropriately administered local anesthesia and sedation, however, the procedure is usually performed under general anesthesia. The most important surgical preparations in either situation are the use of a topical decongestant (oxymetazoline, neosynephrine, or 4% cocaine solution) and submucoperichondrial injection of a local anesthetic mixture containing epinephrine (1:100,000 being the most common concentration).

Under headlight illumination, a #15 scalpel is used to make either a hemitransfixion incision at the caudal edge of septal cartilage or a Killian incision just rostral to it (**Fig. 14.2**); these incisions allow approach to the septum to remove deviations and spurs, or when septal cartilage is needed for grafting purposes. Using a scraping maneuver

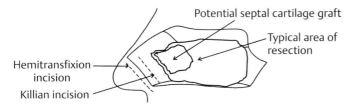

Figure 14.2   Septoplasty incisions.

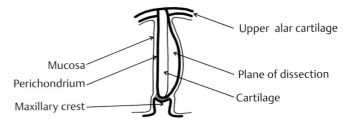

Figure 14.3   A submucoperichondrial flap.

(e.g., with a scalpel, freer, Cottle, or iris scissors), the submucoperichondrial plane is identified as a relatively avascular plane between glistening perichondrium and the more opaque, grainy-textured surface of septal cartilage. Planes should easily separate in this area with sharp then blunt elevation. Establishing the correct plane helps minimize blood loss and prevent septal tears. A nasal speculum is placed in the incision with intermittent use of a Frazier suction to improve visualization.

A submucoperichondrial flap (**Fig. 14.3**) is carefully elevated by advancing a blunt elevator underneath the flap until the bony-cartilaginous junction is encountered. The subperiosteal plane is identified in a similar fashion posterior to the bony-cartilaginous junction on both sides of the PPE and vomer. A Woodson elevator and floor of nose tunnel helps prevent tears raising the flap around bony spurs and the septal-maxillary crest junction. Much of this elevation may need to be performed without direct visualization because of anatomic constraints. If so, maintaining contact between the tip of the Cottle or Woodson elevator and the septal cartilage is important to ensure that the proper plane of dissection is maintained. Bluntly separating the bony-cartilaginous junction with the Freer at this point will often correct any cartilaginous deflection, that is, secondary to abnormalities of the PPE and the vomer. Flaps are widely undermined on both sides of the bony septum. Bony abnormalities are usually resected with a cutting instrument piecemeal (i.e., Jansen-Middleton forceps) or en bloc (i.e., double action scissors and Woodson). Care must be taken to avoid undue torsion on the superior portion of the PPE, which can fracture the cribriform plate and lead to leakage of cerebrospinal fluid or pneumocephalus. Caudal cartilaginous deformities can either be reshaped by scoring the cartilage with a knife on the opposite side of the deflection, or they can be resected being sure to leave at least 1 to 1.5 cm of cartilage as a strut both dorsally and caudally to maintain the support of the nasal tip. Resected cartilage can be carved and placed as a caudal strut to improve the stability of the nasal tip, to increase nasal projection, or to help correct a caudal deflection. Alternatively, cartilage can be banked between submucoperichondrial flaps before closure for potential future procedures if needed. Significant dorsal deflections are important to recognize and address as they can be a significant source of "memory" and redeviation of caudal cartilage. Resection of deviated dorsal cartilage must be maximized without compromising proper support for the nasal dorsum and tip. Alternatively, severe dorsal deviations with obvious external nasal dorsal deformity may be better addressed with an external septorhinoplasty approach, which is beyond the scope of this chapter.

The space between submucoperichondrial flaps is irrigated copiously with antibiotic-infused saline. If there are no holes in either flap, an incision can be made in the posteroinferior portion of elevated flaps on one side for drainage and to prevent hematoma collection. The flaps are reapproximated with a through-and-through quilting stitch of 4.0 plain gut suture on a straight Keith needle, and the incision is reapproximated with interrupted sutures of 4–0 chromic. Slimline merocel packing and reinforced silicone splints are optional for excessive bleeding or flap tears, respectively.

Endoscopic Approach

As endoscopic surgery for treatment of sinus disease has gained a solid foothold in sinus surgery, many patients prefer endoscopic approaches compared with septal surgery. Endoscopy adds certain advantages to the conventional methods of diagnosis and management of nasal septal deviation.[4–7] Nasal endoscopy with 0 degree and angled telescopes allows accurate localization of each of the contributing pathologic factors. Video projection is also a powerful educational tool, providing visualization of the operative field and surgical maneuvers to students, residents, and operating room staff. Some authors suggest operative time required for endoscopic septoplasty is at least equivocal compared with more open approaches.[5,6] One randomized small study also showed no significant decrease in the amount of complications with endoscopic surgery compared with the closed approach when treating limited septal deviations and spurs.[8] Paradis and Rotenberg noted in a large randomized comparison study that endoscopic septoplasty had significantly less complications and operating time compared with closed technique. The outcome patient satisfaction scores, however, did not significantly differ.[9]

The technique is very similar in description to the open endonasal approach to septoplasty, but with the benefit of endoscopic visualization.[7] Using a #15 scalpel or sickle knife a hemitransfixion incision is performed. Under 0 degree endoscopic visualization, the subperichondrial plane is identified in a similar manner as with the open technique. The magnification offered by endoscopy is helpful in establishing this plane. A suction elevator instrument that consists of a suction port at the end of an elevator (i.e., Cottle), can be useful in maintaining visualization. The remaining steps of the procedure are similar to the open endonasal approach with the exception of using an endoscope rather than a speculum and headlight to visualize the dissection.

Directed Endoscopic Approach

In septal surgery, endoscopy allows isolated spurs or septal deflections to be addressed directly.[5,7] The standard local anesthetic mixture with epinephrine is injected in a subperichondrial plane beginning just anterior to the spur.

Under endoscopic visualization an incision is made in an anteroposterior direction through mucosa directly overlying the spur. Submucoperichondrial flaps are raised superiorly and inferiorly over the spur. The bony or cartilaginous abnormality is resected, taking care not to tear the mucosa on the opposite side. The incision is closed and flaps are reapproximated with a single quilting stitch of 4.0 plain gut suture limited to the areas of flap elevation.

Inferior Turbinate Reduction

Inferior turbinate reduction or reshaping is often performed in conjunction with septoplasty. The indications are similar and are primarily for nasal obstruction refractory to medical management. Hypertrophy, particularly of the head of the inferior turbinate, can significantly reduce the cross-sectional area of the internal nasal valve available for airflow. Performed independently or in conjunction with septoplasty, inferior turbinate reduction can be an effective long-term remedy to nasal obstruction.

There are a number of different treatment options for inferior turbinate reduction, although most surgeons only use 1 or 2 of them as part of their standard treatment. These include outfracture, cautery, radiofrequency ablation, cryotherapy, laser reduction, and submucous resection with or without powered instrumentation.[4,5] The goal of each is similar: to reduce the volume of the tissue components obstructing the nasal airway and to minimize blood loss. It is beyond the scope of this chapter to discuss the comparative risks and benefits of each technique. We will outline two common techniques.

Traditional Headlight Approach

The procedure is usually performed under general anesthesia in conjunction with septoplasty. Under headlight illumination through a nasal speculum the head and body of the inferior turbinate are injected with a local anesthetic mixture containing epinephrine (1:100,000 being the most common concentration). After giving adequate time for vasoconstriction (10 to 15 minutes), a steel 18-gauge spinal needle clamped in a hemostat and bent at the hub is inserted in the head of the turbinate and advanced submucosally for the length of the turbinate. Monopolar cautery is applied to the hemostat as it is slowly withdrawn from the turbinate over 8 to 10 seconds. Care must be taken so that the needle does not contact the nasal speculum or vestibule during cautery to avoid cautery burns. This is repeated two to three times. Finally, the inferior turbinate is fractured medially along its entire length using a Freer elevator and then laterally with an out fracture instrument (i.e., speculum). Nasal packing is usually not required, although small amounts of Surgicel may be beneficial to control mild oozing or help prevent synechiae.

Endoscopic Approach

Because inferior turbinate surgery is also often performed in the setting of concurrent sinus surgery, endoscopes and

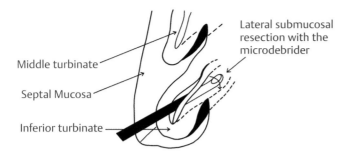

Figure 14.4 Turbinate reduction with a microdebrider.

powered instrumentation are often available and easily adapted to turbinoplasty.[10] A 0-degree scope is positioned at the nasal aperture for visualization of the inferior turbinate. After application of topical decongestant, the head of the turbinate is injected with a local anesthetic mixture containing epinephrine (1:100,000 being the most common concentration). After allowing adequate time for vasoconstriction, a stab incision is made in the head of the turbinate with a #11 scalpel. Submucosal dissection between the medial soft tissue and the turbinate bone is performed with a Cottle elevator. The bone and lateral soft tissue of the turbinate can then be resected submucosally or with the mucosa with Stevens tenotomy scissors or through-cut forceps under endoscopic visualization. Alternatively, a 2.5-cm suction microdebrider blade can be inserted into the stab incision and used both for dissection and submucosal resection of bone and lateral soft tissue with preservation of the turbinate mucosa (**Fig. 14.4**). Healing occurs over the course of 2 to 4 weeks with scarring in the lamina propria layer, which limits the propensity for local venous congestion and recurrent hypertrophy.

Postoperative Care and Complications

Patients are usually followed-up in clinic postoperatively at 1 week, 1 month, and 3 months to remove crusts, help educate patients on proper postoperative care, and observe for any complications. In the immediate postanesthesia period, patients who have sleep apnea should be observed for complications such as respiratory or airway compromise. Often the patient's CPAP is helpful to use in recovery as the patient awakens for anesthesia if the sleep apnea is severe enough. Mild oozing frequently occurs over the first couple of days, and Afrin (oxymetazoline) is often given to stop the oozing. Patients should avoid heavy lifting, sneezing or blowing through the nose, and strenuous activity for 2 weeks. Crusting of the septoplasty incision and turbinates is a common occurrence that can be avoided and treated with saline sprays or rinses and ointment. Splints should be removed after 1 week with antibiotic coverage for staph to prevent toxic shock syndrome.

A hematoma and subsequent abscess can occur up to 2 weeks after surgery or longer if further trauma to the nose occurs postoperatively. This should be quickly recognized and evacuated with drain placement to minimize necrosis of cartilage and nasal support. Bilateral flap tears opposing each other create high risk for septal perforations. This risk (0.4 to 12%) is minimized by approximating tears with closing suture techniques (i.e., endoscopic), stabilizing and covering a cartilage graft in between, and septal splints with ointment to promote healing.[11] Midface growth delay or deficiency is a theoretical risk in young children that prompt some surgeons to wait until after puberty or be cautious with more conservative surgery in the pediatric population.[12]

Overaggressive manipulation or resection of the septum can have significant sequelae. Cerebrospinal fluid leakage at the cribiform can occur from aggressive fracture of the dorsal bony septum. Saddle nose deformity can occur from overresection of dorsal cartilage (0.4 to 3.4% risk).[11] Too high of dissection can cause disruption of the upper lateral cartilage attachment to the septum. Overresection or weakening of the caudal septum can cause nasal tip depression and may be prevented in high-risk patients with a caudal strut graft. Although sometimes required, removal of the anterior maxillary crest or nasal spine can cause numbness of the upper lip and incisors and destabilize the septum at the floor of the nose if not reattached to the periosteum with nonabsorbable suture. Turbinate surgery also contains potential complications, including synechiae with the septum and empty nose syndrome or the sensation of nasal obstruction from overresection of mucosa causing a lack of laminar airflow during respiration.

A more frequent and long-term risk of septal and turbinate surgery is persistent nasal obstruction, which can be caused by several factors.[13] Memory in the cartilage or improper release of septal components from deviating fixed structures, such as a crooked dorsum or dislocated septal maxillary junction, can often "pull" the septum during postoperative healing back to the preoperative deviated position.[3,13] Candidates for open septorhinoplasty need to be properly identified to treat severe dorsal deformities, poor tip support, and lateral nasal valvular collapse simultaneously with the septum.[4] Failure to recognize patients with previous nasal surgery may also compromise the surgeon's ability to reinforce or maintain the integrity of nasal support structures.

Conclusion

Treatment of the septum and inferior turbinates can be effective in patients when performed properly and after examining for other causes of obstruction. Either separately or in combination, these procedures can help relieve nasal obstruction or help with access to the nasal cavity for other procedures. Advances in technology and techniques have added to the surgical armamentarium of the otolaryngologist.

References

1. Standring S, Berkovitz BKB, Hackney CM, Ruskell GL, Collins P, Wigley C. Nose, nasal cavity, paranasal sinuses, and pterygopalatine fossa. In: Standring S, ed. Head and Neck, Gray's Anatomy: The Anatomical Basis of Clinical Practise. New York, NY: Elsevier; 2005:567–579

2. Fettman N, Sanford T, Sindwani R. Surgical management of the deviated septum: techniques in septoplasty. Otolaryngol Clin North Am 2009;42(2):241–252, viii

3. Mlynski G. Surgery of the nasal septum. Facial Plast Surg 2006; 22(4):223–229

4. Dolan RW. Endoscopic septoplasty. Facial Plast Surg 2004; 20(3):217–221

5. Getz AE, Hwang PH. Endoscopic septoplasty. Curr Opin Otolaryngol Head Neck Surg 2008;16(1):26–31

6. Hwang PH, McLaughlin RB, Lanza DC, Kennedy DW. Endoscopic septoplasty: indications, technique, and results. Otolaryngol Head Neck Surg 1999;120(5):678–682

7. Chung BJ, Batra PS, Citardi MJ, Lanza DC. Endoscopic septoplasty: revisitation of the technique, indications, and outcomes. Am J Rhinol 2007;21(3):307–311

8. Bothra R, Mathur NN. Comparative evaluation of conventional versus endoscopic septoplasty for limited septal deviation and spur. J Laryngol Otol 2009;123(7):737–741

9. Paradis J, Rotenberg BW. Open versus endoscopic septoplasty: a single-blinded, randomized, controlled trial. J Otolaryngol Head Neck Surg 2011;40(1)(Suppl 1):S28–S33

10. Gupta A, Mercurio E, Bielamowicz S. Endoscopic inferior turbinate reduction: an outcomes analysis. Laryngoscope 2001;111(11, pt 1): 1957–1959

11. Ketcham AS, Han JK. Complications and management of septoplasty. Otolaryngol Clin North Am 2010;43(4):897–904

12. Christophel JJ, Gross CW. Pediatric septoplasty. Otolaryngol Clin North Am 2009;42(2):287–294, ix

13. Sillers MJ, Cox AJ III, Kulbersh B. Revision septoplasty. Otolaryngol Clin North Am 2009;42(2):261–278, viii

15 Surgery of the Ethmoid, Maxillary, and Sphenoid Sinuses

Edward D. McCoul and Vijay K. Anand

Surgery of the paranasal sinuses is one of the most common procedures in modern otolaryngologic practice, which reflects the high prevalence of chronic rhinosinusitis in developed countries.[1] The widespread use of nasal endoscopy in contemporary practice has resulted in the acceptance of endoscopic sinus surgery (ESS) as the standard of care for the great majority of surgical indications. Moreover, an appreciation of normal sinus anatomy and function, beginning with the work of Messerklinger and Wigand et al, has led to the adoption of ESS in context of functional preservation.[2,3] The principles of functional ESS are based on certain theoretical considerations: (1) sinusitis is rhinogenic in origin and (2) recurrent sinusitis is usually because of stenosis at the ostiomeatal unit. The additional assumption that inflammation most commonly affects the ethmoid sinus implies that the failure to successfully treat pansinusitis is usually because of the inadequate treatment of ethmoidal sinusitis.[4]

A contemporary discussion of paranasal sinus surgery should focus on preserving normal function and limiting dissection to include only diseased structures. The primary goal of functional ESS is the restoration of physiological drainage and ventilation patterns, and is by definition a limited surgery. A secondary goal is to create a pathway for the application of topical intranasal sinus therapy, which is routinely practiced in many patients with chronic rhinosinusitis. This is especially germane for individuals with medical conditions that affect mucociliary flow and mucus formation.

Surgical Principles

Adherence to the principles of sound surgical technique is of central importance to surgery of the paranasal sinuses. Foremost among these principles is a mastery of the pertinent anatomy, which begins with cadaveric study and continues with a stepwise progression of clinical experience. The second principle is obtaining excellent visualization of the surgical target and surrounding structures, which is facilitated by modern fiberoptic endoscopes that provide a view that is both panoramic and microscopic. The third principle is the maintenance of thorough hemostasis throughout the operation. Methods for achieving hemostasis include pressure, pharmacological vasoconstriction, promotion of the clotting cascade, and direct surgical cautery. The fourth principle is minimization of trauma to normal tissue. Unnecessary trauma to nasal mucosa is likely to impair postoperative function and counters attempts at maintaining intraoperative hemostasis.

Nonendoscopic Procedures

As the utilization of ESS has increased, several conventional sinus surgery techniques have fallen out of favor. These operations, developed in the preantibiotic era, were designed to exenterate infections but left a cicatrix-filled sinus cavity without mucociliary function in many patients. Therefore, the following techniques should be reserved for clinical scenarios where ESS is not practicable.

External Ethmoidectomy

External ethmoidectomy remains an acceptable treatment for acute subperiosteal abscess when endoscopic capability is not available. This approach uses a Lynch incision near the medial canthus to access the lamina papyracea through a transorbital route. This is also the traditional approach for ligation of the anterior and posterior ethmoidal arteries. The disadvantages of this technique include an external scar and poor visualization of the adjacent sinuses, and it is not suitable for the routine treatment of chronic rhinosinusitis.

Intranasal Ethmoidectomy

Intranasal ethmoidectomy with a speculum and headlight was the preferred method before the availability of nasal endoscopes.[5] Direct access to the ethmoid sinuses was possible, although visualization was limited without sacrifice of the middle turbinate. This technique is limited by imprecise hemostasis and confinement to one-handed operation while the other hand wields the nasal speculum. In addition, the optics are limited by a narrow view through the nares and a proximal light source, in contrast with ESS, in which the fiberoptic endoscope provides a distal light source. The use of the endoscope enhances visualization of the surgical field and permits the surgeon to operate precisely at the surgical site and recreate normal physiologic function.

Endonasal Inferior Meatal Antrostomy

Inferior meatal antrostomy was historically performed in the routine treatment of acute maxillary sinusitis. However, while the creation of a nonphysiological antrostomy provides ventilation, it does not permit restoration of normal mucociliary clearance. Therefore, it is not a reliable alternative to middle meatal antrostomy in functional surgery for the treatment of chronic rhinosinusitis.[6]

Sublabial Maxillary Antrostomy

This technique, also known as the Caldwell-Luc procedure, requires a sublabial incision with permanent removal of bone over the canine fossa. As with the inferior meatal antrostomy, this operation does not restore the normal physiological condition that is required for the functional treatment of chronic rhinosinusitis. Its use in contemporary practice may be best suited for the extirpation of solid matter, such as a mycetoma or inverted papilloma, which cannot be removed by an endonasal approach.[7]

Operative Planning

Imaging and Navigation

Preoperative computed tomography (CT) imaging is mandatory in the work-up of a patient with rhinosinusitis for whom surgery is being considered. Dedicated coronal, sagittal, and axial views of the paranasal sinuses are preferred. Careful interpretation of the films by the operating surgeon will reveal areas of anatomical variability, bony erosion, and mucocele formation, and will help prevent surgical complications. The preoperative CT scan may be obtained using one of several acquisition protocols for use with a commercially available system for intraoperative navigation.[8]

Instrumentation

Endoscopes

Familiarity with rigid fiberoptic nasal endoscopes is essential for performing ESS. Rigid scopes can be operated with the nondominant hand while surgical instruments can be used simultaneously by the dominant hand. This technique permits the surgeon to dynamically control the field of view during the procedure, which effectively compensates for the absence of stereoscopic vision. The 0-degree endoscope provides a circumferential view and is usually preferred for nasal preparation and the initial surgical steps. Endoscopes angled at 30, 45, and 70 degrees are valuable for providing a direct view of the ostia of the frontal and maxillary sinuses. New endoscopes have also been introduced, which provide variable optical deflection using a single instrument (Acclarent, Menlo Park, California; Karl Storz, Tuttlingen, Germany).

Nonpowered Instrumentation

Surgical instruments for endoscopic surgery generally consist of probes, punches, and forceps. Probes include the angled frontal and maxillary sinus probes, olive-tipped suction cannulas, and the von Eicken antrum cannula. The Freer elevator is a versatile instrument that can be used to medialize or lateralize turbinates and to advance cottonoids

or other adjunctive materials into the desired location. Punches include the straight and angled true-cut punch, the Grunewald punch, mushroom punches, back-biting antrum punches, and Kerrison rongeurs. Forceps include the bayonet, Takahashi, Blakesley-Wilde, and Janson-Middleton.

Powered Instrumentation

Tissue shavers and drills have a role in ESS in certain scenarios. Use of a tissue shaver or microdebrider may aid in shortening operative time in patients with massive polyposis or in whom mucosal edema is severe. Similarly, performance of an uncomplicated ESS may be expedited by the use of powered instrumentation. When hyperostotic chronic rhinosinusitis is present, the presence of thick bony septations may require the use of a high-powered endoscopic drill. While powered instrumentation adds the benefit of speed and internal suction, the potential for propagation of inadvertent intracranial or orbital injury suggests that these instruments should be reserved for use in experienced hands.[9,10]

Electrosurgical equipment has a limited role in ESS. Regardless, a variety of endoscopic attachments are available for use with unipolar and bipolar cautery, which may be useful if bleeding from a discrete arterial vessel is present. Blind cauterization of mucosal bleeding is generally an ineffective enterprise.

Balloon Technology

The recent introduction of specialized balloon catheter systems for sinus dilation has expanded the instrumentation available to the endoscopic sinus surgeon (Acclarent; Entellus Medical, Plymouth, Minnesota). Variable angulation of the catheters permits access to the frontal, maxillary, and sphenoid sinuses under endoscopic guidance. Observational studies have suggested that dilation of sinus ostia without tissue removal is effective in some patients with chronic rhinosinusitis.[11,12] Further study is needed to determine the appropriate role of these instruments in the treatment of paranasal sinus disease.

Adjunctive Materials

A variety of nondurable surgical supplies are available as surgical adjuncts. Cottonoid pledgets can be used liberally throughout the operation to provide focal hemostatic pressure and to apply pharmacological agents. Topical application of thrombin, with or without epinephrine, is a useful strategy to prevent intraoperative and postoperative bleeding. Dissolvable hemostatic agents such as Surgicel (Ethicon Inc., Somerville, New Jersey), Surgiflo (Ethicon), and FloSeal (Baxter, Deerfield, Illinois) may be useful for maintaining hemostasis at the conclusion of the case.[13–15] A variety of dissolvable and nondissolvable packing materials are available, although their necessity has not been well established.[16] Drug-eluting stents have been recently introduced and remain on the horizon of potential adjuncts.

Anesthesia

The majority of individuals undergoing ESS are otherwise healthy and are at low risk for anesthetic complications. Nevertheless, discussion with the practitioner administering anesthesia during the procedure is advisable in the event that unforeseen circumstances arise. In particular, patients with chronic upper airway obstruction, such as from nasal septal deviation or severe nasal polyposis, may have signs of upper airway resistance syndrome. Such patients may benefit from alternate anesthetic regimens, nonnarcotic analgesia, and overnight postoperative monitoring.

General anesthesia is preferred for all forms of paranasal sinus surgery, although monitored sedation with local anesthesia may be considered for limited surgery in patients for whom the risk of general anesthesia is considered unacceptable.[17] Advantages of general anesthesia include efficiency, reduced pain perception, controlled ventilation, and avoidance of aspiration. Endotracheal intubation is the standard for airway control, although use of the laryngeal mask airway has been adopted by some practitioners.[18] Blood pressure should be maintained near hypotensive range to facilitate intraoperative hemostasis.

Endoscopic Techniques

Positioning

The patient is positioned supine on the operative table with one or both of the arms tucked at the side. A slight incline of the head of the bed may be preferred, and the surgeon may choose to sit or stand during the operation. A right-handed surgeon is usually most comfortable standing at the patient's right side and holding the endoscope in the left hand. The video monitor may be positioned across the table from the surgeon, or, in cases where an assistant is present, at the head of the bed along the long axis of the patient's body.

Nasal Preparation

Adequate preparation of the nasal cavity is critical to performing successful ESS. The rich vascularity and reactivity of the intranasal mucosa will obscure the surgical field and increase the risk of complications if the preparatory steps are omitted. Mucosal vasoconstriction is facilitated by the topical application of a sympathomimetic agent, the most commonly used of which are phenylephrine and cocaine. These may be applied to cottonoid pledgets, which should be placed atraumatically using a bayonet forceps and assisted by a nasal speculum and headlamp. A minimum of four pledgets should be used initially, placed superiorly into the bilateral sphenoethmoid recess and inferiorly along the bilateral inferior turbinates.

Local Anesthesia

In cases where septoplasty or polypectomy are being performed concurrent with ESS, injection with a local anesthetic may be performed with a headlamp before applying the surgical drapes. Otherwise, intranasal injection is performed with endoscopic guidance before the surgical start. A short-acting local anesthetic, such as 1% lidocaine is preferred, typically mixed with 1:100,000 epinephrine, and is delivered using a syringe with a long shaft that is angled distally. Key intranasal structures that should be infiltrated with anesthetic include the head and vertical suspension of the middle turbinate, the face of the sphenoid, the uncinate process and the ethmoid bulla. Medialization of the middle turbinate with a Freer elevator will permit access to these latter structures. After injection, a cottonoid pledget with topical decongestant may be placed into the middle meatus. Injection of the sphenopalatine foramen is an important step that reduces intraoperative bleeding and mitigates postoperative pain.[19]

Surgical Steps

Uncinectomy/Infundibulotomy

The technique of functional ESS rests on the assumption that most sinusitis results from obstruction at the ostiomeatal complex. As the anterior ethmoid, frontal, and maxillary sinuses each open into the ethmoid infundibulum, meticulous surgical management of this narrow region is essential to a successful outcome. The goal of surgery is to restore normal paranasal sinus mucociliary function and facilitate adequate sinus ventilation.

The infundibulum is the anterior-most part of the ethmoid sinus. Infundibulotomy is the necessary first step in the great majority of ESS where the intention is treatment of ethmoid and maxillary sinusitis. If the nasal septum interferes with adequate visualization of the ostiomeatal unit, a septoplasty should be performed before continuing. The middle turbinate should be reflected medially and the uncinate process palpated to ascertain the precise site of attachment with the maxillary bone anteriorly (**Fig. 15.1**).[20]

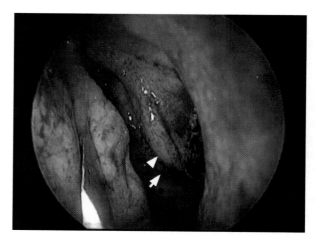

Figure 15.1 Endoscopic appearance of a left nasal cavity showing the uncinate process (arrowhead), which is partially obscuring the ethmoidal bulla (arrow). The middle turbinate is retracted medially with a sickle knife.

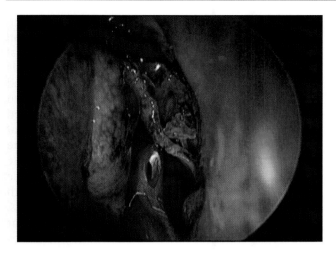

Figure 15.2 Endoscopic appearance after the uncinectomy incision. The middle turbinate has been medialized. An angled Blakesley-Wilde forceps is used to remove the uncinate bone and mucosa.

The uncinectomy incision should be made along this plane of attachment using a sharp instrument such as a sickle knife (**Fig. 15.2**). This incision can be most safely made just lateral to the inferior third of the middle turbinate, which corresponds to the position of the natural ostium of the maxillary sinus; a properly placed incision will typically result in release of a tell-tale air bubble. The uncinectomy is extended inferiorly and posteriorly toward the inferior turbinate and superiorly to the vertical attachment of the middle turbinate. Bony fragments can then be removed using an angled forceps.

Care should be taken to complete the uncinectomy by removing any remnants of uncinate bone, especially at the superior end of the infundibulum near the frontal recess. Miniature Kerrison rongeurs and double-angled fine cutting forceps are ideally suited for these maneuvers. Failure to identify and remove the uncinate process in its entirety can lead to postoperative scarring, obstruction, mucocele, and persistent sinusitis.[21]

Maxillary Sinusotomy

Maxillary sinusotomy, also called maxillary antrostomy, is performed in accordance with the principles of functional ESS by identifying and enlarging the naturally occurring sinus ostium. This is facilitated by performing a complete uncinectomy as described in the preceding section. The maxillary sinus ostium reliably lies in the parasagittal plane at a position lateral to the inferior third of the middle turbinate.[22] Preoperative CT scan will identify the uncommon cases where the maxillary sinus is atelectatic or the natural ostium is oriented in a horizontal plane.

Endoscopic examination may reveal one or more small openings in the lateral nasal wall posterior to the infundibulum. These openings, called fontanelles, are believed to represent the sequelae of previous infectious episodes. Enlargement of these "false" ostia is a pitfall that will fail to reestablish normal mucociliary clearance, and

may cause the surgeon to overlook the correct site at the natural sinus ostium within the infundibulum.[23,24]

Several methods are available for the enlargement of maxillary sinus ostium. These include side-biting punches, straight and angled forceps, and the powered tissue shaver. Over-aggressive bone removal anteriorly should be avoided to prevent injury to the nasolacrimal duct and postoperative epiphora. The extent of posterior enlargement should be gauged by visualizing the posterior maxillary sinus wall, which will prevent disruption of the sphenopalatine artery as it emerges from the pterygopalatine fossa. The surgeon should avoid opening the superior part of the ostium until the location of the bony orbital floor is known with certainty.[25] Visualization of the maxillary sinus lumen with an angled 30- or 45-degree endoscope can yield important information. If sinus polyps or fungal matter is present it can be extracted using angled forceps. Sinus irrigation is not routinely required, but may be performed using an angled catheter, such as in cases of maxillary empyema.

Anterior Ethmoidectomy

Agger Nasi Cells

Pneumatization of the preinfundibular bone can produce narrowing of the frontal outflow tract. Failure to address these cells during surgery can result in frontal sinusitis and persistent ethmoiditis. Safe exenteration of agger nasi cells may be accomplished with upwardly angled forceps and miniature Kerrison rongeurs. Care should be taken to avoid unnecessary tissue removal at the frontal recess, as this may lead to postoperative stenosis and frontal sinus obstruction.

Haller Cells

Pneumatized cells that extend into the maxillary sinus antrum may promote obstruction of that sinus. These cells, called Haller cells, must be distinguished from the orbital floor. Study of coronal CT images is necessary to guide the dissection and avoid inadvertent orbital injury, as well as to prevent a diseased cell from being overlooked.[26] The use of angled endoscopes and instruments is important when opening laterally placed cells. For cells that are positioned completely within the maxillary sinus, medial "uncapping" of the cell may be sufficient rather than complete exenteration, which would require a Caldwell-Luc approach.

Ethmoidal Bulla

The anterior face of the ethmoidal bulla should be visible following adequate uncinectomy. The bulla is entered medially with a full view of the apex of the hiatus semilunaris. Bone is then removed sequentially in an inferolateral and superolateral direction. Dissection should remain posterior to anterior ethmoidal artery, which lies consistently within the posterior wall of the frontal recess. Completion of the anterior ethmoidectomy should result in exposure of the suprabullar and retrobullar recesses. Pneumatization within the sinus lateralis may require additional exenteration laterally, taking care to avoid violation of the lamina papyracea with inadvertent orbital entry.

Concha Bullosa

Pneumatization of the middle turbinate represents an extension of the ethmoid labyrinth that may produce compensatory septal deviation or middle meatal obstruction. Resection of a concha bullosa should be performed so as to preserve the turbinate as a landmark while allowing adequate ventilation. Several techniques have been advocated, including resection of the anterior, inferior, or lateral walls of the concha bullosa. Our preferred method begins with a vertical incision made with a sickle knife in the parasagittal plane. A Struycken nasal cutting forceps is then used to resect the lateral portion of the concha bullosa, facing the middle meatus and the rest of the ethmoid dissection.

Posterior Ethmoidectomy

If a disease is present in the posterior ethmoid sinuses, a posterior ethmoidectomy should be performed. The lateral attachment of the middle turbinate, called the ground lamella, should be entered inferiorly and medially using an upbiting Blakesley-Wilde forceps. Once entry into the posterior ethmoidal sinus is achieved, the surgeon should continue to work in an inferomedial direction, toward the location of the natural sphenoid sinus ostium. The superior and lateral areas are close to the optic nerve and carotid artery and should be avoided. The surgeon must remain constantly aware of the location of the skull base, which in the majority of patients slopes gradually downward in an anterior-to-posterior direction. Study of the sagittal CT scan images will reveal this relationship.

The posterior-most ethmoid cell is referred to as the Onodi cell, and is notable for being in direct association with the orbital apex. The optic nerve typically runs in the posteriosuperior wall of this cell, and in approximately 12% of cases the canal may be dehiscent.[27] For this reason, aggressive dissection within an Onodi cell is not advised.

Sphenoid Sinusotomy

Transnasal Approach

The natural ostium of the sphenoid sinus is found on the sphenoid rostrum just medial to the inferior third of the superior turbinate (**Fig. 15.3**). This corresponds to an approximately 30-degree incline above the horizontal plane of the nasal floor.[28] Meticulous decongestion is required to reveal the sphenoid ostium, and lateralization of the turbinate with a Freer elevator is often necessary. Once the ostium has been identified it is entered initially using a mushroom punch. The sinusotomy is enlarged circumferentially using a Kerrison rongeur or a tissue shaver. Care should be taken to limit the inferior dissection so that the sphenopalatine artery is not injured as it courses above the choana. The inferior portion of the superior turbinate may be resected to improve exposure, although the superior portion should be preserved as a landmark and to prevent inadvertent injury to the skull base.

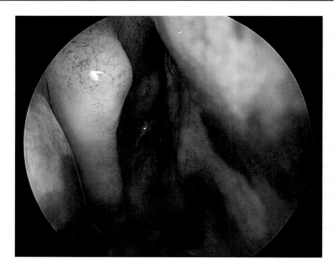

Figure 15.3 Endoscopic appearance of a right nasal cavity showing the sphenoid sinus natural ostium (center) just medial to the inferior third of the superior turbinate.

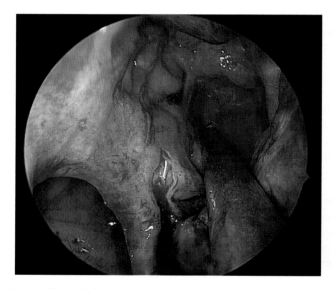

Figure 15.4 Endoscopic appearance of a postsurgical right ethmoid sinus cavity 6 months after primary surgery. The instrument placed against the sphenoid rostrum indicates the site of entry for transethmoidal sphenoidotomy, just lateral to the superior turbinate. The healed maxillary antrostomy is visible at the lower left.

Transethmoidal Approach

Sphenoid sinusotomy may also be performed in conjunction with total ethmoidectomy via a transethmoidal approach. After the last ethmoid cell has been opened, the surgical field should be examined with regard to the height of the skull base and relationship to the level of the maxillary antrostomy (**Fig. 15.4**). Sphenoidotomy is performed by entering the sinus at the inferomedial face of the sphenoid sinus, adjacent to the posterior attachment of the superior turbinate. The sinusotomy is enlarged by circumferential bone removal, which should extend medially to include the natural sinus ostium. Tissue removal or irrigation within the sinus may be appropriate in selected cases, although this is not routinely necessary.

Postoperative Care

ESS is generally performed as an ambulatory surgery from which the patient returns home the same day. While some surgeons advocate postoperative nasal packing for 24 hours or longer, this may not be necessary in every case. We have found that meticulous intraoperative hemostasis combined with the application of an absorbable hemostatic agent at the conclusion of the case is effective prevention against postoperative epistaxis. A small piece of folded nonadherent sponge such as Telfa (Covidien, Mansfield, Massachusetts) placed as a splint into the middle meatus under endoscopic guidance adds a measure of hemostasis as well as effectively preventing lateralization of the middle turbinate during the postoperative period.

Patient should be instructed to anticipate a small amount of mucosanguinous nasal discharge over the first 24 to 48 hours postoperatively. Nose blowing, heavy exercising, and forcible sneezing should be discouraged. The patient should refrain from ingesting compounds that may interfere with normal clotting, including nonsteroidal anti-inflammatory drugs, anticoagulants, vitamin E, and many herbal supplements. The requirement for postoperative analgesia is generally minimal, and may consist of acetaminophen with the addition of a mild narcotic, such as codeine, in selected cases.[29] Oral antibiotics should be continued until the removal of any nonaborsbable surgical material.

Postoperative examination in the office should be performed 5 to 7 days following surgery, at which time any nasal splints may be removed. The sinus cavities are inspected and postoperative crusting is debrided endoscopically. At this time, daily nasal topical therapy may begin, which may include sprays, irrigation or aerosols.[30] Topical therapy may consist of buffered saline solution or may be compounded with antibiotic or steroid agents as deemed clinically necessary. Subsequent examinations occur at regular intervals until the sinuses are well healed and crusting has resolved.

Revision Surgery

The techniques covered previously in this chapter are applicable to cases with intact anatomy that have not had previous sinus surgery. However, a subset of patients with chronic rhinosinusitis experience a long-term relapsing and remitting course of disease that may require additional surgical management. In these cases, important landmarks may have been sacrificed by prior surgical attempts, and active inflammation may obscure anatomic boundaries. The adjunctive use of intraoperative CT navigation may be particularly important for accomplishing the goals of revision surgery and avoiding complications. The components of

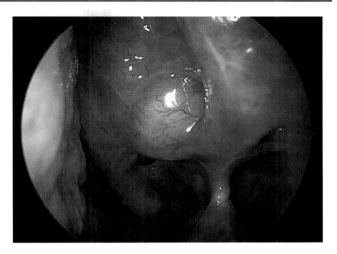

Figure 15.5 Appearance of a mucocele arising from an obstructed ethmoidal cell 1 year after total ethmoidectomy, maxillary antrostomy, and transethmoidal sphenoidotomy.

revision surgery may include lysis of synechiae, resection of polypoid disease, enlargement of stenotic sphenoid or maxillary sinus ostia, and exenteration of isolated ethmoid cells at the skull base or orbital wall (**Fig. 15.5**). Obstruction of the ostiomeatal unit by residual uncinate process is a common reason for surgical failure and should be sought out carefully. Frontal sinusotomy may be required, which is beyond the scope of this chapter. Although certain cases may require extensive revision surgery, in many cases the operative plan calls for target-oriented surgery directed at specific pathology. Each revision ESS should be individualized to the patient with regard to disease process, anatomy, and expected outcome.

Conclusion

Surgery of the ethmoid, maxillary, and sphenoid sinuses is the cornerstone of management for patients with refractory chronic rhinosinusitis. ESS is well established as the technique of choice because of the ability to enhance the natural mucociliary clearance and restore normal sinonasal function. Variability in technique is possible as long as adherence to basic surgical principles is maintained. Attention to detail during ESS is essential to accomplishing the goals of treatment and preventing postoperative complications.

References

1. Anand VK. Epidemiology and economic impact of rhinosinusitis. Ann Otol Rhinol Laryngol Suppl 2004;193:3–5
2. Stammberger H. Endoscopic endonasal surgery—concepts in treatment of recurring rhinosinusitis. Part I. Anatomic and pathophysiologic considerations. Otolaryngol Head Neck Surg 1986;94(2):143–147
3. Wigand ME, Steiner W, Jaumann MP. Endonasal sinus surgery with endoscopical control: from radical operation to rehabilitation of the mucosa. Endoscopy 1978;10(4):255–260

4. Proctor DF. The nose, paranasal sinuses and pharynx. In: Walters W, ed. Lewis-Walters Practice of Surgery. 4th ed. Hagerstown, MD: WF Prior; 1966:1–37

5. Lawson W. The intranasal ethmoidectomy: an experience with 1,077 procedures. Laryngoscope 1991;101(4, pt 1):367–371

6. Lund VJ. The results of inferior and middle meatal antrostomy under endoscopic control. Acta Otorhinolaryngol Belg 1993;47(1):65–71

7. Barzilai G, Greenberg E, Uri N. Indications for the Caldwell-Luc approach in the endoscopic era. Otolaryngol Head Neck Surg 2005;132(2):219–220

8. Fried MP, Parikh SR, Sadoughi B. Image-guidance for endoscopic sinus surgery. Laryngoscope 2008;118(7):1287–1292

9. Graham SM, Nerad JA. Orbital complications in endoscopic sinus surgery using powered instrumentation. Laryngoscope 2003;113(5):874–878

10. Church CA, Chiu AG, Vaughan WC. Endoscopic repair of large skull base defects after powered sinus surgery. Otolaryngol Head Neck Surg 2003;129(3):204–209

11. Bolger WE, Brown CL, Church CA, et al. Safety and outcomes of balloon catheter sinusotomy: a multicenter 24-week analysis in 115 patients. Otolaryngol Head Neck Surg 2007;137(1):10–20

12. Weiss RL, Church CA, Kuhn FA, Levine HL, Sillers MJ, Vaughan WC. Long-term outcome analysis of balloon catheter sinusotomy: two-year follow-up. Otolaryngol Head Neck Surg 2008; 139(3)(suppl 3):S38–S46

13. Chandra RK, Conley DB, Kern RC. The effect of FloSeal on mucosal healing after endoscopic sinus surgery: a comparison with thrombin-soaked gelatin foam. Am J Rhinol 2003;17(1):51–55

14. Shinkwin CA, Beasley N, Simo R, Rushton L, Jones NS. Evaluation of Surgicel Nu-knit, Merocel and Vasolene gauze nasal packs: a randomized trial. Rhinology 1996;34(1):41–43

15. Woodworth BA, Chandra RK, LeBenger JD, Ilie B, Schlosser RJ. A gelatin-thrombin matrix for hemostasis after endoscopic sinus surgery. Am J Otolaryngol 2009;30(1):49–53

16. Orlandi RR, Lanza DC. Is nasal packing necessary following endoscopic sinus surgery? Laryngoscope 2004;114(9):1541–1544

17. Eberhart LHJ, Folz BJ, Wulf H, Geldner G. Intravenous anesthesia provides optimal surgical conditions during microscopic and endoscopic sinus surgery. Laryngoscope 2003;113(8):1369–1373

18. Kaplan A, Crosby GJ, Bhattacharyya N. Airway protection and the laryngeal mask airway in sinus and nasal surgery. Laryngoscope 2004;114(4):652–655

19. Wormald PJ, Athanasiadis T, Rees G, Robinson S. An evaluation of effect of pterygopalatine fossa injection with local anesthetic and adrenalin in the control of nasal bleeding during endoscopic sinus surgery. Am J Rhinol 2005;19(3):288–292

20. Chastain JB, Cooper MH, Sindwani R. The maxillary line: anatomic characterization and clinical utility of an important surgical landmark. Laryngoscope 2005;115(6):990–992

21. Huang BY, Lloyd KM, DelGaudio JM, Jablonowski E, Hudgins PA. Failed endoscopic sinus surgery: spectrum of CT findings in the frontal recess. Radiographics 2009;29(1):177–195

22. May M, Sobol SM, Korzec K. The location of the maxillary os and its importance to the endoscopic sinus surgeon. Laryngoscope 1990;100(10 Pt 1):1037–1042

23. Matthews BL, Burke AJ. Recirculation of mucus via accessory ostia causing chronic maxillary sinus disease. Otolaryngol Head Neck Surg 1997;117(4):422–423

24. Kane KJ. Recirculation of mucus as a cause of persistent sinusitis. Am J Rhinol 1997;11(5):361–369

25. Casiano RR. A stepwise surgical technique using the medial orbital floor as the key landmark in performing endoscopic sinus surgery. Laryngoscope 2001;111(6):964–974

26. Stackpole SA, Edelstein DR. The anatomic relevance of the Haller cell in sinusitis. Am J Rhinol 1997;11(3):219–223

27. Kainz J, Stammberger H. Danger areas of the posterior rhinobasis. An endoscopic and anatomical-surgical study. Acta Otolaryngol 1992;112(5):852–861

28. Kim HU, Kim SS, Kang SS, Chung IH, Lee JG, Yoon JH. Surgical anatomy of the natural ostium of the sphenoid sinus. Laryngoscope 2001;111(9):1599–1602

29. Kemppainen T, Kokki H, Tuomilehto H, Seppä J, Nuutinen J. Acetaminophen is highly effective in pain treatment after endoscopic sinus surgery. Laryngoscope 2006;116(12):2125–2128

30. Miller TR, Muntz HR, Gilbert ME, Orlandi RR. Comparison of topical medication delivery systems after sinus surgery. Laryngoscope 2004;114(2):201–204

16 Endonasal Endoscopic Frontal Sinus Surgery

Amir Minovi and Wolfgang Draf

History of Endonasal Frontal Sinus Surgery

Modern endonasal sinus surgery started roughly around the beginning of the 20th century.[1,2] The endonasal approach to the ethmoid cells was first described by Riberi in 1838, who then reported a case involving the management of the frontal sinus by resection of the lamina papyracea using a chisel.[3] Halle, in 1906, reported on successful endonasal drainage of the frontal sinus using just headlight and the naked eye.[2] However, in the English-speaking literature, Mosher is regarded as the founder of endonasal ethmoid sinus surgery describing a more detailed and structured surgical technique. In 1912, Mosher indicated that the natural ostium of the frontal sinus could be reached more easily through an endonasal approach.[3] At the establishment of this new period in rhinology, only a few surgeons were able to achieve a successful ethmoidectomy and simple drainage of the frontal sinus. In this preantibiotic and pre-endoscopic time, endonasal surgery of the paranasal sinuses performed by less-gifted surgeons was a life-threatening treatment with a high incidence of catastrophic complications including brain abscess, meningitis, and encephalitis. Consequently, despite the early successes of endonasal surgery, Mosher stated that the intranasal ethmoidectomy had "proven to be one of the easiest ways to kill a patient." Lothrop in 1914 described opening of both frontal sinuses using a unilateral external approach for uniting both frontal sinus infundibula and resecting the adjacent upper nasal septum but seriously warning to try this via an endonasal approach.[4] Furthermore, anesthesia techniques were insufficient to provide a satisfactory, bloodless operative field. It was for this reason, that for many decades, most paranasal sinus surgeries were dominated by external approaches.[5]

Therefore, between 1920 and almost 1980, endonasal surgery was generally neglected worldwide and practiced in only a few centers. The new era of endonasal sinus surgery was revolutionized by the introduction of operating microscope(s) and endoscopes in sinus surgery. In the middle of the century, Heermann (1958) introduced the microscope in endonasal sinus surgery.[6] However, it was the advent of endoscopes, mainly associated with the British physicist Harold Hopkins,[7,8] that promoted a renewed interest in endonasal endoscopy as a diagnostic and therapeutic technique.[9,10]

Major steps within rhinology such as the introduction of endoscopic and microscopic visualization techniques and developments in radiology including computer-assisted tomography, magnetic resonance imaging, and interventional radiology facilitated the benefits of endonasal endoscopic frontal sinus surgery (EEFSS).[11,12] These developments have been recently complemented through the use of intraoperative navigation systems and powered instrumentation that have helped to optimize the results.[13]

Between 1980 and 1984, the Fulda school developed a system of endonasal drainage procedures directed to the frontal sinuses.[14] This rebirth of endonasal frontal sinus surgery was also a contribution of general anesthesia, which was, unlike other centers, routinely applied in the Fulda school. The Fulda concept of frontal sinus surgery started as a microendoscopic technique, which developed within the next three decades to an almost exclusively endoscopic approach.

Necessary Technology

For EEFSS, general anesthesia, if necessary, with controlled hypotension is required. In addition, we recommend using a local decongestant and epinephrine to achieve a maximal bloodless operative field. The most important instruments are 0- and 45-degree endoscopes and a pair of straight/curved through-cutting forceps. In experienced hands the shaver allows gentle removal of polyps. In combination with curved diamond and cutting drills, further areas of the frontal sinus can be accessed. Especially in revision surgery of the frontal sinus and in tumor surgery, navigation systems nowadays have gained major importance.[15]

Technical Details of Surgery

EEFSS is performed with the patient under combined local and general anesthesia.[14,15] To reach a bloodless field, a topical decongestant is applied by packing the inferior and middle portions of the nasal meatus with gauze strips soaked in naphazoline hydrochloride and 2 mL of cocaine 10% solution. Xylocaine 1% with 1:120,000 units of epinephrine is injected in the region of uncinate process and agger nasi. Wait for at least 10 minutes to take the effect of local anesthesia and vasoconstriction. Bleeding is a major problem during endoscopic frontal sinus surgery. In many cases, bleeding can be reduced with the help of anesthetic techniques. The anesthesiologist should be informed constantly about the actual bleeding situation and should follow surgery on a monitor. Intraoperative interaction between the surgeon and the anesthesiologist is mandatory. If the comorbidities of the patient provide no contraindication, controlled hypotension at a mean arterial pressure of 60 mm Hg and a heart rate of 50 to 60 bpm is recommended. Arterial hypotension will minimize hemodynamic causes for bleeding.

The influence of various anesthetics on bleeding is continuously under discussion. A total intravenous technique may have advantages with regard to bleeding on the microcirculatory level. In case of diffuse bleeding, adrenaline-soaked pledgets (adrenaline 1:1000) may be applied intraoperatively.[16] We recommend starting the surgery on the right side with the surgeon standing on the same side. The surgical approach is more difficult on the right side than the left, because of the positioning of the surgeon. The EEFSS is performed by using a 45-degree rigid telescope with a suction/irrigation handle. The shaver is very helpful for gentle tissue removal and also for drilling in the frontal sinus. Surgery on the frontal recess is usually preceded at least by an anterior, more often than not by a complete ethmoidectomy. Exceptions are the cases where a complete ethmoidectomy has already been performed. It is important to remove agger nasi cells and to identify the lamina papyracea laterally, the attachment of the middle turbinate medially, and the anterior skull base with the anterior ethmoidal artery superiorly.

Type I: Simple Drainage

Type I drainage is established by ethmoidectomy including the cell septa in the region of the frontal recess (**Fig. 16.1**).[17] The inferior part of Killian infundibulum and its mucosa are not touched. Type I drainage is indicated if there is a minor pathology in the frontal sinus and the patient does

not suffer from "prognostic risk factors" such as asthma and aspirin hypersensitivity, which are associated with reduced quality of mucosa and possible problems in outcome. In the majority of cases, the frontal sinus heals because of the improved drainage via the ethmoid cavity.

Type IIa/b: Extended Drainage

Extended drainage is achieved after ethmoidectomy by removing the floor of the frontal sinus between the lamina papyracea and the middle turbinate (type IIa) or the nasal septum (type IIb) anterior to the ventral margin of the olfactory fossa (**Figs. 16.2** and **16.3**). Hosemann et al[18,19] showed in a detailed anatomical study that the maximum diameter of a neo-ostium of the frontal sinus (type IIa), which could be gained using a curette or a spoon, was 11 mm with an average of 5.6 mm.

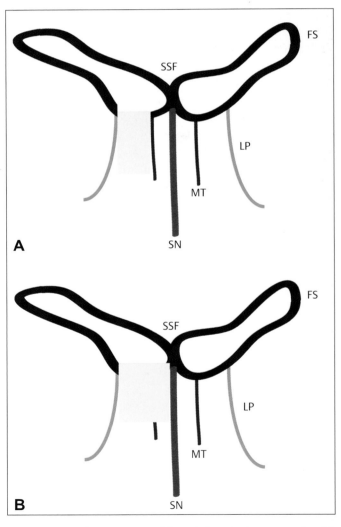

Figure 16.2 Schematic view of frontal sinus drainage type IIa with removal of frontal sinus floor from the lamina papyracea to the middle turbinate (A) or to the nasal septum, which results in type IIb drainage (B). FS, frontal sinus; LP, lamina papyracea; MT, middle turbinate; SSF, interfrontal sinus septum; SN, septum nasi.

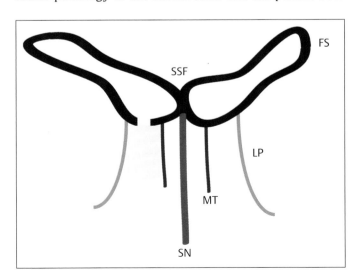

Figure 16.1 Schematic view of frontal sinus drainage type I after complete ethmoidectomy and removal of cell septa in the frontal recess. FS, frontal sinus; LP, lamina papyracea; MT, middle turbinate; SSF, interfrontal sinus septum; SN, septum nasi.

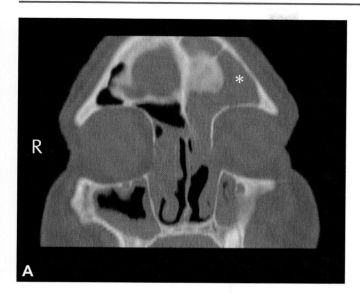

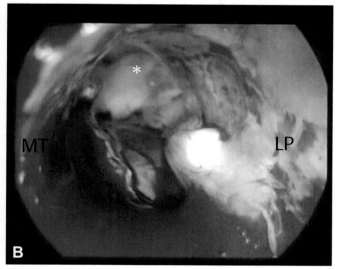

Figure 16.3 (A) Axial computed tomography in a patient with chronic left-sided frontal sinusitis (* indicates total opacification of the left frontal sinus). (B) Intraoperative condition (45-degree endoscope) showing a frontal sinus type IIa drainage. LP, lamina papyracea; MT, middle turbinate.

The bone that goes medially toward the nasal septum increases in thickness; therefore, a drill is needed if one needs to achieve a larger drainage opening such as type IIb. During drilling with the diamond burr in a classic drill hand piece, bone dust may fog the endoscope demanding repeated cleaning. Especially this part of the surgery may become time consuming and needs experienced hands. The endoscopic four-hand technique as an alternative was developed by May in 1990 and has been popularized by several authors.[20] Sinus surgery is performed by the surgeon and an assistant. The rigid telescope is held by the assistant, thereby enabling the surgeon to work with both hands. The surgeon is able to control the suction with one hand and perform dissection with the other hand. Hence, he or she will be able to reach a good visualization when there is more

bleeding. Also, extensive drill working is more comfortable with this technique. A great development for drilling in the frontal sinus is new, straight, and differently curved drill used with the shaver providing simultaneous suction and irrigation, thus minimizing fogging of the endoscopes.

As soon as the frontal recess is identified using the middle turbinate and where identifiable, the anterior ethmoidal artery as landmarks, the frontal infundibulum is exposed and the anterior ethmoidal cells are resected. During surgery, repeated considerations of the computed tomography (CT) will establish the presence of so-called frontal cells,[17] which can develop into the frontal sinus giving the surgeon the erroneous impression that the frontal sinus has been properly opened. Sagittal CT slices and navigation may be helpful in difficult situations. Especially in revision surgeries where extensive work of the frontal sinuses is required, we recommend a navigation system. In the case of frontal cells, a procedure called by Stammberger[21–23] "uncapping the egg" using a 45-degree endoscope may be necessary, resulting in a type IIa drainage.

If, after a type IIa drainage has been performed, further widening to produce a type IIb is required, the diamond burr is introduced into the clearly visible opening in the infundibulum and drawn across the bone into a medial direction along the anterior wall of the frontal sinus.

To be on the safe side, it is recommended to identify the first olfactory fiber just medial to the middle turbinate.

It is important that the frontal sinus opening is bordered by bone on all sides and mucosa is preserved at least on one part of the circumference. If the type IIa drainage appears too small in regard to the underlying pathology, it is better to perform the type IIb drainage. Packing is performed by putting a rubber finger stall into the frontal sinus for approximately 5 days.

Type III: Endonasal Median Drainage

The extended type IIb opening is enlarged by resecting areas of the superior nasal septum in the surrounding of the frontal sinus floor. It is very important that the diameter of this opening should be approximately 1.5 cm (**Fig. 16.4**). Our experience is that most reclosures occur because of not sufficiently removed nasal septum. This is followed by removal of the frontal sinus septum or septa, if there are more than one. We usually carry out this step with a curved diamond drill. Starting on one side of the patient, one crosses the midline along the anterior wall of the frontal sinus until the contralateral lamina papyracea is reached.

To achieve the maximum possible opening of the frontal sinus, it is very helpful to identify the first olfactory fibers on both sides: the middle turbinate is exposed and cut, millimeter by millimeter, from anterior to posterior along its origin at the skull base. After approximately 1.5 mm and just medial to the origin of the middle turbinate, one will see the first olfactory fiber coming out of a little bony hole. The same is done on the contralateral side. After completing

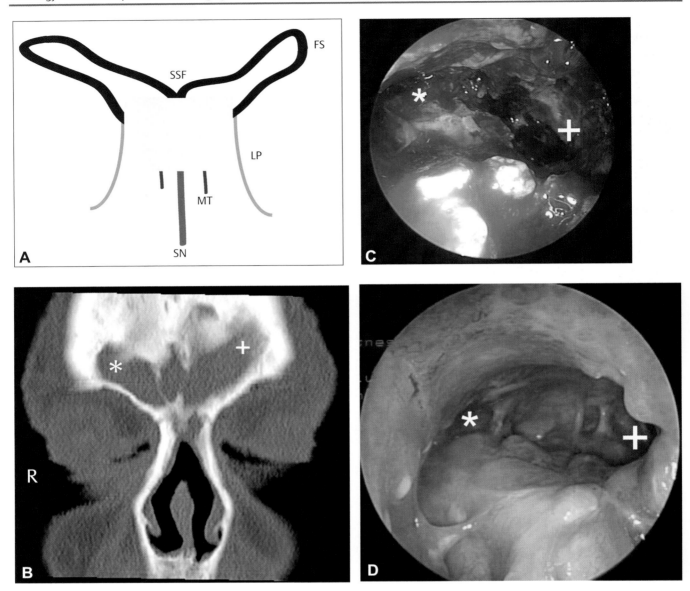

Figure 16.4 (A) Schematic view of frontal sinus drainage type III with removal of the frontal sinus floor from the left to the right lamina papyracea with additional resection of the interfrontal sinus septum and parts of the nasal septum. (B) Axial computed tomography showing recurrent chronic both-sided sinusitis frontalis. (C) Intraoperative condition (45-degree endoscope) after performing type III drainage. (D) Postoperative condition (1 year postoperatively) with wide open frontal sinuses. FS, frontal sinus; LP, lamina papyracea; MT, middle turbinate; SSF, interfrontal sinus septum; SN, septum nasi; *, right frontal sinus; +, left frontal sinus.

the resection of the perpendicular plate back to the first olfactory fibers, the "frontal T,"[5,24] which is a result of surgical dissection, such as the "bridge" in ear surgery, can be identified. Its long crus is represented by the posterior border of the perpendicular ethmoid lamina resection, and the shorter wings on both sides are provided by the posterior margins of the frontal sinus floor resection. After that, the ethmoidectomy on the left side is completed the same way as on the right.

Curved drills of several angles used with the shaver motor are helpful. They allow to go more superiorly with the resection of the interfrontal sinus septum and to be more complete with the resection of an eventual frontal

cell. These measures help create excellent landmarks for the anterior border of the olfactory fossa on both sides, which makes for easier and safer completion of frontal sinus floor resection to its maximum until the first olfactory fiber.

After the upper nasal septum resection is performed, it is possible to work bimeatal from one nasal cavity or the other. It is helpful if the surgeon has learnt to work bimanual, which means to use any instrument with the left or the right hand. This allows reaching for more lateral located areas of the frontal sinus, if working from the contralateral side.

In tricky revision cases, one can start the type III drainage primarily from two beginning points, either from the lateral side as already described or from the medial side. The primary lateral approach is recommended if the previous ethmoidectomy was incomplete and the middle turbinate can be identified as a landmark. One should adopt the primary medial approach if the ethmoidectomy was complete and/ or if the middle turbinate is absent. The medial approach begins with the partial resection of the perpendicular plate of the nasal septum, followed by identification of the first olfactory fiber on each side as already described.

After surgery, the patient is set on antibiotics until the packing is removed on the sixth postoperative day. The rubber finger stall packing allows re-epithelization of most parts of the surgical cavity, which makes the postoperative treatment more comfortable.

The endonasal median drainage is identical with the "modified Lothrop procedure."[25] Lothrop[4,26] warned against using the endonasal route, judging it as too dangerous during his time. In 1906, Halle had already created a large drainage from the frontal sinus directly to the nose using the endonasal approach with no more aids than a headlight and the naked eye.[2]

The endonasal median drainage (type III) is indicated after one or several previous sinus operations have not resolved the frontal sinus problem including an external frontoethmoidectomy. It is also justified as a primary procedure in patients with severe polyposis and other prognostic "risk factors" affecting outcome, such as aspirin intolerance, asthma, Samter triad (aspirin hypersensitivity, asthma, and nasal polyps), Kartagener syndrome, mucoviscidosis, and ciliary dyskinesia syndrome. Its use in patients with severe polyposis without these risk factors is undetermined and needs to be evaluated. It is also useful for the removal of benign tumors in the frontal sinus and the ethmoid as long as the main part of the tumor in the frontal sinus is medial to a vertical line through the lamina papyracea. In addition, the use of type III drainage makes the resection of malignant tumors, which are just reaching the frontal sinus, safer.[27,28]

Indications

Indications for Endonasal Frontal Sinus Drainage Type I to III

Indications for type I drainage are as follows:

1. Acute sinusitis
   a. Failure of conservative therapy
   b. Endocranial and orbital complications
2. Chronic sinusitis
   a. Primary surgery
   b. Revision after incomplete ethmoidectomy
   c. No risk factors (aspirin hypersensitivity, asthma, and nasal polyposis)

Indications for type II drainage are as follows:

1. Type IIa drainage
   a. Good quality mucosa
   b. Medial muco- or pyoceles
   c. Tumor surgery (benign tumors)

d. Serious complications of acute sinusitis
2. Type IIb drainage
   a. All indications of type IIa, if the resulting type IIa is smaller than 5 × 7 mm. For type IIb, usage of drill is necessary.

Indications for type III drainage are as follows:

1. Difficult revision surgery
2. Primarily in patients with prognostic risk factors and severe polyposis, particularly in patients with
   a. Samter triad
   b. Mucoviscidosis
   c. Kartagener syndrome
   d. Ciliary immotility syndrome
   e. Benign and malignant tumors

Postoperative Care

No uniform recommendations concerning postoperative care exist in the literature. We offer some general recommendations for postoperative care and treatment. We have learned by experience that local aftercare should focus on the removal of mobile obstructive material only, not on crusts protecting mucosal wounds.

1. Local aftercare by the ENT surgeon consists of thefollowing after packing removal:
   a. Suction of secretion from the nasal and ethmoidcavity
   b. Removal of mobile fibrin clots and crusts only
   c. Separation of synechiae and adhesions
   d. Continuously expanded visits, based on the patient's needs, over 3 months
2. Daily local care of the operative area by the patient consists of the following:
   a. Inhalation and irrigation of the nose
   b. Application of ointments
   c. Application of topical steroids
   d. Follow postoperative care for a minimum of 3 months
3. Systemic aftercare of the surgical area consists of the following.
   a. *Antibiotics*: They are indicated in the postoperative period for 1 to 2 weeks in cases of acute sinusitis or chronic purulent sinusitis. In type III drainage, we recommend prophylactic antibiotic use, as long as the packing is in place.
   b. *Antiallergic medical therapy*: This is recommended for 6 weeks postoperatively if allergy has been diagnosed by history or by specific tests. In less severe cases, we prescribe day antihistamines. In patients with severe allergy (e.g., Samter triad), the combination of antihistamines with low-dose corticosteroid medication for 6 weeks helps prevent early recurrence of polyps.

Clinical Pearls to Avoid Complications

- Detailed preoperative CT analysis is mandatory for successful endoscopic frontal sinus surgery.

- Early identification of lamina papyracea and middle turbinate as the most important anatomic landmarks.
- If middle turbinate surgery is needed, the superior part should be preserved as an anatomic landmark.
- Always dissect laterally to the middle turbinate, never medially and superiorly.
- If drilling is needed, preserve as much mucosa as possible, especially on the posterior and lateral wall of the frontal recess.
- Control of the eye bulb during whole surgery by the surgeon and the operating nurse.
- Bulb pressing test after Draf and Stankiewicz can be helpful when there is a suspicion of injury to the lamina papyracea.
- Be familiar with techniques of duraplasty when starting to learn frontal sinus type III drainage, because there is a higher risk of dura lesions in beginners of this surgery.
- Perform intensively anatomical dissection trainings before starting difficult frontal sinus cases.

Summary

- With the help of endonasal type I to III drainages, it is possible to adjust frontal sinus surgery to the underlying pathology.
- From type I to III upward surgery is increasingly invasive.
- The type III median drainage is identical to the endoscopic modified Lothrop procedure.[14,25]
- The technique of endonasal drainages of the frontal sinus means preservation of bony boundaries of frontal sinus opening in contrary to the classic external procedures. This means less danger of restenosis with development of muco- or pyoceles. The fronto-orbital external operation is no more indicated for the treatment of inflammatory diseases.

References

1. Spiess G. Die endonasale Chirurgie des Sinus frontalis. Arch Laryngol 1899;9:285–291
2. Halle M. Externe und interne Operation der Nasennebenhoehle-neiterungen. Berl Klein Wschr. 1906;43:1369–1372
3. Draf W. Die chirurgische Behandlung entzündlicher Erkrankungen der Nasennebenhöhlen. Indikation, Operationsverfahren, Gefahren, Fehler und Komplikationen, Revisionschirurgie. Arch Otorhinolaryngol 1982;235(1):133–305
4. Lothrop HA. Frontal sinus suppuration. Ann Surg 1914;59(6):937–957
5. Draf W. Endonasal frontal sinus drainage Type I–III according to Draf. In: Kountakis S, Senior B, Draf W, eds. The Frontal Sinus. New York, NY: Springer;2005
6. Heermann H. Uber endonasale Chirurgie unter Verwendung des binocularen Mikroskopes. Arch Ohren Nasen Kehlkopfheilkd 1958;171(2):295–297
7. Hopkins HH, Kapany NS. A flexible fiberscope. Nature 1954;173:39
8. Draf W. The history and evolution of endoscopic skull base surgery. In: Stamm AC, ed. Transnasal Endoscopic Skull Base and Brain Surgery. New York, NY: Thieme;2011:402–412
9. Draf W. Endoscopy of the Paranasal Sinuses. (German edition 1978: Die Endoskopie der Nasennebenhöhlen). New York, NY: Springer; 1983
10. Messerklinger W. Endoscopy of the Nose. Baltimore: Urban und Schwarzenberg; 1978
11. Leeds NE, Kieffer SA. Evolution of diagnostic neuroradiology from 1904 to 1999. Radiology 2000;217(2):309–318
12. Maroldi R, Ravanelli M, Borghesi A, Farina D. Paranasal sinus imaging. Eur J Radiol 2008;66(3):372–386
13. Klimek L, Mösges R, Schlöndorff G, Mann W. Development of computer-aided surgery for otorhinolaryngology. Comput Aided Surg 1998;3(4):194–201
14. Draf W. Endonasal micro-endoscopic frontal sinus surgery: the Fulda concept. Oper Tech Otolaryngol Head Neck Surg 1991;2:234–240
15. Draf W, Minovi A. Endonasal micro-endoscopic frontal sinus surgery. In: Kountakis S, Önerci M, eds. Rhinologic and Sleep Apnea Surgical Techniques. Berlin: Springer; 2007:83–91
16. Anderhuber W, Walch C, Nemeth E, et al. Plasma adrenaline concentrations during functional endoscopic sinus surgery. Laryngoscope 1999;109(2, pt 1):204–207
17. Lang J. Clinical Anatomy of the Nose Nasal Cavity and Paranasal Sinuses. Stuttgart: Thieme; 1989
18. Hosemann W, Gross R, Goede U, Kuehnel T. Clinical anatomy of the nasal process of the frontal bone (spina nasalis interna). Otolaryngol Head Neck Surg 2001;125(1):60–65
19. Hosemann W, Kühnel T, Held P, Wagner W, Felderhoff A. Endonasal frontal sinusotomy in surgical management of chronic sinusitis: a critical evaluation. Am J Rhinol 1997;11(1):1–9
20. May M, Hoffmann DF, Sobol SM. Video endoscopic sinus surgery: a two-handed technique. Laryngoscope 1990;100(4):430–432
21. Stammberger H. Endoscopic endonasal surgery—concepts in treatment of recurring rhinosinusitis. Part II. Surgical technique. Otolaryngol Head Neck Surg 1986;94(2):147–156
22. Stammberger H. Endoscopic endonasal surgery—concepts in treatment of recurring rhinosinusitis. Part I. Anatomic and pathophysiologic considerations. Otolaryngol Head Neck Surg 1986;94(2):143–147
23. Stammberger H. F.E.S.S. "Uncapping the Egg". The Endoscopic Approach to Frontal Recess and Sinuses. Storz Company Prints; 2000
24. Draf W, Minovi A. The "Frontal T" in the refinement of endonasal frontal sinus type III drainage. Oper Tech Otolaryngol Head Neck Surg 2006;17:121–125
25. Gross WE, Gross CW, Becker D, Moore D, Phillips D. Modified transnasal endoscopic Lothrop procedure as an alternative to frontal sinus obliteration. Otolaryngol Head Neck Surg 1995;113(4):427–434
26. Lothrop HA. The anatomy and surgery of the frontal sinus and anterior ethmoidal cells. Ann Surg 1899;29(2):175–217
27. Bockmühl U, Minovi A, Kratzsch B, Hendus J, Draf W. [Endonasal micro-endoscopic tumor surgery: state of the art]. Laryngorhinootologie 2005;84(12):884–891
28. Minovi A, Kollert M, Draf W, Bockmühl U. Inverted papilloma: feasibility of endonasal surgery and long-term results of 87 cases. Rhinology 2006;44(3):205–210

17 Frontal Sinus Obliteration and Cranialization

Aaron N. Pearlman and Michael G. Stewart

Managing pathology of the frontal sinus has been and remains a complex issue for otolaryngologists. Etiologies such as acute and chronic infection, trauma, mucoceles, tumors, and osteomas may require surgical intervention. Before the advent of antibiotics and, more recently, endoscopy, the majority of frontal sinus pathology was managed surgically through external approaches. The first reports of frontal sinus surgery are from the latter half of the 16th century,[1] but it was not until the 1880s that Ogston and Luc outlined trephination.[2] They described drilling into the frontal sinus and widening the frontal recess using an external anterior ethmoid approach. Breiger and Schonborn, among other surgeons, further described the use of the osteoplastic flap to access the frontal sinus.[2] Riedel detailed frontal sinus ablation by removing the anterior frontal table and supraorbital rim entirely in treating frontal sinus pathology.[3] In the early 20th century, Lothrop described resecting the intersinus septum, medial floor of the frontal sinus, and the superior nasal septum through an external approach described by Lynch.[1,4] Obliteration of the frontal sinus with fat was first described by Tato et al[5] and then performed using an osteoplastic flap procedure by Goodale and Montgomery in 1956.[6]

With the advent of endoscopy and approaches to the frontal sinus through an endonasal approach, the need to obliterate the frontal sinus has become much less frequent. However, it remains a useful tool for various disease processes and this chapter intends to detail the surgical methodology and clinical usefulness of this technique.

Common indications for frontal sinus obliteration or cranialization are as follows:

1. After fracture with posterior table involvement, either comminuted or displaced (**Fig. 17.1**).
2. After neoplasm removal (i.e., large osteoma or inverted papilloma) with extensive mucosal injury, bone loss, or impaired outflow.
3. After failure of endoscopic transnasal management for mucocele, chronically dysfunctional mucosa (i.e., cystic fibrosis and ciliary dysfunction), or persistent chronic infectious sinusitis.

Surgical Anatomy

The frontal sinus is an air-filled space that is usually formed in the later teenage years. It can be thought of as an inverted pyramid with the frontal outflow tract representing the

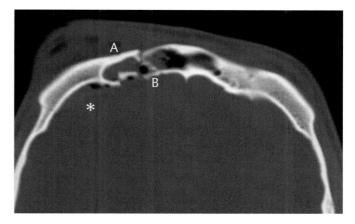

Figure 17.1 Frontal sinus trauma with anterior table (A) and posterior table (B) fractures that are both displaced and comminuted. Note the pneumocephalus (*).

apex. Typically, the sinuses are paired right and left; however, in approximately 10% of people, there will be a variation of this anatomy with either a unilateral frontal sinus only or complete agenesis of both frontal sinuses. Furthermore, the extent of pneumatization of the frontal sinus can vary from a volume occupying the area just superior to the midline to one that may extend laterally past the lateral orbital rim. There may also be variation in the superior extension. The sinus is bordered anteriorly by a bone known as the anterior table and posteriorly, the posterior table. The mucosa of the frontal sinus is ciliated pseudostratified columnar epithelium. Posterior to the posterior table is dura mater. The floor of the frontal sinus is typically adjacent to or part of the superior orbital roof. The mucus produced within the sinus drains through the frontal outflow tract that is located inferomedially. The typical outflow of the frontal sinus is into the middle meatus, posterior to the anterior ethmoid cell known as the agger nasi, anterior to the ethmoid bulla, medial to lamina papyracea, and lateral to the middle turbinate. Variations of this outflow pattern exist. As such, a thorough understanding of a patient's frontal sinus anatomy is imperative before operating.

To preoperatively assess the frontal sinus anatomy, the traditional approach was through radiography. Historically, a 6-foot Caldwell frontal X-ray was taken. A coin would be taped to the X-ray cassette and after developing, this would be used as a size template for the frontal sinus. If the X-ray was performed correctly, then the size match of the frontal sinuses could be used as an exact template for the frontal borders. The X-ray film was sterilized and used during the procedure to aid in the accuracy of osteotomies. Today, however, digital X-rays have made the process of acquiring a Caldwell view with the coin template difficult. Additionally, the wide availability of computed tomography (CT) of the sinuses has made Caldwell views less necessary. CTs allow for a highly accurate assessment of the frontal anatomy. Furthermore, image guidance systems that use the CT for an individual patient in coordination with infrared or electromagnetic localization have allowed for highly accurate mapping of the borders of the frontal sinus. It is important to remember that no technology can replace the surgeon's understanding of the anatomy specific to each patient; and proper preoperative planning is imperative.

Exposing the Anterior Table of the Frontal Sinus

Various surgical approaches to the frontal sinus have been described previously; however, a coronal incision, often referred to as a bicoronal incision, is standard if obliteration or cranialization is being performed. Not only is a coronal flap relatively easy and fast to elevate, it allows for the formation of a pericranial tissue flap that can be fashioned from the overlying periosteum (pericranium) of the frontal skull bone and pedicled inferiorly. Pericranium is especially useful during cranialization as there are often defects in the dura and possible cerebrospinal fluid (CSF) leaks that can be repaired with a high degree of success using this hardy pedicled flap. The pericranial flap receives its blood supply from the deep branches of the supratrochlear and supraorbital vessels and can be harvested up to 40 mm in length.[7]

An incision is planned approximately 2 cm posterior to the hairline with an anterior curve that mimics the natural hairline. The incision is created parallel to the direction of the hair follicles and brought down to the subgaleal plane and elevation is commenced. When elevating the coronal flap great care should be taken not to puncture the pericranium as it may be necessary for dural repair, and holes in the flap may make it unusable. It is important to elevate the flap to the level of the supraorbital rims and nasion. Care is also taken not to damage the supraorbital neurovascular bundles. The lateral extension of the flap should be lateral to the lateral orbital rim and over the zygomatic arches. If there is difficulty getting the proper lateral extension, consider that the incision of the coronal flap may need to be extended inferiorly. As access to the frontal sinus is often needed after frontal sinus trauma, the coronal flap may be tethered in a fracture line. Careful dissection should be performed over the fracture as not to further perforate the pericranium.

If a laceration is present over the brow, the frontal sinus may be approached directly. However, it is important to keep in mind that exposure is key to safely operate in the frontal sinus. It may be necessary to lengthen the laceration surgically to properly expose the anterior table. This may

result in an unsightly scar if the laceration does not lie in a resting skin tension line. If adequate access cannot be achieved through the brow laceration then a coronal flap is still necessary.

Others advocate for a brow incision, especially in males, because of the potential for the coronal scar being readily apparent in patients with male pattern baldness. This incision is placed directly adjacent to the superior brow line and extended over the glabella horizontally. Though brow incisions heal well in some, as a whole, the cosmetic result is poor. Furthermore, as most males are generally taller than females, the vertex scar of a coronal incision, even in bald men, is relatively acceptable to the patient, whereas a horizontal scar over the upper face is not.

Accessing the Frontal Sinus

After the frontal bone has been exposed over the supraorbital rims, attention can be turned to creating the osteoplastic flap to open the frontal sinus. The osteoplastic flap consists of the anterior table of the frontal sinus with the outer pericranium attached inferiorly as a hinge, which will continue to supply blood flow to the bone fragment.

First, the pericranial flap is elevated. If cranialization is planned, or likely, a large flap may be needed and the entire pericranium up to (and even beyond) the coronal incision can be created. However, this is an extensive elevation, which for a standard obliteration will be unnecessary and excessive. Therefore, for obliteration the edge of the pericranial flap is created approximately 2 cm beyond the superior border of the frontal sinus. The flap is partially elevated to a level inferior to the sinus edge, but not all the way to the orbital rim so that periosteum is left attached to much of the anterior table bone to provide continued blood supply.

At this point, the surgeon must precisely mark the borders of the frontal sinus. As discussed previously, CT-image guidance is the contemporary method of choice for this process. Using the image-guided tracking probe, the borders of the frontal sinuses can be easily outlined on the frontal bone using a marking pen or cautery directly on the bone (**Fig. 17.2**). If a radiographic template from a 6-foot Caldwell view is being used, the surgeon will outline it at this time. Another method for viewing the borders of the sinus is to use a light source placed in the patient's nose to illuminate the frontal sinus. This method, however, is less exact as the marrow spaces lateral to the frontal sinus borders may illuminate causing the surgeon to overestimate the size of the sinus.

Once the surgeon is confident on the borders of the frontal sinus, an oscillating saw is used at an oblique angle in a superior to inferior direction to enter the superior aspect of the sinus (**Fig. 17.3**). Some surgeons may choose to use an osteotome. The surgeon should be able to visually confirm that the sinus space has been entered. It is important to be as close to the edge of the sinus as possible and this can be performed either visually or with a vein or nerve retractor to

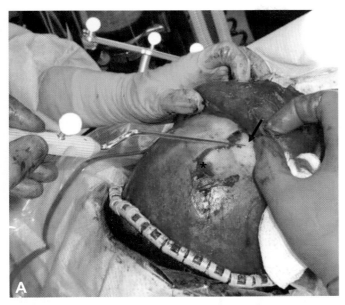

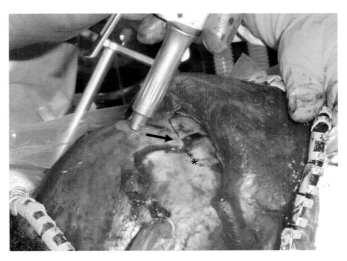

Figure 17.3 Preparing to open the frontal sinus using an oscillating saw. Note the oblique angle (arrow) of the oscillating saw directed at the apex of the frontal sinus. The borders of the frontal sinus have been previously marked (*).

has been successfully raised and the intersinus septum should be removed.

Obliterating the Frontal Sinus

If the purpose of creating an osteoplastic flap is to assess patency of the frontal outflow tract, it can be determined at this time. If obliteration is needed, the mucosa within the sinus must be meticulously removed. A microscope is used to see with certainty that the mucosa has been adequately resected. In addition to magnification, the microscope allows bright illumination and the ability to inspect into the lateral and inferior reaches of the sinus to ensure mucosal removal. Initially, an elevator and curette can be used, but a drill with a diamond burr is always used next. Drilling the bone will remove mucosal remnants within the foramina of Breschet, and the freshly drilled bone provides blood supply to the fat graft that will be used to obliterate the sinus. The mucosa that extends toward the frontal recess can be folded inferiorly and tucked firmly into the recess.

After removal of the sinus mucosa has been achieved, obliteration can be performed. The purpose of obliterating the sinus is to prevent mucosal regrowth and aeration, thus preventing mucocele formation, recurrent sinusitis, or pneumocephalus. The obliteration of the frontal outflow tract is performed by packing temporalis muscle firmly into the outflow tract to seal it. A small piece of fascia can also be placed on top of the muscle graft to further seal the tract and prevent mucosal regrowth. A small amount of sealant may be placed over the graft that will create an airtight seal and secure the graft in place. The obliteration of the sinus comes from the use of a free graft to completely occupy the volume of the sinus. Autologous grafts such as abdominal fat, muscle and bone chips, or bone pate have been used for this purpose. Autologous grafts usually require a donor site,

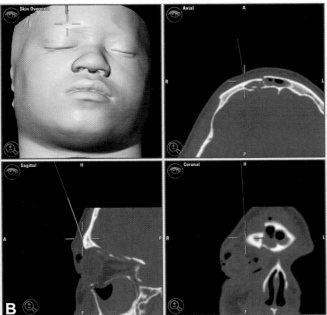

Figure 17.2 Mapping of the borders of the frontal sinus with stereotactic image guidance. Note that the pointer tip (arrow) in (A) corresponds to the lateral border of the right frontal sinus seen in (B). Also evident in (A) is a fracture line (*) through the frontal sinus requiring repair.

palpate the bony overhang present. When the surgeon has confirmed that the sinus edge has been opened, the saw or chisel can be used to open the sinus from superior, moving laterally and then to inferior. Care should be taken to allow the anterior table to remain connected to the pericranium along the inferior portions. Gentle direct chiseling on the inferior border with the sinus floor will detach the bone without lacerating the overlying pericranium. This can also be performed inside the sinus with the osteotome positioned behind the anterior table. At this point, the osteoplastic flap

making a second incision necessary. However, morbidity because of the second operative site is usually low and the incision can often be hidden in the skin folds. Inert material, such as hydroxyapatite, has also been used to obliterate the sinus. Using this material has the benefit of not needing a donor site; however, the long-term follow-up of patients with this material has shown an increased rate of both early and late infections, as well as mucocele formation. Thus, autologous fat is recommended.

The graft of choice for a typical frontal sinus obliteration is abdominal fat or in a very thin patient, buttock fat. A small incision can be made in the bikini line or a natural skin fold of the abdomen. Typically, this incision is made on the left abdomen to avoid mistaking it for an appendectomy scar. Enough fat is needed so that the sinus can be filled with fat with a slight bit of overflow when the anterior bone plate is replaced. It has been demonstrated through postoperative magnetic resonance imaging (MRI) that a significant amount of the fat will remain viable in the sinus for many years following surgery. The remainder of the space is replaced with a fibrous scar. At times, the entire free graft may be replaced with scar, but it still prevents mucosal regrowth or reaeration.

After the fat graft has been placed, the anterior table is replaced, and titanium miniplates and screws are used to secure the bone flap. The pericranium is replaced and closed, and the coronal flap is then relaxed, repositioned, and sutured closed. Some surgeons may choose to place one or two drains under the skin flap to prevent hematoma formation.

Frontal sinus obliteration is not without complications and associated morbidity. Hardy and Montgomery have shown a 19% intraoperative complication rate and postoperative complications consisting of CSF leaks, forehead numbness, and headaches.[8] Others have shown a 10% occurrence rate of mucocele formation as evidenced by MRI over a 5-year period.[9] Rates of recurrent infection in obliterated sinuses ranged from 3 to 10%.[8,10,11] Contour deformities, meningitis, and hematomas have also been reported. Even so, frontal sinus obliteration remains an important tool in addressing pathology of the frontal sinuses.

Cranializing the Frontal Sinus

Cranialization of the frontal sinus refers to removal of the posterior table so that the brain can expand anteriorly against the anterior table. The former volume of the frontal sinus then becomes part of the cranial cavity— "cranialization" (**Fig. 17.4**). There are various indications for this procedure, but the most common is trauma causing severe displacement or comminution of the posterior table. Often, these injuries cause dural tears and a leak of CSF may be present either intranasally or within the frontal sinus. If a dural tear is present, repair will be necessary to seal the CSF leak. A pericranial flap, easily raised during elevation of the coronal flap, is a good material for this repair.

To perform the cranialization, an osteoplastic flap is raised as previously discussed. Typically, there are fragments

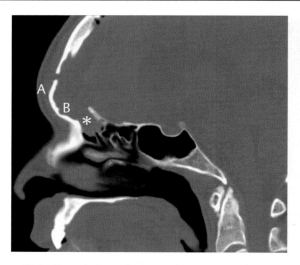

Figure 17.4 Frontal sinus after cranialization procedure. Note the anterior table (A) is intact. The posterior table has been removed and the frontal sinus cavity (B) is occupied by intracranial contents. The frontal recess has been occluded with temporalis muscle (*).

of posterior table that are displaced and should be removed with careful dissection. The remainder of the posterior table is removed with a rongeur or drill. Attention should be paid as to not damage the underlying dura. It is important to drill any sharp edges or bony overhangs to be flush with the inferior and lateral aspects of the frontal sinus. The frontal outflow tract should be occluded tightly with muscle and fascia to prevent communication with the nasal cavity; tissue sealant may also be used. At this time, the pericranial flap can be placed along the floor of the sinus if necessary. The osteoplastic flap is then repositioned and secured in place with titanium mini plates and screws.

Frontal Sinus Ablation

As mentioned above, frontal sinus obliteration is not without complications and long-term sequelae may occur. Anterior table osteomyelitis, chronic infection of the obliterated sinus, or mucocele formation may necessitate the need for further surgery. These patients may benefit from frontal sinus ablation. The procedure, originally described by Riedel, removes the anterior table completely and then the bone overlying the supraorbital rim is drilled flush with the floor of the sinus (**Fig. 17.5**). The skin of the brow is then allowed to rest over the posterior table. The frontal outflow tracts are obliterated with muscle and fascia. The resulting cosmetic deformity requires a second reconstructive procedure at a later date (after all infection has resolved) to improve cosmesis.[1,2] A variation of this procedure was later described by Killian where the supraorbital rim is allowed to remain. This modification can allow for a significant improvement in postoperative cosmesis without the need for additional procedures, depending on the size of the sinus and the patient's anatomy.[1] The Riedel and Killian procedures have been mostly abandoned because of the fear

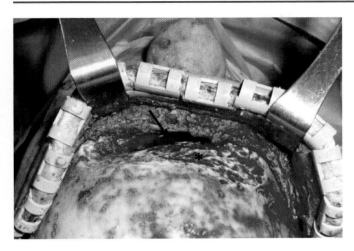

Figure 17.5 Riedel procedure. Note that the anterior table of the frontal sinus has been removed and the posterior table is visible (*). The frontal outflow tract (arrow) will be occluded in this patient who has previously undergone a Lothrop procedure.

of an unacceptable forehead deformity, but are still rarely needed even today.

Summary

Surgical management of pathology of the frontal sinus remains a complicated issue in otolaryngology. Today, endonasal endoscopic techniques have become the primary method of accessing the frontal sinus in the treatment of various etiologies such as acute and chronic infection, mucocele, and tumor. However, there is still a role for external approaches to the frontal sinus when endonasal treatments have failed or frontal sinus trauma requires surgical intervention. Obliteration is a method that has been practiced for more than 100 years and various modifications have made it safer and more reliable. Comminuted or displaced anterior table fractures without injury to the frontal outflow tract are easily treated by reducing and fixating the fracture. However, if the frontal outflow tract

is disrupted, obliteration may be necessary. Furthermore, if the posterior table is displaced or comminuted severely, cranialization is needed. Dural tears causing CSF leak, tumor, or mucocele formation causing dehiscence of the posterior table may also necessitate cranialization. As such, it is important for the otolaryngologist to be familiar with these surgical treatments when considering the management of frontal sinus pathology.

References

1. Donald PJ. Surgical management of frontal sinus infections. In: Donald PJ, Gluckman L, Rice DH, eds. The Sinuses. New York, NY: Raven Press;1995:201–232
2. Bosley WR. Osteoplastic obliteration of the frontal sinuses. A review of 100 patients. Laryngoscope 1972;82(8):1463–1476
3. Raghavan U, Jones NS. The place of Riedel's procedure in contemporary sinus surgery. J Laryngol Otol 2004;118(9):700–705
4. Gross CW, Gross WE, Becker DG. Modified transnasal endoscopic Lothrop procedure: frontal drill out. Oper Tech Otolaryngol—Head Neck Surg 1995;6(3):193–200
5. Tato JM, Sibbald DW, Bergaglio OE. Surgical treatment of the frontal sinus by the external route. Laryngoscope. 1954;64(6):504–521
6. Goodale RL, Montgomery WW. Experience with the osteo-plastic anterior wall approach to the frontal sinus. Arch Otolaryngol 1958; 68:271–283
7. Potparić Z, Fukuta K, Colen LB, Jackson IT, Carraway JH. Galeo-pericranial flaps in the forehead: a study of blood supply and volumes. Br J Plast Surg 1996;49(8):519–528
8. Hardy JM, Montgomery WW. Osteoplastic frontal sinusotomy: an analysis of 250 operations. Ann Otol Rhinol Laryngol 1976; 85(4, pt 1):523–532
9. Weber R, Draf W, Kratzsch B, Hosemann W, Schaefer SD. Modern concepts of frontal sinus surgery. Laryngoscope 2001;111(1):137–146
10. Zonis RD, Montgomery WW, Goodale RL. Frontal sinus disease: 100 cases treated by osteoplastic operation. Laryngoscope 1966;76(11):1816–1825
11. Weber R, Draf W, Keerl R, et al. Osteoplastic frontal sinus surgery with fat obliteration: technique and long-term results using magnetic resonance imaging in 82 operations. Laryngoscope 2000; 110(6):1037–1044

18 Pediatric Sinusitis

Rodney Lusk

Rhinosinusitis (sinusitis) is a common but often misdiagnosed disease in children. It is often confused with upper respiratory tract infections (URTIs), which are primarily caused by viruses. Most viral infections, 80%, will clear on their own without medical intervention. The symptoms are thought as chronic if they persist for more than 3 months. This definition, however, is based on work in adults and may or may not be appropriate for children because of their immature immune systems and the small ostia of the sinuses. For practical purposes, if the child is treated with a prolonged course of a broad-spectrum antibiotic for 20 days and once again is symptomatic within a week, the infection is likely more chronic in nature.

Etiology

Our understanding of sinusitis and predisposing factors continues to evolve. We know that children have an immature immune system and are susceptible to viral infections. Viruses most commonly associated with acute sinusitis are rhinovirus, parainfluenza, influenza, and adenovirus. These viral infections destroy the normal first line of defense—normal ciliary function—resulting in stasis of secretions and inflammation of the mucosa of the nose, ostia, and sinuses. Inflammation is most significant in the ostiomeatal complex where the frontal recess, maxillary, and agar nasi cells drain. This sequence of events results in inflammation and edema of the small ostia, creating an environment appropriate for invasion of bacteria normally residing in the nasal cavity. Chronic ciliary dysfunction, such as Kartagener syndrome, is associated with a very high incidence of unrelenting chronic sinusitis. Children may also be anatomically predisposed to chronic infections because the same amount of edema from an infection will have more of an occlusive effect on the small ostia of the sinuses. We do know, however, that septal deviation, paradoxical turbinates, concha bullosa, and infraorbital cells are not associated with chronic sinusitis.[1,2] Allergies may also be a component of inflammation resulting in recurrent or chronic sinusitis, however, the incidence of sinusitis correlates more concisely with URTI than seasons of significant allergy. In some patients, allergies no doubt play a key role in the etiology of sinusitis. The role of food allergies is not well understood and needs further investigation. The role of gastroesophageal reflux disease (GERD) remains controversial. Barbero[3] noted parallel existence between URTI and reflux and attributed GERD as a possible underlying etiology for chronic sinusitis. GERD could certainly cause inflammation of adenoid and nasal mucosa and interrupt normal ciliary function exposing the mucosa to bacterial colonization. This could in turn be associated with bacterial sinusitis. Objective evidence of this relationship however has not been confirmed. Children with immune deficiencies are unquestionably prone to recurrent and chronic sinusitis and should always be considered as a possible underlying etiology.

The bacteriology of chronic sinusitis continues to evolve because of the pressures of antibiotic therapy. Investigations of acute sinusitis found that *Streptococcus pneumoniae* was the most common organism (30%), followed closely by *Moraxella catarrhalis* and *Haemophilus influenzae* (20%). *H. influenzae* is usually nontypable. Both *M. catarrhalis* and *H. influenzae* have a high incidence of β-lactamase–producing enzymes and are therefore resistant to many antibiotics. Bacteria of chronic sinusitis is very similar, however, Brooks[4] notes a higher incidence of bacteroides and other anaerobes. Resistant strains of *H. influenzae*,[5] *S. pneumoniae* serotype 19A,[6] methicillin-resistant *Streptococcus aureus* (MRSA),[7,8] have markedly increased. Since the introduction of the pneumococcal vaccinations (PCV7), there has been an eradication of *S. pneumoniae* from the adenoids with a shift to more resistant strains of *H. influenzae*.[9]

Signs and Symptoms

Traditionally, nasal congestion, purulent rhinorrhea, headache, irritability, and both daytime and nighttime cough have been followed as indicators of chronic sinusitis. Most pediatric otolaryngologists would be hesitant to diagnose chronic sinusitis without cough as a component. Nighttime cough as a sole symptom would suggest reflux as a cause of cough and not sinusitis. Daytime coughing with nasal congestion and rhinorrhea is highly suggestive of sinus infection and duration of symptoms is a clue to chronicity. Asthmatics appear particularly sensitive to increasing cough with concurrent sinusitis.

Older children are able to articulate where the pain or headache is located. If there is unrelenting pain in the vertex or back of the skull, this is highly suggestive of sphenoid sinusitis and computed tomography (CT) scan should be obtained to rule this out. Younger children cannot articulate where they hurt, and irritability is the primary manifestation of the pain. None of these symptoms however have been validated as a measure of severity of sinusitis. About 78% of the American Society of Pediatric Otolaryngology (ASPO) members are not using validated tools for assessing the outcomes.[10]

Wald differentiates routine sinusitis from more serious sinusitis by noting a high temperature of 103°C rectally and purulent rhinorrhea.[11] The author argues that routine acute sinusitis will clear on its own and does not require antibiotic therapy while more severe sinusitis is associated with higher temperatures and will require antibiotics.

Physical Examination

Children are sometimes a challenge to examine. There is one thing the author has learned over the years; if a child does not want you to look into their nose—you are not going to look in their nose! The author always starts with examination of the ears. If there is a good cooperation then there will be a reasonable chance at looking at the nose. It is recommended to start with an otoscope that is gently inserted into the nose, in a slow nonthreatening manner, bracing the otoscope on the thumb, which is used to slightly rotate the tip of the nose (**Fig. 18.1**). The examiner's fingertips can also gently extend or flex the head. The author cannot emphasize enough that a slow, nonthreatening approach to the child is the key to a successful examination.

Once looking through the otoscope, identify the inferior turbinate and extend the head just a little to identify the middle turbinate. Once the middle turbinate is identified, look laterally to see if the middle meatus can be seen. Purulence can usually be noted if there is a sinus infection (**Fig. 18.2**). It is an unusual child who will tolerate a rigid endoscopy, and it is usually not attempted in the clinic. A flexible scope can be used to examine the middle meatus and adenoid pad in many children. Adequate anesthesia of the nose can be accomplished within a few minutes with a 1:1 mixture of Afrin (oxymetazoline nasal) and 4% lidocaine (lidocaine hydrochloride) sprayed one to two times.

Visualization of the sinuses is beneficial in assessing a child for chronic sinusitis. Several modalities have been recommended. Transillumination in a child is virtually worthless. It only assesses the maxillary sinus, and from the child's perspective, nothing good can be happening in a dark

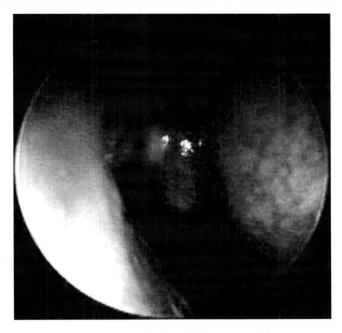

Figure 18.2 Examination of the middle meatus with an otoscope after surgery. Image as seen through the otoscope.

room with a doctor. Plain films are only good for assessing the maxillary sinuses, and inaccurate when compared with CT scans (**Fig. 18.3**).[12,13] A CT scan is clearly the gold standard for assessment of the sinuses. It is not without risk, however, and should not be obtained indiscriminately. Younger children will require sedation or a general anesthetic. There is increasing concern regarding radiation exposure in children. Brenner et al[14] raised concern regarding radiation and increased risk of cancer later in life. This article was highly controversial but sparked further evaluation of how much radiation children were actually getting. Rogers[15] noted that children were getting doses of radiation similar to adults, and because they had smaller heads were actually getting larger doses of radiation. This is of particular concern as 25 to 30% of a child's bone marrow is located in the skull.[16] Pediatric radiologists are now acutely aware of the hazards of radiation and practice "as low as reasonably achievable," doses to obtain the desired results. Imaging of the sinuses to "prove" sinusitis is not necessary, but frequently performed by primary care physicians. If there is purulence in the nose then the sinuses are going to be involved. The author does not recommend obtaining a CT scan unless the Otolaryngologist and parents agree that endoscopic sinus surgery is warranted. Obtaining the CT scan with a protocol for reformatting in the coronal plain can be saved and used for guided imaging in case it is wanted intraoperatively. The primary reason for obtaining a CT scan is to look for anatomical abnormalities, which would increase the risks of surgical intervention and document the extent of ethmoid disease. Magnetic resonance imaging of the sinuses are not of much help unless there is concern about extension of disease into the orbit or cranial cavity.

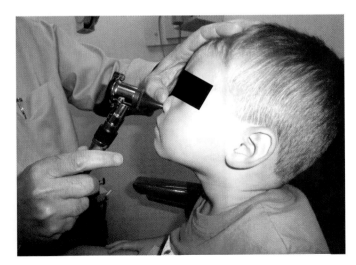

Figure 18.1 Hand position during nasal examination of the nose with an otoscope.

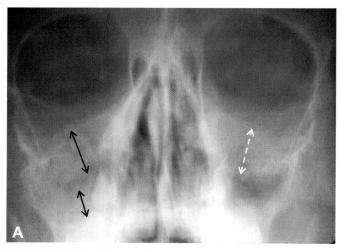

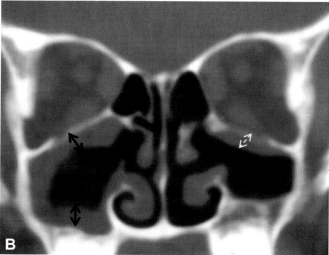

Figure 18.3 Comparison of postoperative plain films and computed tomography (CT) scans, which show greater accuracy and assessment of the sinus with CT. (A) Plain film with markedly thickened mucosa in the right maxillary sinus and markedly thickened opacification along the roof of the left maxillary sinus as marked by the arrows. (B) A CT scan of the same patient within an hour showing much thinner mucosal thickening on the right side, black arrows, and a left hypoplastic sinus with minimal thickened mucosa, white arrows, over the roof of the maxillary sinus.

Work-Up

The initial work-up is variable depending on the symptoms, duration, and age of the patient. If there are recurrent ear infections and purulence over the adenoid pad, an adenoidectomy performed as an initial step is quite feasible. If there are persistent symptoms, more aggressive medical management and evaluation for underlying systemic problems such as allergies, immune deficiencies, GERD, cystic fibrosis, and ciliary dyskinesia are warranted. The order and expertise of the physicians required for these evaluations have to be individualized according to the patient's symptoms and expertise available. It is reasonable to perform allergy and immune screening before CT scanning or endoscopic sinus surgery.

Medical Management

Based on a recent survey of Pediatric Otolaryngologists, there is fairly good agreement of initial medical management of children.[10] Of 158 responding participants, initial therapy would include nasal irrigations in 76%, nasal steroid sprays in 59%, and broad-spectrum antibiotics in 92%. Irrigations are useful, but noncompliance is a real issue in 40% of children.[17] There is good evidence that using irrigation helps chronic sinusitis,[18,19] but is questionable in acute sinusitis.[20] There is a general consensus that buffered normal saline is better for ciliary function than hypertonic solutions.

There are no randomized studies evaluating topical nasal steroid sprays in nonpolyp patients with chronic sinusitis.[21] There is general agreement that steroids are appropriate for allergic rhinitis[22] and does not affect growth in children.[23,24] Evidence of efficacy in chronic sinusitis, however, is lacking but appears to be safe and reasonable.

For chronic sinusitis, most would treat for 20 days with amoxicillin/clavulanate (90 mg/6.4 mg/kg/d), cefpodoxime proxetil, cefuroxime axetil, cefdinir, or clindamycin. If β-lactam hypersensitivity is present, then using trimethoprim/sulfamethoxazole, azithromycin, clarithromycin, or erythromycin should be considered.[25] Combined therapy is rarely appropriate. Examples of combined therapy include high-dose amoxicillin or clindamycin, plus cefixime or rifampin. Rifampin should not be used as monotherapy for longer than 10 to 14 days, as resistance can occur rapidly.[25] There have been no studies systematically looking at the use of prophylactic antibiotics for the treatment of recurrent acute or chronic sinusitis. Based on the experience with wide spread use of prophylaxis and subsequent resistance in treating chronic otitis media with effusion, it would appear that prophylactic therapy would not be appropriate. Topical antibiotic therapy has not been systematically studied. However, there are a few intriguing studies that have looked at mupirocin mixed with irrigations that have effectively treated MRSA and resistant sinusitis.[26,27] This mode of therapy may be particularly helpful in patients who have undergone endoscopic sinus surgery.

Surgical Management

Adenoidectomy

It has long been known that adenoidectomy is successful in clearing some patients of recurrent acute or chronic sinusitis. In a recent metaanalysis by Brietzke and Brigger,[28] a significant improvement in 69.3% ($p > 0.001$) of symptoms after adenoidectomy was found. They concluded that, "Given its simplicity, low risk profile, and apparent effectiveness, adenoidectomy should be considered first line therapy." The exact basis for improvement has not been proven, but may very well be the elimination of biofilms in the crypts of the adenoid pad. Biofilms were first noted adenoid tissue by Zuliani et al[29] in 2005. Coticchia et al confirmed biofilms in children with chronic sinusitis but absent in children with adenoid hypertrophy.[30] These findings have been confirmed by multiple other investigators.[31–33] The presence of biofilms is likely independent of the size of the adenoid pad. Gastric reflux could potentially destroy the mucosa overlying the adenoid pad, resulting in conditions amenable to biofilm formation. Removal of the adenoid pad as a first step therefore seems logical. However, risks of the procedure and anesthetic have to be taken into account for the individual patient.

Antral Lavage

The maxillary sinus can be irrigated through the natural ostium or through another portal with egress of the contents through the natural ostia. The most common other portals are under the inferior turbinate or through the anterior wall of the maxillary sinus. In children this is problematic, as the floor of the maxillary sinus may have not descended inferior enough to allow penetration. The anterior wall of the maxillary sinus is thicker in children and trauma tooth buds of permanent teeth are at real risks. These modalities of treatment are associated with a relatively high incidence of complications and have now been largely abandoned because of their poor success.[34]

There has been renewed interest in antral lavage alone,[35,36] or in association with adenoidectomy,[37] primarily because of the introduction of balloon sinuplasty. So far, these studies have been retrospective and at just a few centers. The tool is intriguing, but requires multi-institution prospective evaluation before it can be accepted as a standard of care in children.

Inferior Meatal Antrostomy and Nasal Antral Window Enlargement

As previously noted, inferior meatal antrostomy is difficult in children because the floor of the maxillary sinus has not descended low enough and is more traumatic than antral window enlargement. If it remains patent, which is unlikely in children, it may aerate the maxillary sinus, but cilia continue to beat toward the natural ostium. If the natural ostium is obstructed, it will continue to result in a diseased sinus. The failure rate is unacceptably high, 60% at 1 month and 73% at 6 month.[34] The procedure may be of use in diseases that have chronic ciliary dyskinesia such as cystic fibrosis and primary ciliary dyskinesia.

Middle meatal antrostomy or enlargement of the natural ostium was first performed by Ostrum as cited by Wilkerson.[38] Hilding studied nine rabbits and noted increased infections if the natural ostium was operated on and it became heresy to perform surgery on the natural ostium until the procedure was revisited by Wilkerson.[38] It

is now generally accepted to be safe and associated with a high rate of patency. Balloon sinuplasty has been proposed as a method of antrostomy but preserving the uncinate process.[39] Further study is required to assess the validity of this argument. The author will not enlarge the maxillary sinus antrum if it is seen as patent after performing an uncinectomy. If the ostium can only be palpated, however, the author will enlarge it approximately twice its normal size into the posterior fontanelle with through biting forceps. The balloon may be a viable option here. It is interesting that 55% of pediatric otolaryngologists have been trained to use balloons, but 92% of them rarely or never use a balloon to enlarge the maxillary sinus.[10]

Ethmoidectomy

Endoscopic sinus surgery was made possible through the advent of the Hopkins rod-lens system. It was first applied by Gross et al[40] and Lusk and Muntz[41] with encouraging results. Polyps are present in children with cystic fibrosis, allergic fungal sinusitis or nonallergic rhinitis with eosinophilia syndrome and more limited initial surgery is the standard. After aggressive medical management and evaluation for systemic disease, most surgeons will perform an anterior ethmoidectomy and maxillary antrostomy as an initial procedure.[10]

A detailed discussion of the techniques of the procedure is beyond the scope of this chapter, but a few helpful tips are listed in **Table 18.1**. Endoscopic sinus surgery is the last but effective treatment. Herbert and Bent[42] performed a meta-analysis and noted 88% improvement among the studies. More recent studies have confirmed these general findings.[43] About 38% of ASPO members stent the cavity but 36% never used a stent. Only 11% now do second looks with a general anesthetic.[10]

There has been concern regarding facial growth based on two studies in piglets,[44,45] where snout growth abnormalities were noted after ethmoidectomy. The findings in piglets however did not match the clinical experience of many investigators. Wolf[46] was one of the first to address facial growth in children after endoscopic sinus surgery and noted no evidence of facial growth abnormalities. Senior et al[47] compared children with unilateral ethmoidectomy for orbital abscess 7 years after surgery and noted no significant variation in the size of maxillary or ethmoid sinuses when compared to adults with and without a history of sinusitis. Bothwell et al[48] examined facial growth in children with a mean age of 3.1 years of age. Forty six children were examined 10 years after endoscopic ethmoidectomy and compared to 21 match children with a history of sinusitis using recognized norms for Caucasian children. Quantitative anthropomorphic analysis was performed using 12 standard facial growth measurements and qualitative facial analysis through standardized photographs. These were assessed by a plastic surgeon blinded to the therapy. These parameters revealed no evidence of facial growth abnormalities in

Table 18.1 Pediatric Endoscopic Sinus Surgery Tips

1. Use Afrin (oxymetazoline nasal) as a vasoconstrictor; there is a little risk of toxicity and works better than cocaine or Neo-Synephrine.
2. Be methodical and meticulous in surgery.
3. Inject the lateral wall with a 27-gauge retrobulbar needle bent 10 degrees toward the bevel.
4. Preserve and minimize trauma to the lateral surface of the middle turbinate and lamina papyracea.
5. Transect the uncinate process with an initial window cut in the midportion with a backbiter and remove the inferior boney portion with a seeker.
6. Trim the remaining mucosa with a small aggressive cutting microdebrider.
7. Examine the maxillary antrum with a 30 degree window and enlarge if the ostium can only be palpated; surgeon preference with cutting forceps, balloon or manual enlargement with a seeker.
8. Remove the anterior bulla sharply by initially creating a perforation with a small curette and then sharply transecting the attachments of the bulla with sharp through biting instruments.
9. Make every effort not to strip mucosa off the lamina papyracea.
10. Follow the lateral surface of the middle turbinate to the basal lamella to ensure complete removal of the uncinate process.
11. Trim remaining bone and mucosa fragments with an aggressive cutting small microdebrider, taking care not to strip the mucosa.
12. Use absorbable stents or packing placed in the middle meatus to keep the surfaces of the middle turbinate and lateral wall separated.
13. About 38% of ASPO members now use stents, but most do not.
14. If packing remains in place for greater than 2 wk it can be a source for increased scarring.
15. Second look procedures under general anesthesia are not warranted.

ASPO, American Society of Pediatric Otolaryngology; wk, week(s).

children with sinusitis or who had endoscopic sinus surgery when compared to the normal population.

Conclusion

The management of pediatric sinusitis requires a stepwise management protocol. The author suggests the following:

- First course of medical management is with broad-spectrum antibiotics, topical nasal steroid sprays, and irrigations if the patient is compliant.
- If this is not effective, then it would be reasonable to perform an adenoidectomy with the expectation that there would be about 65 to 70% improvement.

Appropriate expectations of the parents and referring physician need to be emphasized.

- If adenoidectomy fails, a more in-depth work-up is warranted. One should assess for allergies and immune deficiency. If present, these should be treated before further surgical intervention. Think about gastroesophageal reflux as a potential cause.
- Consider imaging the sinuses after a prolonged course of broad-spectrum antibiotics if the Otolaryngologist and the parents are considering endoscopic sinus surgery as an option. A CT scan is the most effective way to visualize the sinuses but is not required for documentation of sinusitis. Obtain the CT with scan in an image-guided format with coronal reconstructions.
- If the Otolaryngologist's judgment is that significant disease is present, then proceed to anterior ethmoidectomy and maxillary antrostomy. The author recommends using an absorbable stent to keep the two mucosal surfaces of the middle meatus apart. If left in place for greater than 2 week, however, this could be a source of scarring.
- Endoscopic sinus surgery can be expected to result in marked improvement of symptoms in around 85% of children who exhibit symptoms of chronic sinusitis.

References

1. Kim HJ, Jung Cho M, Lee JW, et al. The relationship between anatomic variations of paranasal sinuses and chronic sinusitis in children. Acta Otolaryngol 2006;126(10):1067–1072
2. Sivasli E, Sirikçi A, Bayazýt YA, et al. Anatomic variations of the paranasal sinus area in pediatric patients with chronic sinusitis. Surg Radiol Anat 2003;24(6):400–405
3. Barbero GJ. Gastroesophageal reflux and upper airway disease. Otolaryngol Clin North Am 1996;29(1):27–38
4. Brooks I, Gooch WM III, Jenkins SG, et al. Medical management of acute bacterial sinusitis. Recommendations of a clinical advisory committee on pediatric and adult sinusitis. Ann Otol Rhinol Laryngol Suppl 2000;182:2–20
5. Hsin CH, Su MC, Tsao CH, Chuang CY, Liu CM. Bacteriology and antimicrobial susceptibility of pediatric chronic rhinosinusitis: a 6-year result of maxillary sinus punctures. Am J Otolaryngol 2010;31(3):145–149
6. McNeil JC, Hulten KG, Mason EO Jr, Kaplan SL. Serotype 19A is the most common *Streptococcus pneumoniae* isolate in children with chronic sinusitis. Pediatr Infect Dis J 2009;28(9):766–768
7. McKinley SH, Yen MT, Miller AM, Yen KG. Microbiology of pediatric orbital cellulitis. Am J Ophthalmol 2007;144(4):497–501
8. Huang WH, Hung PK. Methicillin-resistant *Staphylococcus aureus* infections in acute rhinosinusitis. Laryngoscope 2006;116(2):288–291
9. Casey JR, Adlowitz DG, Pichichero ME. New patterns in the otopathogens causing acute otitis media six to eight years after introduction of pneumococcal conjugate vaccine. Pediatr Infect Dis J 2010;29(4):304–309
10. Lusk RP. Current Management of Pediatric Chronic Sinusitis. 2011.
11. Wald ER. Chronic sinusitis in children. [see comments]. [Review] [44 refs] J Pediatr 1995;127(3):339–347

12. McAlister WH, Lusk R, Muntz HR. Comparison of plain radiographs and coronal CT scans in infants and children with recurrent sinusitis. AJR Am J Roentgenol 1989;153(6):1259–1264

13. Lazar RH, Younis RT, Parvey LS. Comparison of plain radiographs, coronal CT, and intraoperative findings in children with chronic sinusitis. Otolaryngol Head Neck Surg 1992;107(1):29–34

14. Brenner D, Elliston C, Hall E, Berdon W. Estimated risks of radiation-induced fatal cancer from pediatric CT. AJR Am J Roentgenol 2001;176(2):289–296

15. Rogers LF. Radiation exposure in CT: why so high? AJR Am J Roentgenol 2001;177(2):277

16. Huda W, Chamberlain CC, Rosenbaum AE, Garrisi W. Radiation doses to infants and adults undergoing head CT examinations. Med Phys 2001;28(3):393–399

17. Kassel JC, King D, Spurling GK. Saline nasal irrigation for acute upper respiratory tract infections. Cochrane Database Syst Rev 2010;(3):CD006821

18. Harvey R, Hannan SA, Badia L, Scadding G. Nasal saline irrigations for the symptoms of chronic rhinosinusitis. Cochrane Database Syst Rev 2007;(3):CD006394

19. Liang KL, Su MC, Tseng HC, Jiang RS. Impact of pulsatile nasal irrigation on the prognosis of functional endoscopic sinus surgery. J Otolaryngol Head Neck Surg 2008;37(2):148–153

20. Shaikh N, Wald ER, Pi M. Decongestants, antihistamines and nasal irrigation for acute sinusitis in children. Cochrane Database Syst Rev 2010;12(12):CD007909

21. Mori F, Barni S, Pucci N, Rossi ME, Orsi Battaglini C, Novembre E. Upper airways disease: role of corticosteroids. Int J Immunopathol Pharmacol 2010;23(1, Suppl):61–66

22. Gawchik SM, Saccar CL. A risk-benefit assessment of intranasal triamcinolone acetonide in allergic rhinitis. Drug Saf 2000;23(4):309–322

23. Agertoft L, Pedersen S. Short-term lower leg growth rate in children with rhinitis treated with intranasal mometasone furoate and budesonide. J Allergy Clin Immunol 1999;104(5):948–952

24. Schenkel EJ, Skoner DP, Bronsky EA, et al. Absence of growth retardation in children with perennial allergic rhinitis after one year of treatment with mometasone furoate aqueous nasal spray. Pediatrics 2000;105(2):E22

25. Anon JB, Jacobs MR, Poole MD, et al; Sinus and Allergy Health Partnership. Antimicrobial treatment guidelines for acute bacterial rhinosinusitis. Otolaryngol Head Neck Surg 2004;130(1, Suppl):1–45

26. Solares CA, Batra PS, Hall GS, Citardi MJ. Treatment of chronic rhinosinusitis exacerbations due to methicillin-resistant *Staphylococcus aureus* with mupirocin irrigations. Am J Otolaryngol 2006;27(3):161–165

27. Laurens MB, Becker RM, Johnson JK, Wolf JS, Kotloff KL. MRSA with progression from otitis media and sphenoid sinusitis to clival osteomyelitis, pachymeningitis and abducens nerve palsy in an immunocompetent 10-year-old patient. Int J Pediatr Otorhinolaryngol 2008;72(7):945–951

28. Brietzke SE, Brigger MT. Adenoidectomy outcomes in pediatric rhinosinusitis: a meta-analysis. Int J Pediatr Otorhinolaryngol 2008;72(10):1541–1545

29. Zuliani G, Carron M, Gurrola J, et al. Identification of adenoid biofilms in chronic rhinosinusitis. Int J Pediatr Otorhinolaryngol 2006;70(9):1613–1617

30. Coticchia J, Zuliani G, Coleman C, et al. Biofilm surface area in the pediatric nasopharynx: chronic rhinosinusitis vs obstructive sleep apnea. Arch Otolaryngol Head Neck Surg 2007;133(2):110–114

31. Galli J, Calò L, Ardito F, et al. Biofilm formation by *Haemophilus influenzae* isolated from adeno-tonsil tissue samples, and its role in recurrent adenotonsillitis. Acta Otorhinolaryngol Ital 2007;27(3):134–138

32. Kania RE, Lamers GE, Vonk MJ, et al. Characterization of mucosal biofilms on human adenoid tissues. Laryngoscope 2008;118(1):128–134

33. Pagella F, Colombo A, Gatti O, Giourgos G, Matti E. Rhinosinusitis and otitis media: the link with adenoids. Int J Immunopathol Pharmacol 2010;23(1, Suppl):38–40

34. Muntz HR, Lusk RP. Nasal antral windows in children: a retrospective study. Laryngoscope 1990;100(6):643–646

35. Ramadan HH, McLaughlin K, Josephson G, Rimell F, Bent J, Parikh SR. Balloon catheter sinuplasty in young children. Am J Rhinol Allergy 2010;24(1):e54–e56

36. Zeiders JW, Dahya ZJ. Antral lavage using the Luma transillumination wire and vortex irrigator—a safe and effective advance in treating pediatric sinusitis. Int J Pediatr Otorhinolaryngol 2011;75(4):461–463

37. Ramadan HH, Terrell AM. Balloon catheter sinuplasty and adenoidectomy in children with chronic rhinosinusitis. Ann Otol Rhinol Laryngol 2010;119(9):578–582

38. Wilkerson WW Jr. Experiments and presentation of cases in which an antral window was made in the middle meatus of the human subject and no additional surgical procedures were performed. Arch Otolaryngol 1949;49(5):463–489

39. Ramadan HH. Safety and feasibility of balloon sinuplasty for treatment of chronic rhinosinusitis in children. Ann Otol Rhinol Laryngol 2009;118(3):161–165

40. Gross CW, Lazar RH, Gurucharri MJ. Pediatric functional endonasal sinus surgery. Otolaryngol Clin North Am 1989;22(4):733–738

41. Lusk RP, Muntz HR. Endoscopic sinus surgery in children with chronic sinusitis: a pilot study. Laryngoscope 1990;100(6):654–658

42. Hebert RL II, Bent JP III. Meta-analysis of outcomes of pediatric functional endoscopic sinus surgery. Laryngoscope 1998;108(6):796–799

43. Terris MH, Davidson TM. Review of published results for endoscopic sinus surgery. Ear Nose Throat J 1994;73(8):574–580

44. Mair EA, Bolger WE, Breisch EA. Sinus and facial growth after pediatric endoscopic sinus surgery. Arch Otolaryngol Head Neck Surg 1995;121(5):547–552

45. Carpenter KM, Graham SM, Smith RJ. Facial skeletal growth after endoscopic sinus surgery in the piglet model. Am J Rhinol 1997;11(3):211–217

46. Wolf G, Greistorfer K, Jebeles JA. The endoscopic endonasal surgical technique in the treatment of chronic recurring sinusitis in children. Rhinology 1995;33(2):97–103

47. Senior B, Wirtschafter A, Mai C, Becker C, Belenky W. Quantitative impact of pediatric sinus surgery on facial growth. Laryngoscope 2000;110(11):1866–1870

48. Bothwell MR, Piccirillo JF, Lusk RP, Ridenour BD. Long-term outcome of facial growth after functional endoscopic sinus surgery. Otolaryngol Head Neck Surg 2002;126(6):628–634

19 Complications in Revision Sinus Surgery

Troy D. Woodard and James A. Stankiewicz

Endoscopic sinus surgery has become increasingly popular and is the standard manner of surgical treatment of sinus disease that is not responsive to medical therapy. Since its inception three decades ago, many technological developments have broadened the surgical scope of the endoscopic approach and have led to better outcomes and less morbidity. Despite the medical and surgical advances, endoscopic sinus surgery is not without risks. The close proximity of sinuses to the orbit, brain, and carotid artery makes sinus surgery one of the most dangerous surgeries within our field. Revision surgery can be even more perilous because many helpful landmarks are not present and heavy scarring and osteitis can increase the difficulty of the surgery (**Fig. 19.1**). Image guidance is particularly helpful in these cases because it can help evaluate the sinus anatomy and recognize altered anatomy that may be problematic during surgery (**Fig. 19.2**). Complications do occur and can be disastrous, resulting in litigation. The endoscopic surgeon must not only be experienced in these techniques, but also have knowledge of the anatomy to help avoid complications. This chapter will provide a closer look at the major complications and provide pearls on how to prevent and manage them.

Classification

There are many types of complications that can occur with endoscopic sinus surgery. They are classified as minor and major complications.[1,2] Minor complications include hyposmia, adhesions, headache, dental/facial pain, epistaxis not requiring blood transfusion, and periorbital ecchymosis or emphysema. Major complications are much more serious and result in more devastating effects. They include orbital hematoma, ocular muscle injury, blindness, carotid injury, and skull base penetrations resulting in cerebrospinal fluid (CSF) leak, meningitis, and/or pneumocephalus.

Orbital Hematoma

The orbit comprises seven bones; the thinnest bone is a portion of the ethmoid bone called the lamina papyracea. This eggshell thick bone forms the lateral border of the ethmoid sinus cavity. Close attention should be paid to this area both preoperatively on computed tomography (CT) scans and intraoperatively for the possibility of bony dehiscence and prolapsed orbital contents into the nasal cavity. Although rare (<1%), orbital complications during sinus surgery do occur.[2–4] They include enophthalmos, emphysema, orbital hematoma, extraocular muscle injury, and optic nerve damage.

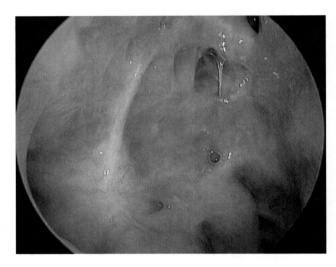

Figure 19.1 Right nasal cavity with excessive scarring and absent middle turbinate.

Orbital hematoma is the most common orbital complication during endoscopic sinus surgery.[2–4] Hematomas can occur when there is damage to the periorbita, orbital fat, and vascular supply to the orbital contents. While there are two types of bleeding that lead to orbital hematomas, immediate and delayed onset, their mechanisms of action are different.[5] Delayed onset hematomas are a result of damage to the orbital veins that lie within the orbital fat and along the lamina papyracea. This low-pressure bleeding results in a gradual accumulation of blood within the orbital cone. While generally considered less catastrophic, this type of bleeding can also result in an increase of intraocular pressure and result in retinal ischemia and blindness.

In contrast with the delayed type, the immediate type is a result of arterial bleeding. When injured, the vessels often retract within the orbit causing rapid accumulation of blood within the tightly spaced orbit. The anterior and/or posterior ethmoidal arteries are usually the culprits. Both arteries are branches of the internal carotid system and ophthalmic arteries. The anterior ethmoid artery runs from a lateral to a medial direction along the skull base just posterior to the frontal recess. While it is usually encased in bone and runs directly along the skull base, it has been shown to be dehiscent and hang below the skull base, making it an easy target during surgery.[5,6] The posterior ethmoid artery is usually more protected. It is encased by bone and runs along the skull base just superior to the sphenoid sinus. Depending on the severity of the sinus disease and extent of nasal polyps, it can be difficult for the surgeon to identify the arteries during surgical dissection.

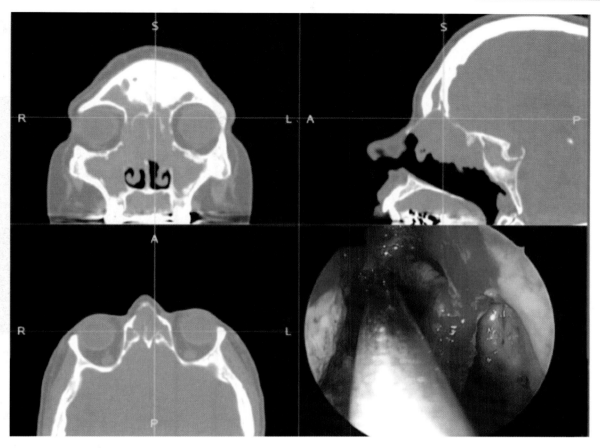

Figure 19.2 Patient with history of previous surgery and extensive nasal polyps. Image guidance is used to help navigate without normal anatomical landmarks.

The first step in prevention is preoperative planning. Preoperative endoscopic examination can not only determine the pathology but can also reveal any altered anatomy in revision cases. Fine CT scans with coronal reconstruction are optimal to study the orbital anatomy. The anterior ethmoidal artery exiting the orbit can be identified by locating the anterior ethmoidal artery peak or "nipple" (**Fig. 19.3**).[7] This is usually located just along the skull base at the confluence of the superior oblique and medial rectus muscles. Any dehiscence or thinning of the lamina papyracea should be noted, especially in a revision surgery.

Another important step is to prepare the patient intraoperatively before beginning the surgery. The eyes should be in the field and taped along the lateral canthal region to allow constant examination and palpation during the surgery. Frequent inspection for periocular bruising and palpation for increased intraocular pressure should be performed during sinus surgery. If orbital bruising, firmness on palpation, and proptosis is discovered, the surgeon must be concerned for a developing hematoma.

Several actions must be preformed simultaneously to prevent a disastrous outcome. The retina is very sensitive to ischemia and blindness has been shown to occur within 90 minutes of hematoma onset.[5,7] The first step is to obtain an intraoperative ophthalmology consult. While awaiting their

arrival, the nasal cavity needs to be inspected for bleeding. Any nasal packing should be removed and hemostasis should be achieved. Intraocular pressures should be evaluated with a tonometer and the source of the bleeding (arterial vs. venous) should be determined. Venous bleeding usually results in a

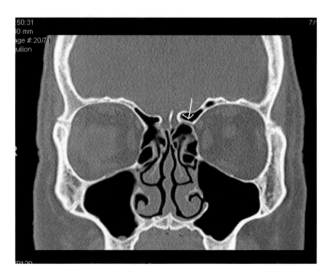

Figure 19.3 Coronal computed tomography scan demonstrating path of anterior ethmoid artery (arrow).

slower build up of hematoma and intraocular pressure. As a result, conservative measures such as intravenous mannitol, steroids, and orbital massage can be given to help lower intraocular pressures. However, close observation should be performed because these methods may fail to lower intraocular pressure. When these fail, surgical intervention should be performed to prevent blindness.

In contrast with venous bleeding, arterial bleeding results in a rapid accumulation of blood within the orbital cone. This results in compromise of the optic nerve vasculature and blindness. Conservative measures are not indicated in this type of bleed because the rise in intraocular pressures is too rapid for the medications to sufficiently lower the pressures. As a result, surgical intervention with a lateral canthotomy and cantholysis or endoscopic orbital decompression is indicated and should be performed promptly to avoid permanent damage to the optic nerve and blindness.

Orbital Muscle Injury

Ocular dysmotility and diplopia result from orbital muscle injury. While the medial rectus is the most commonly injured, the superior oblique and inferior rectus can also be injured.[3,8,9] Damage to the musculature generally occurs in one of the two mechanisms. First, the surgeon can directly enter the orbit during maxillary antrostomy or ethmoidectomy. Care should be given when attempting to remove an uncinate that is adherent to the orbit. Revision surgery is more problematic because of partial uncinectomy or scarring that results in lateralization of the uncinate. Removal can expose the periorbita and predispose it to injury. In addition, the inappropriate use of a rigid backbiter can lead to penetration of the lamina papyracea and inadvertent damage to the medial rectus. Second, muscle injury can result from inadvertent suctioning of orbital fat and muscle through an area of dehiscent bone into the ethmoid cavity with microdebrider. Ocular muscular damage is often associated with visual loss or orbital hematoma.

Preoperative planning is essential for avoiding ocular muscle damage. Thorough examination of axial and coronal CT scans is vital in appreciating a lateralized uncinate, hypoplastic maxillary sinus with a low orbital floor, and a dehiscent lamina papyracea. The eyes should be prepped into the surgical field, taped laterally, and periodically examined for any bruising. Additionally, the orbital press test, also known as the "Stankiewicz maneuver," is a key method that can help prevent orbital injury.[10] This maneuver involves pressing the eye during surgery and looking for transmitted movement along the lamina papyracea, indicating a dehiscent lamina. Surgical dissection with blunt instruments to medialize the uncinate before its removal also reduces the potential for inadvertent orbital entry. Surgery around areas of dehiscence should be done carefully. If a microdebrider is used, the blade should be turned away from the orbit to prevent suction of the orbital contents into the blade.

If the blade enters the orbit accidentally, then further surgical dissection in this area should be halted and the eyes should be immediately inspected. Ophthalmology consultation should be obtained for suspected muscular injury. Proper characterization of the type of injury is imperative to determine the best method of repair: conservative versus surgical reattachment.

Optic Nerve Injury

One of the most devastating orbital complications is vision loss. This can occur from both direct and indirect optic nerve injury. Indirect optic nerve injury occurs from vascular compromise in association with an orbital hematoma. In contrast, direct nerve injury more commonly occurs while performing an endoscopic ethmoidectomy and sphenoidotomy. The optic nerve lies in the superior lateral portion of the sphenoid sinuses and has been found to be dehiscent in 4 to 6% of the population.[3,7,11] Aggressive blind dissection and use of powered instrumentation during sphenoidotomy can directly injure and transect the optic nerve leading to blindness. Similarly, optic nerve damage can also occur while performing a posterior ethmoidectomy. Onodi cells, a posterior ethmoidal cell that lies superior and lateral to the sphenoid sinus, have been found to be present in 8 to 14% of the population and often contain a dehiscent optic nerve.[3,7] Aggressive dissection and manipulation within this posterior cell can also damage the nerve.

Once the optic nerve is transected, little can be done to repair it. Therefore, the best management is prevention. Damage to the optic nerve can be avoided by reviewing the CT scans preoperatively for the presence of dehiscent optic nerves and the presence of Onodi cells, which appear to have a horizontal bony septation within the sphenoid sinus on coronal CT scans (**Fig. 19.4**). In revision surgery, there may be excessive scarring and some of the normal

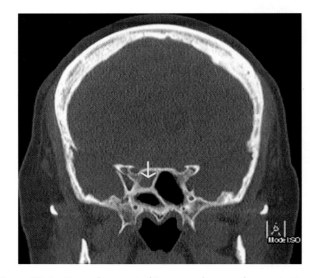

Figure 19.4 Coronal computed tomography scan demonstrating an opacified Onodi cell (arrow).

anatomical landmarks, such as the middle and superior turbinates, may be absent. Therefore, use of image guidance and several other landmarks that tend to remain constant as points of reference can help ensure that one safely enters the sphenoid (**Fig. 19.5**). The natural sphenoid ostium (os) lies 7 cm posterior in a 30-degree angle from the nasal sill.[12,13] In addition, the sphenoid os lies at the same level as the natural maxillary sinus os and should be no higher than the orbital floor. Lastly, once the sphenoid os is identified it should be opened in a medial and inferior direction to avoid vital structures.

Carotid Artery Injury

Ascending to provide blood to the brain, the cavernous portion of the carotid artery runs alongside the sphenoid sinus. As it makes the turn toward the brain, the artery abuts the posterior lateral roof of the sphenoid sinus. The bony wall separating the artery from the sphenoid sinus is very thin. Fujii et al examined 50 carotid arteries in cadavers and noticed that 88% of the specimens had sphenoid bony walls of less than 0.5 mm.[14] In addition, Kennedy et al found that 20% of their cadaveric specimens had a dehiscent intrasphenoid carotid artery.[15] The relationship of the carotid artery to the sphenoid sinus places it at risk during sinus surgery.

Similar to the other complications, review of CT scans is imperative. Axial views of CT scans tend to provide better views to identify the location of the carotid arteries and give an idea of how thick is the surrounding bone.[16] Proper identification and widening of the sphenoid os helps in preventing this devastating complication. The natural os of the sphenoid lies medial to the inferior third of the superior turbinate. In revision cases where that landmark is missing, the os can be found by the use of image guidance, searching at the same level as the natural maxillary sinus os at approximately 1.5 cm above the choana, and 7 cm posterior in a 30-degree direction from the nasal spine. The sphenoid should be opened in a medial and inferior direction. Blind use of powered, biting, and grabbing instruments should be avoided within the sphenoid sinus, as dehiscent carotid artery may get injured. Likewise, penetration of the lateral sphenoid wall can result in carotid artery injury and massive blood loss.

In the event that massive hemorrhage develops during surgery, several steps should be promptly performed by the surgeon and anesthesia staff to keep the patient alive.[16–18] Immediate nasal packing with Foley catheters with inflatable

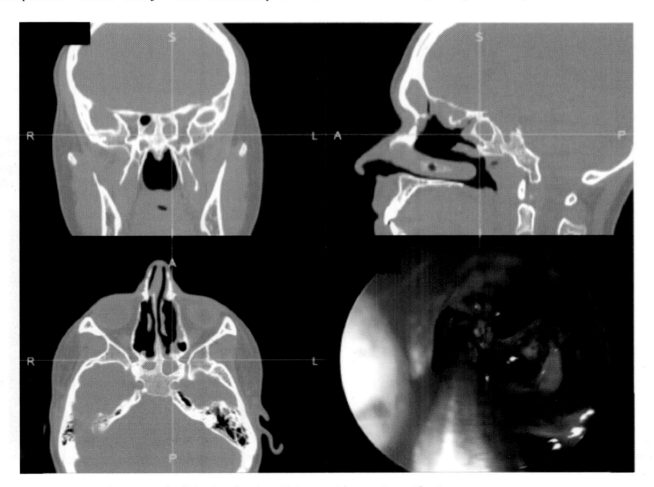

Figure 19.5 Image guidance is used to help identify sphenoid sinuses with extensive ossification.

balloons and gauze placement within the nose and pharynx will help tamponade and slow bleeding. Anesthesia should place several large bore intravenous lines and provide fluid resuscitation. In addition, they should maintain a controlled hypotension to help slow bleeding while still providing cerebral circulation. Next, immediate transportation to the endosvascular suite for definitive management of the hemorrhage is necessary. While stenting is possible, many cases require vessel sacrifice with balloons or coils to stop bleeding.

Cerebrospinal Fluid Leak

Intracranial complications from endoscopic sinus surgery result from penetration of the anterior skull base. This thickness of the skull base varies based on the location. The most medial aspects (cribriform plate and lateral lamella) are the thinnest, while the lateral ethmoid roof tends to be composed of thicker bone. Despite these differences, extreme care should be taken when dissecting all along the skull base because penetration and CSF leak can occur anywhere. In many patients, previous surgery causes an alteration or absence of key skull base structures such as in middle or superior turbinates removal.

Failure to identify the height of the skull base before aggressive surgical dissection is a common cause of intracranial penetration. Coronal CT scans are optimal to determine the height of the skull base. There are several techniques, which can be used to describe the height of the skull base. Keros et al designed a classification system, which is based on the length of the lateral cribriform lamella.[19] The length of the lateral lamella in Keros type I is 1 to 3 mm, Keros type II is 4 to 7 mm, and Keros type III is 8 to 16 mm. A higher Keros stage represents a low-lying skull base and a more dangerous anatomy. As a result, more caution should be displayed during sinus surgery.

Another technique involves comparing the level of cribriform to the orbit. This technique involves dividing the orbit into thirds. A high, safer, skull base is found when the cribriform is at the level of the superior one-third of the orbit. In contrast, when the cribriform is below the level of the superior one-third of the orbit or the medial rectus, the patient has a low-lying skull base (**Fig. 19.6**). This potentially results in a hazardous sinus dissection and requires much caution.[20,21]

Penetration of the cribriform plate and the lateral lamella occurs when dissection is carried too far medial and superior along the middle turbinate. Using drills, which is often the case in revision surgery of the frontal or ethmoid sinus increases the risk of CSF leak. In addition, aggressive manipulation of the middle turbinate should be avoided as it can result in skull base fracture and a resultant CSF leak. In revised cases where the middle turbinate is absent, dissection medially and superiorly along the septum should be performed in a limited fashion and avoided if possible as inadvertent skull base penetration is likely.

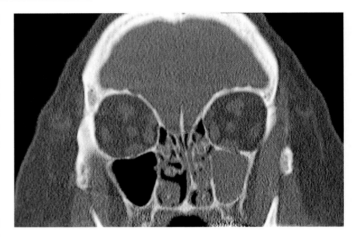

Figure 19.6 Coronal computed tomography scan demonstrating a low lying skull base (line at the level of the cribriform plate).

CSF leaks will manifest with a sudden burst of clear watery fluid that washes away the surrounding blood. When a CSF leak occurs, the surgeon should immediately stop the surgery, identify the location, and repair the defect. The most common sites of injury are the cribriform, lateral lamella, and the ethmoid fovea. These areas need to be fully inspected for a CSF leak and possibly the whitish coloration of dura. If the leak occurs and cannot be identified, the surgeon may get an intraoperative neurosurgical consult for lumbar subarachnoid drain placement and intrathecal fluorescein injection. This fluorescent dye will aid in identifying an active CSF leak and help identify when the leak has been successfully repaired (**Fig. 19.7**).[22] While administration of

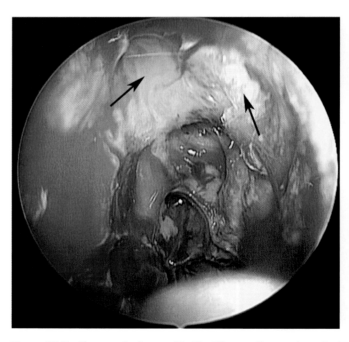

Figure 19.7 Fluorescein dye used to identify an active cerebrospinal fluid leak. The fluorescein can be seen in the superior nasal vault (arrows).

this dye has been associated with causing seizures and other neurological sequelae, very low concentrations have been found to be safe in patients. This dye is mixed at a concentration of 0.01 cm³ in 10 cm³ of the patient's CSF or preservative free saline. It is then slowly injected into the subarachnoid space via the lumbar drain at a rate of 1 cm³/min. Depending on the size of the defect, skull base repair can be performed with a variety of materials including mucosa, muscle, fat, fascia, cartilage, and cadaveric skin. If fluorescein dye is used, one can ensure a tight seal if no more green dye is seen flowing from the defect after repair. Postoperatively, the patient should be awakened very smoothly while minimizing positive pressure ventilation. Neurosurgical consultation should be obtained if there is a suspected cortical injury and for consideration for postoperative imaging.

Conclusion

Revision endoscopic sinus surgery poses a special challenge to the otolaryngologist because of the altered anatomy and fibrous or bony scarring. The close proximity of sinuses to the orbit, brain, and carotid artery makes sinus surgery extremely delicate. While some complications cause little to no permanent sequelae, others are disastrous and can cause extreme morbidity if not death. Thorough preoperative counseling is essential. One must not only be familiar with the sinonasal anatomy, but should also operate cautiously and expect the unexpected. Meticulous review of fine cut CT scans, proper preparation of the patient before surgery, and constant observation during surgery are fundamental elements that will help prevent the development of complications. When complications do occur, prompt intervention and the involvement of appropriate specialists become indispensable.

References

1. Stankiewicz JA. Complications of endoscopic intranasal ethmoidectomy. Laryngoscope 1987;97(11):1270–1273
2. May M, Levine HL, Mester SJ, Schaitkin B. Complications of endoscopic sinus surgery: analysis of 2108 patients—incidence and prevention. Laryngoscope 1994;104(9):1080–1083
3. Bhatti MT, Stankiewicz JA. Ophthalmic complications of endoscopic sinus surgery. Surv Ophthalmol 2003;48(4):389–402
4. Han JK, Higgins TS. Management of orbital complications in endoscopic sinus surgery. Curr Opin Otolaryngol Head Neck Surg 2010;18(1):32–36
5. Stankiewicz JA, Chow JM. Two faces of orbital hematoma in intranasal (endoscopic) sinus surgery. Otolaryngol Head Neck Surg 1999;120(6):841–847
6. Moon HJ, Kim HU, Lee JG, Chung IH, Yoon JH. Surgical anatomy of the anterior ethmoidal canal in ethmoid roof. Laryngoscope 2001;111(5):900–904
7. Welch KC, Palmer JN. Intraoperative emergencies during endoscopic sinus surgery: CSF leak and orbital hematoma. Otolaryngol Clin North Am 2008;41(3):581–596, ix–x
8. Rene C, Rose GE, Lenthall R, Moseley I. Major orbital complications of endoscopic sinus surgery. Br J Ophthalmol 2001;85(5):598–603
9. Huang CM, Meyer DR, Patrinely JR, et al. Medial rectus muscle injuries associated with functional endoscopic sinus surgery: characterization and management. Ophthal Plast Reconstr Surg 2003;19(1):25–37
10. Scianna J, Stankiewicz J. Complications in revision sinus surgery: presentation and management. In: Kountakis S, ed. Revision Sinus Surgery. Heidelberg, Germany: Springer; 2008:223–234
11. Yanagisawa E. The optic nerve and the internal carotid artery in the sphenoid sinus. Ear Nose Throat J 2002;81(9):611–612
12. Kim HU, Kim SS, Kang SS, Chung IH, Lee JG, Yoon JH. Surgical anatomy of the natural ostium of the sphenoid sinus. Laryngoscope 2001;111(9):1599–1602
13. Stankiewicz JA. The endoscopic approach to the sphenoid sinus. Laryngoscope 1989;99(2):218–221
14. Fujii K, Chambers SM, Rhoton AL Jr. Neurovascular relationships of the sphenoid sinus. A microsurgical study. J Neurosurg 1979;50(1):31–39
15. Kennedy DW, Zinreich SJ, Hassab MH. The internal carotid artery as it relates to endonasal sphenoethmoidectomy. Am J Rhinol 1990;4(1):7–12
16. Weidenbecher M, Huk WJ, Iro H. Internal carotid artery injury during functional endoscopic sinus surgery and its management. Eur Arch Otorhinolaryngol 2005;262(8):640–645
17. Park AH, Stankiewicz JA, Chow J, Azar-Kia B. A protocol for management of a catastrophic complication of functional endoscopic sinus surgery: internal carotid artery injury. Am J Rhinol 1998;12(3):153–158
18. Solares CA, Ong YK, Carrau RL, et al. Prevention and management of vascular injuries in endoscopic surgery of the sinonasal tract and skull base. Otolaryngol Clin North Am 2010;43(4):817–825
19. Keros P. On the practical value of differences in the level of the lamina cribrosa of the ethmoid [in German]. Z Laryngol Rhinol Otol 1962;41:809–813
20. Stankiewicz JA, Chow JM. The low skull base: an invitation to disaster. Am J Rhinol 2004;18(1):35–40
21. Stankiewicz JA, Chow JM. The low skull base-is it important? Curr Opin Otolaryngol Head Neck Surg 2005;13(1):19–21
22. Seth R, Rajasekaran K, Benninger MS, Batra PS. The utility of intrathecal fluorescein in cerebrospinal fluid leak repair. Otolaryngol Head Neck Surg 2010;143(5):626–632

20 Epistaxis: Surgical and Nonsurgical Management

Steven D. Pletcher and Andrew N. Goldberg

Epistaxis is a common disorder in both pediatric and adult patients. Many episodes are self-limited and do not require medical care. Otolaryngologists are often consulted to treat patients with recurrent or refractory bleeds. Epistaxis is the most common emergent consultation for the otolaryngologists. A broad knowledge of risk factors and anatomy as well as facility with cautery techniques, packing materials, surgical interventions, and adjunctive treatment measures will allow effective and efficient management of these patients.

Anatomy

The nose receives its vascular supply from branches of both the internal and external carotid systems. The anterior and posterior ethmoid arteries are branches of the ophthalmic artery from the internal carotid system (**Fig. 20.1**). The superior labial artery is a branch of the facial artery that, along with the sphenopalatine artery (SPA), originates from the external carotid system.

Distal branches of the anterior ethmoid artery and the superior labial artery anastomose with branches of the SPA to form Kiesselbach plexis, a vascular region of the anterior septum (**Fig. 20.1**). The majority of anterior nasal bleeds, which account for greater than 90% of all nasal bleeds, arise from this anastomotic region. Bleeds from this area are typically easier to manage than posterior bleeds and may be treated with targeted cautery, direct pressure, and nasal moisturization regimens.

The majority of posterior epistaxis arises from branches of the SPA, the terminal branch of the internal maxillary artery (IMA), which is the primary vascular supply to the posterior nasal cavity. Identification of the bleeding site is more difficult with posterior epistaxis and bleeds from this area are more frequently refractory to conservative treatment.

The anterior and posterior ethmoid arteries supply the superior portion of the nasal cavity. Overall, these vessels are less common sources of epistaxis, except in patients with recent facial trauma or recent sinonasal surgery.

Evaluation of Epistaxis

Appropriate treatment for epistaxis depends on the cause and severity of the bleed. Most patients suffer from primary epistaxis or spontaneous bleeds without a clear cause. Primary epistaxis may be exacerbated by medications, herbal supplements, and underlying medical conditions such as hypertension and atherosclerosis. Some patients presenting with epistaxis will have a clear identifiable cause for their bleeding such as a tumor or blood dyscrasia.

Medical History

Initial evaluation of patients requiring treatment for epistaxis should focus on the possible underlying disorders that may result in secondary epistaxis or exacerbate primary epistaxis. Patients with unexplained refractory bleeds should be evaluated for the use of anticoagulant medication (see "Medications") and the presence of leukemia, liver disease, or myelosuppression, all of which can present as epistaxis. Bleeding from other sources such as hematuria and easy bruising can indicate a systemic source for a coagulopathy. A thorough history will also guide laboratory testing, which typically includes a hemoglobin level, platelet count, prothrombin time, and partial thromboplastin time.

A history of nosebleeds including descriptions of the most recent and most severe bleeds will clarify the severity of epistaxis. Anterior epistaxis is commonly related to digital manipulation, blowing the nose, and a drying environment. These episodes are typically unilateral, recurrent, and self-limited lasting less than 5 minutes, though episodes of prolonged bleeding are occasionally seen. Patients will report that bleeding occurs through the anterior nose first and will readily identify the side that commonly bleeds. With posterior epistaxis, bleeding is often noted initially in the back of the throat and episodes are more commonly severe. Although these episodes are frequently profused and prolonged, they stop suddenly related to vascular spasm, only to resume hours later with similar severity.

Medical comorbidities may exacerbate bleeding and increase concern for complications of blood loss. Patients with hypertension may have more difficulty controlling epistaxis. Vascular disease associated with diabetes may result in a loss of vessel contractility and result in prolonged bleeds. Patients with coronary artery disease are at an increased risk of cardiac complications from epistaxis-associated blood loss, and transfusion thresholds should be considered for patients with significant blood loss.

The presence of epiphora (tearing), facial numbness, or diplopia in association with epistaxis should raise concern for tumors of the nose or paranasal sinuses. Patients with nasal tumors or nasopharyngeal carcinoma typically report

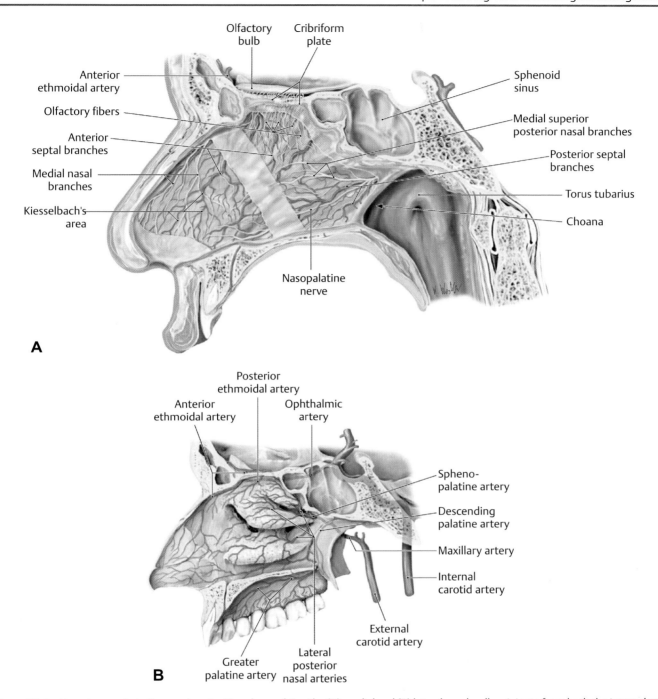

Figure 20.1 Vascular supply to the nasal cavity. Vessels supplying the (A) medial and (B) lateral nasal walls originate from both the internal and external carotid systems.

Printed with permission from: Thieme Publishers. Schuenke M, Schulte E, Schumacher U, Ross LM, Lamperti ED. *Thieme Atlas of Anatomy: Head and Neuroanatomy*. New York and Stuttgart: Thieme; 2007:116; Fig. 7.2 A. Illustrated by Wesker K.

a more indolent course of bleeding and may have other characteristics of malignancy such as cachexia, weakness, and posterior triangle neck adenopathy. Unilateral ear effusion in an adult can be a sign of a nasopharyngeal mass. Family history may be helpful in identifying coagulopathies or other bleeding disorders such as hereditary hemorrhagic telangiectasias.

Medications

Medications that interrupt clotting pathways commonly exacerbate epistaxis. Platelet inhibitors such as aspirin, nonsteroidal anti-inflammatory drugs, and clopidogrel have all been implicated as contributors. A study of 10,241 patients in primary care clinics demonstrated an increased frequency of epistaxis in patients taking aspirin or clopidogrel.[1] Patients taking aspirin have also been demonstrated to experience more severe epistaxis, more frequently require surgical intervention, and have a higher rate of recurrent bleeds.[2] Warfarin treatment, which prolongs the partial thromboplastin time, significantly increases the risk of epistaxis. Although the risk of epistaxis in patients taking warfarin is similar to that of patients taking both aspirin and clopidogrel, nosebleeds in patients taking warfarin are more likely to require hospitalization.[3] Many patients taking warfarin who present to the emergency department with epistaxis have an international normalized ratio above their recommended range.[4]

Along with traditional medication history, patients should be queried regarding their use of complementary and alternative medications or supplements. Many alternative treatments have the potential to directly impair clot formation or alter pharmacokinetics of other medications that impair clotting.[5] Fish oil, gingko biloba, ginseng, ginger, and garlic all inhibit platelet aggregation.

Physical Examination

Vital signs should be taken with specific attention on blood pressure, pulse, and fluid status. Bleeding sites are easier to identify in patients with current or recent bleeding. The extent of blood loss should be evaluated by both the patient's history and ongoing bleeding. Patients with brisk bleeding and significant blood loss should be evaluated and monitored in the emergency department. Fluid resuscitation and transfusions may be required for patients with extensive blood loss.

A close examination of the anterior nasal septum will often identify an area of bleeding. Mucosal prominences and prominent vasculature can be lightly manipulated with a suction or similar device to unmask bleeding sites and identify a target for treatment. Because manipulation of this nature can initiate a bleeding episode, it is helpful to anticipate such bleeding and have appropriate equipment available.

The oropharynx should be evaluated for blood or clots emanating from the nasopharynx. Nasal endoscopy is often helpful in patients with no obvious anterior bleeding. The illumination and magnification provided by an endoscope allows for thorough examination of the posterior nasal mucosa. Tumors of the nasal cavity and paranasal sinuses are often visible on endoscopic examination.

Treatment of Epistaxis

The majority of primary bleeds originate from the anterior septum. Identification of the bleeding sites allows for targeted treatment and increases success rate while minimizing patient morbidity. For patients with active bleeding, careful inspection of this area with appropriate illumination and suction will often reveal the bleeding site. This area can be cauterized with silver nitrate. Use of a topical vasoconstrictor and anesthetic before cauterization allows for a clean field

for cautery and minimizes patient discomfort. Monopolar or bipolar electrocautery may also be judiciously used. Cautery of directly opposing areas of the septum at the same setting creates a risk of septal perforation, as cartilage has no innate blood supply and requires an epithelial covering on at least one side to remain viable.

Clear identification of the bleeding site is the key to successful cautery. For patients who present with recurrent intermittent epistaxis and are not bleeding at the time of presentation, this may be challenging. Using a small suction just adjacent to suspected bleeding areas may elicit bleeding, identifying the target for treatment.

Pediatric patients, in particular, tend to bleed from the anterior septum. Cauterization and use of antibiotic cream decrease the frequency of bleeding in these patients. For patients in whom no obvious bleeding site is identified, use of antibiotic cream alone is a reasonable approach.[6,7] Patients with refractory or heavy bleeds should be evaluated to rule out clotting disorders or sinonasal neoplasms. Patients should also be counseled against local trauma including digital trauma (nose picking).

Cautery may also be used in combination with endoscopy. If an active bleeding site is identified posteriorly in the nose but accessible with the endoscope, a silver nitrate cautery may be performed under endoscopic guidance. Care should be taken not to cause injury to the proximal nasal mucosa while introducing the device used for cautery.

Patients with active bleeding from a source not identified on anterior rhinoscopy or not easily accessible for endoscopic cautery should be considered for nasal packing. Because of the need for removal of nonabsorbable packing materials and associated microabrasions of mucosa, care should be exercised in using nonabsorbable materials in patients with a coagulopathy or with hereditary hemorrhagic telangiectasia.

Multiple options for packing materials exist. Packing the nose with Vaseline ribbon gauze (Covidien Medical, Mansfield, Massachusetts, United States) of 0.25 or perhaps 0.5 in size is a traditional approach. Gauze used in this way is layered in with horizontal rows beginning superiorly, leaving a tag anteriorly for eventual unpacking. This technique is associated with significant patient discomfort and is less commonly used today. Packing Vaseline gauze inside a finger cot or the severed thumb of an examination glove can reduce microabrasions. When the time comes for removal, the internal gauze is extracted and the protective latex slipped out atraumatically.

Multiple commercially available packs have been developed to treat epistaxis. Merocel (Medtronic ENT, Jacksonville, Florida, United States) packs are made of hydroxilate polyvinyl acetate, which expands when exposed to hydration (including blood), to tamponade bleeding sites. Rapid Rhino packs (Arthrocare ENT, Austin, Texas, United States) are inflatable devices coated with a carboxymethylcellulose hydrocolloid compound with hemostatic properties. This device combines the tamponade and hemostatic properties. A comparison of the two devices for patients with anterior epistaxis not amenable to cautery found no difference in efficacy of these devices but did suggest that the Rapid Rhino was easier to insert and remove.[8]

Additional hemostatic materials have been evaluated for treatment of epistaxis. FloSeal (Baxter, Deerfield, Illinois, United States) is composed of a collagen matrix and bovine-derived thrombin. Intranasal application of FloSeal for patients with anterior epistaxis has been compared with standard packing in the emergency department setting. A randomized study of 70 consecutive patients demonstrated higher patient and physician satisfaction as well as increased efficacy with FloSeal.[9] Targeted cautery was not evaluated in this study and only patients with anterior epistaxis were included in the study. FloSeal is significantly more expensive than traditional packing devices, but this increased cost may be balanced by a decreased failure rate and decreased requirement for subspecialty consultation and follow-up. FloSeal has also been successful in treating patients who fail standard packing techniques (Mathiasen and Cruz, Côté et al).[9,10]

While FloSeal has been evaluated primarily in patients with anterior epistaxis, these patients may be often treated effectively with identification of the bleeding site and directed cautery. Hemostatic materials such as FloSeal, Surgicel (oxidized cellulose; Ethicon, Somerville, New Jersey, United States), or Avitene (microfibrillar collagen; Bard Davol Inc, Warwick, Rhode Island, United States) may be used in a targeted fashion under endoscopic guidance to manage the more difficult to treat posterior epistaxis. Use of these materials is often helpful in addition to endoscopic cautery. Posterior packing may be required in patients with refractory bleeding despite attempts at anterior packing and use of hemostatic materials. This may be accomplished by using the balloon of a Foley catheter to occlude the choana and gauze packing in the nasal cavity. Double balloon packs with a long anterior balloon and a smaller spherical posterior balloon that are designed to occlude the choana and nasal cavity are also commercially available (Epistat, Medtronic, Inc., Jacksonville, Florida, United States). Posterior packs are quite uncomfortable and may not be well tolerated by all patients. The success rate for posterior packing is also significantly lower than that of surgery or embolization. It is therefore reasonable to consider surgery or embolization in patients who require placement of a posterior pack.

Close coordination with medical specialists is often required for appropriate treatment of epistaxis. Optimizing blood pressure and adjusting anticoagulant medications are helpful regardless of the treatment approach selected. Patients with underlying liver disease and hematopoietic malignancies also require a team approach.

Treatment of Refractory Epistaxis

Patients with epistaxis refractory to packing require additional intervention. Treatment options for these patients include surgery and embolization.

Surgical Treatment of Epistaxis

The traditional surgical approaches to epistaxis have been largely replaced by endoscopic surgical procedures. Traditional approaches targeted the IMA through a sublabial approach. Endoscopic ligation of the SPA is a less-invasive approach that targets the terminal branch of the IMA. SPA ligation was introduced in the 1990s and multiple clinical series demonstrate the high (> 90%) success rate of this technique.[11–14]

SPA ligation is performed under general anesthesia. Patients often come to the operating room with their nose packed; packing material is left in place until the patient is anesthetized and all surgical instruments are available. Following removal of nasal packing, the nasal cavity is carefully examined using an endoscope. Active sites of bleeding are identified and may be controlled with suction cautery. The SPA is most easily identified at the sphenopalatine foramen. This foramen is located along the lateral nasal wall just beyond the posterior wall of the maxillary sinus. Identifying the natural ostium of the maxillary sinus and opening the sinus posteriorly may assist with SPA identification. In some patients, the impression of the IMA may be seen along the posterior wall of the maxillary sinus and this can help localize the SPA. Alternatively, the vessel can be identified without opening the sinus. The posterior fontanelle of the maxillary sinus may be palpated and a vertical incision is made in the lateral nasal mucosa at the posterior edge of the posterior fontanelle of the maxillary sinus. A suction elevator is then used to elevate mucosa off of the lateral nasal wall in a posterior direction. The crista ethmoidalis, a bony prominence typically located just anterior to the sphenopalatine foramen, is a helpful landmark when looking for the SPA. Wide elevation of mucosa off of the lateral nasal wall is helpful not only for identifying the SPA but also for ensuring that all branches of the SPA are exiting through a single sphenopalatine foramen. Anatomic studies demonstrate that in up to 10% of patients, multiple foramen are present, usually with the posterior septal branch of the SPA exiting through a separate, inferior foramen.[15]

Following identification of the SPA and any secondary branches, the vessel is bluntly dissected from the surrounding soft tissue. The proximal SPA is then ligated using an endoscopic clip applier. Multiple clips may be placed to ensure adequate ligation (**Fig. 20.2**). The clips on the vessel should be closely examined with an endoscope to ensure adequate ligation. Complications from this technique are uncommon and include crusting, pain, and palatal paresthesias. An economic analysis comparing SPA ligation to posterior nasal packing suggests that SPA ligation is a more cost-efficient approach because of the duration of treatment and failure rate associated with posterior packs.[16]

Although the SPA is the dominant vascular supply to the posterior nasal cavity, refractory bleeds may occur from other vessels in the nose. The anterior ethmoid artery

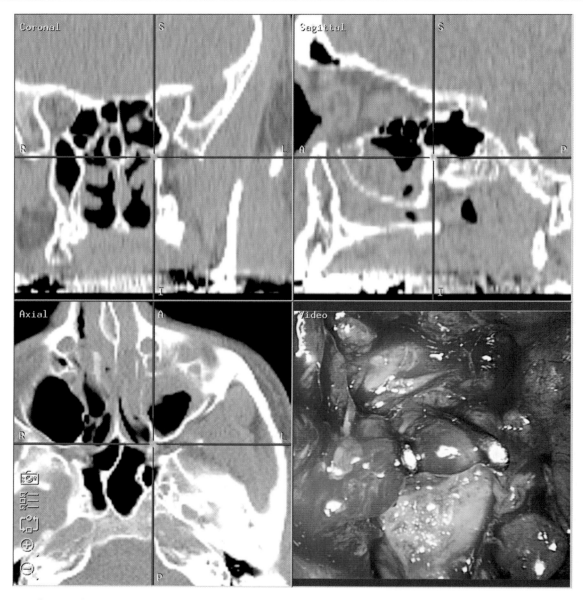

Figure 20.2   Endoscopic ligation of the sphenopalatine artery (SPA). Shown here is the image-guidance view of an endoscopic SPA ligation for epistaxis. Computed tomography image guidance helps confirm anatomy when performing SPA ligation. In the live view frame (right lower corner), the SPA is shown dissected free with an endoscopic clip placed on the proximal SPA.

supplies the superior aspect of the nasal cavity. Injury to this vessel may result in intermittent, high-volume bleeds. This is most frequently seen in patients with recent nasal trauma or sinonasal surgery. Because of its origin from the ophthalmic artery off of the internal carotid system, embolization of the anterior ethmoid artery carries a significant risk of blindness and stroke. Therefore, surgical ligation is the preferred method of vascular control for this vessel. This can be accomplished through an endoscopic transethmoid approach using a miniorbital decompression.[17] Alternatively, an endoscope-assisted transfacial approach may be used to ligate the vessel within the orbit.[18] Vessel ligation may be performed in the same surgical setting as endoscopic cautery and directed packing.

Embolization

Angiography and embolization for the treatment of epistaxis was first described in 1974.[19] This technique involves cannulation of the external carotid system with embolization of the distal branches supplying the nasal cavity. Efficacy of embolization as a treatment for refractory epistaxis is in the 90% range.[20,21] This approach does not require a general anesthetic. Complications of embolization are rare but can be significant. The risk of stroke is reported to be approximately 1%. Soft tissue necrosis, cranial nerve palsy, and persistent facial pain have also been reported.

Embolization requires a skilled interventional neuroradiologist and may not be available at all medical centers. Patients typically receive an arteriogram that includes bilateral internal and external carotid arteries, to gain a complete understanding of the anatomy and bleeding source. Branches of the internal maxillary arteries and facial arteries may be identified as a bleeding source and some or all of these can be embolized at the discretion of the interventional radiologist. The anterior and posterior ethmoid arteries are generally not embolized because of the risk of blindness and stroke.

Conclusion

Epistaxis is a common disorder that is typically self-limited. Most cases occur along the anterior nasal septum. Targeted cautery and nasal moisturization regimens are frequently adequate to control such bleeds. Multiple medical comorbidities and anticoagulant medications may exacerbate epistaxis. Intractable bleeds may be best treated with surgery or embolization.

References

1. Rainsbury JW, Molony NC. Clopidogrel versus low-dose aspirin as risk factors for epistaxis. Clin Otolaryngol 2009;34(3):232–235
2. Soyka MB, Rufibach K, Huber A, Holzmann D. Is severe epistaxis associated with acetylsalicylic acid intake? Laryngoscope 2010;120(1):200–207
3. Shehab N, Sperling LS, Kegler SR, Budnitz DS. National estimates of emergency department visits for hemorrhage-related adverse events from clopidogrel plus aspirin and from warfarin. Arch Intern Med 2010;170(21):1926–1933
4. Smith J, Siddiq S, Dyer C, Rainsbury J, Kim D. Epistaxis in patients taking oral anticoagulant and antiplatelet medication: prospective cohort study. J Laryngol Otol 2011;125(1):38–42
5. Shakeel M, Trinidade A, McCluney N, Clive B. Complementary and alternative medicine in epistaxis: a point worth considering during the patient's history. Eur J Emerg Med 2010;17(1):17–19
6. Kubba H, MacAndie C, Botma M, et al. A prospective, single-blind, randomized controlled trial of antiseptic cream for recurrent epistaxis in childhood. Clin Otolaryngol Allied Sci 2001;26(6):465–468
7. Calder N, Kang S, Fraser L, Kunanandam T, Montgomery J, Kubba H. A double-blind randomized controlled trial of management of recurrent nosebleeds in children. Otolaryngol Head Neck Surg 2009;140(5):670–674
8. Badran K, Malik TH, Belloso A, Timms MS. Randomized controlled trial comparing Merocel and RapidRhino packing in the management of anterior epistaxis. Clin Otolaryngol 2005;30(4):333–337
9. Mathiasen RA, Cruz RM. Prospective, randomized, controlled clinical trial of a novel matrix hemostatic sealant in patients with acute anterior epistaxis. Laryngoscope 2005;115(5):899–902
10. Côté D, Barber B, Diamond C, Wright E. FloSeal hemostatic matrix in persistent epistaxis: prospective clinical trial. J Otolaryngol Head Neck Surg 2010;39(3):304–308.
11. Snyderman CH, Goldman SA, Carrau RL, Ferguson BJ, Grandis JR. Endoscopic sphenopalatine artery ligation is an effective method of treatment for posterior epistaxis. Am J Rhinol 1999;13(2):137–140
12. Kumar S, Shetty A, Rockey J, Nilssen E. Contemporary surgical treatment of epistaxis. What is the evidence for sphenopalatine artery ligation? Clin Otolaryngol Allied Sci 2003;28(4):360–363
13. Wormald PJ, Wee DT, van Hasselt CA. Endoscopic ligation of the sphenopalatine artery for refractory posterior epistaxis. Am J Rhinol 2000;14(4):261–264
14. Asanau A, Timoshenko AP, Vercherin P, Martin C, Prades JM. Sphenopalatine and anterior ethmoidal artery ligation for severe epistaxis. Ann Otol Rhinol Laryngol 2009;118(9):639–644
15. Midilli R, Orhan M, Saylam CY, Akyildiz S, Gode S, Karci B. Anatomic variations of sphenopalatine artery and minimally invasive surgical cauterization procedure. Am J Rhinol Allergy 2009;23(6):e38–e41
16. Miller TR, Stevens ES, Orlandi RR. Economic analysis of the treatment of posterior epistaxis. Am J Rhinol 2005;19(1):79–82
17. Pletcher SD, Metson R. Endoscopic ligation of the anterior ethmoid artery. Laryngoscope 2007;117(2):378–381
18. Douglas SA, Gupta D. Endoscopic assisted external approach anterior ethmoidal artery ligation for the management of epistaxis. J Laryngol Otol 2003;117(2):132–133
19. Sokoloff J, Wickbom I, McDonald D, Brahme F, Goergen TC, Goldberger LE. Therapeutic percutaneous embolization in intractable epistaxis. Radiology 1974;111(2):285–287
20. Christensen NP, Smith DS, Barnwell SL, Wax MK. Arterial embolization in the management of posterior epistaxis. Otolaryngol Head Neck Surg 2005;133(5):748–753
21. Gurney TA, Dowd CF, Murr AH. Embolization for the treatment of idiopathic posterior epistaxis. Am J Rhinol 2004;18(5):335–339

21 Powered Endoscopic Dacryocystorhinostomy

Brendan C. Hanna and Peter-John Wormald

The key concepts for successful, powered endoscopic dacryocystorhinostomy (DCR) are complete opening of the lacrimal sac, mucosa-to-mucosa apposition of the lacrimal sac mucosa to the nasal mucosa, and judicious stenting. This chapter begins with a description of the endonasal anatomy of the lacrimal sac before detailing the indications for powered endoscopic DCR, the procedure itself, the results, and complications.

Anatomy

The endonasal anatomical relationships with the lacrimal sac are the axilla of the middle turbinate, the lacrimal bone, the frontal process of the maxilla, the uncinate process, and the agger nasi cell (**Fig. 21.1**). The axilla of the middle turbinate is the most prominent of these landmarks. It lies close to the opening of the common canaliculus into the lacrimal sac (at an average of 3 mm below the opening). Contrary to older anatomical descriptions, the upper border or fundus of the lacrimal sac projects an average of 8 mm above the axilla.[1] Anterior and medial to the superior projection of the fundus of the sac lies the frontal process of the maxilla, which is composed of thick bone. This bone needs powered instruments to remove and achieve complete exposure of the lacrimal sac during endoscopic DCR. The axilla of the middle turbinate always attaches to the frontal process of the maxilla and not to the lacrimal bone. Thus, it becomes

a medial relation of the upper part of the lacrimal sac as it projects anteriorly. The anterior border of the sac usually remains anterior to the attachment of the axilla.[2] Removal of the axilla of the middle turbinate is, therefore, necessary during endonasal DCR.

Below the axilla of the middle turbinate, the posterior half of the lacrimal sac is covered by the lacrimal bone and the anterior half by the frontal process of the maxilla. The lacrimomaxillary suture also corresponds to the point where the mucosa covering the medial aspect of the uncinate attaches to the lateral nasal wall. This can be visualized as a slight ridge running from the axilla of the middle turbinate to the upper border of the inferior turbinate called the maxillary line.[3] The maxillary line is most exposed just above the upper border of the inferior turbinate so that during surgery, after elevation of a mucosal flap, the junction between the lacrimal bone and frontal process of the maxilla is most easily defined close to the inferior turbinate.

Returning to the more complex anatomy of the lacrimal sac above the level of the axilla of the middle turbinate, the agger nasi cell (when present) will be related to the posterior lacrimal sac. In one study up to 55% of patients had anterior and medial pneumatization of this cell causing the agger nasi cell to overlap the posterior and posteromedial borders of the lacrimal sac.[4] The agger nasi cell is therefore usually entered during complete exposure of the lacrimal sac. Even more medially, the upward projection of the uncinate process to its attachment on the middle turbinate, skull base, or medial border of the agger nasi can also overlap the posterior lacrimal sac above the axilla of the middle turbinate.

Indications

The main indication is epiphora from nasolacrimal obstruction. Nasolacrimal obstruction is classified as either functional or anatomical. Functional obstruction occurs when investigations show no obvious obstruction of the system on dacryocystogram (DCG) investigation. However, lacrimal scintilography, which is a more functional investigation, will show no progression of the isotope from the eye to the nose. Anatomical obstruction is seen when the DCG shows obstruction of the system. If a patient presents with epiphora the eye should be examined for evidence of blepharitis or other causes of excessive tearing, and the eyelids should be checked for ectropion, entropion, and patency of the lacrimal puncta. Such abnormalities do not

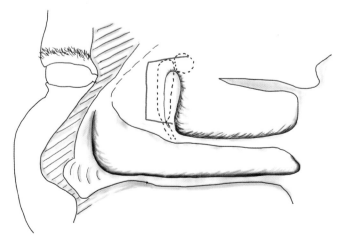

Figure 21.1 Diagram of the lateral wall of the nose showing positions of the lacrimal sac, agger nasi cell, maxillary line, and incisions for raising the initial mucosal flap.

indicate DCR. If patent, the puncta can be cannulated and flushed with saline. Flow of saline through the other puncta indicates patency of the canaliculi, but if obstruction is at the level of the distal common canaliculus or beyond then powered endoscopic DCR is indicated. Reflux through the cannulated puncta indicates blockage of the canaliculus. Some clinicians rely on tactile feedback from probing to determine patency to the level of the lacrimal sac; a hard stop indicates abutment of the probe against the bone of the medial lacrimal sac wall and a soft stop indicates that the probe is stuck in the common canaliculus.

Syringing, however, generates artificially high pressures in the nasolacrimal system that may overcome certain forms of obstruction and produce flow into the nasal cavity without reflux through the canaliculi. This is overcome by lacrimal scintilography where a radioactive dye is introduced into the conjunctival sac and later imaged to produce a lacrimal scintogram that may show failure of the dye to penetrate the lacrimal sac and/or nasal cavity. A combination of DCG and lacrimal scintography in the preoperative work-up for powered endoscopic DCR will determine the most likely area of narrowing and in particular, it will allow identification of common canalicular obstruction that may not be suitable for powered endoscopic DCR.[5] Powered endoscopic DCR can also be used as a treatment for acute dacryocystitis.[6]

Procedure

The endoscopic position of the lacrimal sac rarely varies and is mostly anterior to the orbit. Therefore, preoperative imaging of the nasal anatomy is not required.

DCR begins with inspection of the nasal cavities to determine if a septoplasty is required. If, when using a 0-degree endoscope, the area of the axilla of the middle turbinate is not visible then septoplasty will facilitate surgical access and decrease the chance of postoperative adhesions. It is the senior author's (P.J.W.) experience that a septoplasty is required in approximately 50% of cases. A limited endoscopic submucosal resection of the cartilage and bone in this area is usually sufficient.

The lateral nasal wall, anterior and superior to the anterior border of the middle turbinate, is infiltrated with 2% lidocaine and 1/80,000 adrenaline. The incisions for the mucosal flap determine the extent of exposure of the sac and it is therefore important that these are placed correctly. A superior horizontal incision is made 8 to 10 mm above the axilla of the middle turbinate. As the axilla itself is a medial relation of the lacrimal sac, the incision begins 5 mm posterior to the axilla to allow sufficient access to remove part of the axilla and enter the agger nasi cell. The incision continues horizontally for 10 mm anterior to the axilla of the middle turbinate. If this incision stops short, the flap can easily catch in the suction around the burr during removal of the frontal process of the maxilla and impede visualization. The incision then turns vertically downward

and continues until level with a point corresponding to the junction between the lower one-third and upper two-thirds of the anterior border of the middle turbinate. An inferior horizontal incision is then made at this level and carried posteriorly onto the insertion of the uncinate process (**Fig. 21.1**). A 15-mm scalpel is used for making incisions and a 30-degree endoscope for improved visualization of the lateral nasal wall. The endoscope is held against the upper vault of the vestibule and instruments are introduced to the nasal cavity beneath the endoscope.

The mucosal flap is elevated with a suction Freer elevator. Care is taken when passing over the posterior margin of the frontal process of the maxilla to remain in the plane between the mucosa and the thin lacrimal bone. The flap is elevated to the posterior extent of incisions and then tucked between the middle turbinate and nasal septum.

The junction between the lacrimal bone and frontal process of the maxilla (lacrimomaxillary suture) is now sought. The lacrimal bone ends approximately 5 mm below the axilla of the middle turbinate and just above the upper insertion of the inferior turbinate. A round knife from the ear tray is used to gently flake the lacrimal bone off the posterior inferior portion of the lacrimal sac. The round knife is then placed around the now free posterior margin of the frontal process of the maxilla and used to push the lacrimal sac away from this bone. The forward biting Hajek–Kofler punch is then engaged on the frontal process and closed. Before removing the bone, the jaw of the punch is opened to allow the release of any of the lacrimal sac that may have been pinched by the punch. Removal of the frontal process continues upward in this manner until the bone is too thick to be engaged. This is usually well short of the axilla. The powered endoscopic microdebrider with a rough diamond 2.5 mm DCR Burr (Medtronic Xomed, Jacksonville, Florida, United States) is then used to continue the bone dissection (**Fig. 21.2**). The bone is thinned down before removal with the burr. Care is taken not to allow the burr to fall below the

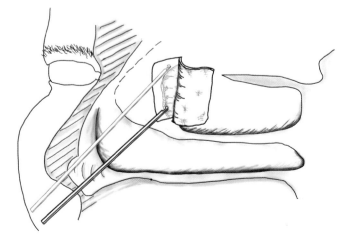

Figure 21.2 The Hajek–Kofler punch removes the bone of the frontal process of the maxilla over the inferior part of the lacrimal sac whereas the diamond burr is required to remove the thicker bone superiorly.

edge of the bone-sac junction, as it will quickly erode the sac wall and cause a perforation. Preservation of the medial wall of the nasolacrimal sac is required so that it can be reflected outward to lie in contact with nasal mucosa at the end of the procedure so that primary intention healing can occur.

Bone removal continues up to the upper border of the initial incision. It is continued anteriorly until the anterior border of the sac is seen. If the periosteum adjacent to skin is exposed then further anterior dissection should stop. Dissection superiorly will involve removal of part of the axilla of the middle turbinate with opening of the agger nasi cell. The mucosa of the agger nasi cell is used to appose the lacrimal sac mucosa to achieve primary intention healing. If there is doubt (when dissecting the bone above the axilla of the middle turbinate) about the location of the lacrimal sac, a DCR light pipe (Medtronic Xomed) can be introduced into the sac and the sac transilluminated.

Following exposure of the nasolacrimal sac any small pieces of bone that are still attached to the sac wall are teased off as they hinder reflection of the medial wall of the sac onto the lateral wall of the nasal cavity. Bowman lacrimal probes are used to cannulate the lacrimal canaliculus after dilatation of the lacrimal puncta with a punctum dilator. Passage of the probe through the common canaliculus is observed intranasally. If the sac has been entered the metal of the probe should be clearly visible through the wall of the sac (**Fig. 21.3**). If the probe is stuck in the common canaliculus it will tent both walls of the sac and the metal tip of the probe will not be seen.

Once the probe is in the sac and tenting the medial sac wall, a lacrimal spear knife (Medtronic Xomed) is used to make a vertical incision through the middle of the medial wall of the sac from top to bottom. The fashioning of anterior and posterior flaps from the medial wall is completed by making upper and lower incisions in the anterior flap with a lacrimal mini sickle knife (to achieve a releasing cut) and similar incisions in the posterior flap are made with

microscissors (**Fig. 21.4**). The flaps are rolled out on the lateral wall of the nose. The mucosa of the agger nasi cell is opened with a standard sickle knife and is apposed to the lacrimal mucosa. The original mucosal flap is trimmed so that it approximates the lacrimal mucosa along the edges of the opened lacrimal sac.

To decide if the common canaliculus needs stenting, the Bowman probe is placed through the common canaliculus. The valve of Rosenmuller patency is assessed by observing how closely the valve grips the probe. Stents should be placed when the valve grips the probe tightly. Research has shown that if the valve is loose there is no additional benefit to placing stents.[7] If the valve is tight, silastic O'Donaghue tubes (B > D > Visitec, Bidford-Upon-Avon, United Kingdom) are placed through the upper and lower canaliculi and brought out through the common canaliculus and out of the nose. The ends of the tube are inserted through a 1.5 by 1.5 cm piece of Gelfoam (Pharmacia and Upjohn Company, Kalamazoo, Michigan, United States), which is slid up the tubes to hold the flaps in place. The Gelfoam needs to be pushed through the vestibule and once in situ the edges of the Gelfoam need to be carefully reflected to ensure that the mucosal flaps have remained in position. A 4-mm wide and a 6-mm long piece of silastic tubing is slid up over the ends of the O'Donaghue tubes to act as a spacer. A loop of the O'Donaghue tube is pulled in the medial canthus to ensure there is no tension on the silastic tubes, which could otherwise erode through the lacrimal punctae. Two ligaclips are then applied below the spacer (**Fig. 21.5**). The O'Donaghue tubes are usually removed at 4 weeks.

Saline nasal wash is commenced the next day following surgery. Broad-spectrum antibiotics are administered for 5 days and antibiotic eye drops for 2 weeks. Gentle nose blowing without closure of the nostril is permitted during the postoperative period. The rhinostomy is inspected for any granulations during the first postoperative visit at 4 weeks and any granulations are removed.

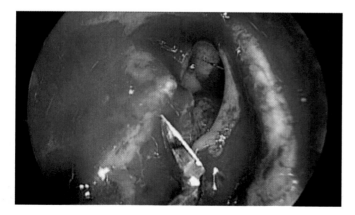

Figure 21.3   Picture of the Bowman probe clearly visible through the medial wall of the lacrimal sac indicating successful cannulation of the common canaliculus. The Spearman knife is in position for incising the sac and the agger nasi cell has been opened posterior to the lacrimal sac.

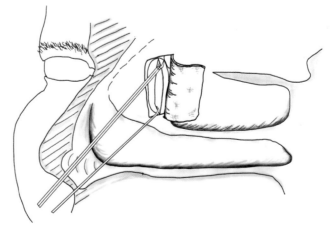

Figure 21.4   A lacrimal mini-sickle knife is used to make the releasing incisions for the anterior lacrimal sac flap and microscissors are used to fashion the posterior flap.

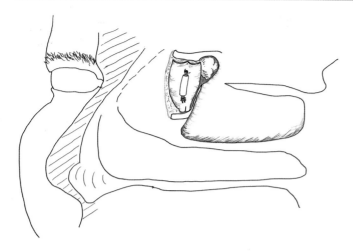

Figure 21.5 The lacrimal flaps have been positioned in contact with the trimmed initial mucosal flap and the mucosa of the agger nasi cell. The O'Donaghue silastic tubes with covering spacer and ligaclips are depicted. The bone forming the original axilla of the middle turbinate has been resected. The piece of Gelfoam applied beneath the spacer is omitted from the diagram to allow visualization of the mucosal flaps.

Special Considerations

Pediatrics

Powered endoscopic DCR can be successfully applied to patients of congenital nasolacrimal duct obstruction but there are several important anesthetic and technical considerations. It should be remembered that all pharmacological agents administered should be adjusted for the child's weight. Septoplasty is relatively contraindicated in growing children to prevent alterations in growth and cosmetic appearance. The small pediatric nasal vestibule and nasal cavity will initially cause difficulty in introducing standard adult-sized instruments but the vestibule will stretch to accommodate a 4-mm endoscope and instrument. The smaller vertical height of the nasal cavity brings the skull base closer to the surgical field increasing the chance of cerebrospinal fluid leak in inexperienced hands. The frontal process of the maxilla is underdeveloped and if the lacrimal bone is not correctly identified orbital penetration may occur. In small children, the frontal process of the maxilla, lacrimal bone and root of the middle turbinate are removed to create a 10 by 10 mm osteotomy and in older children this is enlarged to 10 by 15 mm.

Revision Dacryocystorhinostomy

When using powered endoscopic DCR for revision cases the incisions for the initial mucosal flap should be placed more anteriorly so that the initial incisions are made onto bone. This allows the correct surgical plane to be established anterior to the scar tissue from the previous DCR and allows the nasal mucosa to be sharply dissected off the scar tissue with a scalpel blade. A small and scarred lacrimal sac is often encountered in these cases making the lacrimal ostium smaller. By preserving the nasal mucosal flap, mucosa-to-

mucosa apposition can still be achieved by removing less nasal mucosa during the apposition process.

Results

Powered endoscopic DCR is successful (as judged by free flow of fluorescein into the nose and an asymptomatic patient) in treating anatomical obstruction in up to 97% of cases,[5] which is equivalent to success rates with external DCR.[8] For patients with functional obstruction the technical success of creating a patent lacrimal ostium and dye penetration into the nose is the same as the success of anatomical obstruction but a percentage of these patients that continue to have some epiphora is higher. Success as defined by an asymptomatic patient with a patent ostium in functional obstruction is around 84%.[1]

Complications

Complications in powered endoscopic DCR are uncommon. Hemorrhage (3% in previously published series[9]) is the only event encountered by the authors. A systematic review of the outcome of all DCR procedures revealed periorbital fat exposure to be the second most common intraoperative complication.[10] To prevent this, dissection should not continue posterior to the uncinate process. If orbital fat is exposed it should be left alone and not manipulated. The most common postoperative complications of endonasal DCR in the same review, occurring in less than 5% of cases, were periorbital hematoma and synechia and granulation formation around the ostium.

Conclusion

Endoscopic endonasal DCR is a safe and effective procedure both in adults and children when performed properly in the setting of nasolacrimal obstruction. By adhering to sound principles for diagnosis and surgery, the results are equivalent to open DCR and do not require external incisions. Overall, complications are uncommon in this procedure.

References

1. Wormald PJ, Kew J, Van Hasselt A. Intranasal anatomy of the nasolacrimal sac in endoscopic dacryocystorhinostomy. Otolaryngol Head Neck Surg 2000;123(3):307–310
2. Orhan M, Saylam CY, Midilli R. Intranasal localization of the lacrimal sac. Arch Otolaryngol Head Neck Surg 2009;135(8):764–770
3. Chastain JB, Cooper MH, Sindwani R. The maxillary line: anatomic characterization and clinical utility of an important surgical landmark. Laryngoscope 2005;115(6):990–992
4. Soyka MB, Treumann T, Schlegel CT. The agger nasi cell and uncinate process, the keys to proper access to the nasolacrimal drainage system. Rhinology 2010;48(3):364–367
5. Wormald PJ, Tsirbas A. Investigation and endoscopic treatment for functional and anatomical obstruction of the nasolacrimal duct system. Clin Otolaryngol Allied Sci 2004;29(4):352–356

6. Madge SN, Chan W, Malhotra R, et al. Endoscopic dacryocystorhinostomy in acute dacryocystitis: a multicenter case series. Orbit 2011;30(1):1–6

7. Callejas CA, Tewfik MA, Wormald PJ. Powered endoscopic dacryocystorhinostomy with selective stenting. Laryngoscope 2010; 120(7):1449–1452

8. Tsirbas A, Davis G, Wormald PJ. Mechanical endonasal dacryocystorhinostomy versus external dacryocystorhinostomy. Ophthal Plast Reconstr Surg 2004;20(1):50–56

9. Tsirbas A, Wormald PJ. Mechanical endonasal dacryocystorhinostomy with mucosal flaps. Br J Ophthalmol 2003;87(1):43–47

10. Leong SC, Macewen CJ, White PS. A systematic review of outcomes after dacryocystorhinostomy in adults. Am J Rhinol Allergy 2010; 24(1):81–90

SECTION III: Endoscopic Skull Base Surgery and Related Skull Base Surgery

22 Endoscopic Orbital and Optic Nerve Decompression

Ralph Metson and Jonathan Y. Ting

Endoscopic Orbital Decompression

Graves disease is an autoimmune disorder that primarily affects the thyroid and the orbit. Thyroid manifestations are characterized by the production of autoantibodies to the thyroid-stimulating hormone receptor with subsequent hyperstimulation and resultant hyperthyroidism. Orbital manifestations of Graves disease, known as dysthyroid orbitopathy, occur in up to 80% of patients. This represents an autoimmune process, although the exact antibody target remains unclear. Inflammation associated with infiltration of T cells and deposition of glycosaminoglycan results in the enlargement of orbital fat and extraocular muscles. This increase in volume of contents within the confines of the rigid bony orbit results in increased pressure and resultant proptosis, and/or compression of the optic nerve. Clinical manifestations of dysthyroid orbitopathy range from mild findings such as tearing, photophobia, and conjunctival injection to significant proptosis, diplopia, exposure keratopathy, and visual loss from optic neuropathy. The orbital and thyroid manifestations of Graves disease follow distinct and independent clinical courses.

Graves orbitopathy is characterized by an initial acute inflammatory phase followed by a chronic, fibrotic phase. The acute phase of orbitopathy typically lasts 6 to 18 months and often bears little relation to the degree of thyroid hormone abnormality or its subsequent treatment.[1] Local measures such as eye taping and artificial tears are important if corneal exposure is present. During this initial phase, systemic corticosteroids may reduce orbital inflammation and minimize complications. However, because of the side effects of long-term use and frequent recurrence of symptoms following cessation of treatment, steroids are often used as a temporizing measure or in conjunction with surgical decompression. Low-dose irradiation has also been used during the acute phase to counteract the inflammatory process,[2] but the efficacy of this controversial modality has been challenged by two recent randomized prospective trials.[3,4]

Surgery is rarely done during the acute phase unless vision is directly threatened and refractory to nonsurgical treatments.[5] Fortunately, severe orbital disease is relatively rare and poses a threat to vision in only 3 to 5% of patients with Graves orbitopathy.[6] Eventually, the inflammatory phase gives way to a stable fibrotic phase characterized by statically enlarged extraocular muscles and excess orbital fat. It is during this stable phase, if symptoms persist, that orbital decompression is most commonly performed.

Various open decompression techniques involving removal of each of the four walls of the orbit have been described,[7–10] with the Walsh-Ogura decompression[11] being the favored procedure for most of the 20th century. Initially described in the 1950s, this operation employed the familiar Caldwell-Luc approach to remove the inferior and medial orbital walls, allowing the enlarged orbital fat and muscles to decompress into the ethmoid and maxillary sinus cavities.

Soon after the introduction of transnasal endoscopic sinus surgery in the mid-1980s, surgeons began to experiment with endoscopic orbital surgery. Endoscopic orbital decompression was first described by Kennedy et al[12] and Michel et al[13] in the early 1990s. Enhanced visualization of key anatomic landmarks allowed for safe and thorough decompression of the entire medial orbital wall as well as the medial portion of the orbital floor. This improved visualization is most notable in the region of the orbital apex, a critical area of decompression in patients with optic neuropathy. These advantages have allowed the endoscopic approach to supplant the Walsh-Ogura procedure as the technique of choice for orbital decompression.

Technique

Initial vasoconstriction of the nasal passages is achieved with topical oxymetazoline (0.05%) or cocaine pledgets. The eyes are maintained within the surgical field and protected with scleral shells. Local injection of lidocaine 1% with 1:100,000 epinephrine is administered along the lateral nasal wall in the region of the maxillary line. The entire medial orbital wall, the medial portion of the orbital floor, and the underlying periorbital fascia are removed during endoscopic decompression.

Surgery begins with a complete uncinectomy and maxillary antrostomy. With orbital decompression it is important to widely open the maxillary sinus to achieve adequate access to the orbital floor and prevent blockage of the ostium from orbital fat, which protrudes following decompression. Using a 30-degree endoscope, the wide antrostomy allow easy visualization of the infraorbital nerve as it courses along the floor of the orbit.

An endoscopic sphenoethmoidectomy is performed in a standard fashion. We advocate removal of the middle turbinate during orbital decompression to optimize exposure of the medial orbital wall and facilitate postoperative cleaning. An image-guidance system may be used at this point to confirm the removal of all ethmoid cells along the medial orbital

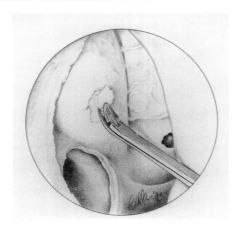

Figure 22.1 View of the right nasal cavity during endoscopic orbital decompression. The lamina papyracea is visible along the medial orbital wall with the enlarged maxillary ostium seen below. Once the lamina papyracea has been opened with a small spoon curette, bony fragments are removed with a Blakesley forceps.

Printed with permission from: John Wiley & Sons. Metson R, Dallow RL, Shore JW. Endoscopic orbital decompression. *Laryngoscope* 1994;104(8, pt 1):950–957.

wall and to ensure complete dissection to the sphenoid face and posterior skull base.

The skeletonized medial orbital wall is then carefully penetrated with a spoon curette or periosteal elevator. The thin bone of the lamina papyracea is elevated while preserving the underlying periorbita. Bone fragments are removed using Blakesly forceps (**Fig. 22.1**). Orbital fat should not be visible at this point if the underlying periorbital fascia is left intact. Bone removal proceeds superiorly toward the ethmoid roof, posteriorly to the face of the sphenoid, inferiorly to the orbital floor, and anteriorly to the maxillary line. Bone in the region of the frontal recess drainage pathway is intentionally left intact as herniated orbital fat may obstruct drainage of the frontal sinus resulting in iatrogenic frontal sinusitis or mucocele formation.

As dissection proceeds posteriorly, thick bone is encountered in the region of the orbital apex within 2 mm of the sphenoid face. This bone corresponds to the annulus of Zinn, from which four of six extraocular muscles originate and through which the optic nerve passes. This landmark represents the posterior limit of a standard decompression. For patients with optic neuropathy, experienced surgeons may consider continuing the decompression posteriorly into the sphenoid sinus. However, the benefits of incorporating an optic nerve decompression into standard orbital decompression are unclear and the procedure may lead to inadvertent injury to the nerve.

Removal of the orbital floor can be technically challenging, depending on its thickness. Only that portion of the floor which is medial to the infraorbital nerve is removed, beginning about 1 cm posterior to the orbital rim. A spoon curette is used to engage the orbital floor along its medial extent and down-fracture the bone (**Fig. 22.2**). The bone of

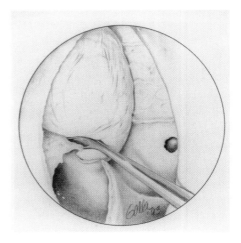

Figure 22.2 A spoon curette is used to down-fracture the medial portion of the orbital floor.

Printed with permission from: John Wiley & Sons. Metson R, Dallow RL, Shore JW. Endoscopic orbital decompression. *Laryngoscope* 1994;104(8, pt 1):950–957.

the orbital floor is thicker than that of the medial orbital wall and significant force may be required for this maneuver. If the spoon curette is not sturdy enough for this portion of the procedure, the heavier mastoid curette may be used. The bone may fracture in one large piece (at a natural cleavage plane along the canal of the infraorbital nerve) or, more frequently, into several small pieces. A 30-degree endoscope and angled forceps may facilitate bone removal while preserving the infraorbital canal as the lateral limit of dissection.

Once the lamina papyracea and medial orbital floor have been removed, the periorbita is fully exposed. A sickle knife is then used to open this fascial layer (**Fig. 22.3**). Care must be taken to avoid "burying" the tip of the sickle knife

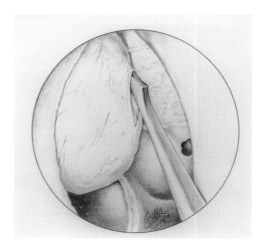

Figure 22.3 The exposed periorbital fascia is incised with a sickle knife in a posterior-to-anterior direction.

Printed with permission from: John Wiley & Sons. Metson R, Dallow RL, Shore JW. Endoscopic orbital decompression. *Laryngoscope* 1994;104(8, pt 1):950–957.

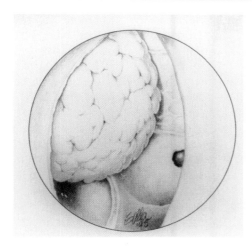

Figure 22.4 At the conclusion of decompression, orbital fat protrudes into the right ethmoid and maxillary sinuses.
Printed with permission from: John Wiley & Sons. Metson R, Dallow RL, Shore JW. Endoscopic orbital decompression. *Laryngoscope* 1994;104(8, pt 1):950–957.

and potentially injuring the underlying orbital contents, including the medial rectus muscle. The periorbital incision should be initiated at the posterior limit of decompression (just anterior to the sphenoid face) and brought anteriorly so that prolapsing fat does not obscure visualization. Parallel incisions are performed along the ethmoid roof and orbital floor. To minimize the risk of postoperative diplopia, a 10-mm wide sling of fascia overlying the medial rectus muscle may be preserved whereas the remainder of the periorbita is removed using angled Blakesley forceps.[14] In patients with optic neuropathy or severe proptosis, this fascial sling technique is not used to allow for maximal decompression. A ball-tipped probe and sickle knife may be used to identify and incise remaining fibrous bands that often course superficially between lobules of orbital fat. On completion of the procedure, the surgeon should observe for a generous prolapse of fat into the opened ethmoid and maxillary cavities (**Fig. 22.4**).

Depending on the clinical scenario and desired degree of decompression, a subsequent lateral decompression may be performed through an external approach that may result in a more balanced decompression. When performed immediately following medial decompression, the orbital contents are easily retracted in a medial direction allowing for excellent exposure of the lateral bony wall. Bilateral decompressions may be performed concurrently or in a staged procedure.

Nasal packing is avoided to ensure maximal decompression and to avoid compression of exposed orbital contents. The patient is discharged the morning after surgery with a prescription for oral antistaphylococcal antibiotics and instructions to begin twice daily nasal saline irrigations. At the first postoperative visit 1 week following surgery, crusts are debrided from the surgical site under endoscopic guidance.

For patients who are at high risk for general anesthesia or those with an only seeing eye, decompression may be performed under local anesthesia with sedation.[15] This approach allows the surgeon to monitor the patient's vision throughout the procedure. Local anesthesia is administered initially with 4% cocaine pledgets followed by an injection of lidocaine 1% with 1:100,000 epinephrine. Patients may report discomfort during removal of the lamina papyracea. This sensation may be relieved by infiltration of a small amount of additional anesthetic solution along the medial orbital wall.

Results

The goals of orbital decompression vary depending on the indication for the procedure. In patients with compressive optic neuropathy, restoration of visual deficits is the key outcome, whereas in patients with corneal exposure or severe proptosis, ocular recession may be the primary endpoint. The reported incidence of improvement following endoscopic orbital decompression for Graves orbitopathy ranges from 22 to 89%.[1,12,16] This wide variation in results reflects the diverse patient populations and definitions of improvement. Postoperative deterioration of visual acuity occurs in less than 5% of patients.[1,13,16] Ocular recession as a result of endoscopic decompression alone averages 3.5 mm (range 2 to 12 mm). The addition of concurrent lateral decompression to the endoscopic procedure provides an additional 2 mm of globe recession.[1]

Complications

The most common complication following orbital decompression is new-onset diplopia or worsening of pre-existing diplopia. This finding occurs in 15 to 63% of patients and is thought to result from the altered vector of pull postoperatively in already abnormal extraocular muscles.[1,13,15,17–19] Decompressive surgery rarely alleviates pre-existing diplopia. All patients should be warned that diplopia may persist or worsen after decompression surgery and that strabismus surgery may be necessary.

Several methods to decrease postoperative diplopia have been reported. Multiple authors have described the preservation of a strut of inferomedial bone between the decompressed floor and medial wall.[16,20] When this strut is maintained, however, it is technically difficult to remove the orbital floor through a purely endoscopic technique. The maintenance of a facial sling in the region of the medial rectus has also been demonstrated to decrease the incidence of postoperative diplopia.[14] This technique provides similar support as the medial strut technique, but allows for endoscopic access to decompress the medial orbital floor. The concept of a balanced decompression (concurrent medial and lateral decompression) has also been suggested as a means to decrease postoperative diplopia.[17,21,22] Although these procedures lower the postoperative diplopia rate by providing a balanced decompression, extraocular muscle enlargement is often asymmetric making it difficult to achieve perfect balance. When operating for compressive optic neuropathy, techniques designed to limit diplopia may also limit the extent of decompression and postoperative diplopia is often accepted as a concession to improved visual acuity.

The incidence of epistaxis following orbital decompression is similar to that following routine endoscopic sinus surgery. The most common site for bleeding is the posterior remnant of the middle turbinate. Postoperative bleeding following decompression is best managed through endoscopic identification and direct cauterization of the bleeding site. Nasal packing is generally not used to avoid pressure on the exposed orbital apex and optic nerve. Orbital hematoma is unlikely as removal of the periorbital bone and fascia prevents focal accumulation of blood.

Postoperative infection is minimized through the use of postoperative antibiotics with staphylococcal coverage. A large maxillary antrostomy and limited bone removal in the frontal recess region minimize the risk of developing postoperative sinusitis. Epiphora may develop if the maxillary antrostomy is extended too far anteriorly with transection of the nasolacrimal duct. This complication is treated with an endoscopic dacryocystorhinostomy. Leakage of cerebrospinal fluid (CSF) and blindness are very rare complications that have been reported following nonendoscopic decompression techniques.

Endoscopic Optic Nerve Decompression

The benefits of endoscopic instrumentation for orbital decompression can be similarly applied when operating in the vicinity of the optic nerve. Decompression of the optic nerve involves complete removal of the bone that forms the medial wall of the optic canal. Although the surgical techniques and indications for orbital decompression are fairly well established, controversy exists regarding both the indications and extent of surgery necessary for optic nerve decompression.

The optic nerve may be divided into three segments: the intraorbital, the intracanalicular, and the intracranial segment. Optic nerve decompression aims to relieve compressive forces within the intracanalicular portion of the nerve. The canal of the optic nerve is formed by the two struts of the lesser wing of the sphenoid and carries both the optic nerve and the ophthalmic artery. At the orbital apex is the annulus of Zinn, a thick, fibrous layer that is the least expandable tissue surrounding the optic nerve. This site has been suggested to be the most likely location for pathologic compression of the optic nerve.[23]

Compression of the optic nerve may result from neoplastic, inflammatory, or traumatic processes. Initial theories of vascular compromise from external compression have been largely discarded. Conduction block and focal demyelination are the favored pathophysiologic explanations for compressive optic neuropathy. Rapid recovery following optic nerve decompression results from relief of a manual compression block, whereas a delayed recovery occurring over a period of weeks to months is attributed to remyelination.[24] Possible indications for optic nerve decompression include traumatic optic neuropathy (TON) and nontraumatic optic neuropathy (NTON).

TON can be attributed to direct and indirect etiologies. Direct TON includes penetrating injuries such as stab/bullet wounds and orbital fractures that lacerate the nerve. Indirect TON generally results from blunt trauma (with or without associated fracture), which results in hematoma, perineural edema, or shearing injury to the microvasculature or axons, with subsequent disruption of axonal transport. Historically, this has been the most common, and perhaps most controversial, indication for optic nerve decompression, with the efficacy of decompression in this setting unclear.

A significant amount of controversy surrounds the treatment of TON. Often, concurrent intracranial injuries are present, which complicate management and prevent optimal ophthalmologic examination. The main treatment options for TON include systemic corticosteroids, surgical optic nerve decompression, or observation. Analysis of the literature is confounded by the variability in management and a lack of randomized, controlled studies. The International Optic Nerve Trauma Study (IONTS) was initially designed to address this question in a randomized fashion, but enrollment was slow and the study design ultimately abandoned in favor of a nonrandomized comparative study.[25] A total of 133 patients were enrolled with no difference between observation, corticosteroids, or surgical decompression. Currently, observation or steroid treatment is advocated. Steroids have been used in TON based on significant improvement in motor and sensory function in patients with acute spinal cord injury who were treated with megadose corticosteroid therapy.[26] However, a more recent randomized study was stopped early because of the significantly increased risk of death in patients who received megadose steroids at their 6-month follow-up when compared with those in the placebo group.[27] In addition, differences may exist between the repair mechanisms of the optic nerve (pure white matter tract) and the spinal cord (mixed gray and white matter tract) and no animal study has demonstrated a beneficial effect of steroid therapy for TON. If severe visual impairment remains despite medical treatment, one could consider a surgical decompression. Contrary to the findings of the IONTS, a single center retrospective study of TON patients demonstrated that patients treated with surgical decompression following failed megadose steroid therapy fared significantly better than patients treated with megadose steroids alone.[28]

NTON may result secondary to pathologic entities that develop slowly over time and exert direct pressure on the optic nerve. Such entities include benign fibro-osseous lesions, Graves orbitopathy, mucopyocele, and orbital meningiomas. NTON may have an insidious onset resulting in delayed diagnosis. Patients' initial symptoms are often vague including mild blurry or "fuzzy" vision without a significant loss of visual acuity and with normal funduscopic examination. More rigorous examination often reveals variable, limited visual field defects, a decrease in color vision, and an afferent pupillary defect on the affected side. Unfortunately, these symptoms may go unnoticed until the more advanced stages of compression result in decreased visual acuity. In these cases, orbital decompression has been shown to be safe and effective in restoring visual acuity in properly selected patients.[29]

Technique

Traditional surgical approaches for optic nerve decompression include transorbital, extranasal transethmoid, transantral, intranasal microscopic, and craniotomy approaches. Endonasal endoscopic decompression of the optic nerve offers many advantages over these approaches including excellent visualization, preservation of olfaction, rapid recovery time, a lack of external scars, and less operative stress in patients who may be suffering from multisystem trauma.

Patients are prepared for surgery in a similar manner to those undergoing orbital decompression. A standard sphenoethmoidectomy is performed. The sphenoid face is widely opened and the bulge of the optic canal is identified along the lateral wall of the sphenoid sinus, superior to the carotid artery. In some patients, the optic canal may be initially identified in the lateral aspect of a posterior sphenoethmoid or Onodi cell, which can be seen on preoperative computed tomography scan.[30] Identification and opening of the Onodi cell is important to provide adequate surgical exposure and allow full access to the optic canal.

Following exposure of the medial orbital wall, a spoon curette is used to fracture the lamina papyracea approximately 1 cm anterior to the optic canal. The lamina is then carefully removed in a posterior direction to expose the annulus of Zinn and the optic canal. Care must be taken to avoid penetration of the periorbita as subsequent herniation of orbital fat will obscure the surgical field. As the optic canal is approached, the thin lamina will be replaced with the thick bone of the lesser wing of the sphenoid. This bone must be thinned before removal. A long-handled drill with a diamond burr is used to methodically thin the medial wall of the optic canal (**Fig. 22.5A**). While drilling, care must be taken to prevent contact of the drill bit with the prominence of the carotid artery located just inferior and posterior to the optic nerve. Care should also be taken to avoid excess generation of heat while drilling this bone as it may result in thermal damage to the optic nerve. After the bone is appropriately thinned, a microcurette is used to fracture the thinned bone in a medial direction, away from the optic nerve. Bone fragments are then removed from the decompressed nerve using Blakesly forceps (**Fig. 22.5B**), with resultant medial decompression of the optic nerve.

Controversy exists regarding the length of optic canal that should be decompressed and the necessity for decompression of the optic sheath. With compressive optic neuropathy secondary to neoplasms, the extent of decompression is dictated by the size and location of the neoplasm. For cases

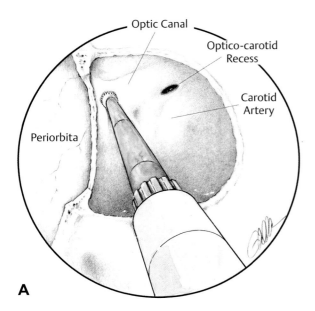

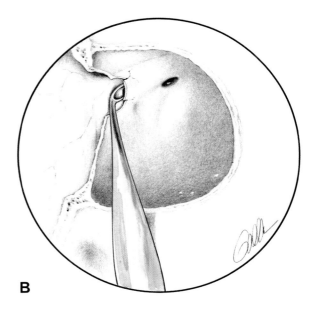

Figure 22.5   (A) Endoscopic view of the right posterior nasal cavity following wide sphenoidotomy. The lamina papyracea has been removed to reveal periorbita near the orbital apex. A diamond burr is used to thin bone along the optic canal. (B) A curette is used to elevate bony fragments and expose the underlying optic nerve.

Printed with permission from: Thieme Medical and Scientific Publishers. Pletcher SD, Sindwani R, Metson R. Endoscopic orbital and optic nerve decompression. *Otolaryngol Clin North Am* 2006;39(5):943–958, vi.

of TON and dysthyroid orbitopathy, removal of bone for a distance of 1 cm posterior to the face of the sphenoid sinus is generally thought to be sufficient.

Incision of the sheath has been advocated by some authors to further decompress the nerve itself; however, this maneuver may be unnecessary and risks damage to the underlying nerve fibers and ophthalmic artery as well as CSF leak with a resultant risk of meningitis. However, the fibrous annulus of Zinn is a tough fibrous layer that may contribute to nerve compression in cases of nerve swelling or intrasheath hematoma. With clear risks and absence of data to suggest benefit for sheath decompression, we do not advocate this maneuver for most patients undergoing optic nerve decompression. However, in cases of demonstrated intrasheath hematoma or significant nerve swelling with papilledema, incision of the optic nerve sheath is considered. When opening the optic nerve sheath, a sickle knife is used to incise the periorbita just anterior to the annulus of Zinn, a tough fibrous layer that may contribute to nerve compression in cases of nerve swelling or intrasheath hematoma. The incision is carried through the annulus of Zinn with a sickle knife or microscissors.

Results

As mentioned previously, the efficacy of optic nerve decompression in TON is unclear. Much of the difficulty in determining the success of surgical intervention arises from the relatively high rate of spontaneous recovery from TON. To date, well-controlled studies with significant power have not been possible because of the rarity of this condition and inherent difficulties in studying trauma victims.[25] Given this situation, it seems prudent in most cases to proceed with observation or corticosteroid therapy, reserving surgical decompression for refractory cases.

In cases of NTON, however, the natural course of disease is not one of spontaneous resolution. Most patients who undergo optic nerve decompression for compressive NTON will have significant improvement in visual acuity. An immediate improvement in visual acuity is frequently observed, probably from relief of a mechanical conduction block. Further improvement may occur over a period of weeks to months as remyelination of the nerve leads to more efficient conduction.[24] In our recent experience with endoscopic optic nerve decompressions for NTON, an improvement in visual acuity greater than two lines on the Snellen chart was seen following 7 of 10 decompressions at a mean follow-up of 6.1 months. One patient required multiple decompressions because of progression of her fibrous dysplasia with recurrent impingement upon the optic nerve.[29]

Complications

Potential complications of optic nerve decompression include CSF leak, meningitis, and worsening or complete loss of visual function. It is possible that these risks are greater than that with standard endoscopic sinus surgery or orbital decompression. The IONTS and another recent study reported several cases of CSF leak, some with associated meningitis and visual decompensation.[17,31] However, in the IONTS series, it is not clear whether these were endoscopic or external decompression cases, with endoscopic decompression representing less than 40% of patients in their series.[25] Similar to orbital decompression, antistaphylococcal antibiotics should be employed to prevent postoperative infections and intranasal packing is avoided to prevent undue compression on the nerve.

Conclusion

The endoscopic transnasal approach lends itself well to orbital and optic nerve decompression because of excellent visualization of the orbital apex, optic canal, and skull base. Outcomes of endoscopic decompression are comparable with those of open, external techniques without the need for facial or intraoral incisions. These operations represent advanced endoscopic techniques and should be performed only by experienced endoscopic sinonasal surgeons.

References

1. Metson R, Dallow RL, Shore JW. Endoscopic orbital decompression. Laryngoscope 1994;104(8, pt 1):950–957
2. Wakelkamp IM, Tan H, Saeed P, et al. Orbital irradiation for Graves' ophthalmopathy: Is it safe? A long-term follow-up study. Ophthalmology 2004;111(8):1557–1562
3. Gorman CA, Garrity JA, Fatourechi V, et al. A prospective, randomized, double-blind, placebo-controlled study of orbital radiotherapy for Graves' ophthalmopathy. Ophthalmology 2001; 108(9):1523–1534
4. Mourits MP, van Kempen-Harteveld ML, García MB, Koppeschaar HP, Tick L, Terwee CB. Radiotherapy for Graves' orbitopathy: randomised placebo-controlled study. Lancet 2000;355(9214):1505–1509
5. Wakelkamp IM, Baldeschi L, Saeed P, Mourits MP, Prummel MF, Wiersinga WM. Surgical or medical decompression as a first-line treatment of optic neuropathy in Graves' ophthalmopathy? A randomized controlled trial. Clin Endocrinol (Oxf) 2005;63(3): 323–328
6. Bahn RS. Graves' ophthalmopathy. N Engl J Med 2010;362(8): 726–738
7. Kronlein R. Zur Pathologie und operativen Behandlung der Desmoid Cysten der Orbita. Beitr Klin Chir 1889;4:149–163
8. Sewall E. Operative control of progressive exophthalmos. Arch Otolaryngol Head Neck Surg 1936;24(5):621–624
9. Hirsch O. Surgical decompression of exophthalmos. Arch Otolaryngol Head Neck Surg 1950;51:325–331
10. Naffziger HC. Progressive exophthalmos. Ann R Coll Surg Engl 1954;15(1):1–24
11. Walsh TE, Ogura JH. Transantral orbital decompression for malignant exophthalmos. Laryngoscope 1957;67(6):544–568
12. Kennedy DW, Goodstein ML, Miller NR, Zinreich SJ. Endoscopic transnasal orbital decompression. Arch Otolaryngol Head Neck Surg 1990;116(3):275–282
13. Michel O, Bresgen K, Rüssmann W, Thumfart WF, Stennert E. Endoscopically-controlled endonasal orbital decompression in malignant exophthalmos. Laryngorhinootologie 1991;70(12):656–662

14. Metson R, Samaha M. Reduction of diplopia following endoscopic orbital decompression: the orbital sling technique. Laryngoscope 2002;112(10):1753–1757

15. Metson R, Shore JW, Gliklich RE, Dallow RL. Endoscopic orbital decompression under local anesthesia. Otolaryngol Head Neck Surg 1995;113(6):661–667

16. Schaefer SD, Soliemanzadeh P, Della Rocca DA, et al. Endoscopic and transconjunctival orbital decompression for thyroid-related orbital apex compression. Laryngoscope 2003;113(3):508–513

17. Shepard KG, Levin PS, Terris DJ. Balanced orbital decompression for Graves' ophthalmopathy. Laryngoscope 1998;108(11 Pt 1):1648–1653

18. Wright ED, Davidson J, Codere F, Desrosiers M. Endoscopic orbital decompression with preservation of an inferomedial bony strut: minimization of postoperative diplopia. J Otolaryngol 1999;28(5):252–256

19. Eloy P, Trussart C, Jouzdani E, Collet S, Rombaux P, Bertrand B. Transnasal endoscopic orbital decompression and Graves' ophtalmopathy. Acta Otorhinolaryngol Belg 2000;54(2):165–174

20. Goldberg RA, Shorr N, Cohen MS. The medical orbital strut in the prevention of postdecompression dystopia in dysthyroid ophthalmopathy. Ophthal Plast Reconstr Surg 1992;8(1):32–34

21. Unal M, Leri F, Konuk O, Hasanreisoğlu B. Balanced orbital decompression combined with fat removal in Graves ophthalmopathy: do we really need to remove the third wall? Ophthal Plast Reconstr Surg 2003;19(2):112–118

22. Graham SM, Brown CL, Carter KD, Song A, Nerad JA. Medial and lateral orbital wall surgery for balanced decompression in thyroid eye disease. Laryngoscope 2003;113(7):1206–1209

23. Anand VS, Sherwood C, Al-Mefty O. Optic nerve decompression via transethmoid and supraorbital approaches. Oper Tech Otolaryngol Head Neck Surg 1991;2:157–166

24. McDonald WI. The symptomatology of tumours of the anterior visual pathways. Can J Neurol Sci 1982;9(4):381–390

25. Levin LA, Beck RW, Joseph MP, Seiff S, Kraker R. The treatment of traumatic optic neuropathy: the International Optic Nerve Trauma Study. Ophthalmology 1999;106(7):1268–1277

26. Bracken MB, Shepard MJ, Collins WF, et al. A randomized, controlled trial of methylprednisolone or naloxone in the treatment of acute spinal-cord injury. Results of the Second National Acute Spinal Cord Injury Study. N Engl J Med 1990;322(20):1405–1411

27. Edwards P, Arango M, Balica L, et al; CRASH trial collaborators. Final results of MRC CRASH, a randomised placebo-controlled trial of intravenous corticosteroid in adults with head injury-outcomes at 6 months. Lancet 2005;365(9475):1957–1959

28. Kountakis SE, Maillard AA, El-Harazi SM, Longhini L, Urso RG. Endoscopic optic nerve decompression for traumatic blindness. Otolaryngol Head Neck Surg 2000;123(1, pt 1):34–37

29. Pletcher SD, Metson R. Endoscopic optic nerve decompression for nontraumatic optic neuropathy. Arch Otolaryngol Head Neck Surg 2007;133(8):780–783

30. Allmond L, Murr AH. Clinical problem solving: radiology. Radiology quiz case 1: opacified Onodi cell. Arch Otolaryngol Head Neck Surg 2002;128(5):596, 598–599

31. Rajiniganth MG, Gupta AK, Gupta A, Bapuraj JR. Traumatic optic neuropathy: visual outcome following combined therapy protocol. Arch Otolaryngol Head Neck Surg 2003;129(11):1203–1206

23 Cerebrospinal Fluid: Physiology and Endoscopic Leak Repair

Alkis J. Psaltis, Zachary M. Soler, and Rodney J. Schlosser

Although the Roman physician of antiquity Galen first described cerebrospinal fluid (CSF) rhinorrhea in 200 AD, the first recorded description in modern medicine was not until 1682 by Willis. This was later confirmed on autopsy by Miller in 1862. Grant is credited with the first transcranial repair in 1923, while Dohlman (1948) and Hirsch (1953) described the first extracranial and transnasal approaches, respectively. The evolution of surgical repair of CSF leaks has followed the desire to reduce morbidities associated with open approaches: the invasive nature of the approach, high failure rate, external scars, anosmia, seizures, cerebral hemorrhage, loss of memory, and personality deficits. With the advent of endoscopic sinus surgery (ESS) and advances in instrumentation, Wigand completed the first successful endoscopic CSF leak repair in 1981. The results of multiple institutional series have confirmed the superior efficacy and lower morbidity of the endoscopic approach, making it now widely accepted as the current standard of care.[1]

Anatomy and Physiology

A sound understanding of CSF production and circulation is critical in the management of CSF leaks. CSF is a colorless transcellular fluid produced predominantly by the ventricular choroid plexi with minor contributions from their ependymal lining, the external pial-glial membrane, and blood vessels within the pia-arachnoid. Production occurs through active transport (70%) and capillary ultrafiltration (20%) with 10% occurring as a product of metabolic water production. CSF is produced at a rate of 20 mL/h with a total volume of 125 to 150 mL unevenly distributed between the ventricles (20%), the subarachnoid (SA) space of the cranium, and spinal cord (80%) at any one time. A pulsatile wave, generated by cerebral arterial flow and the associated expansion of the vascular compartment in the cranial vault, propels CSF in a craniocaudal direction. This travels from the two lateral ventricles into the single midline third ventricle via the interventricular foramen of Monro. From there it passes into the fourth ventricle via the cerebral aqueduct of Sylvius and ultimately into the SA space by way of three openings in its roof: two foramina of Lushka and the foramen of Magendie. CSF pressure is typically less than 200 mm H_2O in adults and is primarily regulated through absorption. Approximately 90% of CSF absorption occur via unidirectional, size-limited, vesicular transport in the arachnoid villi, with the remaining 10% passing directly into the cerebral venules. Absorption of CSF increases linearly above pressures of 70 mm H_2O until approximately 110 mm H_2O, when the rate of secretion and absorption become equal. Being a product of plasma filtration and membrane secretion, CSF is almost completely acellular with a very low protein concentration of 0.3% (20 to 40 mg/dL). Glucose concentration ranges between 50 and 80 mg/dL, with a low CSF to serum ratio of 0.6 because of its use by the ependymal cells and active removal by arachnoid villi and capillaries.[2]

Classification of Cerebrospinal Fluid Leaks

CSF leaks can be classified by etiology, size, or location. Etiological classification remains popular because of the ease with which it can be obtained from the patient history. Har-El[3] classified CSF leaks into traumatic and nontraumatic. Traumatic leaks are more common and occur through accidental or iatrogenic injury. Iatrogenic fistulae have increased in recent times with the widespread practice of ESS and endoscopic skull base surgery.

Nontraumatic causes can be further subclassified into congenital, tumor related, and spontaneous leaks. **Table 23.1**

Table 23.1 Sites of Cerebrospinal Fluid Leaks in Decreasing Order of Frequency according to Etiology

Iatrogenic Trauma	Accidental Trauma	Spontaneous		Tumor	Congenital
Ethmoid roof	Sphenoid	Cribriform plate		Sphenoid	Ethmoid roof
Cribriform plate	Frontal	Sphenoid lateral pterygoid recess		Ethmoid roof	Cribriform plate
Frontal	Ethmoid roof	Ethmoid roof		Posterior frontal	
Sphenoid	Cribriform plate	Central sphenoid			
		Frontal			

lists the common sites of CSF leaks involved in each group.

Traumatic—Iatrogenic Leaks

Unintentional iatrogenic CSF leaks occur in the range of 1/1000 to 2/1000 ESS procedures. Leaks occur more frequently on the right side with the most common sites injured being the lateral lamella of the cribriform plate and the ethmoid roof (**Fig. 23.1**).[4] Injury to the paper-thin lateral lamella can occur during a frontal recess clearance or during high resection of the middle turbinate. Posterior ethmoid injuries often occur when excessively pneumatized maxillary sinuses expand superolaterally reducing the

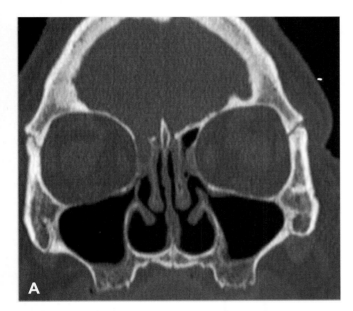

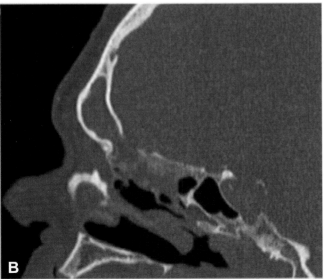

Figure 23.1 (A) Coronal and (B) sagittal computed tomography scans showing an iatrogenic cerebrospinal fluid leak in the anterior ethmoid roof location.

height of the ethmoid complex. If the leak is witnessed intraoperatively every effort should be made for immediate repair. Additionally, iatrogenic leaks often occur during endoscopic skull base surgery. This is becoming a more frequent occurrence as rhinologists and neurosurgeons continue to push the envelope of minimally invasive skull base surgery. Often these defects can be quite large and extend up into the ventricles, resulting in high volume CSF leaks. It is imperative that skull base reconstruction is done in a meticulous fashion in these patients.

Traumatic—Accidental Leaks

Closed head injuries have replaced projectiles as the most common accidental cause with 1 to 3% resulting in fistula. The sphenoid and cribriform plate are the most common sites with up to one-third of patients having multiple sites.[5] CSF rhinorrhea usually presents within 48 hours. Most traumatic leaks spontaneously close (50 to 90%) likely as a consequence of the sealant effect provided by blood products and localized inflammation.[6] Historically, conservative management with bed rest and lumbar drains has been the mainstay of treatment. Surgical intervention is advocated after 7 to 10 days for persistent leaks to reduce the risk of developing ascending meningitis (30 to 40%), although some argue that earlier surgical repair may reduce the risk further. The use of prophylactic antibiotics in traumatic CSF leaks remains controversial, with two meta-analyses on the subject that provided conflicting evidence on their effectiveness in reducing the rate of ascending meningitis.[7,8] Both studies had methodological flaws however, and in 2011, a Cochrane Database review was performed to address the deficiencies of these meta-analyses. This extensive review of more than 20 randomized and nonrandomized trials concluded that there was insufficient evidence supporting the role of prophylactic antibiotics in CSF leaks associated with traumatic base of skull fractures.[9]

Nontraumatic—Congenital Leaks

Congenital encephaloceles with leakage of CSF can be subclassified into sincipital (frontoethmoidal) and basal types. Basal types tend to be encountered more commonly by rhinologists. This type most often presents as a nasal mass but may also present with rhinological symptoms, meningitis, and craniofacial deformities. Most commonly, congenital encephaloceles occur near the middle turbinate's attachment to the cribriform plate. They pose a challenge to the repairing surgeon, both technically and with regard to timing. The potential for telecanthus to occur over time has been described in cases that are left untreated.[10]

Nontraumatic—Tumor Leaks

Intracranial and sinonasal tumors can be responsible for CSF leaks through direct invasion and erosion of the skull base by the tumor. Indirectly, defects can also occur when chemotherapy and radiotherapy treatments are used to shrink these tumors; this can lead to devitalization of the bony skull base. Additionally, tumors may block the CSF pathway, resulting in obstructing hydrocephalus. Repairing the CSF leak without relieving the raised intracranial pressure (ICP) may further exacerbate the intracranial hypertension and is likely to fail.

Nontraumatic—Spontaneous Leaks

Spontaneous CSF leaks occur in the absence of a discernible cause, although increased ICP is thought to play a central role in most cases. They represent a distinct entity with differing demographic, radiographic, and clinical manifestations. Patients are typically obese, middle-aged women who often present with symptoms of benign intracranial hypertension (BIH). Radiologic features include empty sella, arachnoid pits, dural ectasia, optic nerve changes, widespread skull base attenuation, and pneumatization of the lateral sphenoid recess.[11] Surgeons should identify these patients as they often have multiple leak sites, coexistent meningoencephaloceles, and are more likely to recur following repair without management of the underlying intracranial hypertension.

Preoperative Work-Up

Essential to the successful management of CSF leaks is the definitive diagnosis of a leak and the precise localization of its site.

Diagnosis

The detection of β-2 transferrin in nasal secretions using immunoelectrophoresis remains the most commonly used diagnostic test for confirmation of CSF leaks. Beta-2 transferrin is found only in CSF, perilymph, and aqueous humor. This results in a high diagnostic sensitivity (97%) and specificity (93%).[12] Only 0.17 mL is needed for testing and β-2 transferrin is stable for up to 7 days regardless of collection site or storage temperature.[13] False-positive results are uncommon but can occur in patients with liver cirrhosis or contamination with neuraminidase secreting bacteria. Beta-trace protein is commonly used in Europe with similarly high specificity and sensitivity.

Localization

Precise localization of the CSF leak is one of the critical factors in the success of fistula repair. A summary of localization methods can be seen in **Table 23.2**.

Imaging

Imaging is useful in all cases of CSF repair for identifying potential sites, delineating the bony anatomy, and sizing the osseous defect. Imaging modalities commonly used include axial and direct coronal standard CT, high-resolution

multidetector helical CT with multiplanar coronal and sagittal reconstruction, CT cisternography with iodinated and nonionic contrast agents, and magnetic resonance imaging (MRI) with and without intrathecal gadolinium. The sensitivity of high-resolution CT in leak localization when compared with intraoperative endoscopic findings has been shown to be > 90%. Furthermore, when submillimeter collimation is available, very accurate radiologic sizing of the osseous defect is demonstrated.[14] Although utilized commonly in the early days of CSF leak repair, CT cisternograms are now used less because of their invasiveness and lower sensitivity. With this said, they may still have a role in select cases of very low volume/intermittent leaks or in localization of the dural defect in cases with multiple or broad-based osseous defects.[15]

MRI has also been shown to be sensitive (75 to 90%) for CSF leak identification with a specificity close to 100%.[16] Its decreased ability to visualize osseous detail and subtle defects as well as the high cost makes high-resolution, thin-section CT still the initial investigation of choice. MRI, however, may still prove a useful adjunct to CT in difficult to localize or recurrent leaks, or in those with suspected meningoencephaloceles. Studies have shown that when combined with CT, the CSF leak detection sensitivity approaches 97%.[15]

Intrathecal Fluorescein

Preoperative intrathecal injection of sodium fluorescein (IF) has become an important tool in the accurate intraoperative localization of CSF leaks. A recent survey of American rhinologists showed that dosage ranged between 0.5 and 1.0 mL of 10% IF, although much lower doses of 0.1 mL of 10% IF can be equally efficacious.[17] Seth et al's review highlighted that surgeons tend to use IF more commonly in leaks of an iatrogenic nature and spontaneous leaks typically associated with multiple leak sites. This study also showed

Table 23.2 Methods Used to Localize Cerebrospinal Fluid Leaks

Localization Method	Strengths	Weakness
Communication with primary surgeon	Noninvasive Good for iatrogenic injury	Recall accuracy Leak site change
Endoscopic examination	Easy to perform	Subjective Low sensitivity Questionable in low pressure leaks
Imaging	High sensitivity High specificity	Radiation exposure Cost
Intrathecal fluorescein	High sensitivity 100% specificity	Off-label use Rare but serious complications
Valsalva maneuver intraoperatively	Noninvasive	Often low yield

that although IF improved site localization, a false-negative rate of 26% still exists. This reflects an overall sensitivity of around 74%.[18] Reasons for negative results have been postulated to include a transient reduction in CSF volume during the intrathecal catheter/injection placement, delayed transfusion of fluorescein to the fistula site across meningeal adhesions, inadequate time allowed for IF to reach the site of the leak, and increased clearance of the colorant from replacement of CSF volume or metabolism of the dye. **Fig. 23.2** demonstrates the key steps and amount of IF used in the intrathecal instillation. It takes up to 30 minutes postinjection for IF to diffuse to the site of the leak. Additional measures to improve visualization may be used and include Trendelenburg positioning, modified Valsalva maneuver, and use of a blue light filter. Despite its widespread use, intrathecal instillation remains "off-label," with the U.S. Food and Drug Administration neither specifically prohibiting nor endorsing it. This is because of the infrequent yet serious complications including cardiac arrhythmias, peripheral

neuropathies, opisthotonos, seizures, and death. These are almost invariable due to erroneous overdosage resulting in direct chemical/irritant meningeal trauma.[19] Although large studies do exist documenting the safety profile of IF when used in concentrations of < 50 mg/total dose, all surgeons should be aware of the "off-label" classification for this indication, and inform patients of the reported complications.[18–20]

Cerebrospinal Fluid Leak Repair

Surgical Approach

Identification of Normal Landmarks

Identification of and working from known landmarks toward the leak provides a methodological and safe approach that allows the surgery to progress in a timely fashion. Useful landmarks are the skull base, often identified in the sphenoid or posterior ethmoid sinuses, the lamina papyracea,

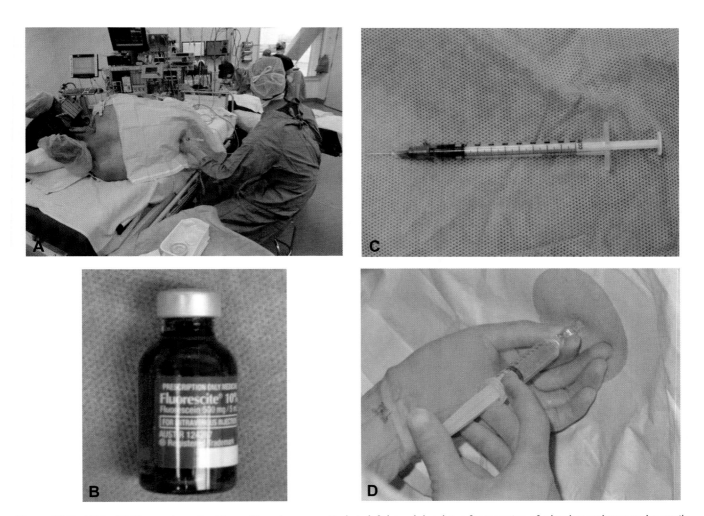

Figure 23.2 (A) to (D) The awake patient is positioned preoperatively in left lateral decubitus for insertion of a lumbar catheter under sterile conditions. About 10 mL of cerebrospinal fluid (CSF) is slowly withdrawn, with regular communication with the patient of the progress and feedback of any neurologic sequelae. Withdrawn CSF is mixed with 0.1 mL of sterile 10% fluorescein sodium and then reinstilled into the patient over a 10-minute period.

often identified in the ethmoid and the frontal sinus ostia as an anterior boundary.

Preservation of Sinus Drainage

Every attempt should be made to preserve the sinus outflow pathways and augment them if needed. Failure to do so may lead to iatrogenic sinusitis and possibly mucoceles. This may require further surgery and disrupt the initial repair.

Wide Exposure of the Bony Defect

Approaching CSF leaks on a broad multidirectional front will achieve wide exposure. Extent of surgery is dependent on the exact site of the leak as localized preoperatively.

Leaks in the ethmoid roof or cribriform plate can be usually approached with standard transnasal endoscopic techniques. Usually a complete ethmoidectomy and maxillary antrostomy are required for adequate exposure of the underlying defect. Sphenoidotomies, frontal sinusotomies, and in some cases middle or superior turbinate resection can be performed for additional exposure or to ensure proper sinus drainage.

Central sphenoid defects can be addressed using a transethmoid or a direct parasagittal approach. To increase exposure, a posterior nasal septectomy and/or resection of the sphenoid intersinus septum can be performed. To address difficult to visualize lateral sphenoid defects, an endoscopic transptyergoid approach may be more appropriate (**Fig. 23.3**).[21] In this technique, a wide sphenoethmoidectomy and large maxillary antrostomy (to the palatine bone) is

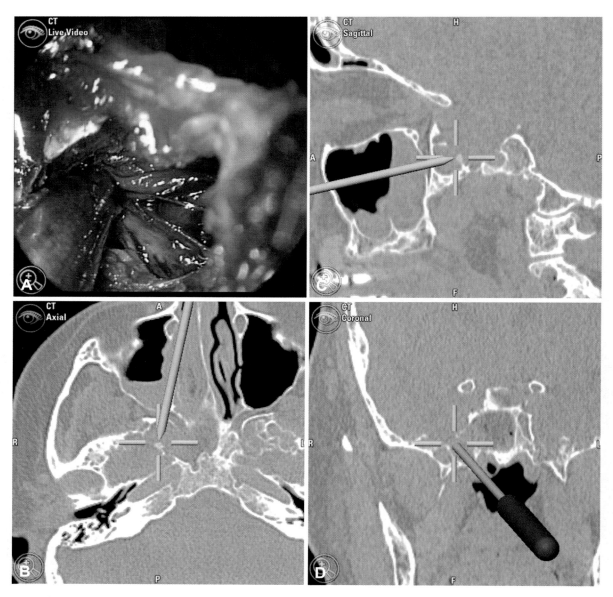

Figure 23.3 A lateral sphenoid recess cerebrospinal fluid (CSF) leak requiring a transpterygoid approach. (A) Endoscopic view of the right lateral sphenoid recess CSF leak and associated encephalocele. (B to D) Axial, sagittal, and coronal image-guidance sequences showing the corresponding computed tomography scan localization of the CSF leak.

performed. The posterior maxillary sinus wall is removed and the pterygopalatine fossa is entered. Control of the internal maxillary artery, maxillary nerve, vidian nerve, and the sphenopalatine ganglion then occurs. The anterior sphenoid sinus wall and pterygoid plates are then removed for direct visualization.

CSF leaks of the frontal sinus can be divided into three sites, each with different surgical implications. Leaks in the ethmoid roof/cribriform plate, adjacent to but not involving the frontal recess, still require a complete frontal recess clearance to maintain frontal sinus drainage. Leaks directly involving the frontal recess are typically the most difficult

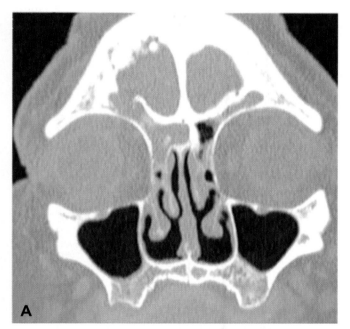

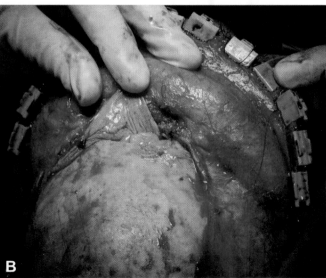

Figure 23.4 (A) Coronal computed tomography image demonstrating a posterolateral frontal sinus cerebrospinal fluid leak. (B) Picture shows a bicoronal flap with an osteoplastic flap and fat obliteration required to close this leak.

sites to approach, often requiring either extended endoscopic approaches, such as the modified Lothrop, or a combined external and endoscopic approach. High superior and lateral defects of the posterior table usually require external procedures. This involves a trephination procedure or osteoplastic flap, with or without fat obliteration (**Fig. 23.4**).

Preparation of the Recipient Bed

Preparing the recipient bed for grafting is crucial to a successful repair. Following circumferential exposure of the bony margins, accurate sizing with an instrument of known dimensions (e.g., curette) occurs. Meticulous removal of approximately 4 to 5 mm of surrounding mucosa proceeds. Some surgeons advocate curetting or drilling bone to stimulate osteoneogenesis, in the hope that this will improve graft take. Bone fragments and prolapsed intracranial contents should be addressed. Bipolar diathermy is commonly employed to shrink meningoencephaloceles in a controlled hemostatic manner. This should be used at the lowest effective setting to avoid intracranial transmission and potential complications (**Fig. 23.5**). The excessive heat and potential collateral damage precludes the use of monopolar diathermy, especially around critical structures. At this point, in cases where a lumbar drain has been placed preoperatively, the drain can be opened to siphon off approximately 10 to 15 mL of CSF and decrease ICP. Drainage of this small volume of CSF will further reduce the encephalocele and prevent reprolapse while the repair material is being harvested.

Repair of the Cerebrospinal Fluid Leak and Reconstruction of the Skull Base Defect

Many factors influence the choice of repair (**Table 23.3**). The interplay of such factors makes each CSF leak unique, and so this section aims to provide the surgeon with general principles rather than dogmatic dictum on factors that may influence decision-making.

Size of the defect is important in the initial planning process of leak repair. In general, small defects up to 3 mm in diameter make the placement of underlay grafts in the epidural space extremely difficult. Consequently, Wormald and McDonogh[22] describe the effective use of fat in his "bath-

Table 23.3 Factors Influencing Choice of Repair

Etiology
Site of bony defect
Size of dural and bony defect
Failed previous leak repair
Availability and state of neighboring tissues
Access to synthetic grafts
Surgeon's preference and experience
Patient comorbities, e.g., raised ICP, BIH, and obesity

ICP, intracranial pressure; BIH, benign intracranial hypertension.

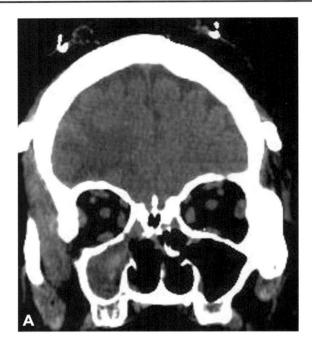

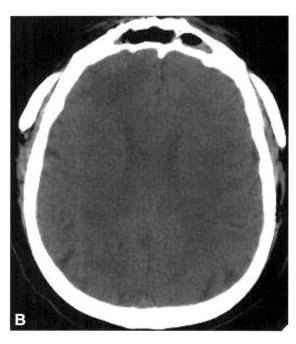

Figure 23.5 (A) Coronal and (B) axial computed tomography scans demonstrating right frontal lobe edema secondary to extracranial bipolar diathermy of a prolapsed encephalocele.

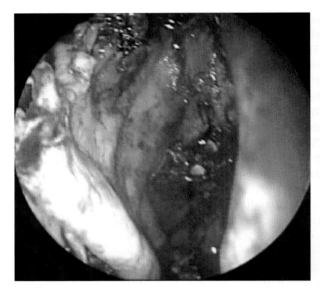

Figure 23.6 Transnasal view of an overlay mucosal graft.

lay graft. Before placing the underlay graft, it is essential to carefully elevate the dura as much as possible over the intracranial bony surface. The choices of graft material are numerous (**Table 23.4**). Tabaee et al[23] listed the following features as critical for graft selection: (1) availability, ade-

Table 23.4 Types of Grafts

Autologous		Heterologous	Synthetic
Free grafts	Vascularized pedicled		
Fat • Ear lobe • Abdominal	Nasoseptal	Bovine • Collagen • Pericardium	Collagen fleece
Mucosa • Septal • Turbinate • Nasal floor	Inferior turbinate	Porcine • Dermis	Hydrogel
Fascia • Tensor facial lata • Temporalis	Tunneled transpterygoid	Cadaveric • Dermis (acellular) • Fat • Fascia • Pericardium • Rib	Mesh • Titanium • Vicryl
Cartilage • Septal • Conchal	Rescue • Palatal mucosal • Middle turbinate		Patches • Polyester urethane • Vicryl/PDS
Bone • Septal • Ethmoid • Mastoid • Iliac crest • Calvarium			

PDS, polydiaxanone sutures.

plug" technique. Ear lobule fat is preferred over abdominal because of the fibrous septae that knit the fat tightly together. After placement, the fat plug is covered by a mucosal graft that sits free or is rotated in. The use of overlay soft tissue grafts without underlying fat have also been advocated by some surgeons for these small defects (**Fig. 23.6**). For defects larger than 4 mm in size, a multilayered reconstruction is preferred with the use of an underlay and an over-

quacy, and easy harvesting of the graft; (2) biocompatibility with minimal chance of resorption, rejection, or infection; (3) low cost; (4) minimal interference with future imaging; and (5) free from potential disease transmission. Prickett et al[24] highlighted the importance of postoperative healing at the donor and graft sites when choosing a graft material. Their study demonstrated that mucosal and allogenic grafts had similar overall success rates when used in endoscopic CSF leak repair. However, allogenic grafts had longer time to mucosalization and more graft crusting, while mucosal grafts had more donor site crusting.

An overlay mucosal graft is typically placed after the underlay graft. Overlay grafts include free mucosal grafts from neighboring tissue such as the septum, inferior or middle turbinate, or nasal floor. Composite free mucosa or bone grafts harvested from the septum and turbinate tissue can be used. Free grafts serve as a scaffold for connective tissue migration and typically adhere to bone at 7 days. By 21 days they are almost completely replaced by fibrous connective tissue. When harvesting such grafts, provision should be made for possible contracture that occurs with the connective tissue ingrowth. In our experience, free mucosal grafts allow for more precise placement and increased contact with the skull base than the composite grafts. It is often useful to mark the mucosal surface of the graft following harvest so as to not confuse it with the undersurface. This will reduce the chance of placing the wrong surface in contact with the bone. When placing the graft, caution must again be exerted to avoid obstruction of the surrounding sinuses. Following placement, attempts should be made to support the graft from below. Gelfoam (Baxter, California, United States) and other absorbable dressings are applied directly to the graft in a careful manner to avoid these substances tracking beneath the graft where they may theoretically interfere with its adherence. More rigid removable supports, such as gloved Merocel packs or inflated balloons, are added for additional short-

term support during the early stages of graft take (**Fig. 23.7**). Smooth emergence from the general anesthetic is preferable to avoid increases in ICP and subsequent graft dislodgement.

Postoperative Management

Antibiotics

The authors recommend the use of broad-spectrum antibiotics with good CSF penetration (e.g., ceftriaxone, trimethoprim/sulfamethoxazole, or levofloxacin) on anesthetic induction with continuation postoperatively for 5 to 7 days. The rational for this is to reduce the risk of CNS infection from the nasal cavities' high bacterial content, as well as limit the chance of toxic shock syndrome from the foreign packing material.

Management of Intracranial Pressure

Bed Rest/Activity

Strict bed rest is essential while lumbar drains are in situ, with the head of bed elevated at 15 to 30 degrees to decrease CSF pressure in the anterior skull base. Once the lumbar drain has been removed, progressive elevation to sitting then ambulation can occur over the next 24 hours. Patients should be educated on avoiding procedures that can increase ICP (e.g., breath holding, bending over, or heavy lifting) and should only perform light activities for the next 6 weeks.

Lumbar Drains

About 67% of otolaryngologists surveyed routinely use lumbar drains as part of their management of CSF leaks, with 4 days being the average duration of use.[17] If inserted preoperatively, they can be used for intrathecal fluorescein instillation as well as maintenance of a reduced meningoencephalocele following cautery. Clear indication for their use remains controversial; not only do they increase the risk of

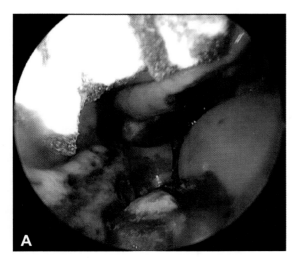 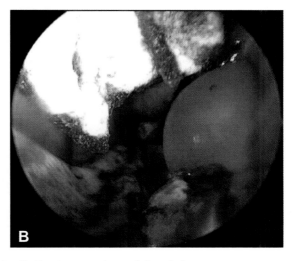

Figure 23.7 (A) Partial and (B) full inflation of a balloon under endoscopic visualization to support a graft from below.

complications (pneumocephalus, lumbar radiculopathies, nausea, vomiting, and dural headache), but numerous studies exist quoting equally high success without their use. The authors' preference is for their utilization in patients with known or suspected increased ICP, recurrent CSF leaks, or when intrathecal fluorescein is going to be used. Postoperatively, if the surgeon is confident in the repair and there is no underlying increased ICP, the drains can be removed immediately. If the repair is tenuous or the patient has elevated ICP, the drains are elevated to maintain a drainage rate of 5 to 10 mL/h for the first 24 to 48 hours to counteract any postoperative elevations in ICP. On postoperative day 2 or 3, the drain is typically closed but left in place. It is removed after 6 to 8 hours if there is no CSF leak.

Long-Term Measures

Acetazolamide, a carbonic anhydrase inhibitor that reduces CSF production, can be used in patients with documented increased postoperative ICP, BIH, or previous failed repair. The precise dosing and duration regimen remains unclear but electrolytes should be monitored while on this therapy. Alternatively, if increased ICP remains an issue or leak recurrence ensues, a ventriculoperitoneal shunt may be considered.

Irrigation/Debridement

This can vary based on surgeon's preference and patient's circumstances. The authors use the following protocol. Patients should be encouraged to irrigate their nose with saline using low-pressure, low-volume devices such as mists and nasal sprays. Surgeons typically review patients at 1 or 2 weeks for gentle debridement of clots to ensure sinus and nasal cavity patency. The graft site should be visualized but left relatively undisturbed during these visits.

Conclusion

The treatment of CSF leaks requires an understanding of the anatomy and pathophysiology of these leaks. The use of preoperative imaging is important to localize the leak. Although it is an off-label use, intrathecal fluorescein is important to consider for localization when needed. The site of the leak, defect size, and patient comorbid factors will influence the steps taken in repair and in the patient's postoperative care.

References

1. Schlosser RJ, Bolger WE. Endoscopic management of cerebrospinal fluid rhinorrhea. Otolaryngol Clin North Am 2006;39(3):523–538, ix
2. Han CY, Backous DD. Basic principles of cerebrospinal fluid metabolism and intracranial pressure homeostasis. Otolaryngol Clin North Am 2005;38(4):569–576
3. Har-El G. What is "spontaneous" cerebrospinal fluid rhinorrhea? Classification of cerebrospinal fluid leaks. Ann Otol Rhinol Laryngol 1999;108(4):323–326
4. Bumm K, Heupel J, Bozzato A, Iro H, Hornung J. Localization and infliction pattern of iatrogenic skull base defects following endoscopic sinus surgery at a teaching hospital. Auris Nasus Larynx 2009;36(6):671–676
5. Locatelli D, Rampa F, Acchiardi I, Bignami M, De Bernardi F, Castelnuovo P. Endoscopic endonasal approaches for repair of cerebrospinal fluid leaks: nine-year experience. Neurosurgery 2006;58(4)(Suppl 2):ONS-246–ONS-256, discussion ONS-256–ONS-257
6. Friedman JA, Ebersold MJ, Quast LM. Post-traumatic cerebrospinal fluid leakage. World J Surg 2001;25(8):1062–1066
7. Brodie HA. Prophylactic antibiotics for posttraumatic cerebrospinal fluid fistulae. A meta-analysis. Arch Otolaryngol Head Neck Surg 1997;123(7):749–752
8. Villalobos T, Arango C, Kubilis P, Rathore M. Antibiotic prophylaxis after basilar skull fractures: a meta-analysis. Clin Infect Dis 1998;27(2):364–369
9. Ratilal BO, Costa J, Sampaio C, Pappamikail L. Antibiotic prophylaxis for preventing meningitis in patients with basilar skull fractures. Cochrane Database Syst Rev 2011;10(8):CD004884
10. Woodworth BA, Schlosser RJ, Faust RA, Bolger WE. Evolutions in the management of congenital intranasal skull base defects. Arch Otolaryngol Head Neck Surg 2004;130(11):1283–1288
11. Wise SK, Schlosser RJ. Evaluation of spontaneous nasal cerebrospinal fluid leaks. Curr Opin Otolaryngol Head Neck Surg 2007;15(1):28–34
12. Abuabara A. Cerebrospinal fluid rhinorrhoea: diagnosis and management. Med Oral Patol Oral Cir Bucal 2007;12(5):E397–E400
13. Bleier BS, Debnath I, O'Connell BP, Vandergrift WA III, Palmer JN, Schlosser RJ. Preliminary study on the stability of beta-2 transferrin in extracorporeal cerebrospinal fluid. Otolaryngol Head Neck Surg 2011;144:101–103
14. La Fata V, McLean N, Wise SK, DelGaudio JM, Hudgins PA. CSF leaks: correlation of high-resolution CT and multiplanar reformations with intraoperative endoscopic findings. AJNR Am J Neuroradiol 2008;29(3):536–541
15. Cui S, Han D, Zhou B, et al. Endoscopic endonasal surgery for recurrent cerebrospinal fluid rhinorrhea. Acta Otolaryngol 2010;130(10):1169–1174
16. Lloyd KM, Del Gaudio JM, Hudgins PA. Imaging of skull base cerebrospinal fluid leaks in adults. Radiology 2008;248(3):725–736
17. Senior BA, Jafri K, Benninger M. Safety and efficacy of endoscopic repair of CSF leaks and encephaloceles: a survey of the members of the American Rhinologic Society. Am J Rhinol 2001;15(1):21–25
18. Seth R, Rajasekaran K, Benninger MS, Batra PS. The utility of intrathecal fluorescein in cerebrospinal fluid leak repair. Otolaryngol Head Neck Surg 2010;143(5):626–632
19. Felisati G, Bianchi A, Lozza P, Portaleone S. Italian multicentre study on intrathecal fluorescein for craniosinusal fistulae. Acta Otorhinolaryngol Ital 2008;28(4):159–163
20. Placantonakis DG, Tabaee A, Anand VK, Hiltzik D, Schwartz TH. Safety of low-dose intrathecal fluorescein in endoscopic cranial base surgery. Neurosurgery 2007;61(3 Suppl):161–165, discussion 165–166
21. Bolger WE. Endoscopic transpterygoid approach to the lateral sphenoid recess: surgical approach and clinical experience. Otolaryngol Head Neck Surg 2005;133(1):20–26
22. Wormald PJ, McDonogh M. 'Bath-plug' technique for the endoscopic management of cerebrospinal fluid leaks. J Laryngol Otol 1997;111(11):1042–1046
23. Tabaee A, Anand VK, Brown SM, Lin JW, Schwartz TH. Algorithm for reconstruction after endoscopic pituitary and skull base surgery. Laryngoscope 2007;117(7):1133–1137
24. Prickett KK, Wise SK, Delgaudio JM. Choice of graft material and postoperative healing in endoscopic repair of cerebrospinal fluid leak. Arch Otolaryngol Head Neck Surg 2011;137(5):457–461

24 Endoscopic Surgery of the Infratemporal and Pterygopalatine Fossae

Steven D. Pletcher and Ivan H. El-Sayed

Tumors and lesions of the infratemporal fossa (ITF) and pterygopalatine fossa (PTF) can be addressed surgically through open and endoscopic surgical approaches. Recent experience using expanded endonasal approaches (EEAs) has increased endoscopic access to lesions of the skull base. Although the endonasal "corridor approach" has been well described for midline skull base lesions,[1–3] several different endoscopic techniques providing varying degrees of access have been described to access the lateral skull base. These include a trans-septal approach,[4,5] a combined Caldwell-Luc/transnasal approach,[6] and an endoscopic anterior maxillotomy (EAM) approach.[7] Approach selection depends on the anatomic location of surgical target, the type of lesion, the goal of surgery, and the skill set of the surgeon.

From an endonasal perspective, the lateral corridor includes any lesion lying lateral to the plane of the medial maxillary wall. Lateral lesions can be located in the medial maxillary wall, the maxillary sinus, or more posteriorly in the lateral sphenoclival bone (vidian nerve), pterygoid fossa, or ITF (**Fig. 24.1**). Lesions involving the mandibular ramus or arising from the skin or parotid gland lateral to this landmark are best managed through open approaches. More anteriorly positioned lesions of the medial PTF are typically easier to access than those in the lateral and posterior regions of the ITF.

Surgical indications include biopsy for histologic diagnosis, surgical debulking, or complete resection. Currently, there are no widely accepted anatomically based staging systems to guide approach selection for lesions of the ITF and PTF. In the authors' practice, lesions that may be amenable to endoscopic approach include (in order of increasing difficulty) lesions of the medial maxillary wall, the V2 nerve to foramen rotundum, the pterygoid fossa, and the ITF. Approach selection is determined on a case-by-case basis and is defined by the tumor pathology and anatomic location as well as the goal of surgery.

Experience and preference of the surgeon are also key factors in approach selection. Successful endoscopic approach to the PTF and ITF requires a detailed anatomic understanding of the region, appropriate instrumentation, and knowledgeable support staff. The surgeon must have enough access to apply effective hemostatic techniques while maintaining an adequate endoscopic view and avoiding inadvertent injury to surrounding structures. The EEA corridor uses a two-surgeon technique to allow three to four hands operating simultaneously. This maintains

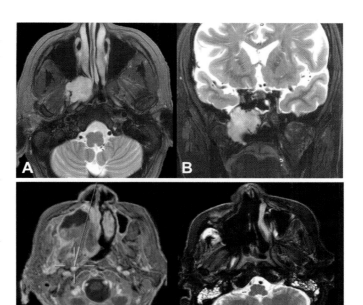

Figure 24.1 Lateral lesions include lesions of the pterygoid fossa and infratemporal fossa. (A, B) Axial and coronal view of schwannoma in pterygoid fossa, abutting the middle cranial fossa through the greater sphenoid wing. (C, D) Squamous cell carcinoma of the maxillary sinus invading the pterygoid fossa and infratemporal fossa. (C) Endoscopic resection revealed positive microscopic margins on the carotid artery (green image-guidance probe). (D) Postoperative imaging 1 year after surgery reveals no recurrence. The patient has no evidence of the disease 5 years after surgery.

endoscopic visualization with potential for hemostatic control using a bipolar cautery, endoscopic vascular clip applier, or by packing hemostatic agents.

Careful preoperative analysis of multiplanar imaging helps determine the feasibility of an endonasal approach. There is a wide variation in the degree of aeration of each of the paranasal sinuses and anatomic relations that impacts endoscopic exposure. Review of images in the coronal, axial, and sagittal planes allows an evaluation of the anatomic constraints of an endonasal approach. Multiplanar imaging also provides an understanding of the three-dimensional boundaries of the underlying pathology and surrounding critical structures. Magnetic resonance imaging (MRI) and computed tomography (CT) provide complementary information when evaluating this region: MRI is often helpful in evaluating the soft tissue extent of tumors or lesions, whereas CT imaging provides a detailed view of the bony anatomy. Overlaying them on an intraoperative image-guidance system is useful during surgery. When lesions approximate the carotid artery, magnetic resonance arteriography or CT angiogram can be added for use with image guidance.

Anatomic Considerations

Pterygopalatine Fossa

The PTF is the anatomic space posterior to the maxillary sinus. The PTF extends to the pterygoid plates posteriorly, the posterior wall of the maxillary sinus anteriorly, and opens into the ITF laterally. Vascular structures including the internal maxillary artery and its terminal branches course through the anterior aspect of the PTF, whereas nerves including the vidian nerve, the sphenopalatine ganglion, and the origin of V2 reside in the posterior aspect of the PTF. The PTF can be approached through the posterior maxillary sinus wall.

Infratemporal Fossa

The ITF is an anatomic space below the middle cranial fossa, posterior to the maxilla, and medial to the ramus of the mandible. The ITF must be considered in three planes when considering the optimal approach. The ITF contains both the parapharyngeal space (medially) and the masticator space (laterally). In the axial plane, the parapharyngeal space (PPS) can be divided into pre- and poststyloid compartments. The prestyloid PPS has fewer critical structures, containing primarily fat and an extension of the deep lobe of the parotid gland. The poststyloid PPS contains the internal carotid artery, internal jugular vein, and lower cranial nerves (IX to XII). The medial and lateral pterygoid muscles are located within the masticator space along with the tendon of the temporalis muscle and proximal segment of the internal maxillary artery. The internal maxillary artery courses from a lateral to medial direction and posterior to anterior until it terminates in the pterygoid fossa to form the sphenopalatine artery. The maxillary artery passes lateral to the lateral pterygoid muscle, but it can divide the superior and inferior heads of the muscle and course medial to the inferior head in about 40% of cases.[8] The maxillary artery gives several relevant branches within the musculature of the ITF. Notably, the inferior alveolar artery courses medially to the ramus of the mandible laterally, whereas the middle meningeal artery proceeds superiorly, lateral to the V3 nerve. Following the lateral pterygoid plate from anterior to posterior leads directly to the foramen ovale that transmits V3 nerve. This is a safe trajectory of dissection within the pterygoid muscles and extending laterally into the ITF as the carotid artery reliably enters the skull base posterior to foramen ovale. The ITF extends well below the plane of the

maxillary sinus floor and nasal cavity floor. This is visualized well on coronal images through this region. Endoscopic access to the inferior aspect of the ITF is quite limited.

Nasal Cavity and Paranasal Sinuses

The variable anatomy of the nasal cavity and paranasal sinuses may impact endonasal access to PTF and ITF lesions. EEAs rely on creating an adequate working corridor to manipulate instruments while maintaining a clear view of the operative field. These approaches typically begin with a wide maxillary antrostomy and total ethmoidectomy. Sphenoidotomy is frequently performed and the middle turbinate may be resected to improve access. The floor and medial wall of the orbit are clearly defined to avoid inadvertent injury. The width of the nasal cavity (determined by the location of the septum and lateral nasal wall and piriform aperture) may compromise mobility of instruments and limit access to the lateral PTF. Septal deviations may be addressed surgically. Removal of the lateral aspect of the medial maxillary wall and inferior turbinate may be required to increase the surgical field, accommodate additional instruments, and improve lateral exposure.

A lateral corridor often requires working through the maxillary sinus. The anterior wall of the maxilla transmits the anterior superior alveolar nerves and vessels that supply sensation and blood to the incisors. The posterior wall opens into the pterygoid plates and pterygoid fossa, whereas more laterally it opens into the ITF. The roof of the maxillary sinus forms the orbital floor.

Poor pneumatization of the maxillary sinus may compromise access to the superior and lateral regions of the PTF and ITF. The relationship of the maxillary sinus floor with the nasal floor is critical in evaluating endoscopic access to the inferior aspect of the PTF and ITF. A superior position of the hard palate and nasal floor relative to that of the maxillary sinus floor will limit access to the inferior portions of these fossae. The floor of the maxillary sinus descends into the alveolar ridge of the maxilla, below the level of the nasal cavity floor, in about one-third of patients and is at the same level in about one-third of patients.[9] The ITF extends significantly below the floor of the maxillary sinus and, even in cases with favorable anatomy, access to inferior aspect of the ITF is limited using an endoscopic approach.

Variations of the sphenoid sinus anatomy can also impact surgery in this region. Lateral aeration of the sphenoid sinus into the sphenoid bone may provide an aerated space behind the PTF. Pathology of this variably present lateral sphenoid recess (frequently encephaloceles) may be accessed by removing the posterior wall of the maxillary sinus, displacing the PTF contents, and opening into the lateral sphenoid recess. Careful evaluation of preoperative imaging is critical in identifying variations in paranasal sinus anatomy that may impact endoscopic access to the PTF and ITF. The vidian canal carries the vidian artery and nerve and runs along the floor of the sphenoid sinus (**Fig. 24.2**), entering the PTF in the

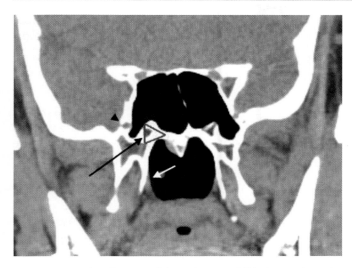

Figure 24.2 Identification of the vidian canal (black arrow) on the anterior face of the sphenoid superior-medial to the pterygoid plate in the pterygoid wedge (red triangle). The vidian canal typically occupies the 6-o'clock position and the foramen rotundum with the V2 nerve (black arrowhead) the 9- (right) or 1-o'clock (left) position.

superomedial portion of the fossa. The vidian canal defines a safe plane of entry into the skull base because of its consistent relationship to the carotid artery. The canal runs just inferior to the anterior border of the second genu of the carotid artery as the vessel transitions from its petrous horizontal segment to the paraclival vertical segment.[10,11] Endoscopic vidian neurectomy at this site has been reported as a treatment for refractory rhinorrhea.[12,13] This technique is controversial and is not a widely accepted practice.

Endonasal Approach to Pterygopalatine Fossa and Infratemporal Fossa

A step-wise approach can be used to select the appropriate surgical technique for lesions of the PTF and ITF. In general, a lesion should be approached using the least-invasive technique that provides adequate exposure. Surgical approaches from least to most invasive include the following: transnasal, transeptal, anterior maxillotomy with medial maxillectomy, sublabial incision, and open transfascial approach. Despite the approach selected, consent for a possible open approach is routinely obtained. Conversion to an open approach is rarely required but may prove useful in the event of uncontrollable hemorrhage or inability to achieve an adequate surgical resection.

Control of bleeding during endoscopic surgery of the PTF and ITF is an important consideration. Hemorrhage of the internal maxillary artery is brisk, but it is controllable with pressure and hemostatic clips. Rupture of internal jugular vein may be problematic, but it is likely controllable. Carotid artery injury has a much higher risk of serious morbidity or mortality. The availability of appropriate vascular and interventional radiologic services should be considered when determining whether to approach a lesion endoscopically.

Transnasal Approach

The simplest endoscopic approach to the PTF involves performing a standard maxillary antrostomy and ethmoidectomy, then removing either some part or complete posterior wall of the maxillary sinus to access the PTF. This technique provides an excellent exposure of the internal maxillary artery and its branches including the sphenopalatine artery. The vidian nerve may also be accessed through this approach at its location in the posteromedial aspect of the PTF. The vidian nerve can also be identified on the anterior wall of the sphenoid immediately as it exits from the vidian canal (**Fig. 24.2**). Internal maxillary or sphenopalatine artery ligation may be performed through this approach for refractory epistaxis.

The transnasal approach allows access to the medial PTF. The inferior access of the approach may be increased by creating a "mega-antrostomy" of the maxillary sinus by resecting the inferior turbinate and the inferior portion of the lateral nasal wall from the natural ostium back to the posterior maxillary sinus wall. Biopsy of lesions extending into the medial PTF or complete resection of those masses confined to the medial PTF may be achieved through this technique.

When more extensive surgery is required, it is often helpful to employ a two-surgeon, four-handed technique. The transnasal approach alone does not provide an adequate corridor for multiple instruments and multiple surgeons. The transnasal approach also provides limited access to the lateral PTF and the ITF. Enhanced exposure to these regions and a larger working corridor may be obtained with an expanded endoscopic approach.

Transnasal and Sublabial Transmaxillary Approach

Combining the endoscopic transnasal technique with a sublabial transmaxillary approach provides a moderate increase in lateral access to the PTF and a second working corridor for instruments. However, angulation of instruments through this second working corridor is limited by bone of the piriform aperture in the anterior maxillary window. If there is a narrow nasal aperture or the maxillary sinus floor is significantly lower than the nasal cavity floor, the access may be limited to the PTF and ITF. Coordination of instruments through two separate portals can be challenging and limits this approach.

Transnasal and Transeptal Approach

This technique is commonly used to provide enhanced access to the PTF and ITF.[5] A significant increase in lateral exposure is achieved by entering through the contralateral nasal passage and passing instruments through the septum, allowing for increased angulation of instruments and greatly enhanced lateral exposure. The use of angled endoscopes through the ipsilateral nasal passage provides clear visualization of the PTF and ITF, and pathology in these areas can be approached and addressed using straight or gently curved instruments passing through the septum. Working through each nostril allows a four-handed technique. To achieve wide exposure, the mid-portion of the inferior turbinate is resected and the maxillary antrostomy is enlarged inferiorly to the level of the nasal floor. Anterior and lateral exposure is attained by opening to the maxillary sinus anteriorly, transecting the nasolacrimal duct.

Possible concerns using this approach include the risk of creating a septal perforation and the potential for postoperative epiphora or dacryocystitis. Risk of a septal perforation may be mitigated by using a vertical incision through the mucoperichondrium on one side of the septum and a horizontal incision on the other side and carefully closing the incisions at the completion of surgery. It is our experience that a clean cut through the nasolacrimal duct rarely results in stenosis of the duct with subsequent epiphora. The duct is filleted open or a silastic stent tubing can be placed at the time of surgery to mitigate this risk.

Despite the access achieved with the transeptal approach, movement of the endoscope and all instruments is still limited by a window created by the nasal septum and the bone of the nasal vault. This can result in crowding of instruments, limiting freedom of movement distally.

Endoscopic Anterior Maxillotomy Approach

The EAM approach widens the proximal diameter of the working corridor at the nasal entrance by removing the piriform aperture. Compared to the transeptal approach, EAM allows an increased lateral exposure of the posterior maxillary wall and improves access anterolaterally (**Fig. 24.3**). Performing an EAM widens the nasal aperture by about 40% from the anterior maxillary wall to the nasal septum and allows four instruments to be used comfortably through either one or two nostrils.[7] Removing this proximal bony restriction also provides less crowding of instruments and results in improved distal-tip instrument control. Furthermore, larger caliber instruments such as standard bayonet bipolars, endoscopic clip appliers, and extended cautery devices may be used through this opening, reducing the reliance on specialized instrumentation.

Compared with the transeptal approach in which the nasolacrimal duct had already been sacrificed, our clinical series revealed an increase angulation of 29% on the ipsilateral side and 18% on the contralateral side, which is adequate to reach the anterior most maxillary sinus and the lateral posterior aspect of the ITF.[7] Using aradiographic analysis of the approach, Prosser et al also compared the EAM with the transeptal approach and found that to obtain equivalent access posteriorly using a 1-cm Denker's approach, 44% of patients would require a very anterior septotomy that did not maintain a 1.5-cm septal strut (increasing risk of saddle nose deformity).[14] The increased angulation allows for enhanced access to the maxilla and ITF compared with the transeptal approach. The EAM is the preferred approach of the authors for complex endoscopic procedures in the lateral PTF and ITF.

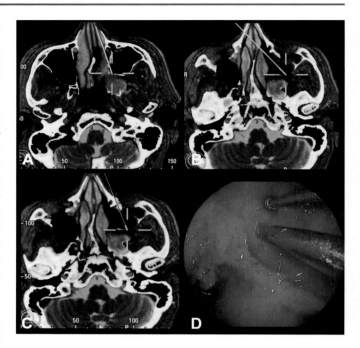

Figure 24.3 Comparison of transeptal, transnasal, and endoscopic anterior maxillotomy (EAM) approach. (A) Image guidance demonstrates lateral access allowed through an endonasal approach. (B) Passing instruments transeptally allows increased lateral access and can be combined with ipsilateral endonasal approach. (C) Removal of piriform aperture and medial anterior maxillary wall (EAM approach) increases the ipsilateral diameter of the endonasal approach. This allows more instruments to be passed freely into the nose and increases the working range of motion distally. (D) Demonstrates drill, suction, and endoscope passed through ipsilateral EAM approach.

This approach does result in anesthesia of the ipsilateral nasal ala and upper incisor. Postoperative anesthesia can be reduced by minimizing the amount of the anterior wall removed and is generally well tolerated and frequently improves months to 1 year after surgery. Approximately 50% of patients will develop mild (2 mm) alar retraction (superior and posterior), which can result in asymmetry of the nasal base and deepening of the nasolabial fold, and preoperative assessment should determine if patients already have an alar asymmetry. With transection of the nasolacrimal duct, there is a risk of postoperative epiphora, although this is uncommon in our experience and can be addressed later if it occurs with standard dacryocystotomy. The authors rarely stent the duct at the time of surgery and have found cases of migration of the stent into adjacent soft tissue when postoperative radiation was delivered. Opening the nasolacrimal duct widely may avoid this result. Mild epiphora may actually offset decreased lacrimal secretions in patients receiving radiation therapy.

Surgical Technique

A total ethmoidectomy and ipsilateral sphenoidotomy are performed to define the plane of the medial orbit wall. A wide maxillary antrostomy is performed and, if necessary, the ipsilateral middle turbinate resected. If a septal flap is required for closure, it is usually harvested at this time and a posterior septectomy is performed. This sequence of procedures is often tailored to each lesion, but this approach allows a clear identification of the key anatomy including the medial orbit wall, the inferior orbit wall, the vidian canal, and carotid artery. The location of the sphenopalatine artery is clearly identified emitting from the sphenopalatine foramen and seen as a bulge in the superior two-thirds of the posterior maxillary sinus wall.

Next, the EAM is performed (**Fig. 24.4**). A vertical endonasal incision is made over the ipsilateral nasal bone extending from the floor of the nose to the height of the maxillary ostium. The mucosal incision is then carried back to the maxillary ostium. After local elevation of soft tissues, a drill is used to remove this inferior portion of the nasal bone and nasofrontal bar and enter the maxillary sinus at its anteromedial apex. The inferior turbinate and lateral nasal wall are then removed below the level of the orbital floor and the nasolacrimal duct is transected.[7]

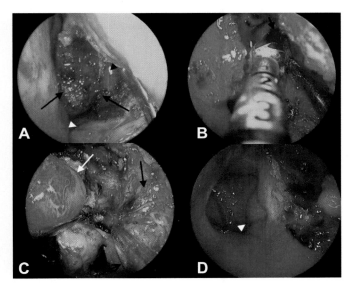

Figure 24.4 Intraoperative dissection through an endoscopic anterior maxillotomy. (A) Incision is made at the anterior edge of inferior turbinate (left black arrow) along the rim of the piriform aperture (right black arrow). The floor of nasal cavity (white arrowhead) and anterior maxillary wall (black arrowhead) are visible. (B) The piriform aperture is drilled away with 1 to 3 mm of the anterior maxillary wall revealing the opening into the maxillary sinus (black arrow). (C) After removal of medial maxillary wall back to the posterior maxillary wall and removal of posterior maxillary wall, the lesion is dissected from lateral to medial. The mass (white arrow) is retracted medially and a clean tissue plane is dissected. In this case, a carbon dioxide laser (black open arrow) is used to dissect away from pterygoid fat (black filled arrow). The internal maxillary artery requires control with a vascular clip. (D) Final defect reveals relation of mass superior and posterior to eustachian tube. The eustachian tube is a landmark for the carotid artery that runs in the carotid canal posterior–superior to it.

The posterior maxillary wall is widely exposed and demucosalized. The bone of the posterior maxillary wall is then thinned with a diamond burr using an extended, high-speed, endoscopic drill. The remaining bone is then removed using a 2-mm Cloward rongeur. Medially the posterior maxillary wall is often fused with the pterygoid plates and requires drilling to identify the plates clearly. The bone is elevated off the underlying periosteum, which provides an excellent border between the pterygoid fat. The periosteum is then incised. If the lesion is in the PTF, the surgeon then angles out laterally to normal tissue beyond the lesion. Fat of the pterygoid fossa opens up laterally to the ITF. Dissection is carried back to identify the medial pterygoid muscle.

At this point, if the internal maxillary artery is encountered in the tissue entering from posteriorly laterally, it should be clipped with endoscopic clips before incising. Tissue is dissected from lateral to medial direction, keeping in mind the level of the V2 nerve and the orbit. The pterygoid plates often fuse with the posterior maxillary wall and require drilling to enter the attachments of the lateral and medial pterygoid to the pterygoid plates. Following the medial pterygoid plate, plane medially leads to the anterior wall of the sphenoid. Removal of the lateral pterygoid plate leads to foramen ovale and V3 nerve, which is the posterior limit of safe dissection before encountering the carotid artery.

If further dissection is necessary, the V2 nerve is followed posteriorly to foramen rotundum. The inferior orbital fissure is identified and the vidian nerve and foramen rotundum are clearly identified. Posterior to the medial pterygoid plate lies the eustachian tube that can be resected. The superior–posterior aspect of the eustachian tube is in contact with the dense fibers of the carotid canal and care should be taken not to cause injury to the carotid directly or via thermal injury secondary to proximate cautery.

Tumors anterior to the level of the medial pterygoid muscle can be safely dissected in this manner. The inferior edge of the tumor should be inspected preoperatively, as it may be difficult to remove tumors extending beyond the floor of the maxillary sinus. Tumors extending beyond the medial pterygoid muscle can reach out laterally toward the mandibular ramus or even internal jugular vein. If further access is needed than provided by an EAM, converting to an open approach with a sublabial incision and removal of the anterior maxillary wall improves access significantly.

The pterygoid muscles are encased with the pterygoid plexus, a network of veins that may bleed copiously and is best controlled by packing with hemostatic agents. Following the plane along the medial pterygoid muscle leads to the fat pad in the lateral ITF and then the mandibular ramus.

For tumors reaching beyond the pterygoid muscles, the senior author (Dr. El-Sayed) has found the lateral pterygoid plate as the main landmark to V3 and the carotid artery. The lateral pterygoid plate angles obliquely toward laterally and leads to the foramen ovale that transmits the third division of the cranial nerve V. Posterior to the V3 lays the foramen spinosum that transmits the middle meningeal

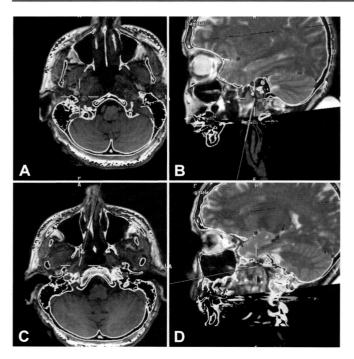

Figure 24.5 Carotid artery exposed through a transcervical approach in axial (A) and sagittal view (B) up to the level of skull base. The computed tomography scan (yellow) overlaid a magnetic resonance image and a magnetic resonance arteriography that demonstrates the carotid artery (red). After transcervical exposure, the lesion, an adenoma of the eustachian tube, is approached through a transeptal and endoscopic anterior maxillotomy for resection. This endoscopic access is demonstrated in the axial (C) and sagittal (D) images.

artery, and posterior to this is the carotid artery in the ITF as it enters the skull base. Medial to this the carotid travels superior the eustachian tube in the carotid canal. The lateral pterygoidplate thus serves as an excellent landmark for the V3 nerve and carotid artery. When a tumor rests anterior to the carotid artery, the carotid can be exposed transcervically first and protected with a pledget and then dissected endoscopically (**Fig. 24.5**).

Summary

Multiple approaches exist for surgery of the PTF and ITF. Recent advances in endoscopic techniques have resulted in increased enthusiasm for endoscopic treatment of these lesions. Although endoscopic approaches can provide an excellent exposure and visualization of lesions in this area, a detailed knowledge of PTF and ITF and familiarity with endoscopic techniques are required for successful surgery in this region. Ultimately, approach selection depends on the anatomic location of surgical target, the type of lesion, the goal of surgery, and the skill set of the surgeon.

References

1. Pirris SM, Pollack IF, Snyderman CH, et al. Corridor surgery: the current paradigm for skull base surgery. Childs Nerv Syst 2007; 23(4):377–384
2. Kassam A, Snyderman CH, Mintz A, Gardner P, Carrau RL. Expanded endonasal approach: the rostrocaudal axis. Part I. Crista galli to the sella turcica. Neurosurg Focus 2005;19(1):E3
3. Kassam A, Snyderman CH, Mintz A, Gardner P, Carrau RL. Expanded endonasal approach: the rostrocaudal axis. Part II. Posterior clinoids to the foramen magnum. Neurosurg Focus 2005;19(1):E4
4. Wormald PJ, Oo iE, van Hasselt CA, Nair S. Endoscopic removal of sinonasal inverted papilloma including endoscopic medial maxillectomy. Laryngoscope 2003;113(5):867–873
5. Robinson S, Patel N, Wormald PJ. Endoscopic management of benign tumors extending into the infratemporal fossa: a two-surgeon transnasal approach. Laryngoscope 2005;115(10):1818–1822
6. Har-El G. Combined endoscopic transmaxillary-transnasal approach to the pterygoid region, lateral sphenoid sinus, and retrobulbar orbit. Ann Otol Rhinol Laryngol 2005;114(6):439–442
7. El-Sayed I, Pletcher S, Russell M, McDermott M, Parsa A. Endoscopic anterior maxillotomy: infratemporal fossa via transnasal approach. Laryngoscope 2011;121(4):694–698
8. Hollinshead WH. Anatomy for Surgeons: The Head and Neck. Philadelphia, PA: Lippincott-Raven; 1982
9. Donald PJ. Anatomy and histology. In: Donald PJ, Gluckman JL, Rice DH, eds. The Sinuses. New York: Raven Press; 1995:25–48
10. Vescan AD, Snyderman CH, Carrau RL, et al. Vidian canal: analysis and relationship to the internal carotid artery. Laryngoscope 2007; 117(8):1338–1342
11. Kassam AB, Vescan AD, Carrau RL, et al. Expanded endonasal approach: vidian canal as a landmark to the petrous internal carotid artery. J Neurosurg 2008;108(1):177–183
12. Robinson SR, Wormald PJ. Endoscopic vidian neurectomy. Am J Rhinol 2006; 20(2):197–202
13. Lee JC, Kao CH, Hsu CH, Lin YS. Endoscopic transsphenoidal vidian neurectomy. Eur Arch Otorhinolaryngol 2011;268(6):851–856
14. Prosser JD, Figueroa R, Carrau RI, Ong YK, Solares CA. Quantitative analysis of endoscopic endonasal approaches to the infratemporal fossa. Laryngoscope 2011;121(8):1601–1605

25 Benign Tumors of the Nasal Cavity and Paranasal Sinuses

Patrick C. Walz, Bradley A. Otto, Daniel M. Prevedello, and Ricardo L. Carrau

This chapter gives a general overview of benign tumors of the sinonasal cavity. With the exception of osteomas, the neoplasms discussed here are relatively rare in occurrence when compared with inflammatory sinonasal disorders such as rhinosinusitis. Although there is quite extensive histopathologic diversity among this group of neoplasms, their presentation, work-up, and management are generally uniform. Two of the most commonly discussed benign sinonasal neoplasms, juvenile nasopharyngeal angiofibroma (JNA) and inverting Schneiderian papilloma, have been covered in Chapter 27 and will not be discussed here in detail.

Prevalence

Osteoma is the most common benign sinonasal neoplasm with an annual incidence of up to 80 per 100,000.[1] Eller and Sillers identified osteomas in up to 3% of routine head computed tomography (CT) scans.[1,2] Hemangioma represents the most common soft tissue neoplasm, and inverted papilloma, which represents up to 4% of all nasal tumors, is the most common epithelial neoplasm.[3] The majority of sinonasal neoplasms, however, are rare, with most references in the literature existing as case reports or small case series.

Clinical Presentation

Presentation varies and is attributable to a combination of factors, most notably aggressiveness of the lesion and location. The most common presentation is that of unilateral nasal obstruction, reported in up to three-quarters of patients.[1] Chronic sinusitis, epistaxis, headache, or an incidental finding on examination/imaging are other common presenting complaints for these uncommon tumors. Progression and extension beyond the confines of the sinonasal cavity, typically late in the disease process, can also lead to less common presenting complaints such as external nasal mass/deformity, globe displacement, epiphora, vision loss, diplopia, oral cavity obstruction,[4] meningitis, subarachnoid hemorrhage, or even pneumocephalus.[5]

Diagnostic Work-up

The diagnostic work-up for any nasal mass begins with a thorough history, noting length, location, severity, and change-over time of symptoms. As noted above, presenting symptoms will vary, but tend to parallel those of inflammatory sinonasal disorders, such as rhinosinusitis.

A complete head and neck examination including nasal endoscopy should be performed. When possible, a biopsy of unilateral nasal masses should be done. Vascular tumors or encephaloceles, as suggested by clinical picture or imaging, should not be biopsied. Signs indicative of advanced tumors, such as cerebrospinal fluid rhinorrhea, globe displacement, external nasal deformity, and numbness, should be identified. Furthermore, superimposed paranasal sinus infections should be identified and addressed before surgical intervention.

Imaging studies generally include CT and magnetic resonance imaging (MRI) scans. CT scans best characterize the bony anatomy and can suggest intracranial or orbital extension. However, in cases with extensive paranasal sinus opacification or with skull base erosion, MRI better distinguishes tumor from adjacent secretions or neural tissue. When indicated by the extent of the lesion, referral to ophthalmology, neurosurgery, or oral and maxillofacial surgery, or dentistry should be made.

Treatment

In general, complete excision of most benign sinonasal tumors is curative. Currently, minimally invasive, endoscopic approaches are the mainstay. However, strategically placed incisions, such as brow, eyelid, or gingivobuccal sulcus incisions, may improve access and extirpation of difficult-to-reach tumors, as discussed in Harvey et al.[1] For more advanced disease or for improved access, traditional "open" approaches may be necessary. Close postoperative surveillance is required not only to detect recurrent tumors but also to assess the physiologic function of the sinonasal cavity following treatment.

Specific Neoplasms

Table 25.1 provides a complete list of tumors, organized in the fashion of the World Health Organization guidelines.[6] The following is a brief description of some of the more common benign tumors found in the sinonasal cavity.

Table 25.1 Benign Neoplasms of the Nose and Paranasal Sinuses

Tissue of Origin	Tumor
Epithelial	Schneiderian papilloma
	Inverted
	Exophytic
	Oncocytic
	Salivary tissue
	Pleomorphic adenoma
	Myoepithelioma
	Oncocytoma
Neuroectodermal	Schwannoma
	Neurofibroma
	Meningioma
	Glioma
Dental	Ameloblastoma
	Odontogenic keratocyst
Muscle	Rhabdomyoma
	Leiomyoma
	Inflammatory myofibroblastic tumor[a]
Vascular	Hemangioma
	Lobular capillary hemangioma
	Cavernous hemangioma
	Juvenile nasopharyngeal angiofibroma
	Paraganglioma
	Angiomyolipoma
	Sinonasal hemangiopericytoma[a]
Bone	Osteoma
	Fibrous dysplasia
	Ossifying fibroma
	Giant cell tumor
	Osteoid osteomas
Cartilage	Chondroma
	Chondroblastoma
	Chondromyxoid fibroma
	Osteochondroma
	Nasal chondromesenchymal hamartoma
Others	Hamartoma (REAH, CORE, and others)
	Fibroma
	Myxoma
	Plasmacytoma
	Lipoma
	Desmoid-type fibromatosis[a]
	Solitary fibrous tumor[a]
Germ cell	Dermoid cyst
	Mature teratoma
	Chordoma

[a]Tumors of increased malignant potential.
REAH, respiratory epithelial adenomatoid hamartoma; CORE, chondroosseous respiratory epithelial hamartoma.

Tumors of Epithelial Origin

Schneiderian Papilloma

Inverted

Inverted papilloma is the most common of the epithelial benign tumors. Refer to Chapter 26 for further details.

Exophytic

Exophytic papilloma (EP) is the second most common Schneiderian papilloma and is located almost exclusively on the nasal septum.[6,7] Also referred to as everted or fungiform papilloma, these lesions exhibit a histologic pattern of branching exophytic proliferations with fibrovascular cores covered by epithelial hyperplasia varying from squamous to transitional to respiratory in addition to occasional mucin-filled microcysts.[6,7] EPs are more common in males by a factor of 2:1 to 10:1 and are typically diagnosed in the third to sixth decades.[6,7] There is strong evidence associating the development of EP with human papilloma virus (HPV) infection, primarily subtypes 6 and 11. In Lawson's recent meta-analysis of HPV in all Schneiderian papillomas, the adjusted prevalence of HPV in the setting of EP ranged from 45 to 86%.[8] Physical examination reveals small (0.1 to 1.5 cm) yellow-tan or gray verrucous exophytic lesion affixed to underlying mucosa by a narrow stalk.[7] Unlike inverted papilloma, malignant transformation is exceedingly rare.[7] Complete resection, including a small margin of healthy tissue at the point of attachment, is curative, but incomplete resection can lead to recurrence rates of 22 to 50%.[6,7]

Oncocytic

Oncocytic Schneiderian papilloma (OSP), or cylindrical cell papilloma, is the least common Schneiderian papilloma, representing 3 to 7% of papillomas.[3,7,9] OSPs are equally distributed among males and females and are diagnosed most frequently in the sixth decade.[6] Like inverted papilloma, OSPs are rarely identified on the septum and localize to the maxillary, ethmoid, or rarely sphenoid sinuses.[3] Physical examination typically reveals a polypoid pink, gray, or tan lesion emanating from the lateral aspect of the nasal cavity.[6,9] Oncocytic papillomas are highly metabolically active and have also been identified on positron emission tomography scan in the process of metastatic evaluation, raising concern for potential metastasis.[10] No association between OSP and HPV has been identified.[6,8] Histologically, OSPs demonstrate exophytic fronds in addition to endophytic areas with oncocytic change and seromucinous glands with frequent microabscesses.[6,7] Although malignant transformation to squamous cell carcinoma, mucoepidermoid carcinoma, sinonasal undifferentiated carcinoma, and small cell carcinoma has been identified in 4 to 17% of cases,[3,6,9] the reported rate is controversial and based on a small population.[3] Nonetheless, complete resection with attention to the point of attachment is indicated to minimize recurrence, which has been reported at the rates of 33 to 40%,[3,10] necessitating careful long-term follow-up.

Glandular Tumors

Pleomorphic Adenoma

Glandular tumors identified in the sinonasal tract are nearly all of salivary gland origin and are benign in 25%.[6] Diagnosed in the third to seventh decades, pleomorphic adenoma demonstrates no sex preponderance and is thought to arise from minor salivary glands or ectopic rests of tissue and are primarily located in the submucosal tissues of the septum in 90% of cases,[6,11] though origin within the maxillary sinus[12] and lateral nasal wall[13] has been reported. Several hundred cases of sinonasal pleomorphic adenoma have been reported,[14] making this the most common benign sinonasal salivary gland tumor. Histologically, sinonasal pleomorphic adenomas appear similar to their major salivary counterparts with unencapsulated epithelial and myoepithelial ductal components in a chondromyxoid stroma, though reports have indicated that sinonasal tumors demonstrate less stromal component.[12] Surgical excision is indicated and curative, with recurrence rates of 5 to 7.5%.[11,13] Risk of malignant transformation is low and proportional to the length of time for which the tumor has persisted.[12] Additional salivary gland tumors reported less frequently in the sinonasal tract include myoepthelioma[15] and oncocytoma.[6] These are managed in a similar fashion.

Tumors of Bone, Cartilage, and Odontogenic Origin

Osteoma

Usually identified between the second and third decades,[2,16,17] osteomas demonstrate a male preponderance of 1.5:1 to 3:1. Osteomas are predominately identified in the frontal (60 to 70%)[2,18] or ethmoid (20 to 55%)[16] sinuses, with a minority identified in the maxillary (less than 5%) and sphenoid (rare) sinuses.[2] Although histologically these tumors may exhibit an eburnated (ivory), spongy, or mixed appearance,[2,6,16] they have a characteristic radiodense, sharply demarcated appearance with polypoid or sessile projection of bone into the affected sinus[5,6,16] (**Fig. 25.1**). Osteomas are uniformly benign with no reports of malignant transformation,[2] so asymptomatic lesions may be followed with serial imaging. Resection is indicated if the tumor is symptomatic or at risk for becoming symptomatic because of its location and growth potential. Recurrence rates are very low.[2,6] Osteomas can be associated with Gardner syndrome, especially if multiple osteomas are identified. As only 7% exhibit multifocal osteomas in the absence of Gardner syndrome,[16] the finding of multiple osteomas should trigger review of imaging to identify supernumerary teeth and referral for gastrointestinal evaluation to identify colonic polyposis, the third characteristic manifestation of Gardner syndrome.[1,2]

Fibrous Dysplasia

Fibrous dysplasia (FD) is a neoplasm characterized by bone remodeling and can have disfiguring consequences.

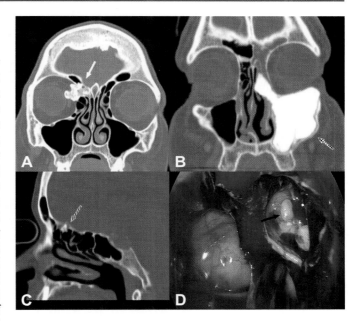

Figure 25.1 Sinonasal osteoma. (A, B) Coronal noncontrasted computed tomography (CT) images of two sinonasal osteomas (white and checkered arrows) with increased density characteristic of osteomas. The right frontal osteoma (white arrow) has extended into the orbit and is contacting the right globe. The left maxillary osteoma (checkered arrow) fills the maxillary sinus and extends to obstruct the middle meatus. (C) A representative ethmoid osteoma (striped arrow) in a sagittal noncontrast CT image that was incidental and asymptomatic in this case. (D) An intraoperative photograph of a left supraorbital ethmoid osteoma (black arrow) lying immediately superior to the optic canal.

Presentation is location dependent, but it may include painless mass, nasal obstruction, epiphora, headache, pressure, vision changes, or cosmetic changes.[4,6,19,20] Monostotic FD is equally distributed between the sexes and six times more common than polyostotic FD, which has a 3:1 female predominance. FD is primarily a disease of youth, affecting patients in their second and third decades with three-quarters of cases diagnosed before 30 years of age.[2,4,6] Within the nose and sinuses, FD affects the maxilla with greatest frequency, followed by the frontal, sphenoid, and ethmoid bones.[20] FD demonstrates a characteristic ground-glass appearance on CT imaging[1] (**Fig. 25.2A**), and histologic findings of fibrous stroma with spindle cells and collagen fibers perpendicular to trabeculae of bone without osteoblastic rimming confirm the diagnosis.[6] FD rarely undergoes malignant transformation (0.5% of polyostotic FD), typically in the setting of McCune-Albright syndrome.[2,6] However, the diffuse nature of bony involvement, potential morbidity associated with complete excision, and typical course of regression or stabilization with skeletal maturity favor a conservative approach to treatment. Partial resection for function and cosmesis along with close observation are the mainstays of treatment. Of note, FD has been associated with the development of aneurysmal bone cysts, which follows a more locally aggressive course and may require additional

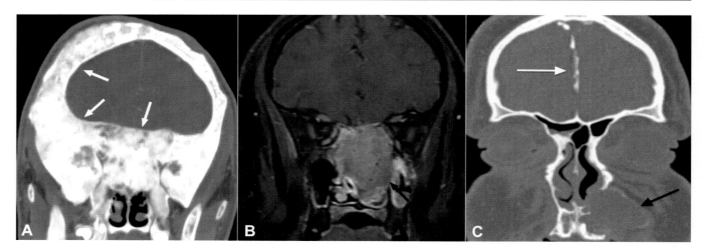

Figure 25.2 Destructive bone lesions. (A) Coronal computed tomography (CT) image of extensive fibrous dysplasia involving the sphenoid, bilateral temporal, and parietal bones (white arrows). Note the characteristic ground-glass appearance of the lesion. (B) T1-weighted magnetic resonance image with a left nasal giant cell tumor (black arrow) with erosion of the bony septum and multiple loculations visible within the substance of the lesion. (C) Coronal CT image of keratocystic odontogenic tumor with its sclerotic rim and scalloped appearance (black arrow). Also seen is extensive falx calcification (white arrow), a characteristic finding of nevoid basal cell carcinoma syndrome.

resection.[19] As mentioned above, FD can be associated with McCune-Albright syndrome, defined by polyostotic FD, café-au-lait spots, and precocious puberty.[2,4,19]

Giant Cell Tumor

Giant cell tumor of bone or soft tissue represents another rare sinonasal neoplasm. Of bone origin, these lesions occur more commonly in the mandible, but maxillary sinus,[6] nasal cavity,[21,22] and sphenoid[23] presentations have also been identified. Most commonly identified in patients less than 30 years of age,[6] there is a female predominance of 1.5:1 to 2:1. Giant cell tumors are locally aggressive, expansile, and bone erosive, often with multiloculated appearance as illustrated in **Fig. 25.2B**.[6,21] Treatment is surgical, with characteristic uniformly spaced clusters of osteoclast-like giant cells with areas of hemorrhage, bone, and collagen deposition identified histologically.[6] Mitoses are not uncommon. Ruling out hyperparathyroidism is crucial in distinguishing this lesion from brown tumor,[6] and evaluation of phosphate status is also to be considered, as giant cell tumors have been associated with hypophosphatemic oncogenic osteomalacia.[22] Long-term surveillance is required because of recurrence risk if resection is incomplete, but prognosis is excellent.

Keratocystic Odontogenic Tumor

Keratocystic odontogenic tumor (KCOT), formerly known as odontogenic keratocyst, is another odontogenic tumor that can rarely localize in the sinonasal region, with 1% of KCOTs reported in the maxilla.[24] More common in males, these locally aggressive tumors occur most frequently in the second and third decades.[6,24] KCOTs may be single or multiple and, if multiple, are more likely to be associated with nevoid basal cell carcinoma syndrome (Gorlin syndrome).[6,24] Radiographically, KCOTs appear as rounded radiolucencies with sclerotic borders that may be unilocular or scalloped

(**Fig. 25.2C**). Histologically, KCOTs are identified by five to eight layers of parakeratin on a well-defined basophilic basal cell layer.[6,24] In the setting of inflammation, however, these characteristics are often obscured.[24] Treatment is surgical, but long-term follow-up is required as recurrence rates are increased because of incomplete resection or the presence of daughter cysts.

Ossifying Fibroma

Arising from the periodontal ligament, ossifying fibroma (OF) is a rare but locally aggressive and destructive sinonasal tumor.[2,6] OF typically demonstrates a more abrupt presentation with increased frequency of proptosis, facial swelling, and visual or oculomotor disturbance as presenting symptoms.[25] There are three subtypes of OF: juvenile psammomatoid OF (JPOF), conventional OF, and juvenile trabecular OF (JTOF). JPOF and JTOF present in the first and second decades, have a male predominance, and are usually located in the nontooth-bearing paranasal sinuses, orbit (JPOF), or maxillary sinus (JTOF). Radiographically these lesions are lytic with a sclerotic rim and locally aggressive[6,26] (**Fig. 25.3**). Histologically, JPOF demonstrates psammomatoid bodies in a fibrous stroma of parallel strands and whorls of collagen with osteoblast-rich lamellar bone, whereas JTOF lacks psammomatoid bodies. Conventional OF typically presents in the second and third decades with a slight female predilection and is predominately found outside the sinuses with only 25% identified in the maxilla and maxillary sinus.[26] Complete resection is required because of the locally aggressive nature of the disease. Both malignant transformation and recurrence risk are low.[2,6]

Ameloblastoma

Although ameloblastoma is among the most common odontogenic tumors, second only to odontoma,[24] it is

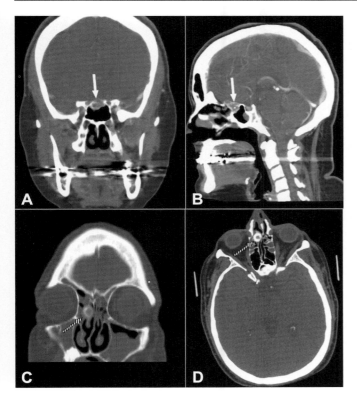

Figure 25.3 Ossifying fibroma. Computed tomography (CT) images in the (A) coronal and (B) sagittal planes. The white arrows indicate the ossifying fibroma in the planum sphenoidale. (C) Coronal and (D) axial CT images of another patient with ossifying fibroma (striped arrow) in which the sclerotic rim characteristic of this disease is well visualized.

very rare in the sinonasal cavity. About 15 to 20% of ameloblastomas originate in the maxilla and can extend to the maxillary sinus or nasal cavity secondarily. This subtype affects a slightly younger population (third to fifth decades)[6,24,27,28] than the more uncommon primary ameloblastoma of the sinonasal cavity, which is thought to be secondary to the shared embryogenesis of the oral and nasal cavities[27] and is most frequently identified in the sixth decade.[28] Ameloblastomas localized to the posterior maxilla typically present as a painless swelling. Imaging most frequently reveals multilocular radiolucencies, occasionally surrounding an unerupted tooth, with resorption of neighboring dentition and erosion of adjacent cortical bone with invasion of adjacent marrow spaces.[6,28] Complete excision of the entire lesion with margins of up to 15 mm is suggested by some authors[29] because of the infiltrative nature of the disease to minimize recurrence. Completeness of resection is also imperative as multiple cases of metastases from ameloblastoma have been reported.[6,29]

Vascular and Other Soft Tissue Tumors

Hemangioma

Hemangiomas are relatively common in the head and neck region, and 10% of these are present in the sinonasal cavity.

Lobular Capillary Hemangioma

The most commonly identified hemangioma is lobular capillary hemangioma (LCH), also referred to as pyogenic granuloma.[1,6] Distribution of LCH varies with age, with LCH being more common in children and adolescent males and females of reproductive age with equal gender distribution beyond 40 years of age. Associations have been made with injury and hormonal levels.[6] It is estimated that up to 2% of pregnant females will develop LCH, most commonly in the second or third trimesters.[30] LCH is found most commonly on the vascular plexus of the septum, the anterior tip of the inferior turbinate, and less commonly in the sinuses.[1,6] Presenting symptoms in this entity are more commonly unilateral epistaxis or unilateral nasal obstruction when located in the nasal cavity or physical deformity from expansile mass when arising in the sinuses.[1,6,31] Symptoms typically arise abruptly because of LCH's rapid development over a period of weeks.[32] Examination reveals a vascular appearing red-blue, smooth, lobulated submucosal mass that is frequently ulcerated.[1,6] The expansile nature of these lesions can lead to resorption of the surrounding bone.[31] Histologically, LCH appears as a lobulated network of capillary-sized vessels with hypercellular endothelium and copious pericytes.[1,6] Surgical resection is curative when complete, but increased recurrence rates are reported with presentation in the pediatric population and with incomplete resection, frequently attributed to larger, bloodier tumors.[6] Malignant transformation to angiosarcoma is exceedingly rare but reinforces the need for long-term surveillance.[1,6]

Cavernous Hemangioma

Less common than LCH, cavernous hemangiomas are more commonly identified on the middle turbinate, lateral nasal wall, or within the paranasal sinuses[1,6,31] and appear similar to LCH on examination, but with less frequent ulceration.[6] These lesions have no gender preponderance and are most commonly diagnosed in the fifth decade.[6] As lateral nasal wall and sinus involvement is more common in these lesions, presentation is more commonly late, with sinus opacification or physical deformity.[6,31] These lesions can produce significant bony destructive changes on examination and CT imaging, raising a concern for malignancy[33] (**Fig. 25.4**). Phleboliths, calcifications of thrombi in the vascular network, are seen occasionally on CT and can assist with diagnosis.[33,34] Biopsy of cavernous hemangiomas may lead to significant blood loss, so preoperative angiography to characterize vascular supply and embolize large feeding vessels should be considered.[33,34] Cavernous hemangioma is histologically characterized by sinusoidal cavities filled with blood with hypercellular endothelial lining.[31] Treatment and recurrence are similar to LCH.

Juvenile Nasopharyngeal Angiofibroma

JNA represents an uncommon but clinically challenging vascular sinonasal tumor. Refer to Chapter 27 for further details.

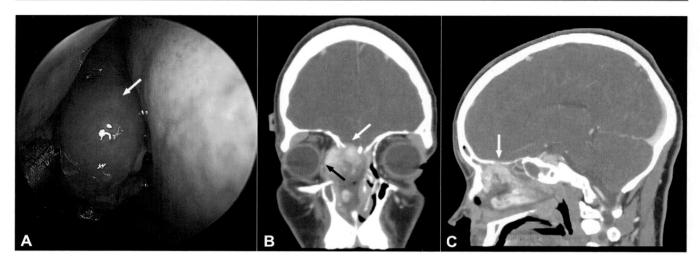

Figure 25.4 Hemangioma. (A) An intraoperative photograph of a right anterior nasal cavernous hemangioma. Computed tomography images in the (B) coronal and (C) sagittal planes, demonstrating the locally aggressive nature of cavernous hemangioma with erosion of the ethmoid roof (white arrows) and orbit (black arrow).

Glomangiopericytoma

Glomangiopericytoma, also known as sinonasal-type hemangiopericytoma, represents less than 0.5% of all sinonasal neoplasms, but the sinonasal cavity is the primary location of presentation.[35] These lesions arise from the pericytes of Zimmerman and have been associated with trauma, steroid use, and hypertension.[36,37] Presenting at any time period, diagnosis peaks in the seventh decade and is more common in females.[6,35] These tumors typically originate in the nasal cavity and may have secondary extension into the sinuses, but they rarely originate in the ethmoid or sphenoid sinus.[6,37] Examination reveals a beefy, red to gray, polypoid, fleshy to friable mass with occasional hemorrhage.[36,38] Histopathology demonstrates a well-delineated but unencapsulated submucosal tumor of closely packed cells with various patterns (fascicular, storiform, whorled, and palisading) with many vascular channels that open to antler-like configurations and are lined by uniform oval neoplastic cells with spindle-shaped nuclei.[6] Recurrence is high (17 to 30%) and can be delayed in presentation. Aggressive variants exist and may be identified by imaging findings of bone invasion and pathologic markers (proliferation index and mitotic rate)[6,36]; however, metastasis has been identified even in histologically benign specimens.[38] Despite a high recurrence rate, survival is excellent, with greater than 90% of patients surviving at 5 years of follow-up.[6] As metastases from glomangiopericytomas have been reported in up to 15% of patients,[36,38] this is likely better characterized as a tumor of low malignant potential rather than a benign tumor; thus, life-long surveillance is requisite.

Schwannoma

Schwannoma is a tumor of perineural Schwann cells that is common in the head and neck. However, less than 4% of these manifest in the nose or paranasal sinuses.[39,40] Several hundred sinonasal schwannomas have been reported in the literature, predominantly located in the ethmoid and maxillary sinuses and less commonly in the nasal cavity (primarily), near the fifth cranial nerve or near autonomic nerve branches.[6,39,41] Rarely, schwannomas arise in the sphenoid and frontal sinuses.

Schwannomas are equally prevalent in males and females and are diagnosed in middle age most frequently. Presenting symptoms are nonspecific, related to the obstructive nature of the tumor. Histology of schwannomas is typically described as a more hypercellular Antoni A or less cellular Antoni B patterns with fusiform cells with spindled nuclei and nuclear palisading. S100 immunostaining is strongly positive.[6] These tumors can extend intracranially, intraorbitally, or to the pterygomaxillary fossa, so imaging is essential for operative planning.[40,42] Recurrence and malignant transformation are extremely rare and complete surgical excision is curative.[6,39,42]

Meningioma

Meningiomas primarily arising within the sinonasal cavity are extremely rare, comprising less than 0.5% of nonepithelial sinonasal tumors.[6] More commonly, an intracranial meningioma may present with extracranial extension into the nasal cavity or sinuses. Sinonasal meningiomas are slightly more common in females and may present throughout life, with a mean age of 42 years at diagnosis.[43] These lesions are thought to arise from arachnoid cap cells that are located in nerve sheaths.[6,43] Sinonasal meningiomas typically arise within the nasal cavity, but can extend into the paranasal sinuses in at least one-third of cases.[6,43] Presenting symptoms include nasal obstruction, headache, vision changes, and physical deformity.[6,43] Symptom duration is prolonged, averaging about 4 years.[6] Physical examination typically reveals a polypoid mass, often with ulceration of the overlying mucosa. Imaging with CT and/or MRI will demonstrate the extent of orbital or intracranial involvement and reveal any bony changes, as meningiomas can infiltrate bone.[6,43] Calcifications and bone fragments within the mass are frequently identified,[6,43] aiding in diagnosis. Histologically, meningiomas appear as lobules of whorls of cells with indistinct borders, intranuclear pseudoinclusions, and possibly psammoma bodies. Multiple variants exist including meningothelial (most common in the sinonasal tract), transitional, metaplastic, atypical, and psammomatous.[6,43] Complete resection is the management of choice, but recurrence rates range widely and are likely a reflection of incomplete resection. Larger series report recurrence rates of 23 to 30%,[6,43] a similar rate to that of intracranial meningiomas, possibly because of their bone-infiltrating nature. Because of this high recurrence rate, long-term surveillance is necessary. Despite this high recurrence rate, the slow-growing nature of this tumor leads to excellent long-term survival.[6,43]

Leiomyoma

Leiomyoma is a benign tumor that occurs very rarely in the sinonasal tract and is thought to arise from smooth muscle of blood vessel walls, erector pili muscles, or rests of mesenchymal tissue.[44,45] Typically diagnosed in the sixth decade, leiomyoma is 3.5 times more common in females, but diagnosed one decade earlier in males.[6] The only known risk factor for leiomyoma development is previous radiation. Most frequently identified in the turbinates, these tumors have also been reported arising within the sinuses or on the lateral nasal wall.[6] The most frequent presenting symptom is nasal obstruction, with rhinorrhea, headache, and pain also being commonly reported.[6,44] Epistaxis is more common in the more vascular variant, angioleiomyoma.[45] Examination reveals a polypoid or sessile smooth well-circumscribed lesion in most cases.[6] Histologic sections reveal spindle-shaped cells in orderly bundles with eosinophilic cytoplasm with positive staining for smooth muscle actin and vimentin.[6,44] Imaging demonstrates homogeneous, elliptical lesions with well-circumscribed borders without bone erosion but possibly demonstrating expansion with bone remodeling.[44] Treatment consists of surgical excision and recurrence is exceedingly rare.

Hamartomas

Hamartomas are varied in presentation and constituent tissue and comprise a small proportion of benign sinonasal neoplasms. The most common of this group is the respiratory epithelial adenomatoid hamartoma (REAH), though many other hamartomatous neoplasms have been described, including glandular hamartoma and nasal chondromesenchymal hamartoma.[6,7] REAH has a nearly 6:1 male preponderance and affects the adult population from the third to the ninth decades, whereas glandular hamartomas present at a slightly younger age.[7] REAH is located primarily in the posterior septum (**Fig. 25.5**), though lateral nasal and maxillary sinus presentations have also been reported.[6,7,46] Histologically, REAH exhibits widely spaced larger glands lined with respiratory epithelium with eosinophilic basement

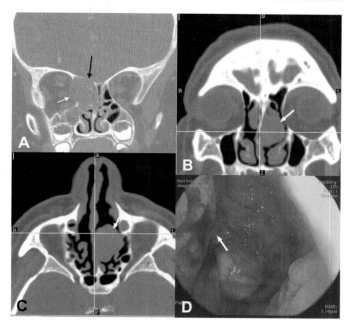

Figure 25.5 Hamartoma. (A) Coronal noncontrasted computed tomography (CT) image of the aggressive nature of some hamartoma, with invasion of this chondromesenchymal hamartoma through the ethmoid roof (black arrow) and lamina papyracea (white arrow). CT images in the (B) coronal and (C) axial planes in addition to an intraoperative photograph (D) of a respiratory epithelial adenomatoid hamartoma (white arrows). Note the common attachment point of the lesion on the posterior septum.

membrane and may have cartilaginous or osseous components.[6,7,47] In contrast, glandular hamartomas demonstrate smaller glands lined with cuboidal epithelium mixed with larger respiratory lined glands,[7] whereas nasal chondromesenchymal hamartomas contain cartilaginous components of varying differentiation, loose spindle-cell stroma, and possible osseous components.[6]

REAH has been identified in the setting of inverting papilloma and solitary fibrous tumor and is frequently identified in the setting of inflammatory polyps.[6,46] Additional associations include nasal chondromesenchymal hamartoma, which has been identified in conjunction with pleuropulmonary blastoma in infants in several cases.[6,48] Hamartomas, especially nasal chondromesenchymal hamartoma, can be locally aggressive, so complete surgical resection is indicated (**Fig. 25.5**). Also in the literature are reports of seromucinous hamartomas harboring rests of squamous cell carcinoma, highlighting the need for careful complete extirpation.[49] A complete resection, which may require multiple attempts,[48] leads to a favorable prognosis.

Conclusion

Benign sinonasal neoplasms are, in general, rare entities occurring in the nasal cavity and paranasal sinuses. Despite their benign moniker, these tumors may demonstrate locally aggressive behavior, bone erosion/invasion, and locoregional recurrence. Furthermore, if left untreated, erosion into the orbit or intracranial cavity may lead to morbidity outside the confines of the sinonasal cavity. The anatomic complexity of the sinonasal cavity, orbit, and skull base necessitate prompt, accurate diagnosis followed by complete, definitive resection with minimal morbidity. Ongoing surveillance will detect recurrence at an early stage and optimize postoperative paranasal sinus function.

References

1. Harvey RJ, Sheahan PO, Schlosser RJ. Surgical management of benign sinonasal masses. Otolaryngol Clin North Am 2009;42(2): 353–375, x

2. Eller R, Sillers M. Common fibro-osseous lesions of the paranasal sinuses. Otolaryngol Clin North Am 2006;39(3):585–600, x

3. Kaufman MR, Brandwein MS, Lawson W. Sinonasal papillomas: clinicopathologic review of 40 patients with inverted and oncocytic schneiderian papillomas. Laryngoscope 2002;112(8, pt 1):1372–1377

4. Nambi GI, Jacob J, Gupta AK. Monofocal maxillary fibrous dysplasia with orbital, nasal and oral obstruction. J Plast Reconstr Aesthet Surg 2010;63(1):e16–e18

5. Das S, Kirsch CFE. Imaging of lumps and bumps in the nose: a review of sinonasal tumours. Cancer Imaging 2005;5:167–177

6. Barnes L, Eveson JW, Reichart P, Sidransky D, eds. World Health Organization Classification of Tumours. Pathology and Genetics of Head and Neck Tumours. IARC Press: Lyon;2005

7. Perez-Ordoñez B. Hamartomas, papillomas and adenocarcinomas of the sinonasal tract and nasopharynx. J Clin Pathol 2009; 62(12): 1085–1095

8. Lawson W, Schlecht NF, Brandwein-Gensler M. The role of the human papillomavirus in the pathogenesis of Schneiderian inverted papillomas: an analytic overview of the evidence. Head Neck Pathol 2008;2(2):49–59

9. Maitra A, Baskin LB, Lee EL. Malignancies arising in oncocytic schneiderian papillomas: a report of 2 cases and review of the literature. Arch Pathol Lab Med 2001;125(10):1365–1367

10. Lin FY, Genden EM, Lawson WL, Som P, Kostakoglu L. High uptake in schneiderian papillomas of the maxillary sinus on positron-emission tomography using fluorodeoxyglucose. AJNR Am J Neuroradiol 2009; 30(2):428–430

11. Kumagai M, Endo S, Koizumi F, Kida A, Yamamoto M. A case of pleomorphic adenoma of the nasal septum. Auris Nasus Larynx 2004; 31(4):439–442

12. Berenholz L, Kessler A, Segal S. Massive pleomorphic adenoma of the maxillary sinus. A case report. Int J Oral Maxillofac Surg 1998; 27(5):372–373

13. Unlu HH, Celik O, Demir MA, Eskiizmir G. Pleomorphic adenoma originated from the inferior nasal turbinate. Auris Nasus Larynx 2003; 30(4):417–420

14. Yazibene Y, Ait-Mesbah N, Kalafate S, et al. Degenerative pleomorphic adenoma of the nasal cavity. Eur Ann Otorhinolaryngol Head Neck Dis 2011;128(1):37–40

15. Nakaya K, Oshima T, Watanabe M, et al. A case of myoepithelioma of the nasal cavity. Auris Nasus Larynx 2010;37(5):640–643

16. Erdogan N, Demir U, Songu M, Ozenler NK, Uluç E, Dirim B. A prospective study of paranasal sinus osteomas in 1,889 cases: changing patterns of localization. Laryngoscope 2009;119(12): 2355–2359

17. Edmond M, Clifton N, Khalil H. A large atypical osteoma of the maxillary sinus: a report of a case and management challenges. Eur Arch Otorhinolaryngol 2011;268(2):315–318

18. Earwaker J. Paranasal sinus osteomas: a review of 46 cases. Skeletal Radiol 1993;22(6):417–423

19. Terkawi AS, Al-Qahtani KH, Baksh E, Soualmi L, Mohamed Ael-B, Sabbagh AJ. Fibrous dysplasia and aneurysmal bone cyst of the skull base presenting with blindness: a report of a rare locally aggressive example. Head Neck Oncol 2011;3:15

20. Zodpe P, Chung SW, Kang HJ, Lee SH, Lee HM. Endoscopic treatment of nasolacrimal sac obstruction secondary to fibrous dysplasia of paranasal sinuses. Eur Arch Otorhinolaryngol 2007;264(5):495–498

21. Tuluc M, Zhang X, Inniss S. Giant cell tumor of the nasal cavity: case report. Eur Arch Otorhinolaryngol 2007;264(2):205–208

22. Battoo AJ, Salih SS, Unnikrishnan AG, et al. Oncogenic osteomalacia from nasal cavity giant cell tumor. Head Neck 2012;34(3):454–457

23. Company MM, Ramos R. Giant cell tumor of the sphenoid. Arch Neurol 2009;66(1):134–135

24. Press SG. Odontogenic tumors of the maxillary sinus. Curr Opin Otolaryngol Head Neck Surg 2008;16(1):47–54

25. Kasliwal MK, Rogers GF, Ramkissoon S, Moses-Gardner A, Kurek KC, Smith ER. A rare case of psammomatoid ossifying fibroma in the sphenoid bone reconstructed using autologous particulate exchange cranioplasty. J Neurosurg Pediatr 2011;7(3):238–243

26. Noudel R, Chauvet E, Cahn V, Mérol JC, Chays A, Rousseaux P. Transcranial resection of a large sinonasal juvenile psammomatoid ossifying fibroma. Childs Nerv Syst 2009;25(9):1115–1120

27. Guilemany JM, Ballesteros F, Alós L, et al. Plexiform ameloblastoma presenting as a sinonasal tumor. Eur Arch Otorhinolaryngol 2004;261(6):304–306

28. Ereño C, Etxegarai L, Corral M, Basurko JM, Bilbao FJ, López JI. Primary sinonasal ameloblastoma. APMIS 2005;113(2):148–150

29. Zwahlen RA, Grätz KW. Maxillary ameloblastomas: a review of the literature and of a 15-year database. J Craniomaxillofac Surg 2002;30(5):273–279

30. Zarrinneshan AAZ, Zapanta PE, Wall SJ. Nasal pyogenic granuloma. Otolaryngol Head Neck Surg 2007;136(1):130–131

31. Zaki Z, Ouatassi N, Oudidi A, Alami N. Cavernous hemangioma of the maxillary sinus. Fr ORL. 2008;94:387–390

32. Benoit MM, Fink DS, Brigger MT, Keamy DG Jr. Lobular capillary hemangioma of the nasal cavity in a five-year-old boy. Otolaryngol Head Neck Surg 2010;142(2):290–291

33. Kim HJ, Kim JH, Kim JH, Hwang EG. Bone erosion caused by sinonasal cavernous hemangioma: CT findings in two patients. AJNR Am J Neuroradiol 1995;16(5):1176–1178

34. Archontaki M, Stamou AK, Hajiioannou JK, Kalomenopoulou M, Korkolis DP, Kyrmizakis DE. Cavernous haemangioma of the left nasal cavity. Acta Otorhinolaryngol Ital 2008;28(6):309–311

35. Thompson LDR, Miettinen M, Wenig BM. Sinonasal-type hemangiopericytoma: a clinicopathologic and immunophenotypic analysis of 104 cases showing perivascular myoid differentiation. Am J Surg Pathol 2003;27(6):737–749

36. Higashi K, Nakaya K, Watanabe M, et al. Glomangiopericytoma of the nasal cavity. Auris Nasus Larynx 2011;38(3):415–417

37. Lin IH, Kuo FY, Su CY, Lin HC. Sinonasal-type hemangiopericytoma of the sphenoid sinus. Otolaryngol Head Neck Surg 2006;135(6): 977–979

38. Gillman G, Pavlovich JB. Sinonasal hemangiopericytoma. Otolaryngol Head Neck Surg 2004;131(6):1012–1013

39. Wada A, Matsuda H, Matsuoka K, Kawano T, Furukawa S, Tsukuda M. A case of schwannoma on the nasal septum. Auris Nasus Larynx 2001;28(2):173–175

40. Ulu EMK, Cakmak O, Dönmez FY, et al. Sinonasal schwannoma of the middle turbinate. Diagn Interv Radiol 2010;16(2):129–131

41. Melroy CT, Senior BA. Benign sinonasal neoplasms: a focus on inverting papilloma. Otolaryngol Clin North Am 2006;39(3): 601–617, x

42. Kodama S, Okamoto T, Suzuki M. Ancient schwannoma of the nasal septum associated with sphenoid sinus mucocele. Auris Nasus Larynx 2010;37(4):522–525

43. Rushing EJ, Bouffard JP, McCall S, et al. Primary extracranial meningiomas: an analysis of 146 cases. Head Neck Pathol 2009; 3(2):116–130

44. Yang BT, Wang ZC, Xian JF, Hao DP, Chen QH. Leiomyoma of the sinonasal cavity: CT and MRI findings. Clin Radiol 2009;64(12): 1203–1209

45. He J, Zhao LN, Jiang ZN, Zhang SZ. Angioleiomyoma of the nasal cavity: a rare cause of epistaxis. Otolaryngol Head Neck Surg 2009; 141(5):663–664

46. Mortuaire G, Pasquesoone X, Leroy X, Chevalier D. Respiratory epithelial adenomatoid hamartomas of the sinonasal tract. Eur Arch Otorhinolaryngol 2007;264(4):451–453

47. Choi E, Catalano PJ, Chang KG. Chondro-osseous respiratory epithelial hamartoma of the sinonasal tract. Otolaryngol Head Neck Surg 2006;134(1):168–169

48. Priest JR, Williams GM, Mize WA, Dehner LP, McDermott MB. Nasal chondromesenchymal hamartoma in children with pleuropulmonary blastoma—A report from the International Pleuropulmonary Blastoma Registry registry. Int J Pediatr Otorhinolaryngol 2010; 74(11):1240–1244

49. Figures MR, Nayak JV, Gable C, Chiu AG. Sinonasal seromucinous hamartomas: clinical features and diagnostic dilemma. Otolaryngol Head Neck Surg 2010;143(1):165–166

26 Endoscopic Surgery for Inverted Papilloma

John M. Lee and Alexander G. Chiu

Inverted papilloma (IP) is one of the most common benign tumors arising from the sinonasal cavity. First described in the 1850s, the surgical management of sinonasal IPs has always been dictated by the tumor's high recurrence rate and the potential for malignant transformation. To ensure adequate tumor extirpation, open approaches including the Caldwell-Luc, lateral rhinology with medial maxillectomy, and osteoplastic flap have historically been the mainstay of IP surgical management.[1-3] With the introduction of endoscopic sinus surgery (ESS) in the mid-1980s, the management of IP has evolved as endoscopic techniques have enabled improved access to the paranasal sinuses and the skull base with reduced patient morbidity.[4-6] This chapter aims to review the indications, techniques, and outcomes of endoscopic surgery for sinonasal IP.

Epidemiology and Histopathology

IPs account for 0.5 to 4.0% of primary nasal tumors with an incidence of 0.2 to 0.7 cases per 100,000 patients per year. They are primarily unilateral tumors but can be bilateral in approximately 5% of cases. The male to female distribution is 3:1 and most commonly present between the fifth and sixth decade of life.[3,7,8] Histologically, IPs have their origins from the ectodermal, mucosal lining (Schneiderian membrane) of the nose and paranasal sinuses. They are in fact the most common subtype of the Schneiderian papillomas, with the exophytic fungiform and cylindrical cell comprising the other types. Grossly, they appear as fleshy, gray-tan mucosal lesions that can be more vascular than a typical inflammatory nasal polyp. Histologically, the defining characteristic of the IP is the proliferation of nonkeratinizing squamous epithelium that has an endophytic or inverted growth pattern into the underling stroma. While the stroma may have a variable amount of inflammation, fibrosis, and edema, there is an absence of seromucous glands and the basement membrane is preserved. Typically, IPs have a benign histologic appearance with no significant atypia. Malignant transformation into squamous cell carcinoma (SCC) is a known risk of IP and this rate is often reported to be less than 10%.[9] The role of human papillomavirus (HPV) in the pathogenesis of IP has garnered a significant amount of interest over the last several years and remains incompletely defined. In a recent meta-analysis and systematic review, the prevalence of HPV in IP surgical specimens has ranged from 0 to 79%. Overall, the pooled prevalence is approximately 22 to 23% depending on the HPV detection method used. The authors also noted a higher HPV prevalence rate in IPs with dysplasia or malignant transformation.[10]

Presentation and Work-up

The clinical presentation of IP can be quite variable ranging from nasal obstruction, epistaxis, and headaches to the patient being completely asymptomatic. Furthermore, IP can present in the setting of sinusitis and nasal polyps.[3,7,8] Given this nonspecific pattern, a high index of suspicion must be maintained to ensure the correct diagnosis and management. Because the tumor is most often unilateral in nature, any patient presenting with unilateral nasal polyps, unilateral sinusitis, or unilateral sinus opacification on imaging should be investigated thoroughly for the possibility of an IP. The most common sites of involvement are typically the lateral nasal wall (89%), maxillary sinus (53.9%), ethmoid sinuses (31.6%), septum (9.9%), frontal sinus (6.5%), and the sphenoid sinus (3.9%).[3]

Imaging

One of the most important aspects in the diagnostic work-up of a patient with an IP is imaging. Computed tomography (CT) scans can provide valuable information regarding tumor location and extension by examining the pattern of sinus opacification as well as the integrity of the surrounding bony walls including the orbit and skull base. However, it is often difficult to distinguish between tumor and postobstructive secretions on a CT scan. Recently, it has been found that areas of bony sclerosis or hyperostosis on CT imaging may help identify the site of tumor attachment, an important target during surgical removal (**Fig. 26.1**). Lee et al in 2007 identified the presence of focal hyperostosis in 48 out of 76 patients with IP. More importantly, these areas of bony thickening identified on CT scan had an 89% positive predictive value for the true tumor surgical attachment, a finding that was corroborated by a similar study performed by Wright et al in 2007.[11,12] However, it is important to recognize that these radiologic changes may not be highly specific since bony osteitis is commonly found on CT scans of patients with chronic rhinosinusitis.[13]

Finally, the role of magnetic resonance imaging (MRI) as a diagnostic modality for IP has also been extensively studied. Karkos et al in 2009 found that T2-weighted images could be helpful in distinguishing tumor from inflammatory tissue. Furthermore, MRIs are particularly useful if there is

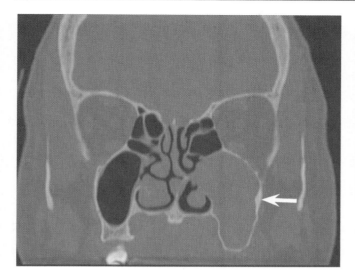

Figure 26.1 Coronal computed tomography scan of a left maxillary sinus inverted papilloma. Note the area of bony hyperostosis on the lateral maxillary sinus wall (a possible area of tumor attachment).

a suspected tumor extension beyond the bony walls of the sinonasal cavity (**Figs. 26.2** and **26.3**). However, the utility of the MRI decreases in the setting of recurrent disease as it can be difficult to discriminate IP from scar tissue.[14] Ultimately, CT and MRI are complementary imaging modalities in the work-up of patient with suspected IP. The authors experience that the combination of the two is invaluable for preoperative planning. Knowing what inspissated secretions versus solid mass is, it will often be the differentiator between a purely endoscopic procedure and the need for an adjunctive external incision (i.e., trephine) to ensure complete tumor removal.

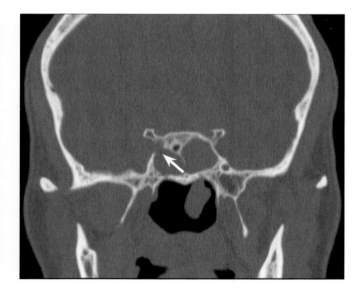

Figure 26.2 Coronal computed tomography scan of sphenoid inverted papilloma. Note the bony dehiscence of the right lateral wall overlying the cavernous carotid artery. It is unclear if there is any extension beyond the sphenoid sinus.

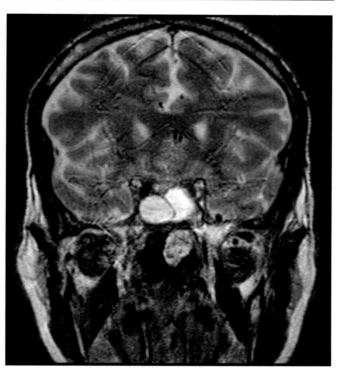

Figure 26.3 Magnetic resonance image of sphenoid inverted papilloma (same patient as in **Figure 26.2**). The T2-weighted images demonstrate tumor within the sphenoid sinus but with no invasion of the cavernous sinus or carotid artery.

Nasal Endoscopy and Biopsy

Nasal endoscopy can be of tremendous utility in the diagnosis of IP. In addition to identifying the presence of a nasal mass or polyp, the endoscope may facilitate a biopsy of the suspected tissue under local anesthetic. The role of biopsy for IP has been examined in several studies. In the setting of unilateral nasal polyps, Tritt et al found a 15.9% prevalence rate of IP in patients undergoing ESS.[15] However, for bilateral nasal polyps, the prevalence of IP is significantly lower ranging from 0 to 0.92%.[16–18] The obvious advantage of a biopsy-proven IP is that it will help in preoperative surgical planning as the extent of surgery will often be different than that for treating inflammatory polyps. This is especially important for patient consent and counseling, particularly if there is any evidence of dysplasia or malignancy. However, clinical biopsies should only be performed if the accessible tissue is not hypervascular and there is clearly no evidence of intracranial extension. The authors' approach has typically been to attempt a clinic biopsy for suspected IP in patients presenting with a unilateral nasal mass after appropriate imaging has been complete. If the patient is not amenable for a clinic biopsy, a frozen section may be performed at the beginning of the surgical case. For bilateral nasal polyps, we do not routinely conduct clinical biopsies unless the tissue is grossly abnormal on endoscopy. However, bilateral nasal polyp samples are always sent for pathological analysis in all cases of ESS.

Table 26.1   Krouse Staging System for Inverted Papilloma

Stage	Appearance
I	Tumors totally confined to the nasal cavity.
II	Tumors involving the ostiomeatal complex, ethmoid sinuses, and/or the medial portion of the maxillary sinus (with or without involvement of the nasal cavity).
III	Tumors involving the lateral, inferior, superior, anterior or posterior walls of the maxillary sinus, the sphenoid sinus, and/or the frontal sinus (with or without stage II criteria).
IV	Tumors with any extranasal/extrasinus extension to involve adjacent structures such as the orbit, intracranial compartment, or the pterygomaxillary space. Tumors associated with malignancy.

Adapted from reference 19.

Staging

The Krouse staging system for IP was first described in 2000 and is still the most commonly used (**Table 26.1**). It attempts to describe the extent of tumor involvement both in the nasal cavity and in the paranasal sinuses. While it is helpful for clinical descriptions of tumor extension, it does not clearly define the indications or limitations of the endoscopic approach for IP tumor removal. Furthermore, while the presence of malignancy (stage IV) is taken into account in this staging system, the issues of tumor attachment and multifocality are not specifically addressed.[19] Other staging systems have subsequently been proposed to better reflect the options for endoscopic treatment.[20,21] However, these systems are not universally used and are not specifically discussed in this chapter.

Endoscopic Surgery for Inverted Papilloma

The underlying principles of surgery for IP remain the same regardless of whether an endoscopic or open approach is undertaken. Given the high recurrence rate and the possibility of malignant transformation, the goals of surgery should include the following:

- Complete tumor removal
- Identifying and adequately treating the site of tumor attachment
- Creating a safe sinus cavity for long-term surveillance
- Minimizing patient morbidity

Regardless of tumor location, the overall indications for an exclusively endoscopic approach have been expanded because the endoscope offers improved direct visualization. Along with the evolution of instruments, such as powered microdebriders and suction irrigation drills, endoscopic techniques now allow surgeons to fully isolate and remove the majority of IPs.

General Endoscopic Surgical Principles for Inverted Papilloma Tumor Removal

Initially, portions of the IP, which are not directly attached to the surrounding sinonasal mucosa can be debulked using a microdebrider. This will help identify the site of tumor attachment while minimizing blood loss and decreasing trauma to the surrounding normal tissues. However, once the site of origin or pedicle is identified, a submucoperiosteal en bloc dissection of the diseased mucosa and tumor should be undertaken. This enables pathologists to fully evaluate the site of origin as one contiguous piece, helping to maintain orientation if dysplasia or malignancy is found. Biopsies are taken of the surrounding mucosa to ensure that complete tumor clearance has been achieved. Finally, after elevating the diseased mucosa, it is important to address the underlying areas of bone. These are the potential sites of bony attachment or invasion, which can be irregular in nature. Chiu et al examined specimens of IP in which the underlying bone had been removed along with the attached tumor. In 17% of these specimens, isolated rests of mucosa were found within the bone itself[22] and continued studies have revealed an IP within the bone (**Fig. 26.4**). As such, we recommend using a diamond drill bit to burr down these areas to minimize the risk of recurrence (**Fig. 26.5**). If these general principles cannot be accomplished endoscopically, the use of an adjunctive open or external approach should be considered. An external procedure is rarely needed for tumor within the maxillary sinus, but is of use for tumors involving the frontal sinus in which the site of attachment is out of reach or attached to dura of the anterior skull base. Finally, it is important to remember that if concurrent malignancy is discovered, standard oncologic surgical principles should be maintained such that negative tumor margins are achieved. The rest of the chapter outlines the specific details of endoscopic surgery for each of the involved sinuses.

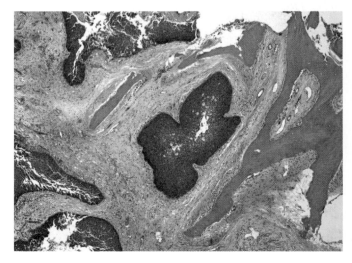

Figure 26.4   A histology slide demonstrating an inverted papilloma within the underlying bone.

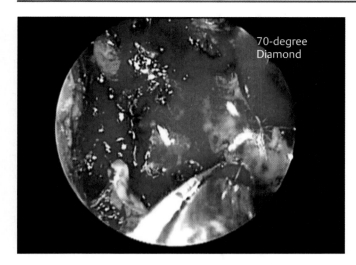

Figure 26.5 Endoscopic image demonstrating the use of a 70-degree diamond burr to drill down the posterior wall of the left maxillary sinus.

Maxillary Sinus

The most common location for an IP is typically the lateral nasal wall followed by the maxillary sinus. As such, the historical approach to remove tumors in this location was a medial maxillectomy via a lateral rhinotomy approach.[2] This concept of removing the medial wall of the maxillary sinus was adapted for endoscopic surgery and was first described by Kamel in 1995.[23] Endoscopically, once the tumor has been debulked from the nasal cavity and middle meatus region, it is then possible to follow the tumor into the maxillary sinus. At this point in the surgery, it is often advantageous to switch to an angled 30- or 70-degree endoscope to fully visualize the site of tumor attachment (**Fig. 26.6**). Endoscopic

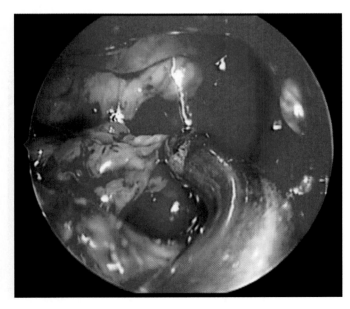

Figure 26.6 A 30-degree endoscopic view demonstrating an inverted papilloma with an anterior wall maxillary sinus attachment.

medial maxillectomy is accomplished by first removing the posterior two-third of the inferior turbinate, and then resecting the medial wall of the maxillary sinus down to the nasal cavity floor with either cutting instruments or a drill. The extent of medial maxillectomy and the need for nasolacrimal duct section again depends on the site of tumor attachment. If the IP is only attached to the posterior medial wall (Krouse stage II), there is no further bone to address. However, if the IP has attachments to any of the other walls of the maxillary sinus (Krouse stage III), additional surgery is required to completely remove the diseased mucosa and drill the underlying bone. While the medial wall may not be directly involved with tumor, the medial maxillectomy is often necessary for adequate access and instrumentation within the sinus.

Given the angulation, a particularly challenging area for endoscopic surgery is the anterior wall of the maxillary sinus. To address this location, we routinely resect the medial maxillary wall anteriorly to the pyriform aperture. This can be done with a variety of instruments, including the backbiter and angled drills. Resection of the medial maxillary wall will require resection of the nasolacrimal duct. Resection of this area is important, as it is a common place for recurrence of IPs originally attached to the anterior wall of the maxillary sinus or the lateral surface of the nasolacrimal gland. By resecting this area, we are ensuring complete tumor removal as well as improving our visualization and ability to instrument the anterior, anterolateral, and anteromedial maxillary walls. This is essentially a modified version of the endonasal Denker operation that has been previously described by Tomenzoli et al.[24] This technique involves elevating the soft tissues over the pyriform aperture and maxilla thus gaining access to resect the anterior wall of the maxillary sinus endoscopically. Because a nasolacrimal duct section is performed concurrently, we routinely marsupialize the nasolacrimal sac at the end of the case to prevent postoperative epiphora. As an alternative, a transseptal approach through the contralateral nostril or a septal dislocation procedure has also been described to allow for greater instrumentation and access of the anterior and lateral maxillary sinus wall.[25,26] Finally, one can always consider an adjuvant Caldwell-Luc procedure if endoscopic access or experience with the above procedures are limited.

Ethmoid Sinuses

Endoscopic surgery for IP of the ethmoid sinuses is often an extension of standard anterior and posterior ethmoidectomy. Again, the key aspect of surgical removal is to debulk the tumor until it is possible to visualize the site of attachment. The standard IP surgical principles apply whereby all the involved mucosa is resected and the underlying bone is smoothed down with a burr. Care must be taken if this attachment is either at the skull base or orbit. The use of a nonaggressive diamond drill bit can help minimize the risk of cerebrospinal fluid (CSF) leak or orbital injury.

Sphenoid Sinus

IP of the sphenoid sinus is relatively rare. Lombardi et al found a 4.2% incidence of sphenoid IP in a series of 212 patients while Guillemaud and Witterick had a 12.7% incidence of sphenoid IP in 71 patients.[27,28] Interestingly, Guillemaud and Witterick found that patients were more likely to present with symptoms of headache and visual disturbance.[28] Endoscopic surgery for sphenoid IP is accomplished via an expanded endoscopic transsphenoidal approach. This will often require removal of the posterior septum and the sphenoid rostrum. The enlarged access is necessary to apply the same surgical principles for IP tumor removal. Perhaps more importantly, the resulting sphenoid sinus opening will be large enough for long-term surveillance.

One area for potential recurrence is in the opticocarotid recess. For obvious reasons, dissection in this region needs to be meticulous. If the IP is benign without any signs of dysplasia, it is of our opinion that prudent management of tumors in this location would be to debulk the bone overlying the carotid and optic nerve. Care must be taken to review the preoperative films closely and to examine for bony dehiscences over the carotid and optic nerve. Careful use of the bipolar cautery may be used to debulk the papilloma in the case of a dehiscent carotid or optic nerve.

Frontal Sinus

The frontal sinus remains one of the most challenging areas for IP resection. Historically, the osteoplastic flap was necessary to ensure complete tumor extirpation. However, the evolution of endoscopic frontal sinus techniques from frontal sinusotomy to Draf II and Draf III (endoscopic modified Lothrop) procedures now enable endoscopic surgeons to tackle a wide variety of frontal sinus pathologies (**Fig. 26.7**). Concerning IP, the key factor in deciding whether the frontal sinus can be managed endoscopically is again determining the extent of mucosal involvement and the site of tumor attachment. From the most recent series by Lombardi et al, 6 out of 11 patients with frontal sinus involvement were managed exclusively by an endoscopic approach. An adjuvant osteoplastic flap was required in the remaining five patients because of extensive mucosal involvement either in a large frontal sinus or in a supraorbital ethmoid cell.[27] Even with an endoscopic modified Lothrop procedure, the main limitation is the far reaching lateral extent of the frontal sinus. With current instrumentation, the ability to fully remove diseased mucosa and drill down the underlying bone in these areas is severely restricted. Similarly, Yoon et al reviewed a series of 18 patients with frontal sinus IP and found that multifocality as well as lateral and anterior wall attachments were the main indications for an osteoplastic flap. In this series, a purely endoscopic approach was achieved in 72% of patients.[29] Unfortunately, the exact surgical strategy for a frontal sinus IP may not be ascertained until during the actual procedure. Limited tumor involvement in the frontal recess may in fact be adequately treated with a Draf IIa or Draf IIb dissection. However, if the tumor involves the frontal sinus proper, the treating surgeon must be prepared to convert to an osteoplastic flap if it is felt that a modified Lothrop procedure will not provide the necessary access for tumor control.

One special situation that may arise is if there is a dehiscence of the posterior table of the frontal sinus. IP adherent to the dura of the frontal lobe is best managed conservatively unless pathology indicates high-grade dysplasia or malignancy. Use of the bipolar cautery and dissection of the tumor off the dura is advised; resection of dura for benign IP can potentially increase patient morbidity as well as allow recurrent tumor to seed the intradural space.

Outcomes of Endoscopic Surgery for Inverted Papilloma

Recurrence Rate

Given that an IP is a benign tumor, the primary outcome of interest is the risk of recurrence. Traditional open approaches have reported recurrence rates ranging from 5 to 30%.[4] In the early years of endoscopic surgery, limited endonasal resections had unacceptably high recurrence rates of 34 to 58%.[30] However, as endoscopic techniques evolved and improved, multiple studies began reporting on much lower recurrence rates that were comparable to the external procedures. Recently, there have been several reviews, which have highlighted the superiority of the endoscopic approach. In 2006, a systematic review of the literature was performed by Busquets and Hwang on the issue of endoscopic resection for sinonasal IP. A "contemporary" cohort of studies from 1992 to 2004 was selected whereby the majority of cases was performed with an endoscopic approach. This was then compared with a "historical" cohort of studies whereby strictly external approaches were used.

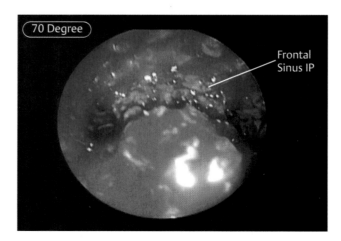

Figure 26.7 A 70-degree endoscopic view demonstrating an endoscopic modified Lothrop procedure (Draf III) to access and reset a frontal sinus inverted papilloma with a medial and posterior wall attachment.

It was found that the contemporary cohort of 32 studies had a statistically significant lower recurrence rate of 15% versus 20% in the historical group of 13 studies ($p < 0.02$). Interestingly, when the contemporary cohort was examined, patients treated endoscopically also had a lower recurrence rate of 12% compared with 20% in patients that were treated nonendoscopically ($p < 0.01$).[6] More recent studies have also corroborated these findings. In 2007, Woodworth et al reported on a series of 114 patients with IP and found that those treated endoscopically had a recurrence rate of 15%.[31] To date, the largest published series on sinonasal IP was performed by Lombardi et al who reported on 212 cases. About 198 patients (93.4%) were treated exclusively with an endoscopic approach and with a mean follow-up of 53.8 months, only 12 patients developed a recurrence (6.1%).[27] With these larger series in the literature, it has been increasingly clear that with the appropriate surgical techniques and indications, endoscopic surgery has now become the gold standard of treatment for sinonasal IP. More importantly, many authors agree that the risk of recurrence appears to be related to the completeness of tumor removal during the primary surgery.[32]

Malignancy

The association between SCC and IP is well documented in the literature. While the rates have ranged from 5 to 32%, most studies report malignancy rate of less than 10%.[9] One study reported a 7.1% synchronous rate and 3.4% metachronous rate between SCC and IP.[33] In the systematic review by Busquets and Hwang where over 1900 patients were reviewed, the overall rate of malignancy was 6.6%.[6] While it is possible that malignancy rates may be overestimated given referral bias at certain institutions, it is necessary to maintain adequate long-term follow-up to monitor both for recurrence as well as for the possibility of malignant transformation.

Complications

For the vast majority of patients with IP, it appears that the endoscopic approach offers a lower recurrence rate than for open techniques. The other obvious advantage of endoscopic surgery is the avoidance of facial incisions and their associated functional or cosmetic complications. However, endoscopic techniques to remove IP are not without their own risks as the extent of bone and tissue removal is often greater than for standard sinus surgery. In the series from Lombardi et al, a complication rate of 9.4% was observed. The immediate postoperative complications included CSF leak and epistaxis whereas delayed problems included mucoceles, frontal sinusitis, and nasolacrimal duct obstruction. Complication rates from other endoscopic series range from 0 to 20% with a mean of 6.5%.[27] Ultimately, while endoscopic approaches are effective in minimizing the risk of IP recurrence, patients must be counseled appropriately on all the potential risks of surgery.

Conclusion

IP is a unique sinonasal tumor that has continued to challenge the skills of the rhinologic surgeon. While the risk of malignancy appears to be low, the challenge has always been to achieve a thorough resection to minimize the risk of recurrence. From the available literature, it appears that with the appropriate indications and techniques, endoscopic surgery should be the first line of treatment for the vast majority of tumors. However, surgeons must be prepared to perform advanced endonasal procedures including medial maxillectomy and extended frontal sinus dissections. Furthermore, adjuvant external approaches including the osteoplastic flap should be in the armamentarium of the surgeon if the disease extends beyond the limit of endoscopic resection.

References

1. Lawson W, Patel ZM. The evolution of management for inverted papilloma: an analysis of 200 cases. Otolaryngol Head Neck Surg 2009;140(3):330–335
2. Myers EN, Fernau JL, Johnson JT, Tabet JC, Barnes EL. Management of inverted papilloma. Laryngoscope 1990;100(5):481–490
3. Melroy CT, Senior BA. Benign sinonasal neoplasms: a focus on inverting papilloma. Otolaryngol Clin North Am 2006;39(3):601–617, x
4. Reh DD, Lane AP. The role of endoscopic sinus surgery in the management of sinonasal inverted papilloma. Curr Opin Otolaryngol Head Neck Surg 2009;17(1):6–10
5. Sautter NB, Cannady SB, Citardi MJ, Roh H-J, Batra PS. Comparison of open versus endoscopic resection of inverted papilloma. Am J Rhinol 2007;21(3):320–323
6. Busquets JM, Hwang PH. Endoscopic resection of sinonasal inverted papilloma: a meta-analysis. Otolaryngol Head Neck Surg 2006;134(3):476–482
7. Krouse JH. Endoscopic treatment of inverted papilloma: safety and efficacy. Am J Otolaryngol 2001;22(2):87–99
8. Lane AP, Bolger WE. Endoscopic management of inverted papilloma. Curr Opin Otolaryngol Head Neck Surg 2006;14(1):14–18
9. Perez-Ordoñez B. Hamartomas, papillomas and adenocarcinomas of the sinonasal tract and nasopharynx. J Clin Pathol 2009;62(12):1085–1095
10. Lawson W, Schlecht NF, Brandwein-Gensler M. The role of the human papillomavirus in the pathogenesis of Schneiderian inverted papillomas: an analytic overview of the evidence. Head Neck Pathol 2008;2(2):49–59
11. Lee DK, Chung SK, Dhong H-J, Kim HY, Kim HJ, Bok KH. Focal hyperostosis on CT of sinonasal inverted papilloma as a predictor of tumor origin. AJNR Am J Neuroradiol 2007;28(4):618–621
12. Yousuf K, Wright ED. Site of attachment of inverted papilloma predicted by CT findings of osteitis. Am J Rhinol 2007;21(1):32–36
13. Lee JT, Kennedy DW, Palmer JN, Feldman M, Chiu AG. The incidence of concurrent osteitis in patients with chronic rhinosinusitis: a clinicopathological study. Am J Rhinol 2006;20(3):278–282
14. Karkos PD, Khoo LC, Leong SC, Lewis-Jones H, Swift AC. Computed tomography and/or magnetic resonance imaging for pre-operative planning for inverted nasal papilloma: review of evidence. J Laryngol Otol 2009;123(7):705–709
15. Tritt S, McMains KC, Kountakis SE. Unilateral nasal polyposis: clinical presentation and pathology. Am J Otolaryngol 2008;29(4):230–232

16. Alun-Jones T, Hill J, Leighton SE, Morrissey MS. Is routine histological examination of nasal polyps justified? Clin Otolaryngol Allied Sci 1990;15(3):217–219

17. Kale SU, Mohite U, Rowlands D, Drake-Lee AB. Clinical and histopathological correlation of nasal polyps: are there any surprises? Clin Otolaryngol Allied Sci 2001;26(4):321–323

18. Diamantopoulos II, Jones NS, Lowe J. All nasal polyps need histological examination: an audit-based appraisal of clinical practice. J Laryngol Otol 2000;114(10):755–759

19. Krouse JH. Development of a staging system for inverted papilloma. Laryngoscope 2000;110(6):965–968

20. Han JK, Smith TL, Loehrl T, Toohill RJ, Smith MM. An evolution in the management of sinonasal inverting papilloma. Laryngoscope 2001;111(8):1395–1400

21. Cannady SB, Batra PS, Sautter NB, Roh H-J, Citardi MJ. New staging system for sinonasal inverted papilloma in the endoscopic era. Laryngoscope 2007;117(7):1283–1287

22. Chiu AG, Jackman AH, Antunes MB, Feldman MD, Palmer JN. Radiographic and histologic analysis of the bone underlying inverted papillomas. Laryngoscope 2006;116(9):1617–1620

23. Kamel RH. Transnasal endoscopic medial maxillectomy in inverted papilloma. Laryngoscope 1995;105(8 Pt 1):847–853

24. Tomenzoli D, Castelnuovo P, Pagella F, et al. Different endoscopic surgical strategies in the management of inverted papilloma of the sinonasal tract: experience with 47 patients. Laryngoscope 2004;114(2):193–200

25. Harvey RJ, Sheehan PO, Debnath NI, Schlosser RJ. Transseptal approach for extended endoscopic resections of the maxilla and infratemporal fossa. Am J Rhinol Allergy 2009;23(4):426–432

26. Ramakrishnan VR, Suh JD, Chiu AG, Palmer JN. Septal dislocation for endoscopic access of the anterolateral maxillary sinus and infratemporal fossa. Am J Rhinol Allergy 2011;25(2):128–130

27. Lombardi D, Tomenzoli D, Buttà L, et al. Limitations and complications of endoscopic surgery for treatment for sinonasal inverted papilloma: a reassessment after 212 cases. Head Neck 2011;33(8):1154–1161

28. Guillemaud JP, Witterick IJ. Inverted papilloma of the sphenoid sinus: clinical presentation, management, and systematic review of the literature. Laryngoscope 2009;119(12):2466–2471

29. Yoon B-N, Batra PS, Citardi MJ, Roh H-J. Frontal sinus inverted papilloma: surgical strategy based on the site of attachment. Am J Rhinol Allergy 2009;23(3):337–341

30. Karkos PD, Fyrmpas G, Carrie SC, Swift AC. Endoscopic versus open surgical interventions for inverted nasal papilloma: a systematic review. Clin Otolaryngol 2006;31(6):499–503

31. Woodworth BA, Bhargave GA, Palmer JN, et al. Clinical outcomes of endoscopic and endoscopic-assisted resection of inverted papillomas: a 15-year experience. Am J Rhinol 2007;21(5):591–600

32. Lund VJ, Stammberger H, Nicolai P, et al; European Rhinologic Society Advisory Board on Endoscopic Techniques in the Management of Nose, Paranasal Sinus and Skull Base Tumours. European position paper on endoscopic management of tumours of the nose, paranasal sinuses and skull base. Rhinol Suppl 2010;(22):1–143

33. Mirza S, Bradley PJ, Acharya A, Stacey M, Jones NS. Sinonasal inverted papillomas: recurrence, and synchronous and metachronous malignancy. J Laryngol Otol 2007;121(9):857–864

27 Endoscopic Surgery for Juvenile Nasopharyngeal Angiofibroma

Candace A. Mitchell, Austin S. Rose, and Adam M. Zanation

Juvenile nasopharyngeal angiofibroma (JNA) is a benign vascular neoplasm, the etiological origin of which remains elusive.[1] Although typically slow growing, these nonencapsulated tumors are locally aggressive, with potential for intracranial or intraorbital extension. JNAs typically arise from the posterolateral wall of the nasopharynx and grow by extrusion via natural ostia. Advanced tumors often assume a dumbbell-shaped configuration, with one portion of the tumor occupying the nasopharynx and the other portion reaching into the pterygopalatine fossa (PPF).[2] Intracranial extension occurs in approximately 10 to 20% of patients.[3–5] JNAs typically derive their blood supply from the ipsilateral internal maxillary artery, a branch off the external carotid artery (ECA); however, bilateral supply and communication with the internal carotid are relatively common. Wu et al describe bilateral vascularity in 36% of patients; with ipsilateral internal carotid artery (ICA) contribution present in 10% of cases.[6] Up to one-third of tumors have contributions from the ascending pharyngeal artery as well. As JNAs expand, they may also recruit additional blood supply from the ophthalmic and contralateral internal maxillary arteries.

JNAs are rare, representing a mere 0.5% of head and neck tumors (approximate incidence = 1:150,000),[2,4,7] and occur almost exclusively in adolescent male patients. Isolated cases of JNAs have been described in female patients and older men.[8,9] The most common presenting symptoms are epistaxis and progressive nasal obstruction; most patients present concurrently with both symptoms.[10] Other presenting symptoms include nasal discharge, pain, sinusitis, otologic symptoms, visual loss, facial deformity, facial hypesthesia, diplopia (from cranial nerve compression or from direct orbital compression), and proptosis. At the time of presentation, a red-to-purple nasal mass may be visible upon gross inspection of the nasal cavity.[11]

Work-up for suspected JNA begins with in-office endoscopy, followed by radiographic imaging typically including both computed tomography (CT) and magnetic resonance imaging (MRI) modalities. CT scans are preferred for assessment of the extent of bony invasion (**Fig. 27.1**), while MRI provides superior visualization of the soft tissue of the tumor itself as well as of adjacent structures such as the ICA, cavernous sinus, and pituitary gland (**Fig. 27.2**).[11] The Holman-Miller sign—anterior bowing of the posterior maxillary wall—is considered pathognomonic for JNA. Angiography provides further confirmation of the diagnosis to allow for concurrent preoperative embolization (**Fig. 27.3**).[11] Biopsy confirmation of the histological

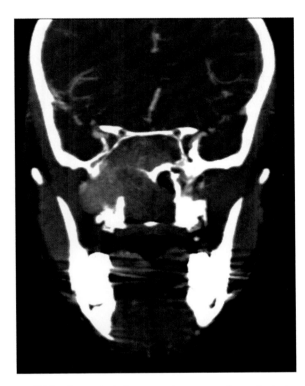

Figure 27.1 Computed tomography scan of a giant juvenile nasopharyngeal angiofibroma. Note the boney destruction of the maxillary sinus with direct extension into the infratemporal fossa.

diagnosis is not performed until in the operating room, after embolization, because of the extensive vascularity of these lesions and the potential for significant bleeding.

Surgical resection is the definitive treatment modality for JNA and is largely considered curative, although recurrence may occur in a minority of patients.[9] Preoperative embolization is typically performed 24 to 48 hours before the scheduled surgery to decrease intraoperative bleeding risk. In the past, resections of JNAs have typically taken place via open approaches. However, endoscopic approaches are quickly becoming a treatment of choice. An incision-free approach obviates the risk of growth center disruption and facial asymmetry in this young population. Furthermore, evidence suggests that endoscopic techniques may decrease operative time, blood loss, and need for transfusion, although definitive data are lacking.[9] This review will focus on endoscopic techniques and outcomes for JNA. We will also discuss potential future adjuncts to surgical treatment through genomic and hormonal translational research.

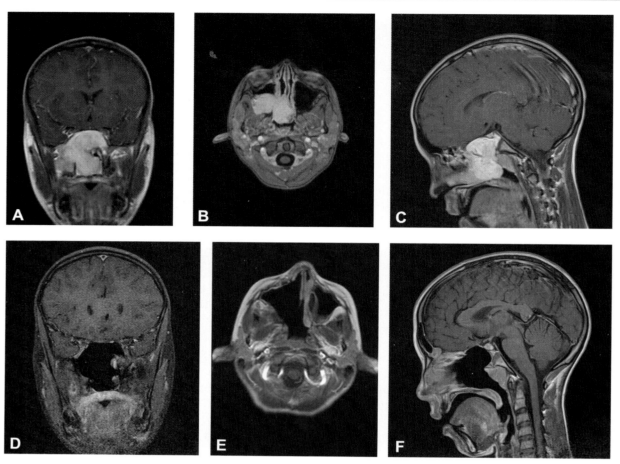

Figure 27.2 Magnetic resonance imaging (MRI) of a giant juvenile nasopharyngeal angiofibroma with infratemporal fossa, sphenoid sinus, orbital, and anterior skull base involvement. (A to C) Preoperative MRIs. (D to F) Postoperative MRIs after endoscopic resection.

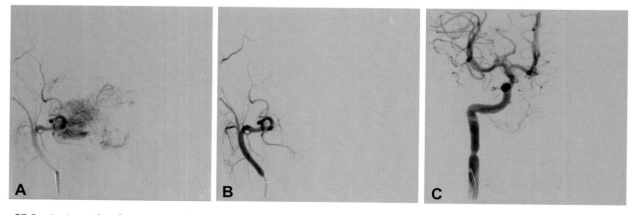

Figure 27.3 Angiography of a giant juvenile nasopharyngeal angiofibroma. (A) Pre-embolization external carotid artery (ECA) with significant tumor blush from the ECA system. (B) Postembolization angiogram with significant decrease in ECA blood supply. (C) Internal carotid artery angiography with inferior-lateral truck blood supply. This could not be embolized because of it being from the internal carotid system. This was controlled with clipping and bipolar cautery intraoperatively.

Staging

Several staging systems have been proposed and modified to classify JNA and most of these are based on the extent and location of the tumor. The three main staging systems are outlined in **Table 27.1**. The Radkowski system is the most widely used system for JNA classification, dividing tumors into three distinct groups (**Table 27.1**). The primary limitation of these older staging systems is that they were not designed for endoscopic approaches. Thus, Snyderman et al at the University of Pittsburgh Medical Center (UPMC) published an endoscopic staging system for JNA.[12] They

Table 27.1   Current Staging Systems for Juvenile Nasopharyngeal Angiofibroma

Study	Stage 1	Stage 2	Stage 3	Stage 4
Onerci et al 2006[37]	Nose, NP, ethmoid and sphenoid sinuses, or minimal extension into PMF.	Maxillary sinus, full occupation of PMF, extension to anterior cranial fossa, limited extension in to ITF.	Deep extension into cancellous bone at pterygoid base or body and GW sphenoid, significant lateral extension into ITF or pterygoid plate, orbital, cavernous sinus obliteration.	Intracranial extension between pituitary gland and ICA, middle fossa extension, and extensive intracranial extension.
Radkowski et al 1996[38]	1a: Limited to nose or NP; 1b: stage 1a with extension into one or more sinuses.	2a: Minimal extension through SPF and into medial PMF; 2b: full occupation of PMF, displacing posterior wall of maxilla forward, orbit erosion, displacement of maxillary artery branches; 2c: ITF, cheek, posterior to pterygoid plates.	Erosion of skull base; 3a: minimal intracranial extension; 3b: extensive intracranial extension with or without cavernous sinus.	N/A
Andrews et al 1989[40]	Limited to NP, bone destruction negligible or limited to SPF.	Invading PPF or maxillary, ethmoid or sphenoid sinus with bone destruction.	Invading ITF or orbit; 3a: no intracranial; 3b: extradural, parasellar involvement.	Intracranial, intradural tumor; 4a: with; 4b: without cavernous sinus, pituitary or optic chiasm infiltration.
Chandler et al 1984[39]	Limited to NP.	Extension into nasal cavity or sphenoid sinus.	Tumor into antrum, ethmoid sinus, PMF, ITF, orbit or cheek.	Intracranial extension.
Synderman et al 2010[12]	1a: Limited to nose and NP; 1b: extension into one or more sinuses.	2a: Minimal extension into PMF; 2b: full occupation of PMF with or without erosion of orbit; 2c: ITF with or without cheek extension.	Intracranial extension.	N/A

NP, nasopharynx; PMF, pterygomaxillary fossa; ITF, infratemporal fossa; GW, greater wing; ICA, internal carotid artery; SPF, sphenopalatine foramen; PPF, pterygopalatine fossa.

noted that tumor size and the extent of sinus disease are less important in predicting complete tumor removal with endonasal surgical techniques. The UPMC staging system for JNA accounts for two important prognostic factors: route of cranial base extension and residual vascularity after embolization (often signifying the presence of internal carotid or bilateral blood supply). Compared with other staging systems, Snyderman asserts that the UPMC system provides a better prediction of immediate morbidity (including blood loss and need for multiple operations) as well as tumor recurrence (**Table 27.1**).[12]

Endoscopic Anatomy

As one considers an anterior endonasal approach, it is crucial to bear in mind the relative anatomic position of the origin, as well as the spread of JNAs (**Fig. 27.4**). JNAs typically originate in the area of the sphenopalatine artery (SPA) and in the area of the PPF. Most commonly, the presenting symptoms are both epistaxis—resulting from the weeping of blood from this vascular tumor supplied by the sphenopalatine arteries—and nasal congestion, related to the blockage of the choana. It is important to understand the complete anatomic relationship of the PPF to be fully able to appreciate complexities involved in the resection of a JNA, as well as to be able to maintain vascular control during the procedure.

The PPF is a small pyramidal space that is limited by the posterior wall of the maxilla on its anterior surface and by the pterygoid plates along its posterior surface. The ascending process of the palatine bone defines the medial boundary and its lateral boundary is the pterygomaxillary fissure, a soft tissue space separating the PPF from the infratemporal fossa along a sagittal plane at the level of the inferior orbital fissure. The pterygomaxillary fissure transmits the internal maxillary artery from the ECA into the PPF. The anterior portion of the PPF contains the terminal division of the internal maxillary artery, the terminal branches being the palatine arteries, SPA, and posterior nasal septal

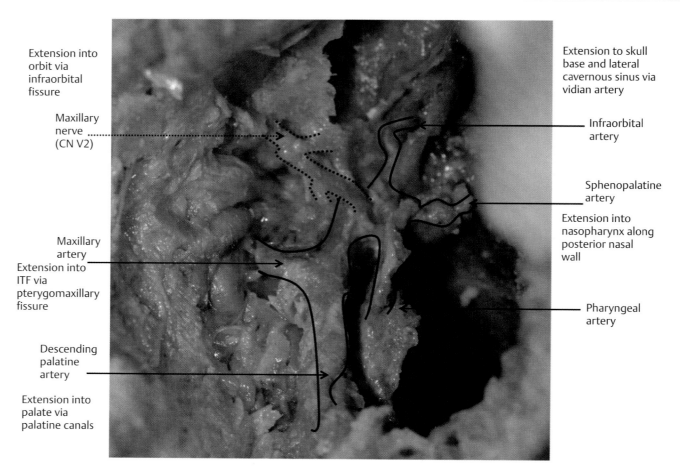

Extension into orbit via infraorbital fissure

Maxillary nerve (CN V2)

Maxillary artery

Extension into ITF via pterygomaxillary fissure

Descending palatine artery

Extension into palate via palatine canals

Extension to skull base and lateral cavernous sinus via vidian artery

Infraorbital artery

Sphenopalatine artery

Extension into nasopharynx along posterior nasal wall

Pharyngeal artery

Figure 27.4 Juvenile nasopharyngeal angiofibroma potential routes of spread via the pterygopalatine fossa (PPF). Shown is a cadaveric dissection of the PPF with arteries and nerves labeled. Extension into the infratemporal fossa, orbit, palate, nasopharynx, and lateral cavernous skull base are shown.

artery. It also gives off an infraorbital artery that runs with the maxillary division of the trigeminal nerve (V2), as well as a small perforating blood supply to the soft tissue components within the PPF. The posterior compartment of the PPF contains V2, the vidian nerve, and the sphenopalatine ganglion and its terminal branches. In an anatomic dissection published in *The Laryngoscope*,[13] all neural structures of the PPF were located posterior to the SPA and lateral to the sphenopalatine foramen. This configuration allows access to the vascular structures of the PPF when dissecting in an anterior to posterior direction from an endonasal approach without direct damage to the nerves residing in the posterior compartment. It should be noted that the number and course of the palatine nerves, as well as the branching pattern of the SPA, are often multiple and variable, ranging from two to seven branches.[14]

Understanding the relative spread outside the PPF for surgical dissection requires a comprehensive grasp of (1) the anatomy of the PPF, (2) the JNAs origin therein, and (3) the propensity of JNAs to spread directly through natural anatomic pathways rather than through destructive invasion. Common routes of direct extension beyond the PPF include:

- Extension into the orbit via the infraorbital fissure,
- Extension into the infratemporal fossa via the pterygomaxillary fissure,
- Extension into the middle cranial fossa (by traveling through the infraorbital fissure to the foramen rotundum or through the foramen ovale from the infratemporal fossa), or
- Extension into the anterior cranial vault via direct extension through the ethmoid cavity.

Tumors invading the anterior cranial vault by this last route often accumulate blood supply from the anterior and posterior ethmoid arteries and extend into the planum sphenoidale or the ethmoid roof. Occasionally, extension into the palate can be seen through the descending palatine canals; however, these very small bony channels tend to be more resistant to direct spread of JNA than the orbit, infratemporal fossa, middle cranial fossa, and anterior cranial vault. Of note, while this tumor type usually pushes boundaries rather than directly invading them, in rare cases it can invade through the periorbita or the dura.

Particular anatomical considerations in the infratemporal fossa include the substantial and variable blood supply coming from multiple branches of the ECA, including the ascending pharyngeal artery and the deep temporal arterial system. Additionally, within the infratemporal fossa feeders can come from the internal carotid, as well as from the foramen lacerum. Dissection laterally into the infratemporal fossa in the coronal plane is possible via an endonasal approach, but often requires an anterior medial Denker type maxillectomy to allow for lateral access for instrumentation.

Special considerations to make when approaching the anterior cranial fossa focus on the potential need for skull base reconstruction. If vascularized reconstruction is to be performed, one must bear in mind that embolization and surgical dissection often disrupts sphenopalatine blood supply to the posterior nasal septum and middle turbinate and inferior turbinates on the side of the tumor; therefore, vascularized flaps should be considered from the contralateral side for dural reconstruction.

If the tumor extends posteriorly into the infratemporal fossa it can disrupt the eustachian tube, causing trismus, and may pick up significant blood supply from the internal carotid system. Anatomic dissections in this area require a thorough understanding of the anatomy and demand surgical dexterity to control the carotid in the carotid canal and foramen lacerum.

Traversing posteriorly from the PPF, we first encounter the pterygoid plates. If the pterygoid plates are removed from medial to lateral then the muscular insertions are encountered, including the lateral pterygoid, medial pterygoid, tensor veli palatini, and levator veli palatini muscles. If the muscular attachments are dissected free and displaced laterally, this approach gives access to more posterior structures. Thus, we achieve direct access to the cartilaginous eustachian tube, which sits between the pterygoid area and pterygoid musculature, and the foramen lacerum. If the eustachian tube is dissected from medial to lateral plane then the dissection follows superiorly toward this attachment at the skull base at the bony–cartilaginous eustachian tube junction. There is an intimate relationship with the carotid canal. The superior and posterior portions of the cartilaginous eustachian tube are often in continuity with the inferior portion of the foramen lacerum, through which passes the carotid artery and the cervical sympathetic chain. Tumors involving this area often pick up significant blood supply from the foramen lacerum portion of the carotid artery, but may also derive blood supply from the paraclival portions of the carotid. Tumors incorporating the clival portions of the carotid often have venous outflow into the clival plexus, which can be difficult to control intraoperatively.

Lateral to the infratemporal fossa, behind the pterygoids, lies the poststyloid parapharyngeal space. This space transmits the carotid sheath with the carotid artery, jugular bulb, and lower cranial nerves. It is rare for a JNA to involve this area. If a JNA were to involve this area, then a combination of endoscopic and lateral approach or a staged endoscopic approach should be considered.

In conclusion, thorough knowledge of the anatomy of the PPF, as well as the surrounding anatomic spaces should be considered essential before performing resections of tumors in this area. Preoperative CT scans and MRIs, as well as preoperative angiography, should be scrutinized by the surgeons to familiarize themselves with the vascular blood supply of the tumor. Additionally, these modalities allow the surgeon to assess for potential spread outside of the PPF and need to dissect critical structures such as the orbit, the infratemporal fossa, or the cranial vault. Posterior extension into the eustachian tube and into the pterygoid and masticator space should alert the surgeon to a more variable blood flow with possible blood flow derived from the ICA, as well as a potential need for a combination endoscopic and open or staged endoscopic resection.

Endoscopic Surgical Techniques

The endoscopic endonasal techniques for the removal of JNA follow the same basic tenets of all endoscopic skull base surgery. After appropriate work-up, patient selection, and patient counseling about the risks and benefits of surgery, the patient is scheduled for surgery.

At the University of North Carolina, patients with JNA are typically admitted for observation following angiography and transcatheter embolization the day before the planned operation. The femoral site is inspected and monitored. A standard array of laboratory studies are obtained as part of the preoperative work-up, including a chemistry panel, complete blood count, coagulation panel, and a type and cross match for two units of packed red blood cells. The angiography and embolization results are then reviewed by the surgical and vascular interventional radiology teams. Steroids are administered, usually dexamethasone at 10 mg every 8 hours, to prevent tumor inflammation. Surgical resection is generally performed on the first or second day following embolization to minimize revascularization as well as to limit the postembolization inflammatory response.

Routine use of CT image guidance with or without MRI fusion should be considered the standard for endoscopic skull base surgery. When the JNA involves both sides of the skull base and nasopharynx, or has significant infratemporal fossa extension, either CT or MR angiography may also be fused with image guidance.

The three basic tenets (in order) of removing a JNA are: (1) making appropriate space in the nasal cavities to allow for a vascular dissection, (2) maintaining vascular control, and (3) removing tumor from the more superior portions of the ventral skull base, such as the orbit and the middle and anterior cranial fossae. If there is significant vascular exposure of the ICA, significant exposure of the dura or creation of a cerebrospinal fluid (CSF) leak, reconstruction must be considered.

Proper preoperative communication with the entire surgical team is paramount in the management of these tumors. This includes maintaining dialogue with the anesthesiologist regarding blood loss and replacement needs. Communication with other members of the surgical team is necessary to have hemostatic agents and Foley catheters—to place pressure on arterial bleeding—readily available in the event of an arterial disaster.

After induction of anesthesia, the patient is registered with the image-guidance system. Thereafter, the operation may proceed once the surgical team and the anesthesia team have a mutual understanding of the potential for significant blood loss, and for complications related to orbital and intracranial structures. Typically, the nasal portion of the tumor must first be debulked to provide better access to the sinonasal structures; this can be done with bipolar cautery and Tru-Cutting instrumentation. Occasionally, tumors are soft enough to be debulked using a tissue debrider.

Once the inferior and middle turbinates can be defined and the choana can be visualized, a medial maxillectomy is usually performed. This involves removing the inferior turbinate and opening the entire lateral wall of the nasal cavity into the maxillary sinus. Sometimes, the middle turbinate must also be removed to reach the lateral ethmoid. This exposure provides direct access to the posterior wall of the maxillary sinus, which is the anterior portion of the PPF. The mucosa should then be removed overlying the posterior wall. The bone should be thinned and removed, providing direct transmaxillary access to the PPF. The tumor usually fills a portion of the PPF; however, it may completely fill the PPF and extend into the infratemporal fossa, superior orbital fissure, and possibly even the middle fossa.

If there is significant extension into the ethmoid cavities or the sphenoid sinus, those areas should be resected before tacking the infratemporal fossa component. However, if there is concern for ICA involvement, it is prudent to tack the portion coming from the ECA first. The basic tenet of "one bleeder at a time" during skull base surgery should be respected. Most commonly, the primary vascular supply derives from the internal maxillary artery as it enters the PPF. Once the fibrotic pseudocapsule of the tumor can be dissected into the PPF, the internal maxillary artery often can be identified, clipped using hemoclips and bipolar, and transected from the lateral edge of the PPF portion of the tumor. Such a maneuver truncates the ECA vascular feed so that the remainder of the dissection has significantly less blood loss. However, it should be noted that certain tumors might also derive vascular supply from the lacerum portion of the ICA, as well as contralateral ECA feeders. Such collateral supply should have been evident on the four-vessel angiogram performed before the surgical procedure.

At this point, removal of the nasal portions of the tumor is complete, and the PPF portion of the tumor is likely disconnected from its blood supply. If the tumor has direct extension into the orbit, the infraorbital fissure may be accessed via the PPF to remove the orbital portion of the fibrotic tumor. If there is significant infratemporal fossa extension, a Denker medial maxillectomy may have to be performed to allow for more lateral access, or a sublabial

Caldwell-Luc type approach may be necessary if maximal lateral access is required. If the tumor does involve the infratemporal fossa it is more likely to have acquired vascular supply significantly more lateral than the PPF. This possibility makes vascular dissection of the infratemporal fossa less predictable, more variable, and technically more difficult than tumors isolated to the PPF.

Tumors involving the middle cranial fossa or anterior cranial fossa should be gently dissected out using a two-surgeon, fourhanded technique. A "dissecting surgeon" dissects while a second experienced endoscopic surgeon drives the endoscope and performs any necessary retraction and suctioning. JNAs usually neither invade the dura nor have a dural transgression and, if there is a skull base involvement it is usually erosive and extradural. Care should be taken to identify the dissection plane between the dura and the tumor and the tumor should be gently dissected from the cranial dura. If there is a CSF leak, the tumor resection should proceed; however, it is crucial to minimize blood exchange with the CSF space. Any CSF leak created should be reconstructed at the end of the procedure. It should be noted that JNAs with middle fossa extension occasionally acquire vascular supply from the middle meningeal artery. Similarly, tumors with anterior cranial fossa extension may have vascular supply from the anterior and posterior ethmoidal arteries. It is reasonable to stage portions of the resections of a JNA if there is excessive blood loss, especially for giant JNAs. Where tumors demonstrate intracranial extension or involvement of the ICA, these areas are dissected in a separate setting. Such staging allows the patient and the anesthesia team to accommodate blood loss and prevents significant surgeon fatigue resulting from sequential dissection of multiple vascular areas.

Special consideration should be given to giant JNAs. A posterior septectomy is at times warranted to allow for a binostril dissection of a large tumor, especially one involving the internal carotid arteries in the clival areas. Having a common cavity in these situations allows for better access for dissection, more mobility for dissection, and a larger reservoir for blood to collect during dissection. When considering septectomy, it must be borne in mind that a septectomy at the beginning of the procedure will destroy any potential nasoseptal flap reconstructive options. Thus, if a septal flap is expected to be necessary for reconstruction, the flap should be harvested and tucked into the nasopharynx on the less involved side. The septectomy can then be performed with the flap safely preserved for utilization at the end of the case.

Once the tumor is completely resected, warm water irrigation (110°F) is copiously performed through the cavity. Any residual bleeding is controlled with bipolar cautery or pressure. FloSeal (Baxter, Deerfield, Illinois) is usually packed into the areas of the PPF and infratemporal fossa compounds. Gelfoam (Pfizer, New York) is then routinely laid over the FloSeal and pressure is applied using a Foley balloon for 24 hours. In cases of a small tumor with minimal blood loss, the patient can be monitored in a standard floor bed; however, if the patient experiences significant blood loss—or for larger JNAs—it is advisable to monitor the patient in the intensive care unit (ICU) while the Foley is in place. The Foley is removed on postoperative day one. The patient is then started on nasal saline sprays for 1 week and is transitioned to nasal saline irrigations after week one. Routinely, the patient is discharged home on this irrigation regimen with instructions to refrain from nose blowing and strenuous activity, including instructions regarding bowel regimens in the setting of constipation. Any events of arterial bleeding should precipitate an endoscopy and possible repeat surgical intervention. If the patient presents with a bleed in the outpatient setting, they should be instructed to report immediately to the emergency room.

Special consideration should be given to reconstruction if there is a CSF leak. Options for skull base reconstruction routinely include the use of vascularized flaps such as the nasal septal flap. In these cases, the flap is then placed over the defect and is bolstered into place with Surgiseal (Adhezion, Wyomissing, Pennsylvania), DuraSeal (Covidien, Mansfield, Massachusetts), and absorbable packing. Nonabsorbable packing is then placed underneath, either in the form of a Foley balloon or finger Cotton-Merocel (Merocel, Mystic, Connecticut) packs. If it is a low-flow leak, packing is left in place for 3 days; for high-flow leaks with a leak into the cistern, packing remains in place for 7 days. Lumbar drainage in the postoperative period should be considered for patients with high-flow CSF leaks, usually performed for 3 days at 10 cm^3/h. If there is a significant CSF leak at the time of the operation a postoperative head CT scan is performed to establish a baseline level of pneumocephalus for future comparisons. The patient is routinely placed in the neurologic ICU and is followed with serial neurologic checks. Broad-spectrum antibiotic coverage using third or fourth generation cephalosporins are used while packs are in place.

In the postoperative setting, patients receive sinonasal endoscopy with debridements in the clinic at approximately 2 weeks, then again at 4 to 6 weeks. Patients usually are well mucosalized within their cavities by 6 to 12 weeks after surgery. Multidisciplinary follow up may be necessary in certain cases. If the patient has significant orbital involvement, postoperative follow-up with ophthalmology for transient double vision may be warranted. If an aggressive Denker medial maxillectomy was performed and the nasal lacrimal duct was transected sharply, postoperative transient epiphora may be expected. Follow up with neurosurgery may be necessary if there was significant intracranial extension or a substantial CSF leak.

Follow-up in the first year is usually after every 3 months. It has become our tendency routinely to obtain a postoperative MRI with contrast in the first 3 months if we believe we achieved a total resection, so that we have baseline imaging for future comparison to detect recurrence. If portions of the tumor might need to be reresected or staged, we obtain an early MRI during the immediate

postoperative hospitalization for planning. Future imaging studies usually consist of MRI at 1 year and clinical follow-up thereafter. Late recurrences are possible and the patients are followed into adulthood.

Discussion

To assess the existing data on endoscopic surgery for JNA, over 350 endoscopic resections of JNAs as described in various case series were analyzed (**Table 27.2**).[8,9,15–32] The vast preponderance of these resections is described without complications (4/352 cases, 1.1%), with minimal persistent disease (12/352, 3.4%), and with similarly low-recurrence rates (16/352, 6.5%). Average blood loss is nearly uniformly described as lower than comparable open surgical approaches, with average blood loss ranging from 168 cm^3—in series with only low-stage tumors—to 1500 cm^3 in series with high-stage (Radkowski stage IIIa or greater) tumors. Average blood loss across studies reporting this data point was 445 cm^3, and average length of hospital stay was 4 days. These numbers compare favorably to generally quoted numbers for open approaches: in a series by Hackman et al, mean blood loss in four patients with open approaches averaged 2500 cm^3 (range: 450 to 7000 cm^3), and all required transfusion.[9]

Admittedly, these data are prone to significant selection bias, as endoscopic approaches tend to be favored in lower stage disease. However, even in series such as Nicolai et al, in which 17/46 (37%) of patients who underwent endoscopic resection had disease of Andrews stage IIIa or greater,[a] no complications and no recurrent disease were reported. Of the four cases persistent disease in that series, three were Andrews stage IIIa or greater.[31] Overall, at least 94/386 (26.6%) of total cases reviewed were documented as high-stage disease (generally Radkowski stage IIIa or greater). Even if all adverse outcomes documented were within this high-stage population (this cannot be determined through the published literature), they would constitute rates of persistent and recurrent disease of 12/94 (12.8%) and 23/94 (24.5%), respectively. With overall recurrence rates for JNA quoted at 13 to 46%,[11,33] even such high estimates of suboptimal outcomes in this high-risk population would be at least comparable, if not superior, to open approaches.

Such evaluation of the available literature, then, suggests that endoscopic approaches have the potential to be as effective and safe as traditional open approaches, even in advanced disease. Combined with the generally accepted advantages of endoscopic surgery, such as favorable cosmetic result and superior intraoperative visualization, this affirmation of the efficacy and safety of endoscopic approaches supports a shift toward endoscopic resection of even the most complicated JNAs.

---

[a]Andrews Type III: Tumor invading inftratemporal fossa or orbital region without intracranial involvement (a) or with intracranial extradural (parasellar) involvement.

Table 27.2 Endoscopic Surgery for Juvenile Nasopharyngeal Angiofibroma—Current Literature

Study	Staging System	Patients in Study	Endoscopic Resections	Advanced Stage Tumors	Complications	Persistent Disease	Recurrences	Blood loss (cm³)	Hospital Stay (Days)	Notes
Roger et al 2002[15]	Radkowski	20	20	9	0	2	0	350		
Onerci et al 2003[16]	Radkowski	12	12	4		2	0	1000		Blood loss reported for low-stage tumors. Blood loss for high-stage tumors: 1,500 cm³.
Hofmann et al 2005[17]		21	21	3		3	3	225	2	
Pryor et al 2005[18]		65	5				0			
Baradaranfar and Dabirmoghaddam 2006[21]	Radkowski	105 (32 JNA)	32	0			2			
de Brito Macedo Ferreira et al 2006[20]	Chandler	9	9	1	0	0	0	1 transfusion	8	Embolization performed average of 4.5 d preoperatively.
Tosun et al 2006[19]	Radkowski	24	9	2	0		0	1 transfusion		
Andrade et al 2007[23]	Andrews	12	12	0	0	0	0	200	3	
Eloy et al 2007[22]	Radkowski	6	6	0			1	575		
Gupta et al 2008[25]	Radkowski	28	28	0	1 intraoperative IMA bleed	1	0	168		Blood loss reported for patients who underwent preoperative embolization. For nonembolized patients, average blood loss = 360 cm³.
Yiotakis et al 2008[24]		20	9	0	0	0	0	248.8	2	
Bleier et al 2009[27]	Andrews	18	10	1	0		1	506	3	4-d hospital stay for open resection.

(Contd)

Table 27.2 *Contd*

Study	Staging System	Patients in Study	Endoscopic Resections	Advanced Stage Tumors	Complications	Persistent Disease	Recurrences	Blood loss (cm³)	Hospital Stay (Days)	Notes
Hackman et al 2009[9]		31	15	3	1 retro-orbital hemorrhage		1	280		
Huang et al 2009[26]	Radkowski	19	19	5			0			
Midilli et al 2009[8]	Radkowski	42	12	1				No transfusions required	5	5 to 7-d hospital stay for open resection.
Ardehali et al 2010[29]	Radkowski	47	47	4	2 ruptures of cavernous sinus		9	770	3.1	Blood loss reported for patients who underwent preoperative embolization. For nonembolized patients, average blood loss = 1,402.6 cm³. Hospital stay for embolized patients: 1.8 d.
Nicolai et al 2010[31]	Onerci/Andrews	46	46	25	0	4	0	580	5	25 advanced tumors by Onerci staging; 23 Andrews.
Renkonen et al 2010[30]	Andrews	27	3	0			0			
Zhou et al 2010[28]	Radkowski	59	59	34			6			All recurrences were in patients with high-stage tumors.
Fyrmpas et al 2011[32]	Radkowski	10	10	2		0		444	5	
Total		548	353	94	4	12	23	445.57 (average)	4.01 (average)	

d, days; JNA, juvenile nasopharyngeal angiofibroma; IMA, internal maxillary artery.

Although radiation for JNA was considered to be a viable alternative to surgery for some time, it was found that involution of tumor took up to 3 years. Additionally, radiation therapy carries the potential for induction of malignancy and inhibition of facial growth, important considerations in this primarily adolescent patient population. Lee et al performed a retrospective analysis of 27 patients who received 3000 to 5500 cGy as the primary treatment modality for JNA. They found that the recurrence rate for this sample was 15% at 5 years. However, at the 2-year mark most cases still had residual tumor present before complete involution.[34]

Cummings et al evaluated secondary malignancies in patients treated with external beam radiotherapy for JNA. They found secondary malignancies in 2 out of the 55 cases evaluated. These were thyroid carcinoma and cutaneous basal cell carcinoma. Both cancers arose in the field of radiation and were considered a result of the treatment.[35] Currently, the treatment of choice is surgical resection. Even in the setting of recurrent disease, additional surgery should be considered before radiation. Radiotherapy should be reserved for symptomatic or progressive tumors with extensive intracranial invasion without available surgical options.

In spite of recent advancements in the surgical treatment of JNA, its exact etiology and potential nonsurgical treatment has yet to be elucidated. A better understanding of this pathophysiology could certainly alter and improve overall treatment. The question of whether the initiating event in the development of these tumors occurs in the endothelium or in the stroma remains unanswered. To date, many studies have been published but no single theory explains all of the characteristics or sex predilection of this disease. Recently, Coutinho-Camillo et al published a comprehensive review of several proposed theories for the origin of JNA, including the possible role of steroid hormones, various growth factors and a description of associated genetic alterations.[1] This translational research will hopefully give us a better armamentarium of nonsurgical and adjunctive treatments, especially for advanced staged tumors. Thus far through the study of genetic, growth hormone and androgen effects on JNA, antiandrogen drugs appear to show clinical promise for the medical adjunctive treatment for JNAs.

Recently, Thakar et al published a prospective, single-arm, study in which 20 patients with advanced staged JNAs were administered flutamide orally for 6 weeks before surgical excision.[36] Pretherapy and posttherapy tumor volumes and responses were measured by MRI. The study yielded interesting results: prepubertal and postpubertal patients responded differently to hormonal therapy. Prepubertal cases had inconsistent and minimal responses, whereas 13/15 (87%) of postpubertal cases demonstrated a partial radiographic response (mean, 16.5%; maximum, 40%). Two cases with symptomatic vision loss and optic nerve compression had visual improvement. Presurgical volume reduction correlated significantly both with serum testosterone level and with postpubertal status. There were minimal side effects from this treatment. This study did not compare the histologic effects of treatment or surgical outcomes to a control group. Flutamide treatment can be considered for presurgical volume reduction, for symptomatic tumor compression, or for advanced tumor stages. However, because no complete responses to the drug were noted, complete surgical removal remains the definitive treatment option.

Conclusion

Many questions remain unanswered regarding the genetics and pathogenesis of JNA. Hopefully continued research efforts will lead to less invasive and specific targeted therapies. One thing now apparent clinically is that resection of these tumors no longer necessitates a large, cosmetically morbid operation. Endoscopic skull base tumor surgery and endoscopic skull base reconstructions now allow for resection of advanced staged and intracranial JNAs at experienced centers. Preliminary data about the outcomes are promising with trends toward decreased blood loss, length of hospital stay, morbidity, and potentially cost. The panoramic visualization of the endoscopic endonasal approach provides more precision when dissecting critical structures even when intracranial, or within the orbit or infratemporal fossa. The tenets of vascular control, staged resections and the possible need to convert to open surgery should be respected with endoscopic resection of JNAs.

References

1. Coutinho-Camillo CM, Brentani MM, Nagai MA. Genetic alterations in juvenile nasopharyngeal angiofibromas. Head Neck 2008;30(3):390–400
2. Mattei TA, Nogueira GF, Ramina R. Juvenile nasopharyngeal angiofibroma with intracranial extension. Otolaryngol Head Neck Surg 2011;145(3):498–504
3. Ungkanont K, Byers RM, Weber RS, Callender DL, Wolf PF, Goepfert H. Juvenile nasopharyngeal angiofibroma: an update of therapeutic management. Head Neck 1996;18(1):60–66
4. Gullane PJ, Davidson J, O'Dwyer T, Forte V. Juvenile angiofibroma: a review of the literature and a case series report. Laryngoscope 1992;102(8):928–933
5. Bremer JW, Neel HB III, DeSanto LW, Jones GC. Angiofibroma: treatment trends in 150 patients during 40 years. Laryngoscope 1986;96(12):1321–1329
6. Wu AW, Mowry SE, Vinuela F, Abemayor E, Wang MB. Bilateral vascular supply in juvenile nasopharyngeal angiofibromas. Laryngoscope 2011;121(3):639–643
7. Batsakis JG. Tumors of the Head and Neck: Clinical and Pathological Considerations. 2nd ed. Baltimore, MD: Williams & Wilkins; 1979:296–300
8. Midilli R, Karci B, Akyildiz S. Juvenile nasopharyngeal angiofibroma: analysis of 42 cases and important aspects of endoscopic approach. Int J Pediatr Otorhinolaryngol 2009;73(3):401–408
9. Hackman T, Snyderman CH, Carrau R, Vescan A, Kassam A. Juvenile nasopharyngeal angiofibroma: the expanded endonasal approach. Am J Rhinol Allergy 2009;23(1):95–99
10. Bremer JW, Neel HB III, DeSanto LW, Jones GC. Angiofibroma: treatment trends in 150 patients during 40 years. Laryngoscope 1986;96(12):1321–1329

11. Blount A, Riley KO, Woodworth BA. Juvenile nasopharyngeal angiofibroma. Otolaryngol Clin North Am 2011;44(4):989–1004, ix

12. Snyderman CH, Pant H, Carrau RL, Gardner P. A new endoscopic staging system for angiofibromas. Arch Otolaryngol Head Neck Surg 2010;136(6):588–594

13. Falcon RT, Rivera-Serrano CM, Miranda JF, et al. Endoscopic endonasal dissection of the infratemporal fossa: anatomic relationships and importance of eustachian tube in the endoscopic skull base surgery. Laryngoscope 2011;121(1):31–41

14. Hosseini SM, Razfar A, Carrau RL, et al. Endonasal transpterygoid approach to the infratemporal fossa: correlation of endoscopic and multiplanar CT anatomy. Head Neck 2012;34(3):313–320

15. Roger G, Tran Ba Huy P, Froehlich P, et al. Exclusively endoscopic removal of juvenile nasopharyngeal angiofibroma: trends and limits. Arch Otolaryngol Head Neck Surg 2002;128(8):928–935

16. Onerci TM, Yücel OT, Oğretmenoğlu O. Endoscopic surgery in treatment of juvenile nasopharyngeal angiofibroma. Int J Pediatr Otorhinolaryngol 2003;67(11):1219–1225

17. Hofmann T, Bernal-Sprekelsen M, Koele W, Reittner P, Klein E, Stammberger H. Endoscopic resection of juvenile angiofibromas—long term results. Rhinology 2005;43(4):282–289

18. Pryor SG, Moore EJ, Kasperbauer JL. Endoscopic versus traditional approaches for excision of juvenile nasopharyngeal angiofibroma. Laryngoscope 2005;115(7):1201–1207

19. Tosun F, Ozer C, Gerek M, Yetiser S. Surgical approaches for nasopharyngeal angiofibroma: comparative analysis and current trends. J Craniofac Surg 2006;17(1):15–20

20. de Brito Macedo Ferreira LM, Gomes EF, Azevedo JF, Souza JR, de Paula Araújo R, do Nascimento Rios AS. Endoscopic surgery of nasopharyngeal angiofibroma. Braz J Otorhinolaryngol 2006;72(4):475–480

21. Baradaranfar MH, Dabirmoghaddam P. Endoscopic endonasal surgery for resection of benign sinonasal tumors: experience with 105 patients. Arch Iran Med 2006;9(3):244–249

22. Eloy P, Watelet JB, Hatert AS, de Wispelaere J, Bertrand B. Endonasal endoscopic resection of juvenile nasopharyngeal angiofibroma. Rhinology 2007;45(1):24–30

23. Andrade NA, Pinto JA, Nóbrega MdeO, Aguiar JE, Aguiar TF, Vinhaes ES. Exclusively endoscopic surgery for juvenile nasopharyngeal angiofibroma. Otolaryngol Head Neck Surg 2007;137(3):492–496

24. Yiotakis I, Eleftheriadou A, Davilis D, et al. Juvenile nasopharyngeal angiofibroma stages I and II: a comparative study of surgical approaches. Int J Pediatr Otorhinolaryngol 2008;72(6):793–800

25. Gupta AK, Rajiniganth MG, Gupta AK. Endoscopic approach to juvenile nasopharyngeal angiofibroma: our experience at a tertiary care centre. J Laryngol Otol 2008;122(11):1185–1189

26. Huang J, Sacks R, Forer M. Endoscopic resection of juvenile nasopharyngeal angiofibroma. Ann Otol Rhinol Laryngol 2009;118(11):764–768

27. Bleier BS, Kennedy DW, Palmer JN, Chiu AG, Bloom JD, O'Malley BW Jr. Current management of juvenile nasopharyngeal angiofibroma: a tertiary center experience 1999-2007. Am J Rhinol Allergy 2009;23(3):328–330

28. Zhou B, Cai T, Huang Q, et al. Juvenile nasopharyngeal angiofibroma: endoscopic surgery and follow-up results [in Chinese]. Zhonghua Er Bi Yan Hou Tou Jing Wai Ke Za Zhi 2010;45(3):180–185

29. Ardehali MM, Samimi Ardestani SH, Yazdani N, Goodarzi H, Bastaninejad S. Endoscopic approach for excision of juvenile nasopharyngeal angiofibroma: complications and outcomes. Am J Otolaryngol 2010;31(5):343–349

30. Renkonen S, Hagström J, Vuola J, et al. The changing surgical management of juvenile nasopharyngeal angiofibroma. Eur Arch Otorhinolaryngol 2011;268(4):599–607

31. Nicolai P, Villaret AB, Farina D, et al. Endoscopic surgery for juvenile angiofibroma: a critical review of indications after 46 cases. Am J Rhinol Allergy 2010;24(2):e67–e72

32. Fyrmpas G, Konstantinidis I, Constantinidis J. Endoscopic treatment of juvenile nasopharyngeal angiofibromas: our experience and review of the literature. Eur Arch Otorhinolaryngol 2012;269(2):523–529

33. Glad H, Vainer B, Buchwald C, et al. Juvenile nasopharyngeal angiofibromas in Denmark 1981-2003: diagnosis, incidence, and treatment. Acta Otolaryngol 2007;127(3):292–299

34. Lee JT, Chen P, Safa A, Juillard G, Calcaterra TC. The role of radiation in the treatment of advanced juvenile angiofibroma. Laryngoscope 2002;112(7, pt 1):1213–1220

35. Cummings BJ, Blend R, Keane T, et al. Primary radiation therapy for juvenile nasopharyngeal angiofibroma. Laryngoscope 1984;94 (12, pt 1):1599–1605

36. Thakar A, Gupta G, Bhalla AS, et al. Adjuvant therapy with flutamide for presurgical volume reduction in juvenile nasopharyngeal angiofibroma. Head Neck 2011;33(12):1747–1753

37. Onerci M, Oğretmenoğlu O, Yücel T. Juvenile nasopharyngeal angiofibroma: a revised staging system. Rhinology 2006;44(1):39–45

38. Radkowski D, McGill T, Healy GB, Ohlms L, Jones DT. Angiofibroma. Changes in staging and treatment. Arch Otolaryngol Head Neck Surg 1996;122(2):122–129

39. Chandler JR, Goulding R, Moskowitz L, Quencer RM. Nasopharyngeal angiofibromas: staging and management. Ann Otol Rhinol Laryngol 1984;93(4, pt 1):322–329

40. Andrews JC, Fisch U, Valavanis A, Aeppli U, Makek MS. The surgical management of extensive nasopharyngeal angiofibromas with the infratemporal fossa approach. Laryngoscope 1989;99(4):429–437

28 Minimally Invasive Pituitary Surgery

Mitchell Ray Gore and Brent A. Senior

Tumors of the pituitary had been described as early as 1641 by Plater, with numerous descriptions of patients with endocrine abnormalities, vision loss, and death associated with pituitary tumors, ultimately leading to the development of surgical approaches to the pituitary.[1] The pituitary was first described as a glandular structure in 1688 by Brunner,[2] whereas the endocrine properties of the gland were detailed in 1886 by Marie.[3] In the early 1900s pituitary surgeons noted a symptomatic improvement in acromegalic patients after pituitary tumor removal.[2] Tumors of the pituitary had been described as early as 1641 by Plater, with numerous descriptions of patients with endocrine abnormalities, vision loss, and death associated with pituitary tumors, ultimately leading to the development of surgical approaches to the pituitary.[1]

Surgical Approaches to the Pituitary

Transcranial and transsphenoidal approaches[3-5] were developed during the early 20th century. Horsley performed a transfrontal approach to the pituitary in 1889,[5] with Paul and Caton attempting resection of a pituitary tumor via a transtemporal approach in 1893.[3,6] In 1906, Horsley published a series of 10 transfrontal or transtemporal approaches.[7] Subsequent modifications and improvements were made by neurosurgeons such as Dandy, Frazier, Heuer, and Cushing.[7] Early transcranial approaches carried a high mortality risk from 20 to 80%,[3] providing an impetus for the development of transnasal approaches. In 1897, a transglabellar approach was proposed by Giordano,[3,8] and his work laid the foundation for Schloffer, who in 1907 originated the transsphenoidal approach to the pituitary,[9] performing a successful resection of a pituitary tumor under cocaine local anesthesia in three stages.[7] This approach[10] resulted in poor cosmesis as well as almost certain ozena, leading others to modify the technique. Cushing performed his first transsphenoidal procedure in 1909 on an acromegalic patient. After a tracheotomy, Cushing performed a modification of the Schloffer technique, making an omega-shaped incision over the forehead and creating a frontal osteoplastic flap. Under headlight illumination, ethmoidectomy was followed by sphenoidotomy, removal of the sellar floor with a chisel, and partial removal of the tumor using a curette. The patient improved and lived another 21 years.[11,12] Cushing modified the technique by incorporating a sublabial incision and submucosal resection of the septum, performing his first sublabial transseptal transsphenoidal approach in 1910 and using a 2-cm sublabial incision, submucosal septal flaps,

and removal of cartilage, perpendicular plate of ethmoid, and vomer with subsequent opening of the sphenoid and sella. Cushing presented his landmark work, *The Pituitary Body and its Disorders*,[10] then reported on 74 operations on 68 patients.[9] Twenty-two patients experienced a slight visual improvement or stabilization of vision over months to years after the operation, whereas 22 experienced a sudden significant visual improvement. Seven deaths occurred for a mortality rate of 9.5% in that early report. Ultimately Cushing reduced the mortality rate to 5.6% later in his career.[3]

Surprisingly, by 1929, Cushing abandoned the sublabial transseptal transsphenoidal approach in favor of transcranial approaches citing concerns of recurrence and mortality.[3,4,13] Because of Cushing's popularity and influence, the majority of neurosurgeons also converted to transcranial approaches. However, during this period the endonasal transsphenoidal approach was maintained by Hirsch, a rhinologist who championed the endonasal transseptal transsphenoidal. Hirsch used a head mirror for lighting with a nasal speculum and a suctioning device to enhance visualization.[4,5] Hirsch performed his first endonasal approach to a pituitary tumor on March 10, 1910, in Vienna, several weeks ahead of Cushing performing his first sublabial transsphenoidal approach. The procedure was a success with the resolution of the patient's headaches and improvement in her vision.[11] Soon after, Hirsch modified his technique into a single stage with incorporation of Kocher submucous resection of the septum and by 1937 Hirsch reported a mortality rate of 5.4% in 277 patients.

With renewed interest in the transnasal approach, Dott, a neurosurgeon from Edinburgh, pioneered novel illumination techniques for pituitary surgery such as a lighted speculum.[3] French surgeon Guiot learned the technique from Dott and performed more than 1000 surgeries, introducing intraoperative fluoroscopy to help define the anatomy of the nasal passages.[3-5,8] Hardy revolutionized the transsphenoidal pituitary surgery by introducing the use of the operating microscope and microsurgical instrumentation in 1967,[3,5] which permitted a more thorough and safer resection of macro- and microadenomas without deaths or major morbidities.[3]

Introduction of Endoscopic Pituitary Surgery

The endoscope and its use by otolaryngologists to treat inflammatory sinus disease as championed by Kennedy,

Stammberger, and others grew in the early 1990s. With its clarity of view and brightness of visualization the endoscope was quickly adopted for transsphenoidal pituitary surgery.[3]

Guiot initially reported the use of the endoscope as a complementary tool during the microscopic sublabial transseptal approach; however, with the exception of Bushe and Halves, no other descriptions of endoscopic transsphenoidal pituitary surgery appeared until 1992 when Jankowski reported the first such procedure in three patients.[3,14] Jho and Carrau in 1997 reported on the first large series of 46 patients managed endoscopically, demonstrating the safety, efficacy, and advantages of this technique[15] and marking the initiation of the modern minimally invasive pituitary surgery (MIPS) era.

Technological advances such as high-resolution computed tomography (CT), magnetic resonance imaging (MRI), and stereotactic navigational guidance systems[16] have significantly improved assessment of the sella, tumor extent, and tumor localization. Endoscopes allow for visualization with close proximity to the operative field and multiple visual angles. Use of endoscopes in MIPS approaches reduces operative time[17–19] with superior illumination and magnification,[19–21] diminished blood loss,[22] enhanced differentiation between normal gland and tumor,[23] better intrasellar and parasellar images,[24] reduced hospital stay, improved patient satisfaction, and decreased need for packing.[25] The MIPS approach alleviates the need for external incisions, while minimizing septal perforations and postoperative nasal obstruction.[19,25] The binocular visualization provided by the microscope is lost in the MIPS technique. Many neurosurgeons have not been trained in the use of the endoscope, which leads to a learning curve for the novice. A joint effort by the otolaryngologist and the neurosurgeon is favored for resection of pituitary tumors; this allows for a safe and rapid approach in which each surgeon performs that part with which they are most comfortable.

Anatomical Considerations

The pituitary gland sits in the sella turcica on the superior aspect of the sphenoid bone. It is located behind the tuberculum sellae, which is located posterior to the optic chiasm. The posterior boundary of the sella is defined by the dorsum sellae and posterior clinoid. Below the dorsum sellae is the clivus, which slopes inferiorly and is continuous with the occipital bone.[26] The lateral extensions of the tuberculum sellae form the anterior clinoid processes. The roof of the fossa is formed by the diaphragm, a dural fold traversed by the pituitary stalk. The lateral extension of the diaphragm forms the roof of the cavernous sinus.[26]

The pituitary gland lies in close proximity to the optic chiasm and nerves, the carotid arteries, cranial nerves III to VI in the cavernous sinus, as well as the basilar artery and brainstem posteriorly. Proper knowledge of this parasellar anatomy is essential to performing these approaches.

The sphenoid sinus is variably pneumatized with three types of sphenoid pneumatization patterns described: conchal (minimal pneumatization with thick bone over the face of the sella), sellar (pneumatized to the face of the sella), and postsellar (pneumatization beyond the face of the sella). The majority of adult sinuses are of the sellar type and postsellar type.[26]

Asymmetry of the two sphenoid cavities is the norm, and multiple septations may be present.[27] The roof of the sinus is formed by the planum sphenoidale anteriorly and the sella posteriorly. The posterior wall corresponds to the clivus and, superiorly, the face of the sella. In the sella, the lateral walls form the medial walls of the cavernous sinus. Intercavernous venous connections usually run inferior to the gland but can run anteriorly and may be a source of bleeding intraoperatively when the dura is incised. The canal of the vidian nerve runs laterally along the sphenoid floor, and the carotid arteries run laterally at about 5- and 7-o' clock position. The optic nerves run superiorly along the lateral walls, at about 2- and 11-o' clock position, with the opticocarotid recess located between the bulges of these two structures.[15]

Surgical Indications

Indications for excision of nonsecreting adenomas include large size or evidence of rapid growth, compressive symptoms, hypopituitarism, visual changes, pituitary apoplexy, or severe headaches. Patients with secreting prolactinomas are referred for surgery after failure of medical management. Patients with acromegaly, hypothyroidism, Cushing disease, Rathke cleft cysts (RCCs), chordomas, and arachnoid cysts are offered primary surgery.

Preoperative Evaluation

Patients are best evaluated by a multidisciplinary team including an endocrinologist, a neurosurgeon, an otolaryngologist, an ophthalmologist, and a radiation oncologist. During the preoperative otolaryngology visit a history and head and neck exam are performed. Flexible endoscopy is used to evaluate the sinonasal anatomy and rule out any infection that may mandate a delay in surgery. The CT scan is reviewed for Onodi cells, asymmetry of the sphenoid cavity, or possible dehiscence of the carotid arteries. At our institution, all patients obtain a fine-cut CT scan for use with the computer-guided navigational system. The preoperative MRI and CT are fused together on the navigational system, allowing for improved intraoperative orientation and visualization of critical structures, such as the carotid artery, particularly essential in revision surgery. The risks and benefits of the procedure are discussed at length and all questions are answered. Preoperative evaluation by an ophthalmologist includes visual acuity and visual field as well as retinal exam, and this serves as a basis for postoperative comparisons to determine improvement, or possibly degeneration, in vision. Preoperative medications prescribed by an endocrinologist are usually continued; hypothyroidism is ideally well controlled, and stress doses of steroids are given preoperatively as necessary.

Surgical Technique

The surgical instruments and 0-, 30-, 45-, and 70-degree 4-mm endoscopes used in the endoscopic endonasal approach are largely the same as those used by otolaryngologists in endoscopic sinus surgery. The 0-degree endoscope is the workhorse for the majority of the procedure. Angled scopes are usually used later in the procedure after the sella is entered and the tumor removed. The use of stereoscopic endoscopes to allow for a three-dimensional view currently remains mostly anecdotal.

The patient is positioned in the "beach-chair" position, with the torso elevated at about 30 degrees and the knees slightly bent for comfort. The head is rotated about 15 degrees toward the surgeon and the patient's head is placed on a foam donut. A computer-guided navigation system is routinely used to facilitate identification of landmarks and orientation in relation to the tumor. The patient's face is left unsterile, as the instruments will be passing through a contaminated nasal cavity. The abdomen is routinely sterilely prepared in case a decision is made to use a sellar fat graft at the end of the procedure for cerebrospinal fluid (CSF) leak repair.

Hemostasis is aided by performing greater palatine blocks by injecting 1.5 mL of 1% lidocaine with 1/100,000 epinephrine transorally into each greater palatine canal. The nasal cavities are decongested with 0.05% of oxymetazoline hydrochloride pledgets, and endoscopic sphenopalatine artery blocks are placed by injecting lidocaine with epinephrine in the region of the sphenopalatine foramen.

Most neurosurgeons are trained to perform pituitary surgery via the midline, trans-septal route. The endoscopic transnasal approach is slightly extra-axial and will result in a somewhat different perspective for sellar visualization. Indeed, because the endonasal approach is a few degrees off the midline, it allows better exposure of the contralateral sphenoid and cavernous sinus. The initial side of approach to the tumor is determined by several factors such as the degree of obstruction of the nasal cavity, though ultimately a bilateral approach is favored improving visualization and allowing for more than one instrument to be inserted in addition to the endoscope. The preoperative endoscopic exam along with review of preoperative CT aids in the assessment of nasal septal obstruction or nasal cavity asymmetry, if present. For smaller pituitary lesions that are off the midline and for those larger tumors extending laterally into the cavernous sinus, the contralateral nasal cavity may present a better angle of initial approach.

The approach to the anterior face of the sphenoid follows the paraseptal corridor medial to the middle turbinate, avoiding the lateral sinuses and minimizing the risk of postoperative sinusitis. Gentle lateralization of the middle turbinate or occasional resection of a concha bullosa may provide better access.

Key to the identification of the sphenoid sinus ostium is the identification of the superior turbinate and the region of the sphenoethmoid recess. The recess is bounded by the skull base, the superior turbinate, and the septum medially and nearly always contains the sphenoid ostium. The ostium can be seen after decongesting the superior turbinate and conservatively resecting its posterior–inferior third. The ostium is located medial to the turbinate, posterior to its inferior edge in the sphenoethmoid recess (**Fig. 28.1**). Dong Jho described using the inferior edge of the middle turbinate as a landmark for orientation to the floor of the sella. This margin leads to the clival indentation, approximately 1 cm below the level of the sellar floor.[15]

The posterior septal branch of the sphenopalatine artery crosses the inferior aspect of the sphenoethmoidal recess on its way to supply the mucosa of the septum. Bleeding from this vessel can be well controlled with bipolar cautery. Vasoconstriction may be obtained by injection of lidocaine or epinephrine solution along the posterior septum, before any incision in the face of the sphenoid is made.

Once the sphenoid sinus ostium is identified the ostium is enlarged in an inferomedial direction, away from lateral wall structures until the ostium is large enough to accept the endoscope to visualize the lateral extent of the sinus. The bone of the sphenoid rostrum is resected until the nasal septum is encountered; occasionally, a high-speed drill is used for this relatively thick bone (**Fig. 28.2**). A partial posterior septectomy is then performed, exposing the contralateral face of the sphenoid. The intersinus septum is resected exposing the sellar face. Great care is taken in resection of the intersinus septum, as it may attach posteriorly over the carotid or optic nerve or both.

Medially, the sella is bordered by the tubercle rostrally and the clivus caudally. Once the sella is entered the optic

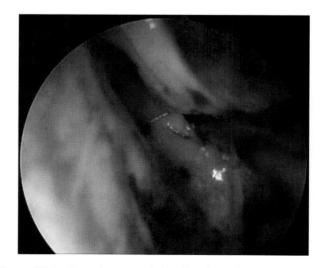

Figure 28.1   Natural ostium of the left sphenoid sinus identified in the sphenoethmoid recess and cannulated using a stapes curette.

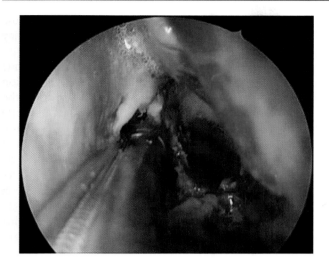

Figure 28.2 Drilling the sphenoid rostrum.

nerves are seen at 11- and 1-o' clock position, whereas the cavernous internal carotid arteries are located at 5- and 7-o' clock position. The carotids are c-shaped with the concavity oriented laterally. Caution must be exercised as carotids can be dehiscent in up to 22% of sphenoid sinuses.[28] We then typically used a four-handed/two-surgeon technique: one surgeon maintains the endoscope while the other bimanually introduces instruments.

The posterior sphenoid mucosa is coagulated and removed. The sella is then entered with a chisel or high-speed drill depending on the thickness of the sellar face and the opening enlarged with a Kerrison rongeur (**Fig. 28.3**). Occasionally, bleeding can be encountered from anterior intercavernous connections; this is controlled with microfibrillar collagen, pressure, or bipolar cautery. The dura is then cauterized and opened. The tumor mass typically bulges through the dural opening at this point, and samples are taken and sent for frozen section and permanent pathology before any suction is used, especially when dealing with microadenomas and

smaller lesions (**Fig. 28.4**). The tumor is then removed with a combination of suction and neurosurgical spatulas and ring curettes with different angulations (**Fig. 28.5**). Tumor tissue is usually easily differentiated from normal yellow pituitary tissue.

Once the bulk of the tumor is removed, the endoscope is inserted into the sella to facilitate more detailed exploration, and angled endoscopes may be used to examine the crevices of the sella. The diaphragm of the sella and normal pituitary tissue often tend to descend into the void created by tumor removal. This can obscure visualization, especially in the lateral and posterior or superior recesses of the cavity.

To improve visualization in this setting, we have developed the technique of "hydroscopy," using normal saline irrigation under several centimeters water pressure attached to the endoscopes. The pressure of the saline expands the soft tissue boundaries of the sella including the diaphragm, washes out small bits of residual tumor, improves visualization, and facilitates inspection of the cavity and ensures as complete a removal of tumor tissue as possible. At the end of the procedure, hemostasis is obtained using a hemostatic substance such as microfibrillar collagen, which is then irrigated out. Reconstruction of the sella is usually only indicated for intraoperative suspicion of a CSF leak.[19] If a leak is identified, reconstruction can be performed using a fat graft, AlloDerm, or a pedicled nasoseptal flap depending on the defect size.

Postoperative Management

Postoperatively, the patient is admitted for routine neurological monitoring and an MRI is obtained on the first postoperative day. Patients are generally discharged home on antibiotics and hormonal replacement as necessary and nose blowing or sneezing is avoided. At the first postoperative visit approximately 3 weeks later, endoscopy is performed to confirm appropriate healing.

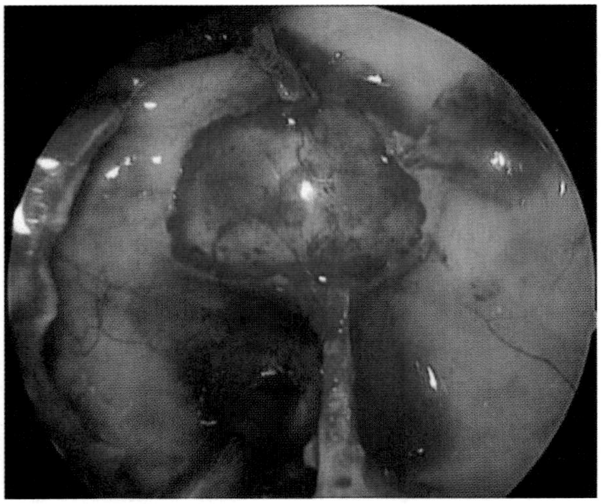

Figure 28.3 Sellar osteotomy exposing the dura over the pituitary mass.

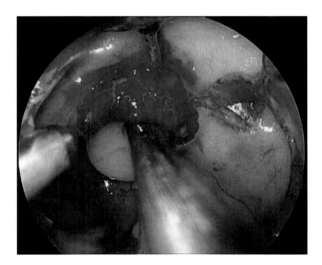

Figure 28.4 Pituitary adenoma being suctioned from the sellar durotomy.

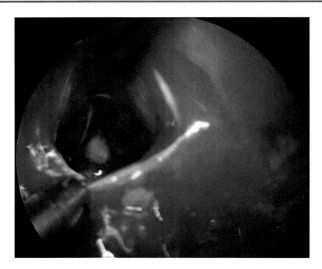

Figure 28.5 Internal view of the sella after removal of the pituitary adenoma.

Outcomes

Senior et al[20] examined the mortality rate in their series of 176 consecutive patients and found a mortality rate of 0.5%, which was similar to the rate in most modern series of 0 to 1.03%. Most mortality reported in the literature is because of medical complications such as pulmonary embolus or cardiac events. Mortality related to the surgery itself is most often secondary to incomplete resection of large, suprasellar tumors that develop significant edema and irreversible neurological insult.

In this same series the overall incidence of diabetes insipidus (DI; deficiency of the pituitary hormone vasopressin causing inappropriately high urine output) was 20.2%, similar to the 3 to 60% rate seen in the literature. The wide range is likely because of the small numbers of patients in some of the other series. Patients with RCCs typically have substantially higher rates of DI in the postoperative period than patients with other tumor types (47.6% for RCCs vs. 20.2% for other types in the Senior et al series[20]; $p = 0.003$).

The rate of vascular complications including intracranial hemorrhage, cerebral vascular accident, epistaxis, and intraoperative hemorrhage was 5.2% in the same series.[20] One instance of intracranial hemorrhage ultimately resulted in the lone mortality in that series. Epistaxis controlled with pressure, cauterization, or anterior packing occurred in six resections (3.1%). One patient with a conchal sphenoid early in the series had significant cavernous bleeding from an anterior communicating sinus that resulted in aborting the procedure. Another patient taking an antiplatelet medication (clopidogrel) perioperatively had 900 mL of blood loss and required blood transfusion. There were no episodes of massive epistaxis, cavernous sinus thrombosis, carotid injury, subdural, or subarachnoid hematoma in any of the 193 procedures.

In the Senior et al[20] series 51 of the 193 (26%) procedures were complicated by a CSF leak. Intraoperative CSF leaks

were seen in 38 resections (19.7%) with 20 patients (10.3%) developing CSF rhinorrhea in the postoperative period. Seven patients (3.6%) experienced both intraoperative and postoperative leaks. Intraoperative CSF leaks were repaired with a fat graft, with four also having lumbar drain placement. Postoperative leaks were managed with lumbar drain ($n = 14$) or endoscopic repair ($n = 6$). One patient with a large arachnoid cyst had two unsuccessful repair procedures after failure of conservative management and eventually required lumboperitoneal shunting.

"Sinusitis" as defined by the presence of extensive inflammation in the sphenoid sinus (with or without frank purulence) occurred after 11 resections (5.7%).[20] All patients were treated with oral and topical antibiotics and no patient developed meningitis as a result of sphenoid sinusitis. One of the 11 patients had a history of chronic rhinosinusitis and previous endoscopic sinus surgery. CSF leak was noted in only 4 of these 11 individuals and was not correlated with the development of postoperative sinusitis. The low rate of sinusitis (5.7%) in this series compared favorably with the rate cited in the literature of 1 to 15%. The nasal anatomy in our approach remains essentially undisturbed, thereby allowing for the sinuses to continue functioning. Only one patient had persistent chronic rhinosinusitis, and this was a pre-existing condition and was not exacerbated by the surgery. Meningitis occurred in 2 of 193 resections (1.0%) in the same series, comparable with the rate of 0.15 to 1.2% reported in the literature. Two patients were asymptomatic, but had positive CSF cultures after removal of the lumbar drain. CSF cultures grew gram-positive organisms such as *Streptococcus viridans*, oxacillin-sensitive *Staphylococcus aureus*, and coagulase-negative staphylococci.

Two neurological complications occurred in the same series,[20] pneumocephalus and cranial neuropathy (1.0%). One patient suffered bilateral abducens palsy in the immediate postoperative course. MRI revealed no hemorrhage, infarct, or cavernous sinus thrombosis and the palsy gradually resolved with no permanent dysfunction. This patient subsequently had a recurrence of his nonsecreting pituitary adenoma, had revision surgery and experienced no cranial neuropathy after the revision surgery. Pneumocephalus was present in one patient, which resolved after repair of the concurrent CSF fistula.

O'Malley et al[21] examined the learning curve in transitioning from traditional microscopic pituitary surgery to MIPS. The authors compared outcomes after purely endoscopic resection versus traditional microscope-aided resection. They examined retrospective data on 25 patients surgically treated for a pituitary lesion, with all procedures performed by the same senior neurosurgeon who was initially unfamiliar with the endoscopic endonasal approach. In the microscopically treated cohort, there were 8 intra- or postoperative complications, 6 intraoperative CSF leaks, 17 (77%) of 22 patients had gross total resection on postoperative imaging, 5 patients underwent two or more operations, and 10 (59%) of 17 reported total symptom resolution at follow-up. The endoscopically treated group had seven intra- or postoperative complications and seven intraoperative CSF leaks. Of the patients who had pre- and postoperative imaging studies, 14 (66%) of 21 endoscopically treated patients had gross total resection; 4 patients had two or more operations, and 10 (66%) of 15 patients reported complete symptom resolution at follow-up. The first nine patients who were treated endoscopically had a mean surgical time of 3.42 hours and a mean hospital stay of 4.67 days. The next eight patients treated had a mean surgical time of 3.11 hours and a mean hospital stay of 3.13 days. The final eight patients treated endoscopically had a mean surgical time of 2.22 hours and a mean hospital stay of 3.88 days. The difference in length of operation between the first nine and the last eight patients treated endoscopically was significantly different. They found a trend toward decreased CSF leaks and other complications from the first two groups treated endoscopically compared with the later endoscopic group. They estimated that the learning curve for endoscopic resection should be 17 or less procedures.

Sonnenberg and Senior[22] also examined the learning curve by examining the first 45 cases of MIPS at their institution. A retrospective review of the first 45 cases of MIPS was conducted and allocated the patients into three groups of 15. The groups were comparable with respect to age, sex, and revision surgery as well as complication rates investigated including death, intracerebral hemorrhage, intraoperative CSF leak, postoperative CSF leak, use of lumbar drain, meningitis, postoperative epistaxis, ophthalmoplegia, visual impairment, and DI. Other factors examined included intraoperative blood loss, length of stay, and tumor histology and were similar between the three groups. Statistically significant ($p < 0.05$) differences in complication rates and other factors between groups were not seen, and the study did not establish a learning curve for the first 45 cases of minimally invasive endoscopic pituitary surgery.

Kabil et al[23] performed a retrospective study of 300 patients who underwent fully endoscopic endonasal pituitary adenoma resection during a 6-year period. Data on outcomes were collected and compared with mean values calculated from several transseptal transsphenoidal reports. From a total of 300 pituitary adenomas treated endoscopically, 139 (46%) were hormonally active, whereas 161 (54%) were nonfunctioning. The mean follow-up period was 38.2 months. The average length of hospital stay was 1.4 days. All patients had postoperative MRI to assess residual or recurrent disease and all patients with hormonally active tumors had additional postoperative hormonal studies. Remission, being defined as no hormonal or radiologic evidence of recurrence within the time frame of the follow-up, was demonstrated in 127/134 (95%) of enclosed and 144/166 (87%) of invasive adenomas. A comparison of fully endoscopic endonasal versus transseptal transsphenoidal remission results revealed an improved outcome using the fully endoscopic endonasal technique for all hormone-

secreting tumor types: adrenocorticotropic hormone (86 vs. 81%), prolactin (89 vs. 66%), and growth hormone (85 vs. 77%). The remission rate for nonfunctioning adenomas was 149/161 (93%). The authors also noted a marked reduction in complications related to the endoscopic procedure, indicating that the fully endoscopic endonasal technique is a safe and effective method for the removal of pituitary adenomas providing more complete tumor removal and reducing complications.

Conclusions

The endoscopic transsphenoidal approach provides a safe, cost-effective, and minimally invasive method for resection of pituitary masses. The use of the natural ostium preserves a functional sphenoid cavity that can be easily monitored postoperatively. The use of this minimally invasive approach has been shown to decrease the length of patient hospital stay, and the two-team approach using an otolaryngological team working in conjunction with a neurosurgical team has a short learning curve and has been shown to have a low rate of postoperative complications.

References

1. de Divitiis E, Cappabianca P, Cavallo LM. Endoscopic Endonasal Transspehnoidal Approach to the Sellar Region. Chapter 7. New York, NY: Springer Wein; 2003:91–123
2. Landolt AM. The pituitary. In: History of Pituitary Surgery: Transcranial Approach. Philadelphia, PA: W.B. Saunders Company; 1996:283–294
3. Liu JK, Das K, Weiss MH, Laws ER Jr, Couldwell WT. The history and evolution of transsphenoidal surgery. J Neurosurg 2001;95(6):1083–1096
4. Lanzino G, Laws ER Jr. Pioneers in the development of transsphenoidal surgery: Theodor Kocher, Oskar Hirsch, and Norman Dott. J Neurosurg 2001;95(6):1097–1103
5. Landolt AM. History of pituitary surgery from the technical aspect. Neurosurg Clin N Am 2001;12(1):37–44, vii–viii
6. Kenan PD. The rhinologist and the management of pituitary disease. Laryngoscope 1979;89(2, pt 2, Suppl 14)1–26
7. Kanter AS, Dumont AS, Asthagiri AR, Oskouian RJ, Jane JA Jr, Laws ER Jr. The transsphenoidal approach. A historical perspective. Neurosurg Focus 2005;18(4):e6
8. Cappabianca P, de Divitiis E. Back to the Egyptians: neurosurgery via the nose. A five-thousand year history and the recent contribution of the endoscope. Neurosurg Rev 2007;30(1):1–7, discussion 7
9. Cushing H. The Weir Mitchell lecture. Surgical experiences with pituitary disorders. JAMA 1914;63:1515–1525
10. Cushing H. The Pituitary Body and Its Disorders: Clinical States Produced by Disorders of the Hypophysis Cerebri. Philadelphia, PA: JB Lippincott; 1912
11. Liu JK, Cohen-Gadol AA, Laws ER Jr, Cole CD, Kan P, Couldwell WT. Harvey Cushing and Oskar Hirsch: early forefathers of modern transsphenoidal surgery. J Neurosurg 2005;103(6):1096–1104
12. Cushing H III. Partial Hypophysectomy for acromegaly: with remarks on the function of the hypophysis. Ann Surg 1909;50(6):1002–1017
13. Welbourn RB. The evolution of transsphenoidal pituitary microsurgery. Surgery 1986;100(6):1185–1190

14. Jankowski R, Auque J, Simon C, Marchal JC, Hepner H, Wayoff M. Endoscopic pituitary tumor surgery. Laryngoscope 1992; 102(2):198–202

15. Jho HD, Carrau RL, Ko Y, Daly MA. Endoscopic pituitary surgery: an early experience. Surg Neurol 1997;47(3):213–222, discussion 222–223

16. Onizuka M, Tokunaga Y, Shibayama A, Miyazaki H. Computer-assisted neurosurgical navigational system for transsphenoidal surgery—technical note. Neurol Med Chir (Tokyo) 2001;41(11):565–568, discussion 569

17. Sheehan MT, Atkinson JL, Kasperbauer JL, Erickson BJ, Nippoldt TB. Preliminary comparison of the endoscopic transnasal vs the sublabial transseptal approach for clinically nonfunctioning pituitary macroadenomas. Mayo Clin Proc 1999;74(7):661–670

18. Ouaknine GSV, Veshchev I, Siomin V, Razon N, Salame K, Stern N. The one-nostril transnasal transsphenoidal extramucosal approach: the analysis of surgical technique and complications in 529 consecutive cases. Oper Tech Otolaryngol--Head Neck Surg 2000;11:261–267

19. Sonnenburg RE, White D, Ewend MG, Senior B. The learning curve in minimally invasive pituitary surgery. Am J Rhinol 2004;18(4): 259–263

20. Senior BA, Ebert CS, Bednarski KK, et al. Minimally invasive pituitary surgery. Laryngoscope 2008;118(10):1842–1855

21. O'Malley BW Jr, Grady MS, Gabel BC, et al. Comparison of endoscopic and microscopic removal of pituitary adenomas: single-surgeon experience and the learning curve. Neurosurg Focus 2008;25(6):E10

22. Sonnenburg RE, White D, Ewend MG, Senior B. The learning curve in minimally invasive pituitary surgery. Am J Rhinol 2004;18(4):259–263

23. Kabil MS, Eby JB, Shahinian HK. Fully endoscopic endonasal vs. transseptal transsphenoidal pituitary surgery. Minim Invasive Neurosurg 2005;48(6):348–354

24. Nasseri SS, McCaffrey TV, Kasperbauer JL, Atkinson JL. A combined, minimally invasive transnasal approach to the sella turcica. Am J Rhinol 1998;12(6):409–416

25. Dew LA, Haller JR, Major S. Transnasal transsphenoidal hypophysectomy: choice of approach for the otolaryngologist. Otolaryngol Head Neck Surg 1999;120(6):824–827

26. Sloan AE, Black KB, Becker DP. Lesions of the sella turcica. In: Donald PJ, ed. Surgery of the Skull Base. Philadelphia, PA: Lippincott-Raven; 1998:555–582

27. Banna M, Olutola PS. Patterns of pneumatization and septation of the sphenoidal sinus. J Can Assoc Radiol 1983;34(4):291–293

28. Kennedy DW. Functional endoscopic sinus surgery. Technique. Am J Rhinol 1985;111(10):643–649

29 Endoscopic Surgery for Clival and Posterior Fossa Lesions

Carl H. Snyderman, Paul A. Gardner, Juan C. Fernandez-Miranda, and Eric W. Wang

Endonasal approaches to the skull base are classified based on their orientation in sagittal and coronal planes.[1] In the sagittal plane, the endonasal approach provides access to lesions of the clivus and posterior fossa from the posterior clinoids to the foramen magnum and upper cervical spine. In the posterior (inferior) coronal plane, the endonasal approach extends laterally below the petrous bone to the medial jugular tubercle and jugular bulb. For centrally located lesions, an endonasal approach provides maximal access with minimal manipulation of normal neural and vascular structures. Limitations of the approach are established by the pituitary gland, the course of the internal carotid artery (ICA) and the cranial nerves, and involvement of intradural structures.

Anatomical Considerations

The clivus is divided into three sections: superior, middle, and inferior (**Fig. 29.1**). The superior clivus is situated posterior to the pituitary gland and extends from the posterior clinoids to the floor of the sella. It is bounded laterally by the cavernous sinus and cavernous segment of the ICA. Intracranially, the superior clivus is associated with the third cranial nerve and the basilar apex. The middle clivus corresponds to the clival recess and extends from the bottom of the sella to the floor of the sphenoid sinus. It is bounded laterally by the paraclival segment of the ICA and the medial petrous apex. Intracranially, the middle clivus is associated with the distal part of the sixth cranial nerve as it passes deep to the paraclival ICA and enters Dorello canal on the superior surface of the petrous bone (**Fig. 29.2**). The inferior clivus extends from the floor of the sphenoid sinus to the foramen magnum. Laterally, it is bounded by the petroclival junction, medial jugular tubercle, and the occipital condyles. Intracranially, the lower third of the clivus is associated with the vertebral arteries, vertebrobasilar junction, and the associated origin of the sixth cranial nerve and the ninth, tenth, and twelfth cranial nerves.

Caudally, the first and second cervical vertebrae (C1 and C2) are situated posterior to the nasopharynx. Access is bounded by the eustachian tubes laterally and the plane of the palate inferiorly (**Fig. 29.1**). The ring of C1 lies just below the level of the hard palate and is superficial to the odontoid process (superior part/peg of C2). The occipital condyles articulate with the lateral mass of C1. The vertebral artery is situated posterolaterally and pierces the dura between the

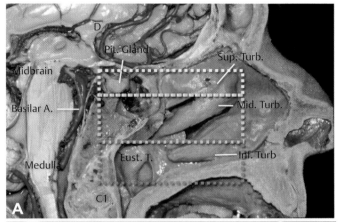

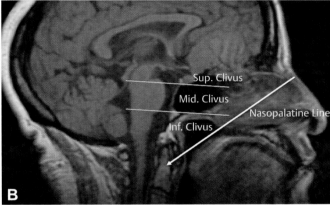

Figure 29.1 Anatomical classification of the clival region. (A) Sagittal cut on a silicon-injected anatomical specimen; the superior clivus (Sup. Turb., yellow interrupted line) corresponds to the dorsum sella (D) and posterior clinoids, and it lies behind the pituitary gland (Pit. Gland). The middle clivus (Mid. Turb., green interrupted line) extends from the sellar floor to the sphenoid sinus floor and relates posteriorly with the prepontine cistern and basilar trunk (Basilar A.). The inferior clivus (Inf. Turb., purple interrupted line) is located behind the nasopharynx and gives access to the premedullary cistern and vertebral (C1) arteries. (B) Sagittal cut of a magnetic resonance image; the transition between superior clivus (Sup. Clivus) and middle clivus (Mid. Clivus) is at the floor of the sella, whereas the transition between the middle and inferior clivus (Inf. Clivus) is at the floor of the sphenoid sinus. The nasopalatine line extends from the inferior margin of the nasal bone to the upper and posterior surface of the hard palate and marks the inferior limit of the endonasal transclival approach.

Source: © 2012 UPMC Center for Cranial Base Surgery.

posterior foramen magnum and lateral lamina of C1 before coursing anteriorly intradurally (**Fig. 29.2**).

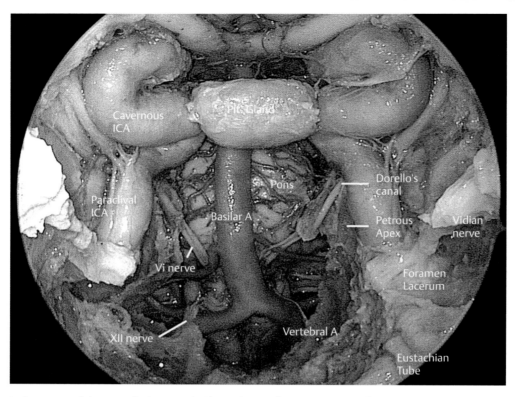

Figure 29.2 Surgical anatomy of the transclival approach. The sixth cranial nerve runs superolaterally in the prepontine cistern and enters the interdural segment just behind the paraclival internal carotid artery (ICA) to reach Dorello canal at the superior surface of the petrous apex. The hypoglossal nerve is the most ventral nerve at the region of the inferior clivus. Note the anatomical relationship of vidian nerve, foramen lacerum, paraclival ICA, and eustachian tube.
Source: © 2012 UPMC Center for Cranial Base Surgery.

An infrapetrous approach to the posterior cranial fossa extends laterally from the inferior clivus to the jugular bulb. It is bounded superiorly by the horizontal petrous and lacerum segments of the ICA and the petrous bone. The hypoglossal canal separates the occipital condyle (inferior) from the jugular tubercle (superior). The jugular bulb is superolateral to the hypoglossal canal. The parapharyngeal segment of the ICA is located lateral to the eustachian tube and the third division of the trigeminal nerve (foramen ovale).

Common Differential Diagnoses and Indications

Lesions of the clivus and posterior fossa are most commonly neoplastic. Tumors may arise from intracranial structures, from the bone, or from extracranial structures. The most common intracranial tumor is a meningioma that may involve any level of the clivus and extend to the petrous bone, craniocervical junction, or other adjacent regions. In particular, petroclival meningiomas can involve the upper, middle, and lower clivus and may have a posterior fossa component that extends posterolateral to the paraclival ICA (**Fig. 29.3**). Meningiomas appear as hypervascular tumors on imaging and usually have a characteristic dural tail. A minority of tumors are completely intraosseous. If incidental,

these are often very slow growing and can be observed initially. Primary bone neoplasms are usually chordomas or chondrosarcomas. Chordomas are more centrally located whereas chondrosarcomas typically originate more laterally, theoretically from the petroclival synchondrosis (**Fig. 29.4**). On imaging, chordomas and chondrosarcomas are osteolytic lesions that are characteristically heterogeneously enhancing and bright and loculated on T2-weighted magnetic resonance imaging. Biopsy is indicated if these tumors are suspected, but if the lesion is more consistent with the more common entity of fibrous dysplasia (which only rarely requires treatment in the setting of progressive cranial neural compression), computed tomography scan should be evaluated for the typical ground-glass appearance of fibrous dysplasia. Extracranial neoplasms that can involve the clivus are most frequently sinonasal malignancies (squamous cell carcinoma, nasopharyngeal carcinoma, adenoid cystic carcinoma, adenocarcinoma, and so on) that arise in the nasopharyngeal mucosa and invade the surrounding soft tissues and bone. All these tumors require biopsy to determine proper treatment, but surgery often plays only a salvage role after radiation and/or chemotherapy. Surgical debulking of the extradural component of sinonasal malignancy before radiotherapy may be considered for relief of symptoms and to enhance the therapeutic effect of radiotherapy.

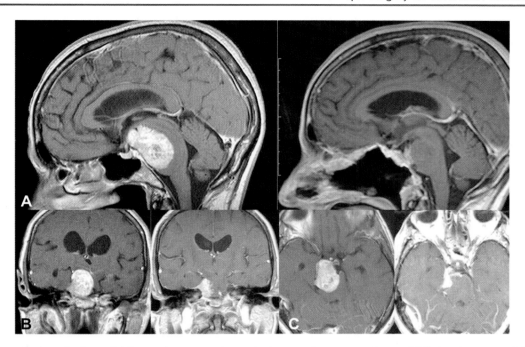

Figure 29.3   Petroclival meningioma. (A) Pre- and postoperative sagittal magnetic resonance image (MRI) showing successful decompression of the brainstem and small tumor remnant through a transclival approach; note the preoperative extension of the tumor behind the sella at the superior clival region and its complete removal on the postoperative imaging. (B) Pre- and postoperative coronal MRI; there is some residual tumor laterally, adjacent to the tentorium. (C) Pre- and postoperative axial MRI; as in (B), there is some residual tumor adjacent to the tentorium; the transclival approach is best suited for removal of tumors with predominant clival component because the petrosal extension of the tumor is less reachable.

Source: © 2012 UPMC Center for Cranial Base Surgery.

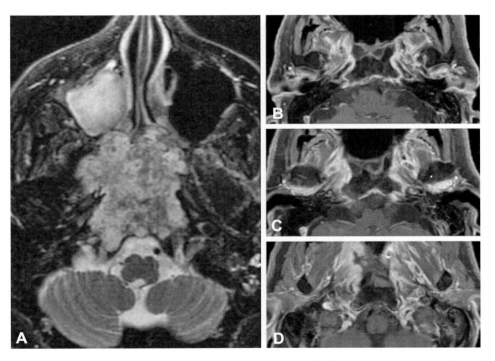

Figure 29.4   Clival chordoma. (A) Preoperative axial magnetic resonance image (MRI) showing a very large chordoma that extends from the superior to the inferior clival region and invades the retro and parapharyngeal spaces as well as the petrous apices and occipital condyles. (B to D) Postoperative axial MRIs at the level of the petrous apex (B), jugular tubercle (C), and occipital condyle (D), demonstrating gross total resection of the tumor.

Source: © 2012 UPMC Center for Cranial Base Surgery.

Inflammatory disease may also involve the clivus and upper cervical spine. In patients with severe osteoarthritis, rheumatoid arthritis, or congenital anomalies, degeneration of the upper cervical spine can result in basilar invagination or inflammatory pannus around the odontoid. The majority of these cases can be treated by fusion to address the underlying instability, but irreducible compression can require an anterior decompression. Osteoradionecrosis of the clivus is a sequela of high-dose radiation therapy for sinonasal cancers and can be difficult to distinguish from recurrent neoplasm. Osteomyelitis of the clivus can be associated with osteoradionecrosis or necrotizing otitis externa and may be present even though the original ear infection has resolved. Biopsy is often necessary to confirm the diagnosis and identify offending bacteria. Drainage of frank abscess or debridement of extensively involved bone can be necessary for resolution.

Operative Preparation

Proper positioning of the patient is necessary to prevent hindrance of surgical instruments, maximize surgeon's comfort, and maintain line of sight for optical navigation systems. For superior transclival approaches, the head is hyperextended to allow instruments to clear the chest and allow reverse Trendelenburg (head-up) positioning to decrease venous congestion, especially in obese patients. Midclival and inferior transclival approaches require a more neutral position because of the low trajectory. This also raises the upper cervical spine relative to the plane of the hard palate.

Neurophysiologic monitoring of cortical function (somatosensory-evoked potentials) and cranial nerves (electromyography) is performed.[2] If dissection of intradural tumor from the brainstem is anticipated, brainstem auditory evoked response monitoring is also performed. Intraoperatively, the use of a nerve stimulator for dissection further decreases the risk of cranial nerve injury.

Antibiotic prophylaxis consists of a third- or fourth- generation cephalosporin with dural penetration (such as ceftriaxone or cefepime). Steroids are not routinely administered unless there is hypopituitarism (hydrocortisone), vision loss (methylprednisolone), or dissection of cranial nerves is anticipated (dexamethasone). Antiseptic prepping of the nasal cavity is confined to the nasal vestibule to avoid mucosal injury and olfactory loss. Topical vasoconstriction is achieved with oxymetazoline-soaked pledgets. Normotensive anesthesia (mean arterial blood pressure greater than 80 mm Hg) is maintained to prevent brain or nerve ischemia, especially when there is neural compromise from tumor compression.

Surgical Techniques

Transclival Approaches

A superior transclival approach provides access to lesions posterior to the pituitary gland and requires a transposition of the pituitary gland. Following a bilateral sphenoidotomy, the sella is decompressed with removal of bone to at least the medial margins of the cavernous sinus. The posterior planum and tuberculum are also removed to provide room for upward displacement of the pituitary gland. The pituitary can be transposed extradurally or intradurally. Extradural transposition merely requires dissection of the sellar dura from the floor of the sella and dorsum sellae. This can provide significantly greater caudal access to the upper clivus and subsequent intradural space while limiting the risk of hormonal dysfunction (**Fig. 29.3**). In contrast, intradural pituitary transposition[3] requires significant pituitary gland dissection, sacrifice of inferior hypophyseal artery supply, and disconnection from venous drainage, all combining for a significant risk of subsequent pituitary dysfunction. The dura of the sella is incised and the diaphragm is cut up to the infundibulum, freeing the gland to swing upward. The pituitary gland is dissected free from loose fibroconnective attachments to the cavernous sinus laterally. One or both inferior hypophyseal vessels can be sacrificed to mobilize the gland. It is important to preserve vascular supply from the superior hypophyseal vessels. The gland can now be displaced superiorly into the suprasellar space. The dura overlying the dorsum sellae and posterior clinoids is now exposed and can be removed, followed by careful drilling of the adjacent bone. To avoid injury to the ICA, torsion of the bone of the posterior clinoids should be avoided because a sharp projection and even a calcified dural ring can extend posterior to the cavernous ICA.

A middle transclival approach provides access to the medial petrous apex and is used to access lesions of the petrous apex such as cholesterol granulomas.[4–6] It may be combined with an infrapetrous approach if the lesion is situated posterior to the petrous ICA. Following a wide sphenoidotomy, the course of the paraclival ICA is identified. In well-pneumatized cases, it is readily apparent but may be partially obscured by lateral septations of the sphenoid sinus. In poorly pneumatized sinuses, the vidian nerve and canal should be identified to provide a rough estimate of the paraclival ICA, keeping in mind that the nerve will ultimately cross laterally over the horizontal petrous ICA to join with the greater superficial petrosal nerve and deep petrosal nerve. The medial surface of the medial pterygoid plate forms a sagittal plane that is shared by the paraclival ICA. Drilling of the bone inferior to the sellar floor and medial to the paraclival ICA exposes cells of the petrous apex. With expansile lesions such as cholesterol granulomas, the lesion often expands into the clival recess and creates the surgical corridor (**Fig. 29.5**). The sixth cranial nerve courses superolaterally in Dorello canal behind the paraclival ICA and is susceptible to thermal injury from drilling or dissection in this area (**Fig. 29.2**). To gain additional access to the petrous apex, it is sometimes necessary to decompress the paraclival ICA by carefully removing the overlying bone. This allows lateral displacement of the artery and can add 3 to 5 mm of exposure. Instrumentation of the deep surface of the ICA should be avoided.

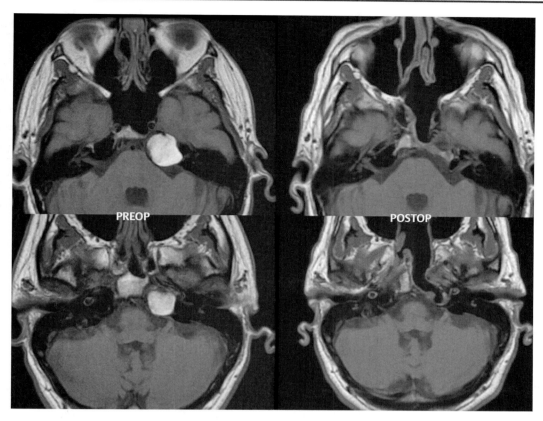

Figure 29.5 Cholesterol granuloma. Preoperative and postoperative axial magnetic resonance image showing complete drainage of the granuloma.

Source: © 2012 UPMC Center for Cranial Base Surgery.

An inferior transclival approach[7] is often combined with a middle transclival approach to provide access from the floor of the sella to the foramen magnum for tumors such as chordomas, meningiomas, and nasopharyngeal cancers. The nasopharyngeal mucosa and underlying rectus capitis and longus capitis muscles are resected to expose the dense pharyngobasilar fascia adherent to the clival bone. This is removed by drilling the cortical surface of the bone. Superiorly, lateral exposure is limited by the paraclival ICAs as detailed above and pars nervosa of the jugular foramen. Inferiorly, removal of clival bone is limited by the occipital condyles and hypoglossal canal (**Fig. 29.6**). The medial half of the occipital condyle can be drilled without the loss of stability. If the dura is to be resected, the dural incision should be placed to avoid injury to the basilar artery, based on preoperative imaging and a Doppler probe. Intradural tumors may also displace the sixth cranial nerves anteriorly, where they can be injured by the dural incision. Intraoperative electromyographic stimulation can be helpful in localizing the nerve after bony removal and before opening of the dura.

A transodontoid approach[8–10] is primarily used for the treatment of basilar invagination, but it may be employed for neoplasms at the foramen magnum and rare traumatic injuries. C1 and the odontoid process of C2 are universally accessible through the nasal cavity and with basilar invagination, they are situated even more superiorly than usual, thereby improving their access. The soft tissues of the nasopharynx are resected between the eustachian tubes and from the sphenoid rostrum to the plane of the soft palate. Tortuous parapharyngeal ICAs may project medially to the fossa of Rosenmüller and are at an increased risk with lateral dissection. To provide an adequate bilateral exposure at the plane of the palate, it is necessary to resect the posterior edge of the nasal septum and drill the midline of the hard palate posteriorly. The ring of C1 is exposed and removed with drilling and bone rongeurs out to the lateral mass. Further removal of bone laterally may put the vertebral artery at risk as the transverse process is approached. The odontoid process is immediately posterior to the ring of C1 and the junction may be indistinguishable with drilling, especially when there is severe degeneration. The central portion of the odontoid can be drilled out and the remaining shell of bone is dissected free from the ligamentous attachments. It is important to not disconnect the tip of the dens from the body of C2 while drilling as this leaves a mobile piece of bone to be disconnected from these sturdy attachments. The underlying pannus is carefully resected until transmitted pulsations from the underlying tectorial membrane or dura are noted. Complete resection of the pannus down to dura is usually not necessary and risks a cerebrospinal fluid leak.

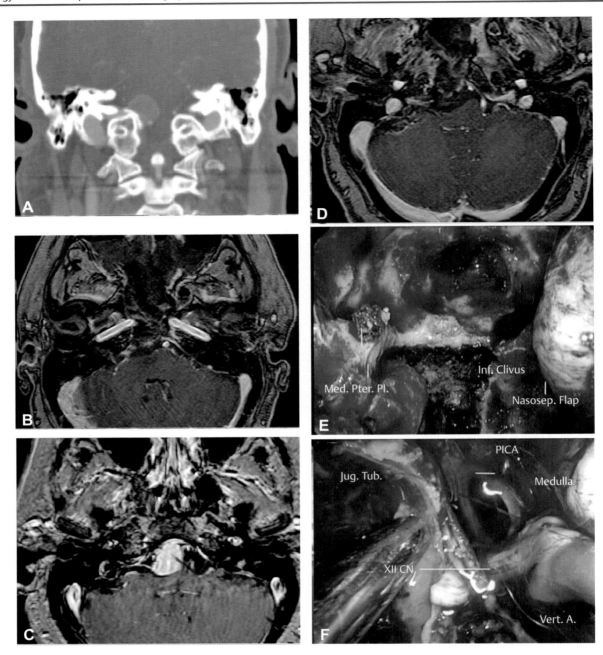

Figure 29.6   Jugular tubercle meningioma. (A) Coronal fine-cut computed tomographic angiography demonstrating a meningioma arising from the right jugular tubercle. (B) Postoperative axial magnetic resonance image (MRI) showing complete removal of the tumor. (C) Preoperative axial MRI. (D) Postoperative axial MRI showing complete removal of the tumor. (E) Intraoperative picture; the approach to the inferior clivus crosses the pharyngobasilar fascia and is limited laterally by the eustachian tubes and medial pterygoid plates. (F) Intraoperative picture; the inferior transclival approach extended to the jugular tubercle has been successfully completed; at the end of the tumor resection we can identify the vertebral artery, the posterior inferior cerebellar artery, and the hypoglossal nerve within the premedullary cistern.

Source: © 2012 UPMC Center for Cranial Base Surgery.

An infrapetrous approach in the coronal plane requires a transpterygoid approach to identify landmarks for exposure of the petrous ICA.[4,7] Following a maxillary antrostomy, the pterygopalatine space is exposed by removing the posterior wall of the maxillary sinus and the sphenopalatine artery is sacrificed. The soft tissues are elevated from the base of the pterygoids in a medial to lateral direction to identify the vidian (pterygoid) canal. Circumferential drilling of the pterygoid base around the vidian nerve and artery defines the genu of the ICA at the junction of the petrous and paraclival segments (**Fig. 29.2**). The medial eustachian tube is resected and the fibrocartilage of the foramen lacerum is carefully transected inferior to the carotid genu. Additional removal of bone inferior to the petrous ICA provides access to the inferior surface of the petrous bone. This approach carries a high risk for ICA injury given its close proximity and dense adherence of the cartilage of foramen lacerum. Lateral dissection is limited by the third division of the trigeminal nerve and the parapharyngeal ICA. Just rostral to the level of the foramen magnum, removal of bone laterally exposes the hypoglossal canal between the occipital condyle and medial jugular tubercle. Identification of the supracondylar ridge, which is the point of attachment of the longus capitis muscles, is helpful as this precisely predicts the hypoglossal canal in the depth.[11]

Reconstruction

Extradural dissections with no evidence of an intraoperative CSF leak do not require reconstruction and the surgical bed is covered with fibrin glue to protect the surgical site and promote healing. Dural defects are repaired with an intradural collagen or fascial graft and transposition of an extradural, onlay septal mucosal flap.[12] Deep clival defects require a wide flap that is oriented horizontally. Alternatively, autologous fat grafts are used to fill the clival defect and then covered with a septal flap. The reconstruction is supported with nasal tampons or a balloon catheter inflated with saline. Packing is necessary only if there is a dural defect or difficulty with hemostasis.

In cases with absent or involved septum, a deep or large defect that cannot be completely covered by the septal flap, or failed repair with a septal flap, an inferior turbinate flap may represent a viable option.[12] The inferior turbinate branch of the sphenopalatine provides the vascular supply for this flap, which can be challenging to harvest given the dense adherence of the bone of the turbinate.

Postoperative Care

Antibiotic prophylaxis is administered as long as nasal packing is in place and may be converted to oral administration after the first postoperative day. Following dural repair, nasal packing remains in place for 5 to 7 days and is removed as an outpatient. Lumbar spinal drains are not routinely used. Indications for lumbar drainage include a large dural defect, arachnoid cistern exposure or dissection, earlier CSF leak, earlier radiation therapy, and morbid obesity. Patients undergoing a transodontoid approach can resume oral feeding on the first postoperative day.

Complications

With use of the vascularized nasal septal flap, postoperative CSF leaks occur in less than 5% of all endonasal skull base surgeries with intraoperative CSF leaks[13,14] but may be higher in posterior fossa approaches and may not be apparent until nasal packing is removed. Early surgical revision is recommended to avoid the risk of meningitis associated with delay. The risk of meningitis remains low with this philosophy, despite an approach through a "contaminated" field (the nasal cavity).[15] In most cases, a small defect at the edge of the flap can be repaired by repositioning of the flap and/or placement of additional fascial and/or fat grafts. Small clival defects can be repaired with an inferior turbinate flap when other tissues are insufficient.

The sixth cranial nerve is the most susceptible to injury during endonasal surgery because of its small size, long course, central location, and frequent involvement with pathology appropriate for this approach (e.g., chordoma and clival meningioma). This results in diplopia with lateral gaze. If the nerve is anatomically preserved, recovery can be anticipated within several weeks to months. Otherwise, functional recovery is aided by oculoplastic surgery to realign the globes.

Vascular injury is the most feared complication of transclival approaches and can be avoided with recognition of anatomical landmarks, good surgical technique, and image navigation.[16] Fortunately, carotid artery injuries are rare (0.3%) with endonasal skull base surgery. In our experience, risk factors for injury include chondromatous tumors (chordomas and chondrosarcomas) with encasement or displacement of the ICA and lack of endoscopic surgical experience. Most carotid injuries will require angiographic sacrifice of the vessel.

Outcomes

There is still a paucity of large series evaluating endonasal surgery. However, at our center, a recent review of endoscopic endonasal resection of 60 chordomas revealed favorable outcomes with 83% gross total resection of primary chordomas.[17] A learning curve was identified with gross total rates improving to 89% for all cases during the past 3 years. A CSF leak rate of 20% was identified, which is comparable to open series. New, permanent cranial neuropathies occurred in only 7% of patients and there were no mortalities, illustrating the low morbidity of the approach.

Endoscopic transpterygoid nasopharyngectomy has been employed to resect a variety of sinonasal malignancies including epidermoid carcinomas, lymphoepithelioma, adenoid cystic carcinoma, adenocarcinoma, mucoepidermoid carcinoma, and sarcoma in 20 patients.[18] Negative microscopic margins were obtained in 95% of patients and no serious complications occurred except a single ICA injury without permanent sequelae. All but one patient received adjuvant therapy (radiotherapy with or without chemotherapy). Overall survival rate was 45% and local control was 65% with a mean follow-up of 33 months (range, 15 to 68 months).

At our center, 17 cholesterol granulomas have been treated endonasally with a transclival (9 patients) and a combination of transclival and infrapetrous (8 patients) approaches.[6] All patients had some improvement of their symptoms. There were two recurrences, both of which were successfully retreated endonasally. There were no major morbidities or mortalities, but 3 out of 17 patients (18%) had complications, including transient abducens palsy, epistaxis, chronic serous otitis media, and eye dryness.

Conclusions

Development of endonasal approaches to the clivus and posterior fossa has been enabled by advances in endoscopic technology, a greater understanding of endonasal skull base anatomy, and surgical team collaboration. An anatomically based, modular approach to the ventral skull base allows adaptation to the patient's surgical needs. Morbidity is acceptable and improved reconstructive techniques have limited the risk of a postoperative CSF leak. A growing body of literature on outcomes of endoscopic endonasal surgery of the clivus and posterior fossa demonstrates the value of these surgical techniques.

References

1. Snyderman CH, Pant H, Carrau RL, Prevedello DM, Gardner PA, Kassam AB. Classification of endonasal approaches to the ventral skull base. In: Stamm AC, ed. Transnasal Endoscopic Skull Base and Brain Surgery. New York, NY: Thieme; 2011:83–91
2. Thirumala PD, Kassasm AB, Habeych M, et al. Somatosensory evoked potential monitoring during endoscopic endonasal approach to skull base surgery: analysis of observed changes. Neurosurgery 2011;69(1, Suppl Operative):ONS64–ONS76, discussion ONS76
3. Kassam AB, Prevedello DM, Thomas A, et al. Endoscopic endonasal pituitary transposition for a transdorsum sellae approach to the interpeduncular cistern. Neurosurgery 2008;62(3, Suppl 1):57–72, discussion 72–74
4. Kassam AB, Gardner P, Snyderman C, Mintz A, Carrau R. Expanded endonasal approach: fully endoscopic, completely transnasal approach to the middle third of the clivus, petrous bone, middle cranial fossa, and infratemporal fossa. Neurosurg Focus 2005; 19(1):E6
5. Snyderman C, Kassam A, Carrau R, Mintz A. Endoscopic approaches to the petrous apex. Operative Techniques in Otolaryngology-Head and Neck Surgery 2006;17(3):168–173
6. Paluzzi A, Gardner P, Fernandez-Miranda J, et al. Endoscopic endonasal approach to cholesterol granulomas of the petrous apex: a series of 17 patients. J Neurosurg 2012;116(4):792–798
7. Gardner PA, Snyderman CH, Tormenti MJ, Fernandez-Miranda JC. Sella and beyond: approaches to the clivus and posterior fossa,

8. Kassam AB, Snyderman C, Gardner P, Carrau R, Spiro R. The expanded endonasal approach: a fully endoscopic transnasal approach and resection of the odontoid process: technical case report. Neurosurgery 2005;57(1, Suppl):E213, discussion E213
9. Nayak JV, Gardner PA, Vescan AD, Carrau RL, Kassam AB, Snyderman CH. Experience with the expanded endonasal approach for resection of the odontoid process in rheumatoid disease. Am J Rhinol 2007;21(5):601–606
10. Gardner P, Kassam A, Spiro R, et al. Endoscopic endonasal approach to the odontoid. In: Mummaneni P, Kanter A, Wang M, Haid R, eds. Cervical Spine Surgery: Current Trends and Challenges. St. Louis, MO: Quality Medical Publishing; 2009
11. Morera VA, Fernandez-Miranda JC, Prevedello DM, et al. "Far-medial" expanded endonasal approach to the inferior third of the clivus: the transcondylar and transjugular tubercle approaches. Neurosurgery 2010;66(6, Suppl Operative):211–219, discussion 219–220
12. Bhatki A, Pant H, Snyderman C, et al. Reconstruction of the cranial base after endonasal skull base surgery: local tissue flaps. Operative Techniques in Otolaryngology-Head and Neck Surgery 2010;21(1):74–82
13. Kassam AB, Thomas A, Carrau RL, et al. Endoscopic reconstruction of the cranial base using a pedicled nasoseptal flap. Neurosurgery 2008;63(1, Suppl 1):ONS44–ONS52, discussion ONS52–ONS53
14. Zanation AM, Carrau RL, Snyderman CH, et al. Nasoseptal flap reconstruction of high flow intraoperative cerebral spinal fluid leaks during endoscopic skull base surgery. Am J Rhinol Allergy 2009;23(5):518–521
15. Kono Y, Prevedello DM, Snyderman CH, et al. One thousand endoscopic skull base surgical procedures demystifying the infection potential: incidence and description of postoperative meningitis and brain abscesses. Infect Control Hosp Epidemiol 2011;32(1):77–83
16. Carrau RL, Fernandez-Miranda JC, Prevedello DM, Gardner PA, Snyderman CH, Kassam AB. Management of vascular complications during endoscopic skull base surgery. In: Stamm AC, ed. Transnasal Endoscopic Skull Base and Brain Surgery. New York, NY: Thieme; 2011:386–391
17. Koutourousiou M, Snyderman CH, Fernandez-Miranda JC, Gardner PA. Skull base chordomas. Otolaryngol Clin North Am 2011;44(5):1155–1171
18. Al-Sheibani S, Zanation AM, Carrau RL, et al. Endoscopic endonasal transpterygoid nasopharyngectomy. Laryngoscope 2011;121(10):2081–2089

petrous apex, and cavernous sinus In: Georgalas C, Fokkens WJ, eds. Rhinology. Stuttgart, Germany: Thieme, 2013:758–771

30 Endoscopic and Endoscopic-Assisted Skull Base Surgery for Anterior Skull Base Malignancy: Management Rationale

Bharat B. Yarlagadda and Anand K. Devaiah

Sinonasal and skull base malignancies (SSBM) are relatively rare and comprise approximately 1 to 3% of all head and neck cancers.[1,2] Proximity of the tumor to vital neurovascular structures and insidious growth patterns result in advanced stage presentation. This can complicate the management of these patients, and necessitates a comprehensive evaluation. The vast majority of cases involve squamous cell carcinoma (SCC). Adenocarcinoma, adenoid cystic carcinoma, sinonasal undifferentiated carcinoma (SNUC), esthesioneuroblastoma, and other histopathologies comprise the remainder of cases.[3-5]

Although the use of an open transfacial or craniofacial approach is a time-honored method, endoscopic methods have been gaining favor for several reasons including but not limited to: increased experience in endoscopic surgery, growing understanding of the surgical outcomes, and the pursuit of reduced patient morbidity. The knowledge gap of our understanding of effectiveness of open approaches and those using endoscopic methods has been closing steadily. It is important to note that while endoscopic techniques are growing, being able to execute an open approach or collaborate with a colleague who can perform them is important for patient care. In the end, the goal is curing or reducing the patient's cancer burden with the least amount of morbidity.

Failure of local control has been established as a primary cause of death,[6,7] underscoring the importance of complete extirpation. The exact approach used depends on the location and degree of spread of the primary tumor and involvement of vital structures. For instance, the anterior craniofacial approach is used for tumors involving the sinonasal cavity and anterior cranial fossa. Treatment using open approaches alongside appropriate adjuvant therapies has been successful in achieving variable 5-year survival rates, in some studies ranging from 40 to 70%.[8-11]

However, open procedures can have undesirable results in terms of postoperative appearance. These patients may suffer loss of function because of alterations of the facial contour, nerve sacrifice, and loss of velopharyngeal competence, among other deficits. Endoscopic approaches have been used to reduce potential morbidities associated with transfacial and other access-related incisions (e.g., oral cavity, and oropharynx) while providing other enhancements to surgical access. Continued refinements

in equipment and technique, as well as ongoing outcomes reporting, have allowed endoscopic surgeons to help create new branch points in the surgical paradigm for SSBM.

Patient Evaluation

History and Physical Examination

A thorough history and physical examination in a patient with sinonasal neoplasm can provide vital clues regarding the extent of the lesion. Nasal obstruction, epistaxis, anosmia, recurrent sinusitis, and facial pain and pressure are common symptoms and may allow the lesion to masquerade as a benign pathology. Endoscopic examination of the nasal cavity is essential (**Fig. 30.1**), but may be obscured by the presence of edema or secretions. The tumor bulk will also obscure the extent of involvement. Oral and oropharyngeal fullness can indicate mass effect from the tumor and extension beyond the sinonasal cavity. Trismus is another

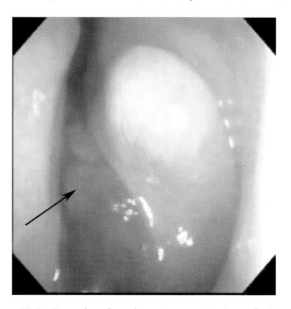

Figure 30.1 Example of endoscopic examination of sinonasal malignancy. Endoscopic examination of the nasal cavity is important in the assessment of sinonasal malignancies. Image shows the clinical examination of a patient with esthesioneuroblastoma (arrow) extending into the left nasal cavity from the anterior skull base.

sign of an advanced lesion, and can signify involvement of the pterygoid fossa, infratemporal fossa, or beyond. Careful palpation of the cervical lymph nodes is also important. The likelihood of cervical lymphadenopathy at presentation varies depending on the pathology but can be as high as approximately 20%, as for esthesioneuroblastoma.[12,13]

Ophthalmological examination should be undertaken in patients with possible or known orbit involvement. Proptosis, decreased visual acuity, reduced ocular motility, epiphora, diplopia, pupil asymmetry, or visual field defects may indicate involvement of the orbit and visual system. These findings can help determine whether preservation of the orbit and its contents is feasible, modify patient counseling, and fine-tune the surgical approach. It can also help determine whether the approach should be open, endoscopic, or endoscopic-assisted. Involvement of the orbit is not necessarily an indication to routinely sacrifice the orbit, as this varies based on patient and disease characteristics.[14]

Neurological examination should be thorough and tailored for the patient. Cranial nerve function should be carefully assessed as deficits may indicate extent of the tumor including the possibility of perineural spread, a poor prognostic sign. Depending on the extent, a full neurological assessment may be necessary, including understanding of the handedness of the patient. With transcranial involvement, early involvement of a neurosurgical colleague in the evaluation and management of the patient will make treatment planning more effective.

Imaging

Imaging is necessary for staging and determining the extent of a lesion. Understanding local, regional, and distant involvement is critical to patient management. Baseline studies are useful to understand a patient's response to treatment. Of the imaging modalities, computed tomography (CT) scan is excellent for delineating bony changes surrounding a neoplasm and assessment of orbital involvement. The use of intravenous contrast permits assessment of tumor vascularity and involvement of the carotid vasculature. Magnetic resonance imaging (MRI) provides superior soft tissue characterization compared with CT, but poor for bony architecture; this is especially useful to understand dural and transcranial involvement, as well as perineural extension. In addition, T2-weighted imaging can differentiate entrapped secretions from tumor to better delineate disease extent. Positron emission tomography (PET) is employed at many centers for staging of regional and distant metastasis. Alternately, this can be accomplished with whole-body CT or MRI.

Biopsy

Tissue diagnosis is essential to management of a sinonasal malignancy. Biopsy with biting forceps under endoscopic vision will generally provide appropriate tissue for pathological analysis. Endoscopic biopsy in the office setting—using local anesthetic and decongestion—should be considered if the patient is amenable to an office-based biopsy and the tumor does not appear to be vascular; vascular tumors can bleed uncontrollably and can be difficult to manage in an office setting. If a vascular tumor is suspected, or the patient is not amenable to an office-based biopsy, then the biopsy should be performed in the operating room where bleeding can be controlled and the patient can be kept comfortable. Depending on the clinical picture, imaging may be obtained first to assess the vascularity and aid in decision making for tissue diagnosis. Having the patient perform a Valsalva maneuver while observing the mass for engorgement can help assess for intracranial or venous connection, and may further help determine the safest place to perform a biopsy. If doubt remains, fine-needle aspiration of the mass may be performed, but success with this method depends on sampling and expertise of the pathologist reading the needle aspirate.

Pathology

There are many histopathological varieties of sinonasal malignancy. With the exception of esthesioneuroblastoma, they share a staging system set forth by the American Joint Committee on Cancer (**Table 30.1**).[15] Recent revisions to the primary lesion staging criterion emphasize the importance of determining the extent of invasion and involvement of adjacent structures.

Squamous Cell Carcinoma

In multiple series, SCC represents the most common variety of sinonasal malignancy.[1,16] Numerous environmental agents have been described as risk factors including aflatoxin, nickel, chromium, and aromatic hydrocarbons.[17] Cervical metastases are present in approximately 10% of patients at initial diagnosis and are an independent prognostic indicator.[1,18,19] SCC may also arise from inverted papillomas of the sinonasal regions; such lesions demonstrate more aggressive local growth and a tendency for distant metastatic spread.[20]

Adenocarcinoma

This histopathology comprises approximately 10% of sinonasal malignancies rendering it the second most common variety.[4] Chronic exposure to various dust particles of wood, leather, and textiles is an associated risk factor. Sinonasal adenocarcinoma is characterized by aggressive local growth and infrequent metastasis.

Sinonasal Undifferentiated Carcinoma

SNUC was previously classified as a form of high-grade epithelial malignancy with possible neuroendocrine differentiation but is now considered a distinct carcinoma

Table 30.1   Staging System for Tumors of the Nasal Cavity and Paranasal Sinuses as Set Forth by the American Joint Committee on Cancer

Primary Tumor (T)	
TX	Primary tumor cannot be assessed.
T0	No evidence of primary tumor.
Tis	Carcinoma in situ.
Maxillary Sinus	
T1	Tumor limited to maxillary sinus mucosa with no erosion or destruction of bone.
T2	Tumor causing bone erosion or destruction including extension into the hard palate and/or middle meatus, except extension to posterior wall of maxillary sinus and pterygoid plates.
T3	Tumor invades any of the following: bone of the posterior wall of the maxillary sinus, subcutaneous tissues, floor or medial wall of orbit, pterygoid fossa, ethmoid sinuses.
T4a	Moderately advanced local disease. Tumor invades anterior orbital contents, skin of cheek, pterygoid plates, infratemporal fossa, cribriform plate, sphenoid or frontal sinuses.
T4b	Very advanced local disease. Tumor invades any of the following: orbital apex, dura, brain, middle cranial fossa, cranial nerves other than maxillary division of trigeminal nerve (V2), nasopharynx, or clivus.
Nasal Cavity and Ethmoid Sinuses	
T1	Tumor restricted to any one subsite,[a] with or without bony invasion.
T2	Tumor invading two subsites in a single region or extending to involve an adjacent region within the nasoethmoidal complex, with or without bony invasion.
T3	Tumor extends to invade the medial wall or floor of the orbit, maxillary sinus, palate, or cribriform plate.
T4a	Moderately advanced local disease—tumor invades any of the following: anterior orbital contents, skin of nose or cheek, minimal extension to anterior cranial fossa, pterygoid plates, sphenoid or frontal sinuses.
T4b	Very advanced local disease—tumor invades any of the following: orbital apex, dura, brain, middle cranial fossa, cranial nerves other than V2, nasopharynx, or clivus.

Adapted from reference 15.

Note: This system does not apply to nonepithelial tumors such as those of lymphoid tissue, soft tissue, bone, cartilage, and mucosal melanoma.

[a]The nasal cavity includes four subsites: septum, floor, lateral wall, and vestibule. The ethmoid sinuses and maxillary sinuses are divided into two subsites each: left and right.

of uncertain histogenesis. The tumor often presents with a rapid onset of symptoms relative to the slow and insidious nature of other sinonasal malignancies. Grossly, SNUC is characterized by a high degree of local invasiveness with involvement of multiple anatomic subsites. Histologically, there is a dense hypercellular proliferation, a high mitotic rate, and a lack of squamous or glandular differentiation.[21] There is no specific characteristic immunohistochemical staining pattern, but these studies are crucial to rule out other entities on the differential diagnosis, namely, esthesioneuroblastoma.

Esthesioneuroblastoma

This uncommon malignancy is thought to arise from the neuroepithelium of the olfactory bulb and is located at the interface of sinonasal cavity and the anterior skull base. The most widely used classification scheme is the Kadish staging system[22] with stage A lesions confined to the nasal cavity, stage B lesions involving the paranasal sinuses, and stage C lesions extending to include regions outside of the sinonasal cavities. The value of the Kadish staging system in prognostication was confirmed by multiple reports and it is highly utilitarian in its simplicity.

Esthesioneuroblastoma can occur at any age but demonstrates a bimodal distribution with peak incidence in the second and sixth decades of life, without a gender predilection.[23] The tumor demonstrates an insidious growth pattern often resulting in presentations at advanced stages with extensive local destruction and tumor involvement. Approximately 5 to 8% of cases have cervical lymphadenopathy at the time of diagnosis and 20 to 25% of patients eventually develop regional metastatic disease. Note that 62% of esthesioneuroblastoma cervical metastases occur 6 months or more after primary treatment.[13] This pattern of delayed regional metastasis may be because of lymphatic micrometastases undetected at the time of initial staging. The ideal treatment of the clinically negative neck in patients with esthesioneuroblastoma is under investigation.

Other Pathologies

Multiple other histopathologies affecting the sinonasal cavity exist including soft tissue and bony sarcomas, adenoid cystic carcinoma, mucosal melanoma, and lymphoma. Reports of these pathologies are usually limited to case series and retrospective reports. The principles of oncological resection used for treatment of more common pathologies are applicable to these lesions as well.

Survival

The American Joint Committee on Cancer describes observed and relative survival rates for sinonasal malignancy of epithelial origin (**Fig. 30.2**). Survival data for nonepithelial tumors of the sinonasal region are often grouped with data from other head and neck subsites given the relatively low incidence, which often confounds survival statistics. SCC is frequent enough to characterize this histopathology with independent survival date based on staging.[1] Prognostic indicators include the T staging, status of lymphatic spread to the neck, pathological characteristics, such as extracapsular spread from lymph nodes, perineural invasion, and tumor thickness.[15] Histopathology is also crucial for prognosis as different tumors have different biological behavior. For example, mucosal melanoma is well known to have much worse prognosis than SCCA or adenocarcinoma.[10] SNUC also has a poor prognosis for overall survival.[24]

Basic Considerations of the Endoscopic Approach

Over the past two decades, advancements in endoscopic technology have allowed for the development of minimally invasive resection techniques via an endonasal approach. Such approaches were initially described for benign sinonasal pathology such as papillomas[25] and juvenile nasopharyngeal angiofibroma.[26] Application to malignancies was spurred by improvements such as instrumentation, hemostatic techniques, image-guidance systems, biological dressings, and advances in reconstruction (**Fig. 30.3**). The application of endoscopic and endoscopic-assisted techniques to the resection of nasal and paranasal sinus malignancies is more controversial, primarily because of the concern about violating oncological principles and en bloc resections.

Practitioners of the endoscopic approach should adhere to the principles of proper visualization of the lesion, oncological resection with appropriate margins, preservation of critical neurovascular structures, and secure reconstruction of defects including those involving the dura (**Fig. 30.4**). With endoscopic visualization, endomicroscopic examination of the patient's anatomy can be done with superior visualization compared with standard microscopy by eliminating line-of-site issues through angled endoscopes. However, if oncological and reconstructive principles cannot be met, an open or combined endoscopic-assisted approach should

be considered. Endoscopic-assisted approaches combine the necessary portion of an open approach (e.g., resection of involved external soft tissue) with the ability to navigate deep into the skull base through smaller access portals.

Endoscopic and endoscopic-assisted surgery is not typically a "single surgeon" procedure for malignancy. Multidisciplinary operative teams are typically needed with the involvement of otolaryngology, neurosurgery, ophthalmology, and others. While there are single-surgeon techniques, two-surgeon techniques are more often employed in the setting of complicated malignancies. This allows a greater ability for surgical manipulation, with one surgeon providing visualization and another performing bimanual surgical dissection. For endoscopic-assisted methods, tumors may be approached through multiple approaches, including combining endonasal and open transcranial approaches if needed.

A way to consider endoscopic surgery is to view the approach and resection as defined by approach corridors. This has been well described in the open literature, with the paradigm shifted because of the use of endoscopic methods; in contrast with open techniques, a wide lateral corridor is not needed to reach deep in the skull base (**Fig. 30.5**). The surgeon can choose a more direct path to a lesion and use the endoscope to reach it. This allows access with the least manipulation of healthy tissue.

The limits of endoscopic resection continue to expand with the improvement in techniques and equipment. Tumors that preclude a completely endoscopic approach include those with involvement of superficial structures such as skin and subcutaneous fat. Furthermore, invasion of the anterior orbit or globe, or lesions superior or lateral to the optic nerve can be difficult to access endoscopically.[26,27] Tumors meeting these criteria should be approached by an open or endoscopic-assisted approach.

The goals of surgery often depend on the histopathology of the lesion. For most tumors, such as SCC, esthesioneuroblastoma, or adenocarcinoma, complete extirpation is desired. In cases of highly aggressive local growth such as tumors that encase the carotid artery or invade the cavernous sinus, surgical excision has a high morbidity and mortality. It is often reserved for salvage after neoadjuvant chemotherapy with or without radiation. For tumors, such as adenoid cystic carcinomas, however, even procedures with curative intent often cannot remove the entirety of the lesion because of the potential for extensive perineural spread into the skull base and intracranial cavity. The goal is to remove as much tumor as possible with as little damage to the cranial nerves, orbit, and other vital structures in preparation for adjuvant therapies. For patient with metastatic disease or those medically unfit for lengthy surgeries, palliative resection is performed to relieve symptoms such as mass effect and pressure, epistaxis, nasal obstruction, and pain. The ease of access to the endonasal corridor makes repeat palliative debulking procedures a possibility.[26,27]

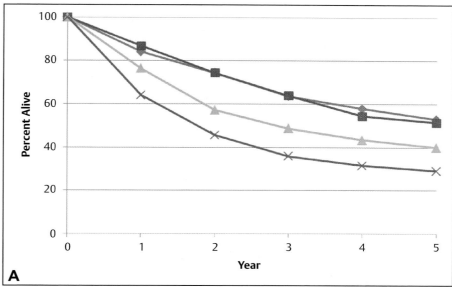

Observed Survival	1	2	3	4	5	95% CIs	Cases
Stage 1 ◆	84.1	74.4	63.6	57.9	53.0	43.2–62.8	144
Stage 2 ■	86.8	74.4	63.9	54.4	51.5	42.7–60.2	159
Stage 3 ▲	76.4	57.1	48.7	43.4	40.0	33.9–46.1	329
Stage 4 X	64.0	45.6	35.9	31.7	29.2	25.7–32.7	798

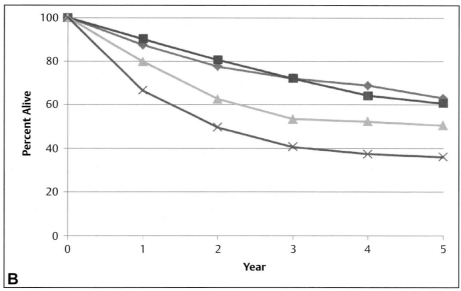

Relative Survival	1	2	3	4	5	95% CIs	Cases
Stage 1 ◆	87.6	77.4	72.1	68.8	62.9	51.2–74.6	144
Stage 2 ■	90.3	80.6	72.1	64.1	60.6	50.3–70.9	159
Stage 3 ▲	79.8	62.4	53.2	52.0	50.3	42.6–58.0	329
Stage 4 X	66.5	49.4	40.6	37.3	35.9	31.6–40.3	798

Figure 30.2 (A) Five-year, observed survival by American Joint Committee on Cancer (AJCC) stage for sinonasal carcinomas (all histologies). The 95% confidence intervals (CIs) correspond to 5-year survival rates. (B) Five-year, relative survival by AJCC stage for sinonasal carcinomas (all histologies). The 95% CIs correspond to 5-year survival rates.

Printed with permission from: American Joint Committee on Cancer (AJCC), Chicago, IL. Nasal cavity and paranasal sinuses. In: Edge SB, Byrd DR, Compton CC, Fritz AG, Greene FL, Trotti A, eds. *AJCC Cancer Staging Manual*. 7th ed. New York, NY: Springer; 2010:69–73.

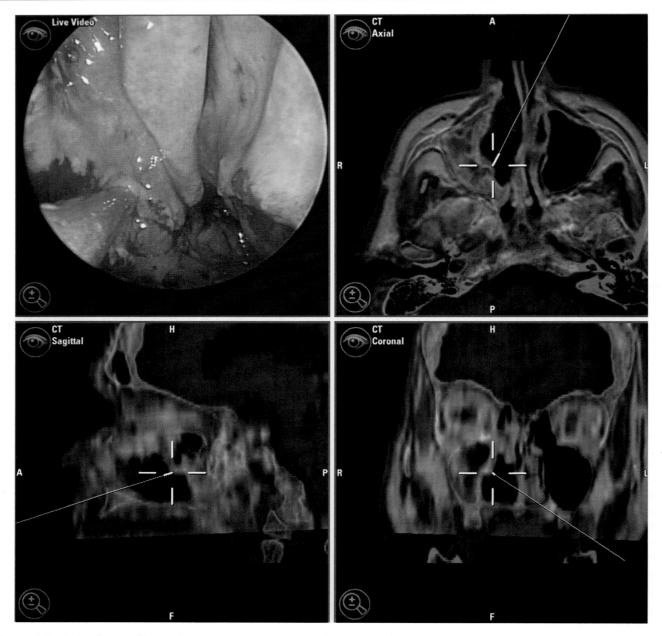

Figure 30.3 Technology enabling endoscopic tumor resections. Different technologies have enabled resection of malignancies through an endoscopic route. A key technology is image guidance, with the ability to fuse computed tomography scan, magnetic resonance imaging, and positron emission tomography images. Image shows an endoscopic view of a sarcoma extending into the infratemporal fossa, localized with image guidance, to allow for intraoperative navigation.

Much of the hesitation to accept the endoscopic or some endoscopic-assisted approaches is centered on the likely inability to preserve the en bloc excision of a tumor. The classic en bloc resection may not be possible because of the size of the lesion relative to the operative portal. As such, it is often necessary to debulk the tumor to gain full access of the lesion, with acquisition of the same margins as one would in an open procedure.[28] There is concern that this could lead to seeding of the tumor into uninvolved tissues and violate the principles of oncological resection. However, in the case of sinonasal lesion, the debulking reduces the volume of tumor growing into the air-filled cavities of the sinuses and does not violate or manipulate normal tissue planes.[27] In addition, large series report that a true en bloc resection is rarely achieved even in the traditional craniofacial and open approaches.[29] There are no data to suggest that en bloc excision provides an advantage in survival or recurrence. Piecemeal excisions have proven successful in various other scenarios including treatment of cutaneous malignancy (e.g., Moh excisions), performance of endoscopic laryngeal surgery, and excision of inverting papillomas. More important than en bloc excision is the

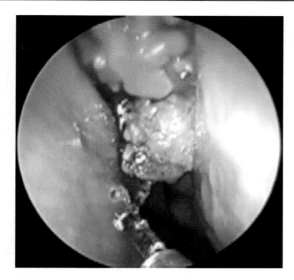

Figure 30.4 Endoscopic resection of a malignant tumor. Image shows a sinonasal undifferentiated carcinoma undergoing carbon dioxide laser-assisted resection. Note the cut below the level of the tumor along the nasal septum to provide a wide margin for resection.

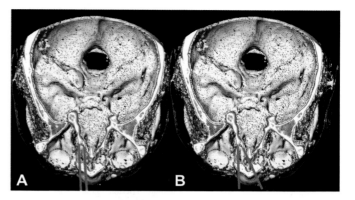

Figure 30.5 Endoscopic versus open corridor approach. An advantage of endoscopic approaches is the reduced surgical corridor aperture required to reach anatomic areas. Image shows an example of (A) the endoscopic corridor versus (B) the analogous open corridor to reach the same anatomic area.

achievement of clear surgical margins confirmed with frozen sectioning no matter what the means. This is underscored by the association of local recurrence and decreased survival with positive surgical margins.[30] Critics of the endoscopic approach state that the nature of the piece meal resection creates difficulty in confidently resecting a tumor with adequate surgical margins and that this risk of residual tumor outweighs the cosmetic benefit of incision-free surgery.[31] Cohen et al performed a retrospective analysis of patients undergoing either endoscopic or craniofacial resections anterior skull base malignancies and found that there was no difference in the rate of positive or close margins.[32] The authors concluded that the endoscopic approach did not compromise the ability to perform safe oncological resection.

Reconstruction, Postoperative Care, and Complications

Key concepts of perioperative care are presented here for the reader's consideration. It is important to note that there is no head-to-head study on reconstruction methods or postoperative management. Hence, there is a significant amount of variability in patient management and success using a variety of methods. Creating a ready-to-heal surface through use of tissue and grafts promotes healing. Surgical reconstruction with exposed fascia, fat, muscle, or bone can often be left to granulate in and mucosalize, but some patients may have a protracted course of healing and nasal crusting. Vascularized tissue or other resilient biological barriers can also help expedite healing and recovery. The use of tissue flaps has expanded the endoscopic surgeon's ability to reconstruct skull base defects with decreased incidence of postoperative cerebrospinal fluid (CSF) leaks.[33]

Other assistive efforts can help with healing postoperatively. Strip gauze, nasal tampons, balloons, or other devices placed intranasally can be used to support the reconstruction. They are removed at variable times postoperatively depending on the reconstruction and the practitioner. The senior author (A.K.D.) generally does not debride any tissue except after such devices are removed. Nasal airflow is maintained by cleaning the lower nasal airway, and then more extensive debridement and gentle sinus irrigation is performed after 1 month. This allows movement of air through the nose without destabilizing the reconstruction located superiorly. Till date, there have been no reconstruction failures in the senior author's practice by using this basic protocol, but other successful protocols exist.

The rate of CSF leakage is reported as low as 5% and the majority can be managed with the use of lumbar drainage catheters, bed rest, and head of bed elevation. Depending on surgeon's preference, lumber drainage catheters can be placed routinely in the perioperative period or can be reserved for cases of postoperative CSF leakage, complicated dural reconstructions, or suspected increased intracranial pressure.[34] Excess drainage of CSF should be avoided as this can lead to pneumocephalus and herniation.[35] CSF leaks are more prone to occur in cases of reconstructive graft or flap migration, movement of brain into excess dead space, previous radiation, and poor vascularity.[27,36,37] Leaks that do not resolve with CSF drainage may require revision surgery with placement of further grafting material through either an endoscopic or craniotomy approach.

Antibiotics are administered while the lumbar drain is in place. They are not typically given for surgical site prophylaxis unless there are concerns regarding preoperative sinonasal infection or seeding of the intracranial space. Reported infection rates are quite low, especially given the presence of sinonasal commensal organisms in the operative field. The risk of infectious complications, such as meningitis and intracranial abscess, increases with necrosis or sloughing of the reconstruction materials. Postoperative acute bacterial sinusitis also may occur and should be treated aggressively with culture-directed antibiosis. The risk of sinusitis can be reduced by unroofing adjacent sinus air cells to allow for adequate drainage.

Other perioperative complications include epistaxis, orbital hematoma, and mental status changes. The patient should follow-up on a close and routine basis for sinonasal debridement and monitoring of the surgical site. In the postoperative healing period, patients may experience dacryocystitis, atrophic rhinitis, and excess crusting. Crusting can be troublesome and is addressed with gentle debridement under direct visualization and nasal saline irrigations.

Outcomes

Perioperative factors related to the endoscopic approach have been reported in the literature. When compared with the craniofacial approach, patients treated with the endoscopic approach have a significantly shorter operative time, intensive care unit stay, and overall hospital stay.[36,37] Blood loss and transfusion rates are lower in the endoscopic approach but the difference is not significant.[37] The reported rate of postoperative complications varies from 6 to 27.8%, with CSF leak as the most frequent adverse outcome.[36,37] In most series, this is equivalent to or lower than the rate of complications in the patients undergoing craniofacial repair. In a large international collaborative series, Ganly et al report a complication rate of 36.3%, the most frequent being wound and central nervous system sequelae, and a mortality rate of 4.7%.[38]

The body of literature reporting oncological outcomes has increased as treatment centers gain experience with the endoscopic approach. Early results were reported by Stammberger et al.[39] About 36 patients with sinonasal and skull base malignancy were treated with a strictly endoscopic approach including 8 patients with esthesioneuroblastoma. The authors report that outcomes were equivalent to open approaches. A portion of patients were treated with adjunctive radiotherapy and all eight esthesioneuroblastoma patients were free of disease at 37 months. Roh et al report an early United States experience with 19 patients managed with an endoscopic approach.[40] Six patients required adjunct craniotomy for adequate resection and 15 patients received radiation therapy with or without chemotherapy either pre- or postoperatively. Patients treated with a curative intent has local recurrence rate of 21.4%, overall survival rate was 85.7% at a mean follow-up of 32.1 months, and the disease-free survival rate was 85.7% at a mean follow-up of 33.1 months. The authors conclude that these rates are comparable to open approaches as well.

Nicolai et al report a large series of patients who underwent endoscopic resection with or without adjunct craniotomy for various histopathologies.[36] In those undergoing a completely endoscopic approach, the rate of recurrence was 18.7%, the overall survival rate was 93.8%, and the disease-free survival was 90%. These numbers were quite favorable compared to the group requiring adjunct craniotomy. Recurrence rates were also stratified by specific histology showing rate of 9% for esthesioneuroblastoma, 23% for epithelial malignancies, and 65% for mucosal melanoma. Hanna et al report similar findings in a study of 93 patients undergoing a completely endoscopic approach and 27 patients with adjunct craniotomy.[41] There was no significant difference in disease-free survival rates or overall survival rates between the groups. Complication rates were similar as well. These findings should be interpreted with several caveats. A direct comparison of endoscopic to endoscopic-assisted procedures is difficult because of changes in technique over the study periods, relatively low number of cases, and variances in tumor staging within individual studies. In addition, many large European studies have a higher proportion of adenocarcinoma patients than would be found in the United States; this histopathology has a more favorable prognosis than, for instance, SCCA and undifferentiated carcinoma.[41]

Although numerous small series exist, meta-analyses have allowed meaningful investigation of outcomes. A meta-analysis of 361 patients from 23 publications of esthesioneuroblastoma studies, ranging from 1992 to 2008, analyzed results of endoscopic versus open methods for the first time in a large series.[35] Statistical analysis showed that surgical therapy has better outcomes than nonsurgical therapy and that endoscopic surgery produced better survival rates than open surgery. This difference was preserved even after stratifying for year of publication. However, when the patients are sorted by Kadish staging, there is a statistically significant finding that higher stage tumors (Kadish C and D) were more often treated with open surgery, which was a caveat of the study and study period. The significance of this difference is unclear, because previous studies have shown no difference in survival rates between T2, T3, and T4 tumors of various histologies, though T1 staging prognosticated a survival advantage.[42] In addition, the authors acknowledge that although there was no difference in median follow-up times, the open treatment groups had more cases of long-term follow-up. This is an important parameter in an entity known for temporally remote local recurrence and regional spread. Regardless, the study established a definite role in endoscopic and endoscopic-assisted treatment of esthesioneuroblastoma.

Meta-analyses for other entities are not available because of aggregation of outcomes data in the published studies without stratification based on histopathology. This is in spite of the higher incidence of histopathologies other than esthesioneuroblastoma. Analysis of available data on endoscopic treatment of sinonasal adenocarcinoma, for example, shows that proper meta-analysis is not possible because of aggregated data reporting and inconsistent follow-up periods.[4] However, overall survival rates for the endoscopic approach for adenocarcinoma range from 53 to 93.5%, and range from 40 to 70% in the open approach, suggesting that two approaches are comparable in outcomes.[4] Further data are needed and meta-analyses will be possible as more studies reach publication.

Multimodality Multidisciplinary Care

The management of SSBM often requires the input of surgeons, radiation oncologists, and medical oncologists. Many patients benefit from the use of radiation with or without chemotherapy in the treatment regimen. This varies according to histologic type. For example, the use of radiation therapy in early stage of esthesioneuroblastoma and use of radiation with chemotherapy for later stage tumors has been advocated.[43] Sinonasal mucosal melanoma also has better control with use of adjuvant radiation.[44] However, adjuvant therapies carry morbidities. Side effects of radiation to this area include atrophic rhinitis, frontal lobe atrophy and necrosis, blindness, cataracts, and hearing loss. Patients with high-risk features, such as dural invasion, adverse histology, or positive margins, obtain a benefit from adjuvant radiation.[45] Studies also show a potential role for induction chemotherapy in some advanced stage neoplasms.[46] Regardless, the treatment regimen should be tailored to the individual patient, taking into account the specifics of their disease and expected tolerance of therapy.

In addition to treatment for the tumor, one must remember to include other professionals who can help with the rehabilitation of the patient posttherapy. This can involve speech therapy, occupational therapy, physical therapy, and others. The return to a cancer-free, functional status is the goal of multidisciplinary care. Involving the necessary professionals in the pre- and posttreatment phases can help patients receive the appropriate, timely treatment needed.

Future Directions

The endoscopic approach continues to gain momentum with the release of encouraging outcomes data and technical improvements. Future developments will focus on advancing technologies and techniques, as well as studying their outcomes. Three-dimensional stereoscopic endoscopes are under study, which may improve depth perception and visualization over the currently used two-dimensional equipment; this may allow the surgeon more confidence in working near the delicate structures of the skull base. Intraoperative image navigation systems continue to evolve to employ better skull base algorithms in navigation, to incorporate CT, MRI, and PET imaging. Real-time intraoperative CT and MRI systems may help surgeons delineate changes in the skull base lesion and patient anatomy to better navigate and resect tumors. Robotic surgical technology may play a role in future treatment strategies, as the increased range of motion of these instruments may be invaluable in the confined spaces of the skull base.

Conclusion

Malignancy of the sinonasal cavity and skull base is not a single entity, but rather a classification of multiple pathologies with unique behaviors and disease trajectories. Improvements in endoscopic methods, technology, and outcome studies demonstrate the value of endoscopic and endoscopic-assisted surgery as another tool in the surgeon's armamentarium.

References

1. Lee CH, Hur DG, Roh HJ, et al. Survival rates of sinonasal squamous cell carcinoma with the new AJCC staging system. Arch Otolaryngol Head Neck Surg 2007;133(2):131–134
2. Orvidas LJ, Lewis JE, Weaver AL, Bagniewski SM, Olsen KD. Adenocarcinoma of the nose and paranasal sinuses: a retrospective study of diagnosis, histologic characteristics, and outcomes in 24 patients. Head Neck 2005;27(5):370–375
3. Cohen MA, Liang J, Cohen IJ, Grady MS, O'Malley BW Jr, Newman JG. Endoscopic resection of advanced anterior skull base lesions: oncologically safe? ORL J Otorhinolaryngol Relat Spec 2009;71(3):123–128
4. Devaiah AK, Lee MK. Endoscopic skull base/sinonasal adenocarcinoma surgery: what evidence exists? Am J Rhinol Allergy 2010;24(2):156–160
5. Katz TS, Mendenhall WM, Morris CG, Amdur RJ, Hinerman RW, Villaret DB. Malignant tumors of the nasal cavity and paranasal sinuses. Head Neck 2002;24(9):821–829
6. Alvarez I, Suárez C, Rodrigo JP, Nuñez F, Caminero MJ. Prognostic factors in paranasal sinus cancer. Am J Otolaryngol 1995;16(2):109–114
7. Porceddu S, Martin J, Shanker G, et al. Paranasal sinus tumors: Peter MacCallum Cancer Institute experience. Head Neck 2004;26(4):322–330
8. Batra PS, Citardi MJ, Worley S, Lee J, Lanza DC. Resection of anterior skull base tumors: comparison of combined traditional and endoscopic techniques. Am J Rhinol 2005;19(5):521–528
9. Dulguerov P, Jacobsen MS, Allal AS, Lehmann W, Calcaterra T. Nasal and paranasal sinus carcinoma: are we making progress? A series of 220 patients and a systematic review. Cancer 2001;92(12):3012–3029
10. Ganly I, Patel SG, Singh B, et al. Craniofacial resection for malignant melanoma of the skull base: report of an international collaborative study. Arch Otolaryngol Head Neck Surg 2006;132(1):73–78
11. Howard DJ, Lund VJ, Wei WI. Craniofacial resection for tumors of the nasal cavity and paranasal sinuses: a 25-year experience. Head Neck 2006;28(10):867–873
12. Cantù G, Bimbi G, Miceli R, et al. Lymph node metastases in malignant tumors of the paranasal sinuses: prognostic value and treatment. Arch Otolaryngol Head Neck Surg 2008;134(2):170–177
13. Zanation AM, Ferlito A, Rinaldo A, et al. When, how and why to treat the neck in patients with esthesioneuroblastoma: a review. Eur Arch Otorhinolaryngol 2010;267(11):1667–1671
14. Essig GF, Newman SA, Levine PA. Sparing the eye in craniofacial surgery for superior nasal vault malignant neoplasms: analysis of benefit. Arch Facial Plast Surg 2007;9(6):406–411
15. Nasal cavity and paranasal sinuses. In: Edge SB, Byrd DR, Compton CC, Fritz AG, Greene FL, Trotti A, eds. AJCC Cancer Staging Manual. 7th ed. New York, NY: Springer; 2010:69–73
16. Luong A, Citardi MJ, Batra PS. Management of sinonasal malignant neoplasms: defining the role of endoscopy. Am J Rhinol Allergy 2010;24(2):150–155

17. Weymuller EA Jr, Gal TJ. Neoplasms. In: Cummings CW, ed. Otolaryngology-Head and Neck Surgery. 4th ed. St. Louis: CV Mosby; 2005:1197–1214

18. Bhattacharyya N. Factors predicting survival for cancer of the ethmoid sinus. Am J Rhinol 2002;16(5):281–286

19. Bhattacharyya N. Factors affecting survival in maxillary sinus cancer. J Oral Maxillofac Surg 2003;61(9):1016–1021

20. Tanvetyanon T, Qin D, Padhya T, Kapoor R, McCaffrey J, Trotti A. Survival outcomes of squamous cell carcinoma arising from sinonasal inverted papilloma: report of 6 cases with systematic review and pooled analysis. Am J Otolaryngol 2009;30(1):38–43

21. Wenig BM. Undifferentiated malignant neoplasms of the sinonasal tract. Arch Pathol Lab Med 2009;133(5):699–712

22. Kadish S, Goodman M, Wang CC. Olfactory neuroblastoma. A clinical analysis of 17 cases. Cancer 1976;37(3):1571–1576

23. Thompson LD. Olfactory neuroblastoma. Head Neck Pathol 2009;3(3):252–259

24. Reiersen DA, Pahilan ME, Devaiah AK. Meta-analysis of treatment outcomes for sinonasal undifferentiated carcinoma. Otolaryngol Head Neck Surg 2012;147(1):7–14

25. Busquets JM, Hwang PH. Endoscopic resection of sinonasal inverted papilloma: a meta-analysis. Otolaryngol Head Neck Surg 2006;134(3):476–482

26. Carrau RL, Snyderman CH, Kassam AB, Jungreis CA. Endoscopic and endoscopic-assisted surgery for juvenile angiofibroma. Laryngoscope 2001;111(3):483–487

27. Snyderman CH, Carrau RL, Kassam AB, et al. Endoscopic skull base surgery: principles of endonasal oncological surgery. J Surg Oncol 2008;97(8):658–664

28. Devaiah AK, Larsen C, Tawfik O, O'Boynick P, Hoover LA. Esthesioneuroblastoma: endoscopic nasal and anterior craniotomy resection. Laryngoscope 2003;113(12):2086–2090

29. McCutcheon IE, Blacklock JB, Weber RS, et al. Anterior transcranial (craniofacial) resection of tumors of the paranasal sinuses: surgical technique and results. Neurosurgery 1996;38(3):471–479, discussion 479–480

30. Patel SG, Singh B, Polluri A, et al. Craniofacial surgery for malignant skull base tumors: report of an international collaborative study. Cancer 2003;98(6):1179–1187

31. Levine PA. Would Dr. Ogura approve of endoscopic resection of esthesioneuroblastomas? An analysis of endoscopic resection data versus that of craniofacial resection. Laryngoscope 2009;119(1):3–7

32. Cohen MA, Liang J, Cohen IJ, Grady MS, O'Malley BW Jr, Newman JG. Endoscopic resection of advanced anterior skull base lesions: oncologically safe? ORL J Otorhinolaryngol Relat Spec 2009;71(3):123–128

33. Hadad G, Bassagasteguy L, Carrau RL, et al. A novel reconstructive technique after endoscopic expanded endonasal approaches: vascular pedicle nasoseptal flap. Laryngoscope 2006;116(10):1882–1886

34. Batra PS. Minimally invasive endoscopic resection of sinonasal and anterior skull base malignant neoplasms. Expert Rev Med Devices 2010;7(6):781–791

35. Devaiah AK, Andreoli MT. Treatment of esthesioneuroblastoma: a 16-year meta-analysis of 361 patients. Laryngoscope 2009;119(7):1412–1416

36. Nicolai P, Battaglia P, Bignami M, et al. Endoscopic surgery for malignant tumors of the sinonasal tract and adjacent skull base: a 10-year experience. Am J Rhinol 2008;22(3):308–316

37. Eloy JA, Vivero RJ, Hoang K, et al. Comparison of transnasal endoscopic and open craniofacial resection for malignant tumors of the anterior skull base. Laryngoscope 2009;119(5):834–840

38. Ganly I, Patel SG, Singh B, et al. Complications of craniofacial resection for malignant tumors of the skull base: report of an International Collaborative Study. Head Neck 2005;27(6):445–451

39. Stammberger H, Anderhuber W, Walch C, Papaefthymiou G. Possibilities and limitations of endoscopic management of nasal and paranasal sinus malignancies. Acta Otorhinolaryngol Belg 1999;53(3):199–205

40. Roh HJ, Batra PS, Citardi MJ, Lee J, Bolger WE, Lanza DC. Endoscopic resection of sinonasal malignancies: a preliminary report. Am J Rhinol 2004;18(4):239–246

41. Hanna E, DeMonte F, Ibrahim S, Roberts D, Levine N, Kupferman M. Endoscopic resection of sinonasal cancers with and without craniotomy: oncologic results. Arch Otolaryngol Head Neck Surg 2009;135(12):1219–1224

42. Goffart Y, Jorissen M, Daele J, et al. Minimally invasive endoscopic management of malignant sinonasal tumours. Acta Otorhinolaryngol Belg 2000;54(2):221–232

43. Oskouian RJ Jr, Jane JA Sr, Dumont AS, Sheehan JM, Laurent JJ, Levine PA. Esthesioneuroblastoma: clinical presentation, radiological, and pathological features, treatment, review of the literature, and the University of Virginia experience. Neurosurg Focus 2002;12(5):e4

44. Moreno MA, Roberts DB, Kupferman ME, et al. Mucosal melanoma of the nose and paranasal sinuses, a contemporary experience from the M. D. Anderson Cancer Center. Cancer 2010;116(9):2215–2223

45. Bentz BG, Bilsky MH, Shah JP, Kraus D. Anterior skull base surgery for malignant tumors: a multivariate analysis of 27 years of experience. Head Neck 2003;25(7):515–520

46. Lee MM, Vokes EE, Rosen A, Witt ME, Weichselbaum RR, Haraf DJ. Multimodality therapy in advanced paranasal sinus carcinoma: superior long-term results. Cancer J Sci Am 1999;5(4):219–223

31 Endoscopic and Endoscopic-Assisted Anterior Skull Base Surgery for Malignancy: Surgical Considerations

Larry A. Hoover and Ashwin Ananth

Anterior skull base malignancies are a challenging problem because of the complex anatomy, vital adjacent and often involved structures, and many skull base fissures and foramina that transmit vessels and nerves and may allow central extension. Until 1960s there were only sporadic cases of transfascial resection of anterior skull base tumors in the United States,[1] and in Germany, by Schloffer (1906) and Hirsch (1910) were reported.[2] Too often these tumors were incompletely excised by isolated attempts from either below or above.

Extensive lesions in this area generally require the combined skills of a team of specialists, including otolaryngology/head and neck/skull base surgeons and neurosurgeons, to successfully resect lesions that extend both intra- and extracranially. Ketcham in 1963, and then subsequently in 1967, first described the combined transcranial and transfascial approach to these tumors.[3] Since then, the technologic developments of computed tomography (CT) and magnetic resonance image (MRI) scanning have significantly improved our ability to evaluate the extent of these tumors and plan surgical approaches preoperatively. When such imaging indicates a tumor is highly vascular, angiographic techniques allow embolization to markedly reduce operative bleeding and enhance tumor visualization. Modern operating room guidance systems allow visual display fusion of preoperative CT, MRI, and magnetic resonance angiography that greatly assists in complete resection with avoidance of excess bleeding.[4]

At our institution, we have organized a skull base surgical team consisting of the previously mentioned surgical specialties, and such a team is highly recommended at any institution performing this type of surgery. We frequently use the services of radiation and medical oncologists who understand our goals and treatment plan. We previously described the importance of the use of endoscopes during these resections and will discuss this use later on in this chapter.[3–5] In this chapter, we will explore important general considerations in the multidisciplinary approach, techniques, and rationale for endoscopic and endoscopic-assisted anterior cranial base surgery.

General Considerations and Institutional Experience

As a backdrop to this discussion, the authors reviewed the experience of the senior author (L.A.H.). During a 21-year time period, the senior author has treated 208 patients with anterior skull base lesions. Of the 208 patients who underwent anterior skull base tumor resection, 100 had sufficient information and follow-up at 5 years to be included in this review. Outcomes were separated into no evidence of disease, active disease, or death. Of the 100 patients included in this analysis, there were 63 (63%) males and 37 (37%) females, with a mean age of 56 years (standard deviation, 17 years). Presentation most commonly included a history of nasal obstruction, sinusitis, or unilateral epistaxis. Resected tumors included three main types: squamous cell carcinoma (29), adenoid cystic carcinoma (14), and esthesioneuroblastoma (26). The other histologic tumor types are shown in **Table 31.1**. When overall results

Table 31.1 Various Malignant Tumors Resected in Our Study Population[a]

Histologic Tumor Type	Patient Numbers
Squamous cell carcinoma	29
Esthesioneuroblastoma	26
Adenoid cystic carcinoma	14
Sarcoma	7
Adenocarcinoma	3
Lymphoma	3
Melanoma	3
Nasopharyngeal carcinoma	3
Sinonasal undifferentiated carcinoma	3
Small cell neuroendocrine carcinoma	3
Ameloblastoma	1
Hemangiopericytoma	1
Meningioma	1
Metastatic renal cell carcinoma	1
Mucoepidermoid carcinoma	1
Neuroblastoma, child	1
Total	100

[a]The tumor types are listed in order of frequency. Of note, ameloblastoma and meningioma are included in this analysis as both neoplasms exhibited high-grade malignant features and were treated with excision.

Table 31.2 Analysis of Survival Following the Resection of Malignant Anterior Skull Base Tumors[a]

Author	Publication Year	No. of Malignancies	Patient Survival		
			Survival	Alive with Disease (%)	Dead (%)
Ketcham and Van Buren[3]	1967	32	4 patients NED 20–59 mo 6 patients NED 5–9 y Total 10 NED 31%	13 patients (40)	28
Shah et al[4]	1997	115	NED 4.7 y 58% NED 10 y 48%	10	40
Kelley et al[9]	2000	29	NED 44%	17	41
Hoover and Ananth	N/A (internal review)	100	NED 5 y 65%	21	14

[a]As transcranial and transfascial approaches have evolved and endoscopy has become an important tool for visualization and evaluation of tumors, outcomes have improved along with postoperative cosmesis.

mo, month(s); y, year(s); NED, no evidence of disease.

of this patient group are compared with published reports in the literature, they compare favorably (**Table 31.2**). The technical considerations in this chapter reflect the experience in treating these patients.

Surgical Planning and Technology

Several technological advancements and tools assist in the execution of endoscopic and endoscopic-assisted surgery, and these are reviewed in detail in other chapters. However, it is important to realize how much technology has enabled the use of minimally invasive methods. The use of preoperative imaging with preoperative endoscopic examination is indispensable to planning and intraoperative execution (**Fig. 31.1**). CT, MRI, and positron emission tomography (PET) are the powerful tools that help the team understand what approaches to a malignancy will be necessary and the resulting defect to reconstruct. The use of image guidance, when combined with endoscopic instruments, has greatly improved our ability to perform delicate microscopic dissections at the skull base. Using instruments that are synchronized to image-guidance systems (e.g., guided-suction debriders and probes) allows for real-time navigation to confirm structures either in direct view or in proximity to the working space. Many systems will also allow for preoperative planning and with mapping of key structures such as the carotid, optic chiasm, and other important anterior skull base landmarks.

Operative Techniques and Rationale

Several different approaches exist in endoscopic and endoscopic-assisted skull base surgery. Most surgeons employing endoscopic methods feel that combining no incision or a cosmetic incision (specifically a sublabial/transmaxillary/facial degloving for access) with endoscopic resection techniques is an effective method to approach skull base malignancies. Endoscopic visualization of these tumors allows an excellent initial assessment of the tumor and a microscopic evaluation of tumor margins at the end of the procedure for complete resection.[5–7] The surgical strategy in this group of patients must be highly individualized because no two tumors are exactly alike. Tumor grade, aggressiveness, and patient health status must also be taken into account when weighing treatment options. Combined wide coronal flap, anterior craniotomy, and lateral rhinotomy (Weber-Ferguson) incisions may still be used for wide exposure and direct tumor visualization in some cases. However, over the years craniotomy size has been reduced and endoscopic instrumentation now allows excellent tumor visualization and removal through small cosmetic incisions or by the transnasal route alone. Often, even large anterior skull base tumors can now be removed by subfrontal craniotomy and endoscopic resection of nasal and sinus extensions.[5–8]

As the endoscopic corridor for operating is generally more restricted, there are several important considerations. The narrow cavities and recesses of the skull base rarely allow classic en bloc resections as are frequently performed in the soft tissue of the neck or oral cavity. The mass of large skull base tumors often obscures their site of origin and areas of invasion. The use of suction debriders, which are the workhorses for polyp removal, now allow the rapid excision of the main bulk of large tumors. Once these tumors are debulked, small nests and rests of residual tumor can be identified endoscopically and removed. Wide surgical margins are generally not possible with skull base tumors. Having a microscopic/endoscopic view can be beneficial in distinguishing subtle differences between normal tissue and those involved with tumor. It also allows identification and resection of all visible tumor from recesses found throughout the anterior skull base.

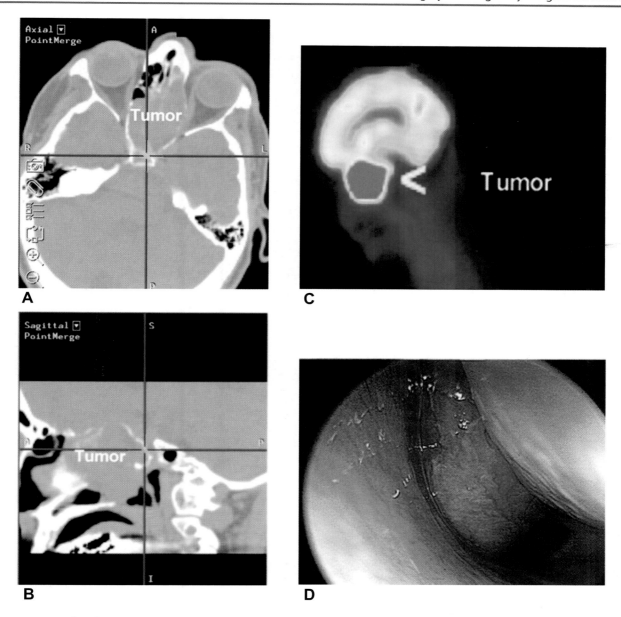

Figure 31.1 Examples of using preoperative technology to aid in surgical execution. (A) Axial computed tomography (CT) scan demonstrating a skull base tumor expanding into the medial orbit and skull base, which allows the surgeon to understand tumor extent and plan accordingly. (B) Sagittal CT scan of skull base tumor showing expansion and erosion into the anterior cranial fossa, which will help the surgeon understand technical needs for both resection and reconstruction. (C) Positron emission tomography (PET) scanning demonstrates this highly metabolic skull base tumor. PET scanning of many types of tumors can reveal metastatic disease in the pre- and postoperative setting and assist in surgical and nonsurgical therapeutic planning. (D) Endoscopic view of a tumor before resection. This tumor is seen obstructing the nasal cavity, showing the vascularity and surrounding structures, which help in planning.

Adjunctive Techniques and Considerations

Endoscopic instruments allow wide drainage of sinuses adjacent to anterior skull base resections. If this is not performed, postoperative sinus obstruction frequently occurs and can be the source of serious postoperative infections.[12] Furthermore, it can cause late complications such as chronic sinusitis and mucoceles.

Angiography and embolization of vascular tumors greatly reduce bleeding and allow a dry field in which to use the microscopic view provided by endoscopic telescopes to assure complete removal is accomplished. Although the invasive nature of aggressive squamous cell carcinomas can result in skull base erosion and central invasion, the anatomy of this area favors tumor expansion by the path of least resistance into the nasal and sinus area before actual skull base erosion occurs. This is especially the case with less aggressive esthesioneuroblastomas and adenoid cystic carcinomas, which made up 40% of the cases in our series. Often, these tumors thin skull base bone by pushing and expanding to the point that the bone cannot be identified on CT scanning, but after removal, the intact skull base or at least the intact dura is identified. Both these structures provide effective barriers to central invasion, as does the periorbital membrane surrounding the soft tissues of the eye and the carotid sheath surrounding these vessels.

Invasion of the dura indicates a very aggressive tumor and is associated with high recurrence and failure rates.[5] Even with the aid of the microscopic view provided by endoscopic telescopes, complete removal of every cell of microscopic disease is often not possible with extensive tumors of the skull base. However, complete resection of the entire "visible" tumor as observed by the microscopic view of endoscopic telescopes is a reasonable goal. Endoscopic techniques allow minimal tissue disruption so that essential postoperative radiation therapy can be instituted within a few weeks of surgery to sterilize any microscopic residual tumor.

Reconstruction

It is important for the reader to realize that there are different ways to achieve the same reconstructive goals in anterior skull base surgery. Although further detailed discussions about reconstruction methods are contained in a different chapter, we present some of our methods in the context of planning and executing endoscopic and endoscopic-assisted anterior skull base surgery in the following text. A significant concern in resection of tumors with large extensions into the anterior cranial fossa is watertight closure of large dural and anterior skull base floor defects. In our experience and others, a hardy, carefully dissected pericranial flap provides a rapid, durable, and reliable solution to this problem.[9,10] Supraorbital and, if possible, superficial temporal, blood supply is cautiously preserved. The pericranial flap is sutured first to the posterior margin of the dural defect, then to the sides, and finally the anterior dural defect margin. This technique provides watertight and airtight closure, which is essential for the prevention of cerebrospinal fluid leaks, meningitis, and pneumocephalus.

Although pericranial flaps provide an excellent closure, protection of the undersurface of these flaps from the hostile environment of the lower nasal cavity is recommended. An option that we favor is a split-thickness skin graft of moderate thickness; this easily adheres to the undersurface of the pericranial flap, provides protection from drying, and over time contracts to provide a stiff layer that prevents transmitted pulsations. We have found split-thickness skin grafts superior to free bone grafts and metal hardware in medial orbital wall and floor reconstruction.[5] When attempts are made to reconstruct the orbital walls with free bone grafts and metal hardware that are exposed to the hostile environment of a crusting skull base cavity, the invariable result is bone necrosis and extrusion of the metal hardware. This is a problem that can delay postoperative radiation therapy. Split-thickness skin grafts, however, can be used by anchoring them to the skull base and orbital bone remnants by sutures sewn through drilled holes. A silk suture "hammock" provides temporary support for the split-thickness skin graft orbital walls until healing of the grafts to orbital soft tissue occurs and contracture pulls orbital structures into their nearly perfect preoperative position (**Fig. 31.2**).

Lumbar drains have been used fairly consistently in this series. In recent years, we have opted for shorter durations and at lower drainage rates (10 cm^3/h) because significant complications can occur. When extensive frontal lobe involvement requiring significant frontal lobe resection and/or frontal retraction and trauma is unavoidable, such drainage is very helpful in preventing increased intracranial pressure. When frontal lobe trauma is minimal, however, such drains are rapidly clamped and removed. In all cases, these drains must be monitored very closely. Patient movement and positioning can rapidly increase drainage to alarming levels, and contamination with resultant meningitis is a constant risk.

We favor the use of a layered support for the reconstruction. We use a 1-cm thick layer of "biologic" abdominal fat packing to reinforce the reconstruction.[10] This aids in the creation of a watertight seal of the defect. A superior portion of this graft will become vascularized and form a permanent portion of the repair. Fibrin glue is used and aids in holding a split-thickness skin graft and the underlying fat graft in place, further supporting the creation of this watertight seal.[4,11] Additional "biologic" abdominal fat packing is placed below this to reinforce the repair, but it will not become vascularized and is slowly removed over the first several weeks postoperatively. Below this, nasal trumpets are placed in the inferior meatus and cut to proper length so that they will just break the seal of the soft palate to the posterior pharyngeal wall and stabilized by suturing to the nasal columella. This allows deflation of positive pressure in the nasal cavity and pharynx, especially during coughing and gagging with awakening and extubation, thereby preventing the development of pneumocephalus and air trapping through the fresh anterior skull base repair (a significant problem early on in the senior author's experience). Closure is often the most critical element and should not be left to the most inexperienced members of the surgical team.

Postoperative Treatment

In skull base tumor surgery, it is imperative that reconstructive techniques that result in rapid healing are used so that essential postoperative radiation therapy can be started in a timely fashion. This treatment should begin within 4 weeks of surgery if microscopic residual tumor is to be sterilized before resistant larger nodules can be formed. Patients are examined endoscopically and debrided during

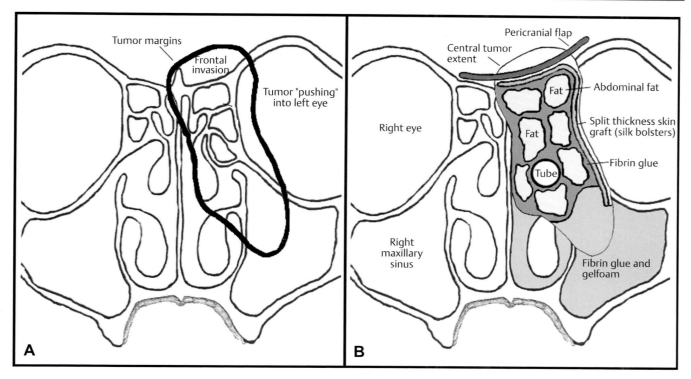

Figure 31.2   An illustration of surgical resection and reconstruction options. (A) Coronal skull base drawing through mid-orbits demonstrating a skull base malignancy involving the nasal cavity, maxillary sinus, pushing into the medial orbit and eroding into the anterior cranial fossa. (B) Coronal skull base drawing postresection demonstrating closure of the skull base defect with first a "vascularized" pericranial flap with an adherent underlying split-thickness skin graft. Underlying this for support and to obtain an initial watertight closure are free abdominal fat grafts held in place with fibrin glue. A nasopharyngeal tube breaks the seal of the palate and prevents air trapping and pneumocephalus.

and near the end of radiation therapy and followed especially closely immediately thereafter. Baseline contrasted CT and MRI scans are obtained 2 to 3 months after the completion of radiation therapy as a baseline for comparison with future scans. PET scanning has been very helpful in revealing recurrences or metastases in metabolically active tumors that have a bright signal on preoperative examination (**Fig. 31.1C**). PET scanning must be performed preoperatively, however, to demonstrate a specific identifiable tumor signal is present. If preoperative PET scanning is not performed a postoperative negative scan means very little, and cannot rule out metastatic disease.

Conclusion

The effective treatment of anterior skull base tumors requires careful pretreatment evaluation. This includes using CT, MRI, PET scanning, and a multidisciplinary approach. Adjunctive techniques can significantly improve the ability to perform a complete resection. Endoscopic endonasal and combined approaches from above and below allow complete tumor removal, even with extensive lesions that involve invasion of brain parenchyma. Watertight closure and prevention of cerebrospinal fluid leaks are paramount when dealing with dural defects. Survival depends not just on the thoroughness of the preoperative evaluation and planning but also on the

skill of the skull base surgical team. The endoscopic surgical techniques and instruments used by our team and others have enhanced tumor visualization and enabled precise endomicroscopic resection.

References

1. Cushing H. III. Partial hypophysectomy for acromegaly: with remarks on the function of the hypophysis. Ann Surg 1909; 50(6):1002–1017

2. Donald PJ. History of skull base surgery. Skull Base Surg 1991;1(1):1–3

3. Van Buren JM, Ommaya AK, Ketcham AS. Ten years' experience with radical combined craniofacial resection of malignant tumors of the paranasal sinuses. J Neurosurg 1968;28(4):341–350

4. Shah JP, Bilsky MH, Patel SG. Malignant tumors of the skull base. Neurosurg Focus 2002;13(4):e6

5. Buchmann L, Larsen C, Pollack A, Tawfik O, Sykes K, Hoover LA. Endoscopic techniques in resection of anterior skull base/paranasal sinus malignancies. Laryngoscope 2006;116(10):1749–1754

6. Stammberger H, Anderhuber W, Walch C, Papaefthymiou G. Possibilities and limitations of endoscopic management of nasal and paranasal sinus malignancies. Acta Otorhinolaryngol Belg 1999;53(3):199–205

7. Walch C, Stammberger H, Anderhuber W, Unger F, Köle W, Feichtinger K. The minimally invasive approach to olfactory neuroblastoma: combined endoscopic and stereotactic treatment. Laryngoscope 2000;110(4):635–640

8. Thaler ER, Kotapka M, Lanza DC, Kennedy DW. Endoscopically assisted anterior cranial skull base resection of sinonasal tumors. Am J Rhinol 1999;13(4):303–310

9. Kelly MB, Waterhouse N, Slade DE, Carr R, Peterson D. A 5-year review of 71 consecutive anterior skull base tumours. Br J PlastSurg 2000;53(3):184–190

10. Scher RL, Cantrell RW. Anterior skull base reconstruction with the pericranial flap after craniofacial resection. Ear Nose Throat J 1992;71(5):210–212, 215–217

11. Chandler JP, Silva FE. Extended transbasal approach to skull base tumors.Technical nuances and review of the literature. Oncology (Williston Park) 2005;19(7):913–919, discussion 920, 923–925, 929

12. Morioka M, Hamada J, Yano S, et al. Frontal skull base surgery combined with endonasal endoscopic sinus surgery. SurgNeurol 2005;64(1):44–49

32 Open Approaches to the Sinuses and Anterior Skull Base

David C. Shonka, Jr. and Paul A. Levine

The adaptation of endoscopic techniques for the treatment of sinonasal and anterior skull base pathology has resulted in a significant change in the management of patients in recent years.[1] However, open approaches to the sinuses and skull base have withstood the test of time and are integral to the comprehensive care of patients with sinonasal pathology. The appropriate selection of an open technique provides the surgeon wide exposure and direct visualization of all aspects of the paranasal sinuses and anterior skull base. This allows identification of the complete extent of tumor before tumor manipulation and enables the surgeon to perform an en bloc resection. These approaches also permit an unrestricted access for reconstructive procedures after tumor extirpation is complete. This chapter will address transfacial and intracranial approaches to the sinonasal region with special attention to the craniofacial resection for the treatment of malignant tumors of the anterior skull base.

Transfacial Approaches

Caldwell-Luc

Caldwell and Luc described the anterior antrostomy separately in the late 1800s. This approach allows access to the entire maxillary sinus, orbital floor, and pterygomaxillary fossa. A sublabial incision is performed leaving enough of a cuff of gingival mucosa to allow later reapproximation. The periosteum is elevated from the front face of the maxilla preserving the infraorbital nerve. After the elevation of periosteum from the medial buttress to the lateral buttress and superiorly to the infraorbital rim, the thin anterior wall of the maxillary sinus is entered sharply at the canine fossa with an osteotome or drill. A rongeur is then used to remove the remainder of the anterior wall of the sinus or as much bone as required to achieve the desired exposure.

The Caldwell-Luc approach for chronic sinusitis has largely been replaced by endoscopic techniques but can still be a useful procedure when endoscopic methods fail.[2–4] Endoscopic sinus surgery has also become the preferred approach for biopsy of maxillary sinus tumors, approaches to the orbital floor, removal of polyps, and approaches to the pterygopalatine fossa because it is associated with decreased morbidity compared with the Caldwell-Luc approach.[5] Despite this, the Caldwell-Luc approach remains useful in certain instances for orbital decompression, removal of benign tumors isolated to the maxillary sinus, foreign body removal, and management of facial trauma and is a tool

that should remain in the repertoire of the head and neck surgeon.[6–8]

Midfacial Degloving

The midfacial degloving approach was described for the removal of tumors from the nasal cavity, paranasal sinuses, nasal septum, and nasopharynx in 1979.[9] The operative technique was originally described in 1974.[10] Bilateral intercartilaginous incisions are performed and extended to a transfixion incision posterior to the medial crura. The upper and lower lateral cartilages are separated and the nasal envelope is elevated off the upper lateral cartilages through the intercartilaginous incisions. The intranasal incision is extended circumferentially around the piriform aperture and nasal floor effectively separating the nasal tip and bilateral lower lateral cartilage from the nasal septum, nasal dorsum, and piriform aperture. Bilateral sublabial incisions are connected across the midline, and the periosteum is elevated to the inferior orbital rim with care taken to preserve the infraorbital nerves (**Fig. 32.1**). A medial maxillectomy is performed by making bone cuts through

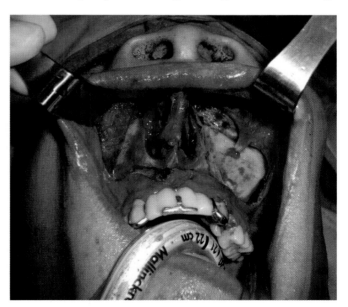

Figure 32.1 Midfacial degloving approach. Sublabial and intranasal incisions allow elevation of the nasal envelope and lower lateral cartilages. The left maxilla has been exposed to the infraorbital rim for medial maxillectomy. Note preservation of the infraorbital nerve on the left.

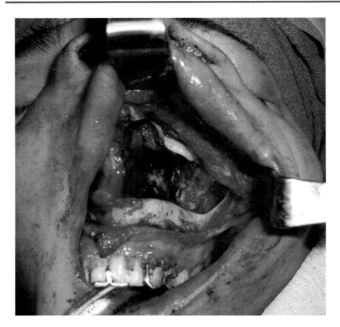

Figure 32.2 Midfacial degloving approach. Medial maxillectomy allows access to the nasal septum, nasopharynx, pterygopalatine fossa, and maxillary sinus. Note surgical clips on distal branches of the internal maxillary artery.

the medial buttress superiorly and inferiorly, and then removing the lateral nasal wall with the attached inferior turbinate. The anterior and posterior walls of the maxillary sinus can also be resected if indicated. This provides access to the nasal septum, maxillary sinus, pterygopalatine fossa, infratemporal fossa, and nasopharynx (**Fig. 32.2**). Exposure to the superior ethmoid sinuses and the frontal sinus as well as the anterior skull base is limited with this approach. After tumor removal, the medial buttress can be plated back into position as a free bone graft. Careful attention should be directed to closure of the circumferential intranasal incisions to prevent vestibular stenosis.

An obvious advantage of this approach is the avoidance of a visible scar. Complications include nasal crusting, vestibular stenosis, and transient hypesthesia in the distribution of the infraorbital nerve.[11] Modifications of the procedure have been described to decrease the incidence of vestibular stenosis, limit intranasal incisions, or avoid exposure of the contralateral midface.[12–16] The midfacial degloving approach can be combined with Le Fort I osteotomies to improve access to the nasopharynx and clivus.[17]

Indications for the midfacial degloving approach include treatment of midfacial trauma, treatment of large septal perforations, resection of benign and malignant tumors of the nasal septum, nasal sidewall, maxillary sinus, and nasopharynx.[18,19] It is ideally suited for large or benign but locally aggressive tumors that are not amenable to resection with endoscopic techniques such as dentigerous cysts, inverted papilloma, or larger juvenile (neuro) angiofibromas as it provides a wide exposure without the need for facial incisions.[11] It can be used in conjunction with intracranial

approaches for large anterior skull base malignancies with invasion of the palate, clivus, or cavernous sinus.[20] Tumors that involve the anterior skull base, medial orbital wall, and ethmoid sinuses are not ideally suited to resection via a midfacial degloving approach alone because exposure and visualization of these areas is limited.[11]

Lateral Rhinotomy

Moure of Bordeaux presented the lateral rhinotomy technique in 1902. Classically, this approach involves a skin incision beginning below the brow and medial to the medial canthus, extending inferiorly in the nasofacial groove. The incision is then taken to the alar groove and curves around to the upper lip. The lip can be split by continuing the incision inferiorly along the ipsilateral philtrum,[21] but a significant exposure can be attained laterally without splitting the lip. Modifications of the classic incision have been described to improve cosmesis. These include placement of the incision between the dorsal and lateral nasal esthetic units instead of in the nasofacial groove, and adding a "V" to the incision opposite the medial canthus to prevent webbing.[22,23] After incising the skin, the dissection continues to the maxilla. The periosteum is elevated from medial to lateral off the maxilla inferiorly and the lamina papyracea superior-laterally. Care is taken to preserve the infraorbital nerve and to leave the skin and periosteum attached to the nasal bone medially. Inferiorly, the nasal cavity is entered along the piriform aperture. To allow access to the superior nasal cavity, low lateral, transverse, and occasionally medial osteotomies are performed. These permit the ipsilateral nasal bone to be elevated with the soft tissue envelope toward the contralateral side (**Fig. 32.3**). This approach exposes the ipsilateral nasal

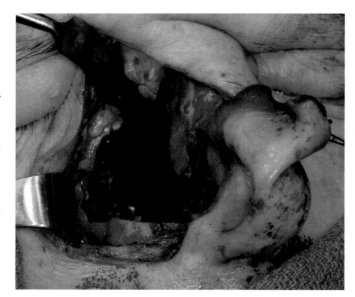

Figure 32.3 Lateral rhinotomy approach. Medial maxillectomy through lateral rhinotomy approach allows access to the nasal septum, maxillary sinus, ethmoid sinuses, sphenoid sinus, nasopharynx, and anterior skull base.

cavity and nasal septum and allows access to the ipsilateral maxillary, ethmoid, frontal, and sphenoid sinuses.

Medial maxillectomy is the most common procedure performed through the lateral rhinotomy approach.[24] The ethmoid and frontal sinuses can be accessed through the superior aspect of this incision for external ethmoidectomy or frontal sinusotomy. It also provides access to the anterior and posterior ethmoid arteries. As will be discussed in greater detail later, the lateral rhinotomy can be combined with intracranial approaches for unparalleled access to the anterior skull base. Although this approach involves an incision on the face, meticulous closure results in an inconspicuous scar that is well tolerated by patients and is minimally visible to observers.[25]

The Weber-Ferguson incision is an extension of the classic lateral rhinotomy incision that involves carrying the inferior incision through the upper lip and gingivolabial sulcus and the superior incision laterally, inferior to the eye. The periosteum is elevated from medial to lateral, raising a laterally based skin flap and exposing the entire maxilla. Although this provides access for total or subtotal maxillectomy, these regions can often be reached without the superior incision. If an orbital exenteration is indicated at the time of total maxillectomy, an additional incision can be made superior to the eye. Modifications of the lateral rhinotomy incision that allow for total maxillectomy—without the Weber-Ferguson extension—have also been described. The Weber-Ferguson extension has been shown to result in lower eyelid complications, unsightly scarring, and poor cosmetic outcome.[26]

For many years, lateral rhinotomy was the approach of choice for the surgical treatment of inverted papilloma.[27] Several studies have demonstrated the effectiveness of endoscopic approaches for inverted papilloma, even for large or recurrent tumors.[28,29] Endoscopic resection of inverted papilloma has become the favored approach.[30–34] Open approaches remain important in selected cases such as those with frontal sinus or supraorbital extension, associated malignancy, or significant scarring.[35–37] The lateral rhinotomy approach has been demonstrated to be a safe and effective approach for the treatment of a variety of sinonasal pathology including benign and malignant tumors, epistaxis, and cerebrospinal fluid leaks.[38]

Intracranial Approaches

Frontal Sinus Osteoplastic Flap

Goodale described the osteoplastic flap for the treatment of chronic frontal sinus disease in 1958, although the use of the osteoplastic flap to access the frontal sinus was described in 1800s.[39,40] The classic approach involves a coronal incision and an inferiorly based bone flap, although this approach can be performed through a mid-forehead or brow incision and a superiorly based bone flap has also been described.[41] The coronal incision is performed and the dissection proceeds

in the subgaleal plane superior to the temporal line and immediately superficial to the deep temporal fascia laterally. The pericranium is incised and elevated separately allowing harvest of a pericranial flap if indicated. Several methods have been described for determining the location of the bone cuts to create an inferiorly based bone flap of the frontal sinus anterior table. This includes transillumination of the sinus, mini burr holes, computed tomography–generated templates, and intraoperative image guidance.[42–45] The senior author (P.A.L.) has extensive experience in using a 6-foot Caldwell-generated sterilized template with excellent accuracy and without complication.[46] Regardless of the technique used to define the limits of the frontal sinus, the bone cut into the sinus should be beveled toward the center of the sinus. This provides a shelf of bone upon which the anterior table bone flap can rest at the end of the procedure, as well as to prevent inadvertent extension beyond the confines of the sinus.

The frontal sinus osteoplastic flap remains a useful approach in select patients.[47] This approach has been described for treatment of chronic frontal sinusitis, frontal sinus mucocele, tumors invading the frontal sinus, and frontal sinus trauma.[48] Obliteration of the sinus can be performed for the treatment of chronic frontal sinusitis refractory to endoscopic approaches with excellent success.[49] This procedure involves careful removal of all mucosa from the sinus and obliteration of the frontal sinus with fat and the frontal sinus outflow tract with a muscle plug. Care must be taken to remove all mucosa to prevent later mucocele formation. The frontal sinus approach also allows access to the anterior skull base.[46] After entering the sinus, a perforating drill is used to gain access to the epidural space through the posterior table of the sinus. After elevation of the frontal lobe and sagittal sinus, the remainder of the posterior table is removed. This exposes the midline skull base from the medial orbital roofs laterally to the tuberculum sella posteriorly. Because the exposure is limited inferiorly and is often dependent on the size of the frontal sinus, by itself, the frontal sinus approach is useful for tumor extirpation only in select cases, but it can be combined with transfacial approaches for larger tumors that extend inferiorly.

Standard Frontal Craniotomy

Frontal craniotomy is rarely used alone for the treatment of anterior skull base pathology but is often used in combination with transfacial approaches. In this approach, a coronal incision is performed and the scalp flap is elevated inferiorly to the level of the supraorbital rims. A pericranial flap can be harvested if indicated. Burr holes are made superiorly under the hair-bearing scalp, and bone cuts are made preserving at least 1 cm of bone superior to the superior orbital rims. Care is taken to separate the dura and the superior sagittal sinus from the bone. After removal of the frontal bone, the frontal lobe of the brain is retracted posteriorly and the dura is incised at the crista galli, severing the olfactory fibers at the cribriform plate. The resulting dural defect can be repaired primarily or with a patch technique. This allows exposure of the frontal sinus, orbital roof, and cribriform plate. Posterior exposure to the planum sphenoidale requires extensive frontal lobe retraction and is facilitated by removal of 30 to 60 cm^3 of cerebrospinal fluid.[50]

The standard frontal craniotomy approach is seldom used alone in the treatment of anterior skull base pathology because it provides limited access posteriorly and inferiorly. Adding the osteotomies performed in a subcranial approach has been shown to significantly improve exposure in these locations in a cadaveric study.[51] Direct comparison of the subcranial with frontal craniotomy approach when each was used alone for anterior skull base tumors found the subcranial approach to be superior.[52]

Subcranial Approach

The subcranial approach was described by Raveh in 1988 for the treatment of facial trauma.[53,54] The steps of the approach have been described in detail in the literature.[55] As with the other intracranial approaches, a coronal incision is performed and the skin flap is elevated to the superior orbital rims. A pericranial flap is harvested and deep temporal fascia is preserved. The flap must be elevated further inferiorly than with the osteoplastic flap and standard frontal craniotomy approaches so that the lateral orbital rims and the nasal bones are completely exposed. This requires dissection of the supraorbital neurovascular bundle out of the supraorbital notch so that it can be preserved and reflected inferiorly with the flap. The next step involves osteotomies to access the skull base. These can be performed at different locations, depending on the extent of the tumor. The widest exposure is obtained by placing the osteotomies superior to the frontal sinuses (across the frontal bone), through the lateral orbital rims and inferior to the nasal bones. This allows removal of the anterior and posterior tables of the frontal sinus, nasal bones, superior nasal septum, anterior 1 to 2 cm of orbital roof, superior orbital rims, and frontal bone as a single piece.

The advantages of the subcranial approach include improved exposure to the paranasal sinuses compared with the frontal craniotomy approach, absence of facial incisions, and limited retraction of the frontal lobe.[17,56] Compared with the frontal craniotomy, the subcranial approach limited anosmia and frontal lobe retraction.[52] It has been demonstrated to be a safe approach with acceptable rates of complications for treatment of sinonasal malignancies, facial trauma, and cerebrospinal fluid leaks.[57–59] Although it compares favorably with the craniofacial resection for treatment of malignant tumors of the anterior skull base, it has not been studied as extensively, and the studies are limited by smaller numbers of patients treated and shorter length of follow-up.[60,61] The exposure afforded by the subcranial approach is limited inferiorly, particularly when there is lateral or posterior extension of a tumor. In these situations, such as when a tumor invades the maxillary sinus,

nasopharynx, clivus, or palate, the subcranial approach can be combined with transfacial approaches to allow for complete extirpation.[17] Drawbacks of this approach include placement of burr holes on the forehead instead of the hair-bearing scalp, the need to correct bilateral telecanthus, and possible ramifications on facial growth in the pediatric and adolescent population.[62]

Craniofacial Resection

A combined intracranial and transfacial approach to the anterior skull base was described initially by Ketcham in 1963.[63] The craniofacial resection classically involves a standard frontal craniotomy to approach the cribriform plate and orbital roof from above with a lateral rhinotomy approach to the nasal cavity, ethmoid sinuses, orbit, and anterior skull base from below. These approaches have been previously described individually. Used in combination, the lateral rhinotomy and frontal craniotomy approaches provide exposure to the nasal cavity, paranasal sinuses, nasopharynx, orbits, nasal vault, frontal lobe, and the anterior skull base (**Figs. 32.4** and **32.5**). This often allows the entirety of the tumor to be visualized before manipulation and facilitates an en bloc resection. The wide exposure of the lamina and orbit also allows a careful assessment of the periorbita, which serves as a barrier to tumor spread allowing preservation of the eye with good oncologic and functional outcomes.[64]

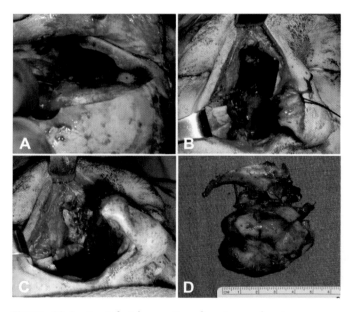

Figure 32.4 Craniofacial resection for sinonasal osteosarcoma. (A) Frontal craniotomy and retraction of the frontal lobe allows wide exposure of the cribriform plate that has been resected. (B) Lateral rhinotomy and medial maxillectomy allows access to the nasal cavity, septum, lateral nasal wall, and maxillary sinus. (C) The anterior skull base can be accessed from below through the lateral rhinotomy. Note the resected cribriform plate and exposed dura. (D) This approach permits en bloc tumor removal.

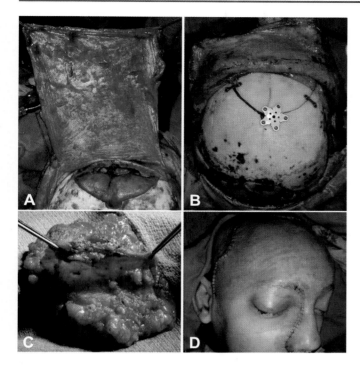

Figure 32.5 Craniofacial resection for osteosarcoma. (A) A pericranial flap is harvested. (B) The flap is placed over the anterior skull base defect and separates the frontal lobe from the nasal cavity. (C) An abdominal fat/fascia graft is harvested and placed in the superior nasal cavity to further separate the brain from the nasal cavity. (D) Incisions are closed and the nasal cavity is packed with Vaseline gauze.

The craniofacial approach has been extensively studied in the treatment of sinonasal malignancies and remains the gold standard against which other techniques should be measured.[65] A collaborative study examining the outcome of craniofacial resection on 334 patients for malignant tumors of a variety of histologies excluding esthesioneuroblastoma showed 5-year overall survival rates of 48.3% and found that margin status, histology of the tumor, and intracranial involvement were the most important predictors of outcome.[66] A broader collaborative study of 1193 patients specifically aimed at evaluating postoperative complications and mortality showed a postoperative mortality rate of 4.7% and a complication rate of 36.3%.[67] The use of a standardized broad-spectrum antibiotic regimen has been shown to decrease the incidence of wound-related complications.[68]

Studies have attempted to compare endoscopic techniques to craniofacial resection, but at this point these suffer from selection bias, limited patient numbers, and lack of long-term follow-up.[69–71] Length of follow-up is particularly important for esthesioneuroblastoma, which has been shown to recur up to 15 years after successful treatment.[72] In a large series of 50 patients with esthesioneuroblastoma at the University of Virginia, excellent outcomes were demonstrated using a regimen of preoperative radiation (Kadish A or B) or preoperative radiation and chemotherapy (Kadish C) followed by craniofacial resection with disease-free survival of 86.5% at 5 years and 82.6% at 15 years. Mean recurrence occurred at 6 years, underscoring the importance of long-term follow-up.[73]

Conclusion

There are several open approaches to the sinuses and anterior skull base. When the appropriate technique is selected, these approaches allow unparalleled access to all aspects of the anterior skull base and paranasal sinuses. Although there have been significant advances in endoscopic sinus surgery that have broadened the range of applications of these techniques for the treatment of sinonasal pathology, open approaches remain an important tool in the armamentarium of the head and neck surgeon. Particularly in the treatment of sinonasal malignant tumors, open approaches have set the standard for survival and recurrence rates by which other techniques should be compared.

References

1. Mehta RP, Cueva RA, Brown JD, et al. What's new in skull base medicine and surgery? Skull Base Committee Report. Otolaryngol Head Neck Surg 2006;135(4):620–630
2. Cutler JL, Duncavage JA, Matheny K, Cross JL, Miman MC, Oh CK. Results of Caldwell-Luc after failed endoscopic middle meatus antrostomy in patients with chronic sinusitis. Laryngoscope 2003;113(12):2148–2150
3. Matheny KE, Duncavage JA. Contemporary indications for the Caldwell-Luc procedure. Curr Opin Otolaryngol Head Neck Surg 2003;11(1):23–26
4. Becker SS, Roberts DM, Beddow PA, Russell PT, Duncavage JA. Comparison of maxillary sinus specimens removed during Caldwell-Luc procedures and traditional maxillary sinus antrostomies. Ear Nose Throat J 2011;90(6):262–266
5. Ikeda K, Hirano K, Oshima T, et al. Comparison of complications between endoscopic sinus surgery and Caldwell-Luc operation. Tohoku J Exp Med 1996;180(1):27–31
6. Barzilai G, Greenberg E, Uri N. Indications for the Caldwell-Luc approach in the endoscopic era. Otolaryngol Head Neck Surg 2005;132(2):219–220
7. Friedlich J, Rittenberg BN. Endoscopically assisted Caldwell-Luc procedure for removal of a foreign body from the maxillary sinus. J Can Dent Assoc 2005;71(3):200–201
8. Ong JC, De Silva RK, Tong DC. Retrieval of a root fragment from the maxillary sinus—an appreciation of the Caldwell-Luc procedure. N Z Dent J 2007;103(1):14–16
9. Conley J, Price JC. Sublabial approach to the nasal and nasopharyngeal cavities. Am J Surg 1979;138(4):615–618
10. Casson PR, Bonanno PC, Converse JM. The midface degloving procedure. Plast Reconstr Surg 1974;53(1):102–103
11. Browne JD. The midfacial degloving procedure for nasal, sinus, and nasopharyngeal tumors. Otolaryngol Clin North Am 2001; 34(6):1095–1104, viii
12. Buchwald C, Bonding P, Kirkby B, Fallentin E. Modified midfacial degloving. A practical approach to extensive bilateral benign tumours of the nasal cavity and paranasal sinuses. Rhinology 1995;33(1):39–42
13. Cansz H, Tahamiler R, Yener M, et al. Modified midfacial degloving approach for sinonasal tumors. J Craniofac Surg 2008;19(6): 1518–1522

14. Jeon SY, Jeong JH, Kim HS, Ahn SK, Kim JP. Hemifacial degloving approach for medial maxillectomy: a modification of midfacial degloving approach. Laryngoscope 2003;113(4):754–756

15. Krause GE, Jafek BW. A modification of the midface degloving technique. Laryngoscope 1999;109(11):1781–1784

16. Kim HJ, Kim CH, Kang JW, et al. A modified midfacial degloving approach for the treatment of unilateral paranasal sinus tumours. J Craniomaxillofac Surg 2011;39(4):284–288

17. Fliss DM, Abergel A, Cavel O, Margalit N, Gil Z. Combined subcranial approaches for excision of complex anterior skull base tumors. Arch Otolaryngol Head Neck Surg 2007;133(9):888–896

18. Maniglia AJ. Indications and techniques of midfacial degloving. A 15-year experience. Arch Otolaryngol Head Neck Surg 1986; 112(7):750–752

19. Berghaus A, Jovanovic S. Technique and indications of extended sublabial rhinotomy ("midfacial degloving"). Rhinology 1991; 29(2):105–110

20. Fliss DM, Zucker G, Amir A, Gatot A. The combined subcranial and midfacial degloving technique for tumor resection: report of three cases. J Oral Maxillofac Surg 2000;58(1):106–110

21. Schramm VL, Myers EN. "How I do it"—head and neck. A targeted problem and its solution. Lateral rhinotomy. Laryngoscope 1978;88(6):1042–1045

22. Hussain A, Hulmi OJ, Murray DP. Lateral rhinotomy through nasal aesthetic subunits. Improved cosmetic outcome. J Laryngol Otol 2002;116(9):703–706

23. Thankappan K, Sharan R, Iyer S, Kuriakose MA. Esthetic and anatomic basis of modified lateral rhinotomy approach. J Oral Maxillofac Surg 2009;67(1):231–234

24. Harrison DF. Lateral rhinotomy: a neglected operation. Ann Otol Rhinol Laryngol 1977;86(6, pt 1):756–759

25. Lueg EA, Irish JC, Katz MR, Brown DH, Gullane PJ. A patient- and observer-rated analysis of the impact of lateral rhinotomy on facial aesthetics. Arch Facial Plast Surg 2001;3(4):241–244

26. Vural E, Hanna E. Extended lateral rhinotomy incision for total maxillectomy. Otolaryngol Head Neck Surg 2000;123(4):512–513

27. Weisman R. Lateral rhinotomy and medial maxillectomy. Otolaryngol Clin North Am 1995;28(6):1145–1156

28. Lee TJ, Huang SF, Lee LA, Huang CC. Endoscopic surgery for recurrent inverted papilloma. Laryngoscope 2004;114(1):106–112

29. Jameson MJ, Kountakis SE. Endoscopic management of extensive inverted papilloma. Am J Rhinol 2005;19(5):446–451

30. Heathcote KJ, Nair SB. The impact of modern techniques on the recurrence rate of inverted papilloma treated by endonasal surgery. Rhinology 2009;47(4):339–344

31. Busquets JM, Hwang PH. Endoscopic resection of sinonasal inverted papilloma: a meta-analysis. Otolaryngol Head Neck Surg 2006;134(3):476–482

32. Lombardi D, Tomenzoli D, Buttà L, et al. Limitations and complications of endoscopic surgery for treatment for sinonasal inverted papilloma: a reassessment after 212 cases. Head Neck 2011;33(8):1154–1161

33. Pagella F, Giourgos G, Matti E, Canevari FR, Carena P. Endoscopic treatment of maxillary inverted papilloma. Rhinology 2011; 49(3):369–374

34. Sautter NB, Cannady SB, Citardi MJ, Roh HJ, Batra PS. Comparison of open versus endoscopic resection of inverted papilloma. Am J Rhinol 2007;21(3):320–323

35. Lawson W, Patel ZM. The evolution of management for inverted papilloma: an analysis of 200 cases. Otolaryngol Head Neck Surg 2009;140(3):330–335

36. Dubin MG, Sonnenburg RE, Melroy CT, Ebert CS, Coffey CS, Senior BA. Staged endoscopic and combined open/endoscopic approach in the management of inverted papilloma of the frontal sinus. Am J Rhinol 2005;19(5):442–445

37. Carta F, Verillaud B, Herman P. Role of endoscopic approach in the management of inverted papilloma. Curr Opin Otolaryngol Head Neck Surg 2011;19(1):21–24

38. Mertz JS, Pearson BW, Kern EB. Lateral rhinotomy. Indications, technique, and review of 226 patients. Arch Otolaryngol 1983;109(4):235–239

39. Goodale RL, Montgomery WW. Experiences with the osteoplastic anterior wall approach to the frontal sinus; case histories and recommendations. AMA Arch Otolaryngol 1958;68(3):271–283

40. Sessions RB, Alford BR, Stratton C, Ainsworth JZ, Shill O. Current concepts of frontal sinus surgery: an appraisal of the osteoplastic flap-fat obliteration operation. Laryngoscope 1972;82(5):918–930

41. Kudryk WH, Mahasin Z. Superiorly based osteoplastic flap for frontal sinus disease. J Otolaryngol 1988;17(7):395–397

42. Maniglia AJ, Dodds BL. A safe technique for frontal sinus osteoplastic flap. Laryngoscope 1991;101(8):908–910

43. Fewins JL, Otto PM, Otto RA. Computed tomography-generated templates: a new approach to frontal sinus osteoplastic flap surgery. Am J Rhinol 2004;18(5):285–289, discussion 289–290

44. Melroy CT, Dubin MG, Hardy SM, Senior BA. Analysis of methods to assess frontal sinus extent in osteoplastic flap surgery: transillumination versus 6-ft Caldwell versus image guidance. Am J Rhinol 2006;20(1):77–83

45. Fung MK. Template for frontal osteoplastic flap. Laryngoscope 1986;96(5):578–579

46. Persing JA, Jane JA, Levine PA, Cantrell RW. The versatile frontal sinus approach to the floor of the anterior cranial fossa. Technical note. J Neurosurg 1990;72(3):513–516

47. Lee JM, Palmer JN. Indications for the osteoplastic flap in the endoscopic era. Curr Opin Otolaryngol Head Neck Surg 2011;19(1):11–15

48. Anand VK, Hiltzik DH, Kacker A, Honrado C. Osteoplastic flap for frontal sinus obliteration in the era of image-guided endoscopic sinus surgery. Am J Rhinol 2005;19(4):406–410

49. Correa AJ, Duncavage JA, Fortune DS, Reinisch L. Osteoplastic flap for obliteration of the frontal sinus: five years' experience. Otolaryngol Head Neck Surg 1999;121(6):731–735

50. Osguthorpe JD, Patel S. Craniofacial approaches to tumors of the anterior skull base. Otolaryngol Clin North Am 2001;34(6):1123–1142, ix

51. Acharya R, Shaya M, Kumar R, Caldito GC, Nanda A. Quantification of the advantages of the extended frontal approach to skull base. Skull Base 2004;14(3):133–142, discussion 141–142

52. Jung TM, TerKonda RP, Haines SJ, Strome S, Marentette LJ. Outcome analysis of the transglabellar/subcranial approach for lesions of the anterior cranial fossa: a comparison with the classic craniotomy approach. Otolaryngol Head Neck Surg 1997;116(6, pt 1):642–646

53. Raveh J, Vuillemin T. The surgical one-stage management of combined cranio-maxillo-facial and frontobasal fractures. Advantages of the subcranial approach in 374 cases. J Craniomaxillofac Surg 1988;16(4):160–172

54. Raveh J, Vuillemin T, Sutter F. Subcranial management of 395 combined frontobasal-midface fractures. Arch Otolaryngol Head Neck Surg 1988;114(10):1114–1122

55. Fliss DM, Zucker G, Amir A, Gatot A, Cohen JT, Spektor S. The subcranial approach for anterior skull base tumors. Oper Tech Otolaryngol-Head Neck Surg 2000;11(4):238–253

56. Raveh J, Laedrach K, Speiser M, et al. The subcranial approach for fronto-orbital and anteroposterior skull-base tumors. Arch Otolaryngol Head Neck Surg 1993;119(4):385–393

57. Kellman RM, Marentette L. The transglabellar/subcranial approach to the anterior skull base: a review of 72 cases. Arch Otolaryngol Head Neck Surg 2001;127(6):687–690

58. Fliss DM, Zucker G, Cohen A, et al. Early outcome and complications of the extended subcranial approach to the anterior skull base. Laryngoscope 1999;109(1):153–160

59. Ross DA, Marentette LJ, Moore CE, Switz KL. Craniofacial resection: decreased complication rate with a modified subcranial approach. Skull Base Surg 1999;9(2):95–100

60. Raveh J, Turk JB, Lädrach K, et al. Extended anterior subcranial approach for skull base tumors: long-term results. J Neurosurg 1995;82(6):1002–1010

61. Moore CE, Ross DA, Marentette LJ. Subcranial approach to tumors of the anterior cranial base: analysis of current and traditional surgical techniques. Otolaryngol Head Neck Surg 1999;120(3):387–390

62. Shlomi B, Chaushu S, Gil Z, Chaushu G, Fliss DM. Effects of the subcranial approach on facial growth and development. Otolaryngol Head Neck Surg 2007;136(1):27–32

63. Ketcham AS, Wilkins RH, Vanburen JM, Smith RR. A combined intracranial facial approach to the paranasal sinuses. Am J Surg 1963;106:698–703

64. Essig GF, Newman SA, Levine PA. Sparing the eye in craniofacial surgery for superior nasal vault malignant neoplasms: analysis of benefit. Arch Facial Plast Surg 2007;9(6):406–411

65. Howard DJ, Lund VJ, Wei WI. Craniofacial resection for tumors of the nasal cavity and paranasal sinuses: a 25-year experience. Head Neck 2006;28(10):867–873

66. Ganly I, Patel SG, Singh B, et al. Craniofacial resection for malignant paranasal sinus tumors: Report of an International Collaborative Study. Head Neck 2005;27(7):575–584

67. Ganly I, Patel SG, Singh B, et al. Complications of craniofacial resection for malignant tumors of the skull base: report of an International Collaborative Study. Head Neck 2005;27(6):445–451

68. Gil Z, Patel SG, Bilsky M, Shah JP, Kraus DH. Complications after craniofacial resection for malignant tumors: are complication trends changing? Otolaryngol Head Neck Surg 2009;140(2):218–223

69. Gallia GL, Reh DD, Salmasi V, Blitz AM, Koch W, Ishii M. Endonasal endoscopic resection of esthesioneuroblastoma: the Johns Hopkins Hospital experience and review of the literature. Neurosurg Rev 2011;34(4):465–475

70. Eloy JA, Vivero RJ, Hoang K, et al. Comparison of transnasal endoscopic and open craniofacial resection for malignant tumors of the anterior skull base. Laryngoscope 2009;119(5):834–840

71. Castelnuovo PG, Delù G, Sberze F, et al. Esthesioneuroblastoma: endonasal endoscopic treatment. Skull Base 2006;16(1):25–30

72. Bachar G, Goldstein DP, Shah M, et al. Esthesioneuroblastoma: The princess margaret hospital experience. Head Neck 2008;30(12):1607–1614

73. Loy AH, Reibel JF, Read PW, et al. Esthesioneuroblastoma: continued follow-up of a single institution's experience. Arch Otolaryngol Head Neck Surg 2006;132(2):134–138

33   Endoscopic Skull Base Defect Repair

Satish Govindaraj, Anthony G. Del Signore, and David W. Kennedy

Because of the technological advancements and a greater understanding of endonasal vascular anatomy, the endoscopic repair of skull base defects has undergone a progressive evolution over the past decade. The authors' initial success with repairing cerebrospinal fluid (CSF) leaks encountered during sinus surgery has evolved to the repair of large defects associated with tumor resection in the anterior, middle, and posterior cranial fossae. Endoscopic techniques were successful because of maintenance of the principles of open skull base reconstruction: (1) multilayer closure, (2) preservation of neurovascular structures, and (3) utilization of vascularized tissue.

CSF leak repair has advanced greatly since the first reported repair by Dandy, who in 1926 sealed a cranionasal fistula using a frontal craniotomy approach. Ultimately, improved instrumentation, enhanced resolution of imaging, and miniaturization of instruments allowed for endoscopic repair of CSF leaks by Wigand in 1981.[1] In his report, he described the use of endoscopes to seal a small CSF leak using fibrin glue. Over the past 20 years, the minimally invasive endoscopic approach has gained widespread acceptance and become the standard of care because of its high success rate and lower morbidity than traditional intracranial techniques.[2–5]

Skull Base Defect Etiology

Skull base defects are secondary to traumatic or nontraumatic etiology. Nontraumatic causes are predominantly spontaneous CSF leaks and skull base erosion secondary to tumor. Traumatic leaks are a result of blunt or penetrating trauma or surgical procedures involving the skull base.

Nontraumatic

Majority of the nontraumatic CSF leaks are of spontaneous or idiopathic origin, where no other discernible etiology is present, with a reported frequency of 15 to 23%.[6,7] These are primarily located at the cribriform plate and lateral recess of the sphenoid sinus, but can also be noted at multiple sites approximately 30% of the time.[8–10] The pathophysiology is thought to involve an elevation in intracranial pressure, exerting a constant pulsatile force at weakened sites in the skull base. Because of the elevated pressures, spontaneous CSF leaks tend to have the highest recurrence rate, which stresses the importance of CSF pressure control at the time of surgical repair.

Congenital causes are extremely rare and difficult to repair. They are often caused by skull base malformation, allowing the herniation of brain and meninges through the defect into the sinonasal cavity. The most common location is the foramen cecum, as noted by Woodworth et al, in 63% of the cases.[11]

Traumatic

Historically accidental trauma was the most common etiology of CSF leaks, occurring in 1 to 3% of all cranial head injuries.[9] These injuries were often classified as penetrating versus nonpenetrating, and depending on the extent of injuries could present as either an acute leak upon presentation or in a delayed fashion. Fracture patterns can be focal or diffuse, with patients most commonly presenting with cribriform plate (23%) and ethmoid skull base defects (20%), while 35% of patients have multiple sites of injury.[12]

Surgical Trauma

Defects secondary to surgery are a result of planned defects from skull base tumor resection or iatrogenic CSF leaks most often associated with endoscopic sinus surgery. Defect size and location often dictates the option for repair. The most common locations for CSF leaks secondary to endoscopic sinus surgery were the ethmoid skull base (35.1%), cribriform (27%), and sphenoid sinus (18.9%).[12] Defect location varies with the type of surgery performed, with the ethmoid roof, cribriform plate, and sphenoid commonly injured during functional endoscopic sinus surgery, while the sphenoid is more frequently injured during neurosurgical cases.[5]

High-Flow Leak versus Low-Flow Leak

With the advent of advanced tumor resection of the skull base, defects requiring repair have advanced in size and complexity. Patel et al introduced the concept of dividing CSF leaks into high and low flow.[13] Low-pressure leaks are seen in cases of encephaloceles with small defect size or in pituitary adenoma resection where the sella diaphragm is thin with weeping of CSF. These cases are distinct from a high-pressure leak where either a ventricle or arachnoid cistern is entered.[13] High-pressure leaks are seen in cases of endoscopic endonasal approaches (EEAs) to the skull base where tumor removal is performed.

EEA to the skull base can be subdivided into the respective regions of repair with vascular flaps that can be utilized for each region (**Table 33.1**). Region I, the anterior cranial fossa, extends anteriorly from the frontal sinus to the anterior border of the planum sphenoidale or roof of the sphenoid sinus. In region II, middle cranial fossa, there is a central and lateral component that is divided by the anterior clinoid process. Defects in a central location are created with approaches to the sella or suprasellar regions. Lesions located lateral to a sagittal plane through the anterior clinoid process involve the pterygopalatine and infratemporal fossae. In region III, the posterior cranial fossa, clival lesions are the predominant pathologic entity seen. Last, region IV accounts for lesions involving the odontoid and cervical spine.

Reconstructive Materials Available

Selection of the appropriate graft materials depends on the many factors encountered during the preoperative and operative stages of repair. The size and location of the defect encountered plays a role in the appropriate graft material to be used. Anatomic considerations and the state of the prepared defect site may also determine the selection of grafting material. Each defect encountered is unique with various confluences of factors influencing the necessary reconstructive material. With a plethora of materials available, algorithms and consensus statements do not presently exist to guide in the selection process. Ultimately, the selection of a specific closure material and technique is based upon the surgeon's familiarity and experience.

Autologous tissues in the form of bone, fascia, fat, cartilage, muscle, and mucosa have been used extensively because of

Table 33.1 Intranasal and Regional Vascular Flap Choices for Skull Base Reconstruction

Flap	Vascular Pedicle	Reconstructive Site
Nasoseptal flap	Posterior septal branch of sphenopalatine artery	Ideal choice for all defects
Inferior turbinate flap	Inferior turbinate artery from posterior lateral nasal artery	Clivus and sella/parasellar
Middle turbinate flap	Middle turbinate artery from posterior lateral nasal artery	Small anterior cranial fossa and sella defects
Temporoparietal fascia flap	Superficial temporal artery	Clivus and parasellar
Pericranium flap	Supraorbital and supratrochlear arteries	Ideal for all defects
Lateral nasal wall flap	Branches of facial and anterior ethmoid arteries	Anterior cranial fossa defects up to planum sphenoidale

their low cost, availability, and ease of transfer. When local tissue is scarce, nonautogenous grafts or tissue engineered matrices can be utilized successfully but with the added cost of manufacturing and processing.[14-16] Below is a discussion on the various reconstructive materials available.

Nonvascularized Autografts

Originally used in the early attempts of skull base reconstruction, nonvascularized autografts provide an excellent source for reconstruction. Bone, fascia, and fat are mainly utilized, acting as a scaffold for viable tissue to be incorporated. Because of the absence of vascularity, a slow resorptive process of the tissue occurs, allowing an influx of native cellular products to be incorporated. Experimental studies have shown free graft adherence to bone by 1 week, fibroblast invasion by 3 weeks, and a substantial amount of postoperative contracture.[17]

Of the free nonvascularized grafts, fat is most commonly used, primarily for its abundance, ease of harvesting, and malleability to conform to a variety of defects encountered. Typically, fat is harvested from a lower abdomen or lateral thigh incision, because of its high availability. For larger defects, fascia from either incision can also be harvested concurrently, as rectus fascia or fascia lata. Reconstructions utilizing free nonvascularized grafts tend to utilize several different layers of alternating consistency, that is, fat plug followed by fascial layer followed by subsequent layers with the eventual goal of creating a water-tight seal.

The success rate for avascular reconstructive techniques in small and idiopathic defects may be as high as 90 to 97%.[18] Unfortunately, the closure rate drops to 50 to 70% in large surgically induced defects. The overall size of the defect encountered and a high CSF leak rate may prevent the utilization of avascular reconstructive techniques.

Vascularized Mucosal Flaps

The development of various vascular pedicled flaps has permitted closure of very large, high-flow defects, with a low CSF leak rate of 3 to 5%.[19-23] The process of harvesting a vascularized flap is considered difficult and technically demanding than that described for nonvascularized tissue. On the contrary, the major advantages of these flaps are a preserved vascular pedicle, a capability to cover large surface areas, and relative resistance to volume loss. Many of the described flaps are based on solely one pedicle and therefore imperative that the vascular supply remains intact.

Many options for vascularized pedicled flaps are available and include the workhorse nasoseptal flap based off the posterior septal branch of the sphenopalatine artery, the inferior turbinate flap based off the inferior turbinate artery, tunneled periosteal flaps based off the superficial temporal artery, middle turbinate flap based off the posterior sphenopalatine branches and finally "rescue" or palatal flaps based off the descending palatine arteries.[22-25] The nasoseptal flap, as described by Hadad et al, is commonly used given its versatility (**Fig. 33.1**). The flap is based on the posterior septal neurovascular pedicle, with the possibility of modifications for flap length and width given the various dimensions of defects encountered. Generally, it is advised that an overestimation of flap harvest takes place, with trimming excess tissue as needed. The mucoperichondrium is elevated in an anterior to posterior fashion with careful dissection along the pedicle. Once elevated, the flap is displaced in the nasopharynx or maxillary sinus until ready to use. This nasoseptal flap has become the workhorse of most skull base reconstructions, given its proximity to most

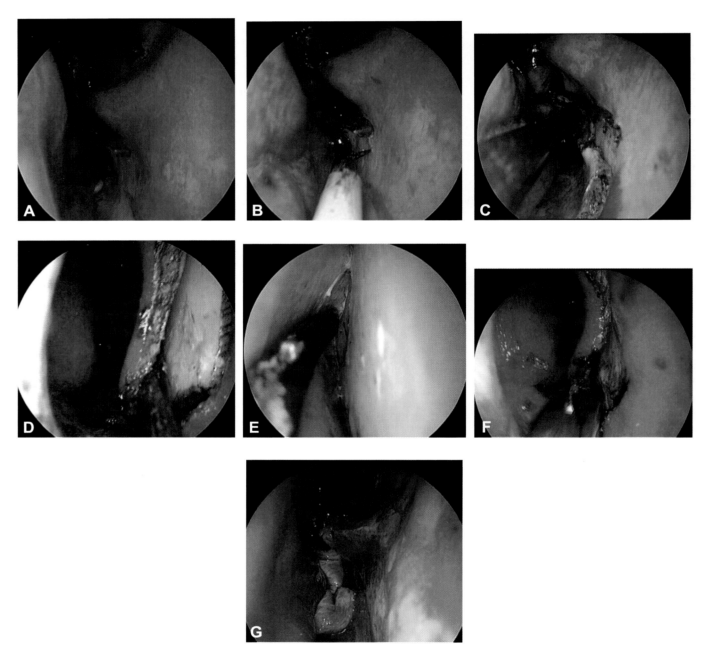

Figure 33.1 Right side of the nasoseptal flap. (A) Make posterior incisions first above and below pedicle and then extend onto the septum. Note the large septal spur of the posterior septum. The presence of a spur may make flap elevation more difficult, but it is still feasible. (B) The inferior vertical incision is then made onto the floor. This can be done with a long needle tip bovie. A similar superior vertical incision is performed next. (C) The inferior incision has been completed from the face of the sphenoid and then brought anteriorly onto the septum. (D) An anterior incision is then made and the flap is elevated in a posterior direction. (E) In the correct plane elevation of the flap will be avascular. The superior and inferior cuts are not made until the flap is elevated to the posterior incisions. (F) The inferior and superior incisions are made last using an endoscopic scissor. Cautery used along the superior incision may result in olfactory dysfunction. (G) Push the flap back into the nasopharynx. Notice that flap elevation was performed despite the presence of a large septal spur.

areas needed to be addressed and its large surface area to be utilized for coverage.[26] Depending on the vascular pedicle isolated during the harvest, the extent of the flap rotation can address defects extending from the lateral, ventral, and anterior skull base.[20]

Patel et al, in a review of the various flaps currently described, provided a list of advantages and limitations associated with each of them.[13] The nasoseptal flap was found to be a versatile flap for many of the defects encountered. The inferior turbinate flap was found to be a great option for small clival and sella/parasellar defects,[23] but is limited in the overall reach within the paranasal sinuses. The middle turbinate flap was a great option for small anterior cranial defects, but it provided little tissue with thin mucosa, which was difficult to elevate. The inferior turbinate flap is more suited for more posterior reconstruction in the region of the sella and clivus. It does not have the reach nor width to reconstruct the anterior cranial fossa.[13] More recently, description of both anterior and posterior pedicle lateral nasal wall flaps have been described as additional options for intranasal vascular flap reconstruction. These flaps are extensions of the inferior turbinate flap with incorporation of the nasal floor mucoperiosteum thus providing greater width and a pedicle that allows reconstruction of the anterior cranial fossa.[27,28] The blood supply of the flaps is derived from branches of the facial and anterior ethmoidal arteries.[27,28] The flap can be utilized to reconstruct anterior cranial fossa defects up to the planum sphenoidale.[28] These pedicled flaps should be utilized for extensive reconstructions.[13]

It is important to consider operative planning and exposure when considering the specific vascular flap to harvest. In many operative cases, obtaining the flap is often in the initial stages of the procedure. Therefore, planning for subsequent endonasal procedures is important, as many could potentially destroy the flap or compromise blood flow. It is recommended that the flap be "safe guarded" in an area of the sinonasal cavity that is convenient and will not be the focus of the procedure.

Reconstruction Techniques

Operative Preparation

With an endoscopic approach, preoperative set up is crucial to the success of the case. Patients should have adequate nasal decongestion with oxymetazoline followed by injection with lidocaine 1% with 1:100,000 epinephrine at the middle turbinate insertion to the lateral nasal wall. Transoral sphenopalatine blocks will also enhance vasoconstriction. We are now using topical epinephrine pledgets (1:1000) in place of oxymetazoline because of the improved vasoconstriction. Topical vasoconstrictive agents are used during the approach and exposure of the defect, however, they are not applied directly to the extradural or intradural skull base.

The patient should be prepped for possible harvest of the appropriate tissue grafts. In cases where a pericranial

or temporoparietal fascia flap or temporalis fascia graft may be needed, the scalp and appropriate areas must be prepped and draped into the field. In addition, the abdomen and thigh should be prepped as well if a fat or fascia graft is needed, respectively.

Endoscopic Approach to Skull Base

In the patient with previous sinus or skull base surgery, visualization may be unobstructed. Alternatively, in those with nonoperated sinonasal cavities, the approach and exposure of the skull base may require clearing the sinuses below the defect, harvest of intranasal vascular flaps, and possible resection of a portion of the nasal septum. The amount of tissue dissection is dependent on the lesion and more importantly its location. In addition, the presence of a high-flow leak versus low-flow leak is important to consider when making a decision regarding the need for vascular tissue reconstruction. In low-flow defects, there is no need for vascular tissue to obtain a successful CSF leak repair.[18,29]

Anterior Cranial Fossa

In unilateral CSF leaks or encephaloceles (low flow) involving the anterior cranial fossa, clearing the sinuses ipsilateral to the CSF leak with preservation of the nasal septum is sufficient. All sinuses on the side of the defect are opened, including the maxillary and sphenoid sinus, clearance of all partitions in the ethmoid cavity, and a frontal sinusotomy. In addition, the middle turbinate is resected at its attachment to the skull base. By doing this, graft placement is facilitated at the skull base and the long-term risk of mucocele formation or frontal recess stenosis is alleviated.

Middle Cranial Fossa

For lesions involving the central middle cranial fossa (sella/suprasellar region), the degree of dissection is dependent on the lesion. For lesions of the planum sphenoidale (i.e., meningioma), bilateral clearance of the ethmoid sinuses, opening of both sphenoid sinuses and a posterior septectomy is performed. The need for vascular grafts is determined before the surgery and either unilateral or bilateral nasoseptal flaps should be elevated and reflected into the maxillary sinus or nasopharynx. An endoscopic drill is needed to reduce the bone of the planum sphenoidale because of its thickness.[30] Once the bone has been thinned a curette is used to expose the dura and a Kerrison rongeur is then used to remove the remaining bone. After lesion removal, reconstruction is performed.

Lesions involving the sella and suprasella are approached in a similar fashion; however, dissection in the ethmoid cavity can be limited. The sphenoid sinuses are opened bilaterally through a direct approach. In cases with limited access, resection of the superior turbinates can be performed and bilateral posterior ethmoidectomies can be done especially in cases with an Onodi cell. For pituitary tumors where a CSF leak may not be encountered and a nasoseptal flap may not be necessary, horizontal incisions at the face of the sphenoid sinus above the posterior septal artery pedicle are made and carried onto the septum. A Freer elevator can be used to reflect this mucoperiosteum inferiorly moving the pedicle away from potential harm. A 2-cm posterior septectomy and lowering of the bony face of the sphenoid can then be performed without violating the pedicle to the nasoseptal flap if needed. In addition, if a hybrid endoscopic/microscopic approach is performed, reflection of the pedicle inferiorly protects it from injury with speculum placement during the microscopic portion.

Lateral lesions of the middle cranial fossa skull base will require a wide opening of the maxillary sinus in addition to clearance of the ethmoid and sphenoid sinuses. Once this is done, the posterior wall of the maxillary sinus is removed to expose the pterygopalatine fossa. The periosteum is incised to expose the contents of the fossa. Fat is first encountered and can be reduced with gentle bipolar cautery. Identification of the internal maxillary artery and its terminal branch, the sphenopalatine artery, is performed. The vessels can be reflected inferiorly before the removal of bone at the skull base if an ipsilateral nasoseptal flap is needed. If the pedicle is violated or the lesion involves the pedicle and must be sacrificed as with a juvenile nasopharyngeal angiofibroma, a contralateral nasoseptal flap can be elevated.

Posterior Cranial Fossa

Lesions involving the posterior central skull base, more specifically the clivus, are approached similar to an approach to the sella. The sphenoid sinuses are opened widely and if needed nasoseptal flaps are elevated. For defects in the area, the anterior incision for the nasoseptal flap does not need to be brought to the columella. In general, an anterior vertical incision at the anterior head of the middle turbinate provides sufficient length. The flap is reflected into the nasopharynx and the rostrum or face of the sphenoid sinus is reduced and brought flush with the mucoperiosteum overlying the clivus. The bone of the clivus requires drilling to expose the underlying dura. Once this bone has been thinned, a Kerrison rongeur is used to remove the underlying bone.

Repair Techniques

The repair techniques are plentiful and versatile. In general, an underlay technique is combined with an overlay when feasible. In cases where there is a bony ledge to place an underlay graft, the options consist of fascia, AlloDerm (LifeCell, Bridgewater, New Jersey), DuraGen (Integra LifeSciences, Plainsboro, New Jersey), or a fat plug technique. After this layer is placed either a free mucosal graft in case of low-flow leaks or a vascularized flap in case of a high-flow leak is placed in an overlay fashion and secured with tissue glue and bolstered in place with Gelfoam (Pfizer, New York, New York) soaked in gentamicin and then non-absorbable packing.

An overlay graft requires preparation of the recipient site by the removal of mucosa from the edges of the bony skull base defect. This is critical for stability and adequate acceptance of the graft at the recipient site. The amount of exposed bone varies, but typically 5 mm is sufficient.

Anterior Cranial Fossa

In defects involving the anterior cranial fossa, an underlay and overlay technique is often utilized (**Fig. 33.2**). In some low-flow leaks involving the cribriform plate, an underlay technique is not always feasible because of an inadequate medial bony ledge and repairs may require an overlay graft of free mucosa. In high-flow leaks of the anterior cranial fossa, an underlay technique is often utilized when there are sufficient bony ledges around the perimeter of the defect. The graft material, usually avascular fascia can be placed either deep to the dura or between the dura and the overlying bone. If there is a dural defect with adequate edges, a fascial synthetic (DuraGen) or AlloDerm graft can be sutured in place as the initial step in repair.[27,28]

Nitinol u-clips (Coalescent Surgical, Inc., Sunnyvale, California) are used because they permit suturing in a confined space and are self-tying (**Fig. 33.3**). Originally devised for cardiovascular anastomoses, the technique was modified by Gardner et al for securing tissue grafts to the surrounding native dura.[19] The novel technique uses a specially designed, needle driver to place suture through the graft and dura, and then a hemoclip applier is used to tighten and coil the clip. This step can be both time consuming and technically demanding. In addition, if sufficient dural edges are not available, this initial layer of closure will not be feasible. Preparation of the inlay site, involves adequately separating the adherent brain and dura from the overlying bone to allow acceptance of the graft material. Of note, any remaining mucosal tissue must be removed from the repair site to prevent delayed mucocele formation. The choice of graft as mentioned is usually autologous fascia or an allograft such as DuraGen or AlloDerm. Germani et al have reported success with a single layer AlloDerm closure of anterior cranial fossa defects with the placement of the graft as an underlay–overlay technique (**Fig. 33.4**).[14] The graft lies in an intracranial location with its edges extending extracranially to cover (overlay) the bony edges of the defect. The authors use Gelfoam to "tuck" and stabilize the underlay component of the graft. There was a CSF leak rate of less than 4% and a subset of these patients underwent adjuvant radiation therapy with graft survival.

After placement of the underlay graft, in high-flow leaks a vascularized flap is placed as an overlay graft. A nasoseptal flap is the vascularized graft of choice because of the ease of harvest, graft durability, and the ability to cover any size skull base defect. One exception is sphenoid sinuses with increased postsellar aeration where a portion of the flap length is lost as it covers the sphenoid sinus before extending anteriorly onto the anterior cranial fossa skull base. The rostrum of the sphenoid sinus can be reduced to the clivus to alleviate some of this loss of length. It is recommended that for large

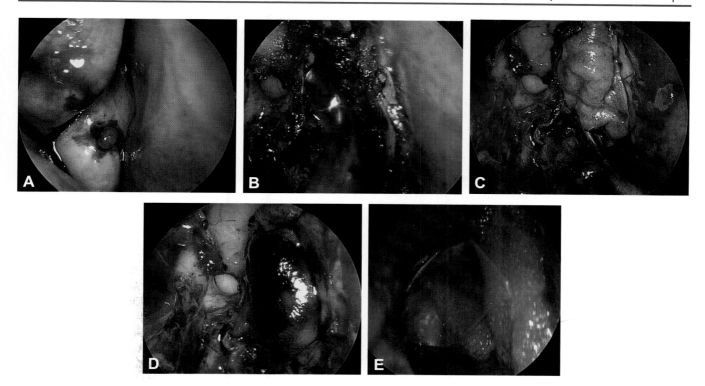

Figure 33.2 Anterior cranial fossa reconstruction with underlay and overlay technique. Figure shows a right anterior cranial fossa encephalocele, with key aspects of reconstruction after removal. (A) Right endoscopic view of large encephalocele medial to right middle turbinate. (B) After fulgurating encephalocele to the level of the bony defect, the dura around the defect is elevated. Here, a curette is used to elevate the dura around the lateral aspect of the defect. (C) AlloDerm underlay graft in place. Note the exposed area of bone on the superior septum around the defect. (D) Overlay graft harvested from ipsilateral middle turbinate is placed and then secured with fibrin tissue sealant. (E) A frontal sinus stent is placed over gentamicin-soaked Gelfoam to stabilize the graft and maintain patency of the frontal sinus.

defects extending to the posterior table of the frontal sinus and extending from orbit to orbit, the anterior limb of the incision be made at the septum–columella junction, and extend onto the floor of the nose to insure adequate length and width of the graft. Batra et al demonstrated that the average dimensions of the anterior cranial fossa window are 33.7 mm from anterior to posterior and 23.5 and 19.1 mm from orbit to orbit at the anterior and posterior ethmoid arteries, respectively. In the preoperative planning, imaging can be reviewed and distance measured to determine if the nasoseptal flap would have sufficient length and width to cover the anterior skull base.

In the setting where a nasoseptal flap is not feasible (i.e., septal perforation, previous septectomy, vascular pedicle compromised), the main options are the pericranial flap or the lateral nasal wall flap recently described if vascularized tissue is needed. Otherwise, reconstruction must be performed in multilayer fashion or using the technique described by Germani et al with AlloDerm or fascia.[14] The pericranial flap requires a glabelar incision on the face using the technique described by Zanation et al.[31] An alternative if there are no reconstructive options is a conventional bicoronal approach with elevation onto the glabella in the midline, which would alleviate the need for a facial incision, as well as provide an easier surgical field to harvest the pericranial flap.

Middle Cranial Fossa

A common repair technique used in sphenoid sinus defects is obliteration, often with harvested autologous fat. The cavity or sinus is prepared by meticulous removal of sinus mucosa, to prevent the development of subsequent mucocele. The sinus is then packed with the autologous fat completely obliterating any dead space. Although this is a reconstructive option, technique advancements have fat obliteration of the sphenoid sinus as a last resort. The best way to avoid mucocele formation is to maintain a functional sinus.

Composite and layered closure is the reconstructive technique of choice in the central skull base of the middle cranial fossa. One such method, as described by Hadded et al, frequently used in conjunction with the aforementioned nasoseptal flap, is construction of a multilayer scaffold. The multiple layers are placed in sequence, allowing a water-tight seal to be formed. Initially, a collagen matrix is positioned as an inlay, followed by a fascial graft or abdominal fat placed as an overlay to obliterate the associated dead space. The nasoseptal flap is then placed as the next layer, secured in place using fibrin glue and placement of packing to support the repair during the healing period.[20] Abdominal fat should not be placed intracranially to obliterate dead space in the setting of an open ventricle to avoid the risk of iatrogenic hydrocephalus.[32]

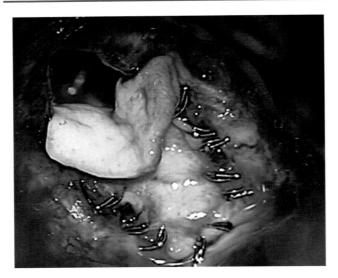

Figure 33.3 ᴜ-clip closure of an anterior cranial fossa defect.

graft is stabilized in place with the placement of vomer or a miniplate to "wedge" the edges of the graft in place and create a water-tight seal. A nasoseptal flap can then be placed over this repair in an overlay fashion.

Another method as described by Briggs et al, utilizes the layered technique of fat allograft plug and reinforced mucoperiosteal graft. In the described technique, the defect bed is prepared by removing all surrounding mucosa, bone fragments and prolapsing dura. The fat is harvested either from the ear lobe or abdomen, to match the size of the defect. Once harvested, the graft is placed in the defect as a plug occupying both the intracranial and intranasal sides. Once the fat plug is secured in place, a bone graft can be used to provide additional support, before laying the mucoperiosteal graft. The final layer utilizes a fibrin glue to secure all layers in place. After a 27-month follow-up, 90% of the patients experienced primary repair with a 100% closure rate after a second procedure.[33]

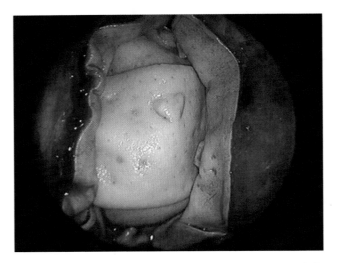

Figure 33.4 A single layer closure of AlloDerm placed as an underlay–overlay technique to reconstruct an anterior cranial fossa defect. *Image Courtesy* of Dr. Jean Anderson Eloy, Vice-Chairman and Associate Professor, Department of Otolaryngology, University of Medicine and Dentistry of New Jersey, Newark, New Jersey.

For approaches to the sella, reconstruction of the skull base is determined by the presence of a CSF leak. In the absence of a leak with an intact arachnoid, repair of the sella defect is done with vomer harvested from the nasal septum, which can be secured in place with fibrin sealant and collagen matrix. In the presence of a CSF leak, a water-tight closure is needed and can be done in two ways (**Fig. 33.5**). First, is a multilayer closure with an underlay graft of free tissue (fascia, AlloDerm, and DuraGen) and then an overlay graft with septal mucosa or in the presence of a high-flow leak, a nasoseptal flap. The second option is a gasket-seal closure with the use of a free tissue graft placed in an underlay–overlay fashion similar to that described by Germani et al for anterior cranial fossa defect repair. The

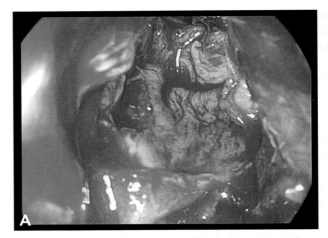

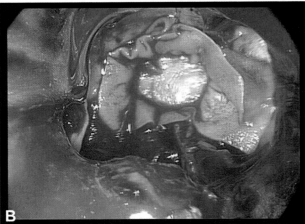

Figure 33.5 Reconstruction of a middle cranial fossa. (A) The naso-septal flap is placed in an overlay fashion after the mucosa from the sphenoid sinus is removed. A fibrin sealant is then applied around the edges of the flap followed by gentamicin-soaked Gelfoam and nonab-sorbable Merocel packing. (B) Gasket-seal closure of skull base defect using septal bone and AlloDerm as the initial layer of repair. This alone resulted in a water-tight seal.

Posterior Cranial Fossa

Lesions of the posterior cranial fossa, more specifically the clivus, are closed with either the use of a nasoseptal or inferior turbinate flap. A short flap is needed in these cases and before the posterior septectomy that is often required in approaching this area, the nasoseptal flap can be elevated and reflected into the nasopharynx. The graft is secured in place with fibrin sealant and collagen matrix. A transnasal approach serves best to address lesions involving the upper one-third of the clivus.

Frontal Sinus

As with functional endoscopic sinus surgery, the approach to frontal sinus defects poses a significant problem. Access is often difficult and hindered by the natural anatomical barriers. Again, location of the leak determines the appropriate approach and restrictions for repair. Typically with superior and laterally based leaks, there is an increased difficulty for endonasal access and may require a trephination or osteoplastic approach. Inferior-based leaks, found near the frontal recess and frontal outflow tract, may be amenable to a combined endoscopic and external approach or sole endoscopic approaches.

Authors have described the repair of frontal sinus defects, superior and lateral, via complete endoscopic approaches. Originally described by Gross et al for the treatment of chronic rhinosinusitis, the endoscopic modified Lothrop procedure, allows adequate visualization of frontal sinus leaks.[34] Becker et al reported the treatment of two "difficult to access" superolateral CSF leaks utilizing this technique with complete resolution of symptoms.[35]

Postoperative Management

The immediate postoperative period is especially important in the repair of skull base defects. Adequate control of local and systemic factors, are essential in facilitating an adequate seal to be formed. Precise control of intracranial pressure during this period is of utmost importance. As advocated by Hegazy et al, the use of lumbar drains in the immediate postoperative period allows for accurate measurement and control of pressures.[18] Lumbar drains are not placed on a routine basis and there are no clear criteria as to what cases would benefit from postoperative lumbar drain placement. The exception is the spontaneous CSF leak patient where there is an underlying elevation in intracranial pressure and control of this pressure in the immediate postoperative period can be beneficial as the free tissue graft undergoes the critical period of imbibition. This process nourishes the graft until neovascularization begins to take place in 36 hours. As noted by Schlosser et al, another method used in conjunction with lumbar drains includes the use of diuretics, such as acetazolamide and furosemide to decrease CSF production.[9]

Other patient modifiable behaviors that increase intracranial pressure and place undue stress on the repair should also be addressed. Counseling patients on the avoidance of nose blowing, strenuous activities, and straining should be a part of the preoperative discussion and postoperative care. For those receiving narcotic pain control, an adequate bowel regimen should be instituted with stool softeners. Upon discharge from the hospital, it is imperative that these recommendations are followed. The avoidance of heavy activity and lifting should be in place for 4 to 6 weeks postsurgery. Patients should also be followed at 1, 4, and 8 weeks after surgery for endoscopic debridement if needed. Endoscopic debridement in these cases is less aggressive to avoid manipulation of the graft. Sterile saline sprays are used in the first 4 weeks and then irrigations are initiated. Antibiotics may be needed to treat any evidence of sinusitis because of the mucous stasis and crusting. With more extensive resections, crusting and debridement may be needed for up to 3 to 4 months. The resumption of normal activity is usually cleared at postoperative week 8 but is case-dependent.

Conclusion

The endoscopic repair of skull base defects has evolved over the last decade because of the advent of vascularized intranasal and regional flaps that have decreased postoperative CSF leak rates to the same level as that seen in open surgical repairs. Lesions that were traditionally treated with an open approach are now managed through extended EEAs. The critical factor in approaching these lesions is not only the challenge of resection, but also the ability to reconstruct these defects in a fashion that provides similar structural support and durability to that seen in an open approach. Numerous free tissue options are available for low-flow leaks and all have met with a success of greater than 90%. The options are more limited in large defects with high-flow leaks where vascularized tissue is important in maintaining an acceptable postoperative CSF leak rate. In addition, an understanding of the sinonasal anatomy is critical to avoid long-term sequelae of chronic rhinosinusitis and mucocele formation in this patient population. The complexity of the central skull base and its accessibility through a multitude of endonasal corridors requires the combined expertise of both neurosurgery and otolaryngology.

References

1. Wigand ME. Transnasal ethmoidectomy under endoscopical control. Rhinology 1981;19(1):7–15
2. Stankiewicz JA. Cerebrospinal fluid fistula and endoscopic sinus surgery. Laryngoscope 1991;101(3):250–256
3. Burns JA, Dodson EE, Gross CW. Transnasal endoscopic repair of cranionasal fistulae: a refined technique with long-term follow-up. Laryngoscope 1996;106(9, pt 1):1080–1083
4. Mattox DE, Kennedy DW. Endoscopic management of cerebrospinal fluid leaks and cephaloceles. Laryngoscope 1990;100(8):857–862

5. McMains KC, Gross CW, Kountakis SE. Endoscopic management of cerebrospinal fluid rhinorrhea. Laryngoscope 2004;114(10):1833–1837

6. Lindstrom DR, Toohill RJ, Loehrl TA, Smith TL. Management of cerebrospinal fluid rhinorrhea: the Medical College of Wisconsin experience. Laryngoscope 2004;114(6):969–974

7. Lee TJ, Huang CC, Chuang CC, Huang SF. Transnasal endoscopic repair of cerebrospinal fluid rhinorrhea and skull base defect: ten-year experience. Laryngoscope 2004;114(8):1475–1481

8. Kirtane MV, Gautham K, Upadhyaya SR. Endoscopic CSF rhinorrhea closure: our experience in 267 cases. Otolaryngol Head Neck Surg 2005;132(2):208–212

9. Schlosser RJ, Bolger WE. Nasal cerebrospinal fluid leaks: critical review and surgical considerations. Laryngoscope 2004;114(2):255–265

10. Schlosser RJ, Wilensky EM, Grady MS, Bolger WE. Elevated intracranial pressures in spontaneous cerebrospinal fluid leaks. Am J Rhinol 2003;17(4):191–195

11. Woodworth BA, Schlosser RJ, Faust RA, Bolger WE. Evolutions in the management of congenital intranasal skull base defects. Arch Otolaryngol Head Neck Surg 2004;130(11):1283–1288

12. Locatelli D, Rampa F, Acchiardi I, Bignami M, De Bernardi F, Castelnuovo P. Endoscopic endonasal approaches for repair of cerebrospinal fluid leaks: nine-year experience. Neurosurgery 2006; 58(4, Suppl 2):ONS-246–ONS-256, ONS-256–ONS-257

13. Patel MR, Stadler ME, Snyderman CH, et al. How to choose? Endoscopic skull base reconstructive options and limitations. Skull Base 2010;20(6):397–404

14. Germani RM, Vivero R, Herzallah IR, Casiano RR. Endoscopic reconstruction of large anterior skull base defects using acellular dermal allograft. Am J Rhinol 2007;21(5):615–618

15. Lorenz RR, Dean RL, Hurley DB, Chuang J, Citardi MJ. Endoscopic reconstruction of anterior and middle cranial fossa defects using acellular dermal allograft. Laryngoscope 2003;113(3):496–501

16. Esposito F, Cappabianca P, Fusco M, et al. Collagen-only biomatrix as a novel dural substitute. Examination of the efficacy, safety and outcome: clinical experience on a series of 208 patients. Clin Neurol Neurosurg 2008;110(4):343–351

17. Gjuric M, Goede U, Keimer H, Wigand ME. Endonasal endoscopic closure of cerebrospinal fluid fistulas at the anterior cranial base. Ann Otol Rhinol Laryngol 1996;105(8):620–623

18. Hegazy HM, Carrau RL, Snyderman CH, Kassam A, Zweig J. Transnasal endoscopic repair of cerebrospinal fluid rhinorrhea: a meta-analysis. Laryngoscope 2000;110(7):1166–1172

19. Gardner P, Kassam A, Snyderman C, Mintz A, Carrau RL, Moossy JJ. Endoscopic endonasal suturing of dural reconstruction grafts: a novel application of the U-Clip technology. Technical note. J Neurosurg 2008;108(2):395–400

20. Hadad G, Bassagasteguy L, Carrau RL, et al. A novel reconstructive technique after endoscopic expanded endonasal approaches: vascular pedicle nasoseptal flap. Laryngoscope 2006;116(10):1882–1886

21. Harvey RJ, Sheahan PO, Schlosser RJ. Inferior turbinate pedicle flap for endoscopic skull base defect repair. Am J Rhinol Allergy 2009;23(5):522–526

22. Fortes FS, Carrau RL, Snyderman CH, et al. Transpterygoid transposition of a temporoparietal fascia flap: a new method for skull base reconstruction after endoscopic expanded endonasal approaches. Laryngoscope 2007;117(6):970–976

23. Fortes FS, Carrau RL, Snyderman CH, et al. The posterior pedicle inferior turbinate flap: a new vascularized flap for skull base reconstruction. Laryngoscope 2007;117(8):1329–1332

24. Prevedello DM, Barges-Coll J, Fernandez-Miranda JC, et al. Middle turbinate flap for skull base reconstruction: cadaveric feasibility study. Laryngoscope 2009;119(11):2094–2098

25. Oliver CL, Hackman TG, Carrau RL, et al. Palatal flap modifications allow pedicled reconstruction of the skull base. Laryngoscope 2008;118(12):2102–2106

26. Pinheiro-Neto CD, Ramos HF, Peris-Celda M, et al. Study of the nasoseptal flap for endoscopic anterior cranial base reconstruction. Laryngoscope 2011;121(12):2514–2520

27. Rivera-Serrano CM, Bassagaisteguy LH, Hadad G, et al. Posterior pedicle lateral nasal wall flap: new reconstructive technique for large defects of the skull base. Am J Rhinol Allergy 2011;25(6):e212–e216

28. Hadad G, Rivera-Serrano CM, Bassagaisteguy LH, et al. Anterior pedicle lateral nasal wall flap: a novel technique for the reconstruction of anterior skull base defects. Laryngoscope 2011;121(8):1606–1610

29. Senior BA, Jafri K, Benninger M. Safety and efficacy of endoscopic repair of CSF leaks and encephaloceles: a survey of the members of the American Rhinologic Society. Am J Rhinol 2001;15(1):21–25

30. Batra PS, Kanowitz SJ, Luong A. Anatomical and technical correlates in endoscopic anterior skull base surgery: a cadaveric analysis. Otolaryngol Head Neck Surg 2010;142(6):827–831

31. Zanation AM, Snyderman CH, Carrau RL, Kassam AB, Gardner PA, Prevedello DM. Minimally invasive endoscopic pericranial flap: a new method for endonasal skull base reconstruction. Laryngoscope 2009;119(1):13–18

32. Tabaee A, Anand VK, Brown SM, Lin JW, Schwartz TH. Algorithm for reconstruction after endoscopic pituitary and skull base surgery. Laryngoscope 2007;117(7):1133–1137

33. Briggs RJA, Wormald PJ. Endoscopic transnasal intradural repair of anterior skull base cerebrospinal fluid fistulae. J Clin Neurosci 2004;11(6):597–599

34. Gross WE, Gross CW, Becker D, Moore D, Phillips D. Modified transnasal endoscopic Lothrop procedure as an alternative to frontal sinus obliteration. Otolaryngol Head Neck Surg 1995;113(4):427–434

35. Becker SS, Duncavage JA, Russell PT. Endoscopic endonasal repair of difficult-to-access cerebrospinal fluid leaks of the frontal sinus. Am J Rhinol Allergy 2009;23(2):181–184

34 Nasopharyngeal Carcinoma

William I. Wei and Daniel T. T. Chua

Nasopharyngeal carcinoma (NPC) is an uncommon pathology in the West but endemic in Southern China, South Asia, and Sub-Saharan Africa. NPC is highly aggressive; it has a propensity to invade surrounding tissues such as the paranasal sinuses and skull base and tends to spread to cervical lymph nodes. The undifferentiated type of NPC is the predominant histological type in endemic regions, and it has a high propensity for distant metastases. Radiotherapy with or without chemotherapy is the primary treatment modality for newly diagnosed NPC, whereas surgery is usually reserved for management of residual or recurrent disease. In patients with locoregional recurrence, salvage surgery should be considered if technically feasible. Patients who are not candidates for surgery can receive reirradiation. In patients with advanced recurrence and distant metastases, palliative chemotherapy can often achieve durable control of symptoms and disease. Less frequently, long-term survivors are seen after aggressive chemotherapy and targeted therapy.

Symptoms and Signs

The symptoms of NPC are related to the location of the tumor in the nasopharynx, extension to surrounding structures, and regional metastasis. Unilateral nasal obstruction with blood-stained nasal discharge is the most common nasal symptom. Hearing loss and tinnitus are related to the tumor affecting eustachian tube function and resulting in serous otitis media. Patients with advanced disease may present with cranial nerve palsies that are the result of superior extension of the tumor to the skull base. Cranial nerves III, IV, and VI are frequently involved. The commonest mode of presentation is a painless upper neck unilateral mass, and this is a metastatic cervical lymph node. Symptoms of early stage disease are usually nonspecific and minor, thus frequently ignored by the patient and even the physician, resulting in most patients presenting at the late stage of disease.

Diagnosis

Clinical Examination

Examination of the nasopharynx can be performed under local anesthesia with either a rigid or a flexible endoscope. The rigid 0- or 30-degree Hopkins rod endoscopes provide an excellent view of the nasopharynx (**Figs. 34.1** and **34.2**). When a suspicious lesion is seen, a biopsy can be taken with a pair of forceps inserted along the endoscope. The use of flexible fiberoptic endoscopes allows a more thorough

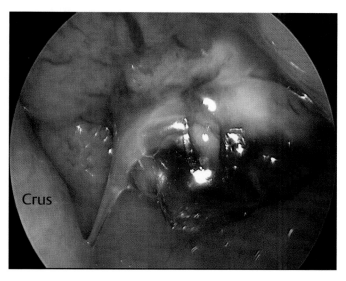

Figure 34.1 Endoscopic view of a nasopharyngeal carcinoma situated at the posterior wall of the nasopharynx with the 0-degree endoscope inserted through the right nasal cavity. The medial crus of the right eustachian tube are marked.

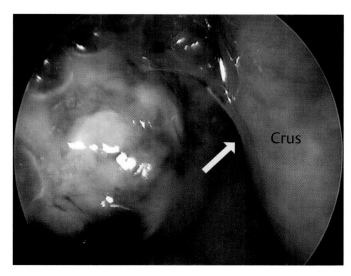

Figure 34.2 Endoscopic view of the same nasopharyngeal carcinoma situated at the posterior wall of the nasopharynx with the 0-degree endoscope inserted through the left nasal cavity. The medial crus of the left eustachian tube are marked. The left fossa of Rosenmüller is shown (arrow).

examination of the whole nasopharynx; the tip of the endoscope can be manipulated behind the nasal septum to see the entire nasopharynx with the scope inserted through one nasal cavity.

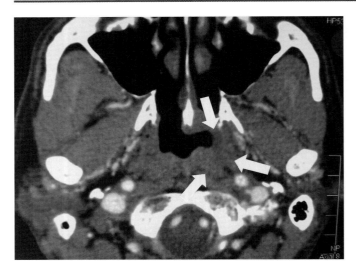

Figure 34.3 Axial computed tomography showing a recurrent nasopharyngeal carcinoma (arrows) at the posterolateral wall of the nasopharynx.

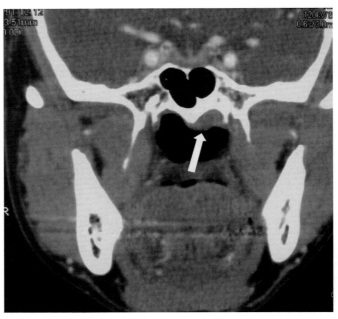

Figure 34.4 Coronal computed tomography showing the same recurrent nasopharyngeal carcinoma (arrow) attached to the skull base.

Serology

As Epstein-Barr virus (EBV) has a strong association with NPC, the level of antibodies against EBV is related to the stage of the tumor, which is proportional to the tumor burden. The antibodies (IgA) for the viral capsid antigen and early antigen have been used widely to screen for early NPC. In recent years, circulating free EBV DNA can be detected by polymerase chain reaction assay in patients suffering from NPC; this has been shown to be more accurate than measuring the antibody titers against the various EBV antigens.[1]

Imaging Studies

Cross-sectional imaging contributes to the assessment of the tumor. This includes the involvement of the musculature of the nasopharyngeal wall and the erosion of bone at skull base. Computed tomography (CT) is useful in detecting skull base bone erosion and tumor extension into the paranasopharyngeal space. These findings provide information for accurate staging of this malignancy (**Figs. 34.3** and **34.4**). When a biopsy of an enlarged retropharyngeal node is required and it cannot be visualized with an endoscope, then the CT navigation system is applicable. Under the guidance of the navigation system, the surgeon can insert forceps through the wall of the nasopharynx accurately into the retropharyngeal node for the biopsy.

Magnetic resonance imaging (MRI) cannot demonstrate subtle bone erosion, but it has better tissue specificity and distinguishes tumor from inflammation. It also has multiplanar capabilities and is useful in evaluating the extent of cervical nodal metastases; this includes the retropharyngeal nodes of Rouviere. Cross-sectional imaging modalities, such as CT and MRI, complement each other and display the extent of the primary tumor precisely.

Positron emission tomography can reveal NPC at the primary site and the metastatic lymph nodes. However, it does not improve the diagnostic rate or affect the staging.[2] Although it can detect distant metastasis, it has been shown to be less sensitive than whole body MRI. Its real value is the ability to detect residual and recurrent tumors in the nasopharynx.[3]

Treatment

Radiotherapy

Radiotherapy is the primary treatment modality for locoregionally confined NPC. The outcome of patients after radiotherapy for NPC has improved significantly from a 5-year survival rate of 25% in the 1950s,[4] to 50% in the 1970 to 1980s,[5] and to 75% in the 1990s.[6] This improved outcome is because of multiple factors including earlier stage disease at presentation, improved imaging technique, use of conformal radiotherapy technique, and combined chemoradiotherapy. In designing radiotherapy for NPC, a large target volume is needed to cover the nasopharynx and potential sites of spread, which includes the paranasopharyngeal space, oropharynx, base of the skull, sphenoid sinus, posterior ethmoid sinus, and posterior half of maxillary antrum. Extension of treatment field to cover cavernous sinus and cranial fossa may be needed in advanced disease. Cervical nodal irradiation is mandatory even in node-negative patients because of the high incidence of neck relapse in the absence of prophylactic nodal irradiation.[7] A dose of 65 to 70 Gy is normally given to the primary tumor, 65 to 70 Gy to the involved neck nodes, and 50 to 60 Gy to node-negative neck. In recent years, intensity-modulated radiotherapy (IMRT) has become the preferred technique for the treatment of NPC. IMRT is a radiation technique that allows the delivery of highly conformed dose distribution to the target and critical structures through optimization of intensity of multiple beams. The treatment design is based on the computer algorithm to calculate the best result that matches the user-defined parameters in a process called inverse planning. The advantages of IMRT include the ability to deliver highly conformal radiotherapy to irregular target, the ability to treat primary and regional lymphatic in one volume, and the ability to deliver simultaneous integrated boost in the same setting. IMRT has already achieved excellent local control rates for newly diagnosed NPC, with a reported local control rate of 92 to 97% at 3 to 4 years.[8,9] Apart from improvement of tumor control, IMRT also reduces the risk of late complications such as xerostomia in early stage disease.[10]

Combined Chemoradiotherapy

Combining chemotherapy and radiotherapy has been used increasingly for the treatment of NPC, especially for those with advanced disease. The high incidence of distant metastases, despite successful locoregional control with radiotherapy alone, helps support this strategy. NPC has a high response rate to most chemotherapeutic agents, and these agents also have a radiosensitizing effect when used in combination with radiotherapy. Many randomized trials have been conducted to explore the benefits of combined chemoradiotherapy in NPC. Four randomized phase III studies comparing induction chemotherapy followed by radiotherapy versus radiotherapy alone in NPC have been reported.[11–14] None of these studies have demonstrated survival benefits when adding chemotherapy to radiotherapy. However, two of these studies were recently updated and the data pooled for analysis; a significant improvement in disease-free survival in the chemotherapy arm was observed, but the overall survival was not improved.[15] Only two adjuvant chemotherapy phase III studies have been reported, and both showed no survival benefits.[16,17] These studies showed that induction chemotherapy alone has a limited role in NPC, whereas the role of adjuvant chemotherapy remains undefined.

In recent years, concurrent chemoradiotherapy has emerged as the treatment of choice for locoregionally advanced NPC. This is largely because of the positive findings of the Intergroup 0099 trial. This was the first randomized trial to demonstrate survival benefit with the use of chemotherapy in this disease.[18] The Intergroup trial employed both concurrent and adjuvant chemotherapy in the study arm and reported an absolute survival improvement of 31% at 3 years. Subsequent randomized trials conducted in endemic regions have largely confirmed the benefits of concurrent chemoradiotherapy for advanced NPC, although different regimens and schedules were used in these studies.[19–22] Only one study employed the same chemotherapy regimens used in the Intergroup study. The final report from that study showed no survival benefits, although there was an improvement in progression-free survival.[23] Nevertheless, current evidence indicates that concurrent chemoradiotherapy has a major role in advanced stage NPC, but the optimal regimen/schedule remains to be defined. On the basis of current evidence, the doctors should advise chemoradiotherapy to all patients with nodal disease or T3 to T4 disease, whereas radiotherapy alone should be reserved for those with T1 to T2 N0 disease.

Residual or Recurrent Disease

Incidence

Despite the use of concurrent chemoradiation with improved outcomes, there are still patients who have persistent or recurrent locoregional tumors. The incidence of local residual or recurrent was around 8.3%[24] and regional recurrences in the cervical nodes was around 4.7%.[24] Endoscopic examination of the nasopharynx with biopsy of suspicious lesions is the standard procedure to confirm the presence of residual or recurrent disease. Elevated copies of EBV DNA in blood and imaging studies such as CT and MRI are useful adjunct tests to raise the suspicion of possible persistent or recurrent disease. This is particularly so with increasing number of EBV copies and progressive enlarging masses. Positron emission tomography scan has also been shown to be better than the conventional imaging studies in the diagnosis of residual disease.[25]

Residual or recurrent tumor in the cervical lymph nodes after radiotherapy is however more difficult to confirm. Fine needle aspiration is not helpful because only clusters of tumor cells are present in some of the pathological lymph nodes, and it is difficult to get a cytological diagnosis.[26] The increasing size of the lymph nodes on clinical examination or sequential imaging is worrying. The definitive diagnosis still depends on histological examination and occasionally this becomes available only after salvage surgery.

For localized disease in the nasopharynx or the neck, salvage therapy should be offered if possible. Survival after salvage therapy for extensive disease remains poor, but it is still higher than that in patients receiving only supportive treatment.[27]

Disease in the Cervical Lymph Node

With a second course of external radiotherapy to treat cervical lymph node metastases, the 5-year actuarial control rate of local nodal disease was 51% and the overall 5-year survival rate was 19.7%.[28] Some report that the excision of these lymph nodes followed by a second course of radiotherapy was not promising,[29] and the second course of radiotherapy was associated with significant morbidity.

The optimal management of localized metastasis in the neck lymph nodes depends on the pathologic behavior of the tumor. Radical neck dissection is recommended as the salvage treatment of choice for cervical nodal metastasis after radiotherapy. Serial sectioning study of radical neck dissection specimens revealed there were more tumor-bearing lymph nodes than clinically evident, and 46% of these nodes exhibited extracapsular spread.[30] With radical neck dissection as salvage surgery, the 5-year rate of control of disease in the neck was 66%, and the 5-year actuarial survival for this group of patients was 38%.[31] A recent review showed that neck nodes in level I were infrequently affected in these patients, and that a less extensive neck dissection sparing level I might be applicable in patients.[32]

When the residual or recurrent cervical lymph node has extensive involvement, such as affecting the floor of the neck or the overlying skin, then brachytherapy should be applied in addition to the radical neck dissection for salvage. The skin over the metastatic cervical node is removed with the specimen, and hollow nylon tubes are positioned over the operative site for after loading brachytherapy with iridium wires. The cutaneous defect in the neck is covered with either a deltopectoral flap or a pectoralis major myocutaneous flap. With this form of therapy, local tumor control rate of more than 60% has been reported.[33]

Disease in the Nasopharynx

If a patient develops residual or recurrent tumor only in the nasopharynx following radiation or concurrent chemo-radiation, then salvage therapy is sometimes possible. The decision depends on the extent of tumor, the condition of the patient, and the expertise of the treating clinicians.

Reirradiation of Residual or Recurrent Tumor

Reirradiation of NPC is challenging, because of the large numbers of critical structures in the vicinity of target. These have already been irradiated to a high dose in primary treatment. For patients with small volume disease or tumor confined to the nasopharynx, brachytherapy or stereotactic radiosurgery is preferred. External beam reirradiation is reserved for those with bulky tumor or disease extended beyond the nasopharynx. Important prognostic factors for patients receiving external reirradiation for recurrent NPC include T stage, time to recurrence, and reirradiation dose for local control and survival. The most consistent prognostic factor being reported was recurrent T stage; patients treated for advanced T stage had poor local control and survival after reirradiation. There appears to be an important relationship between reirradiation dose and treatment outcome, with most series reporting poor tumor control with a dose less than 60 Gy.[34,35] However, the optimal dose is yet to be defined.

External Beam Reirradiation

The reported 5-year survival rates after external beam reirradiation using conventional technique ranged from 8 to 36%.[36,37] Toxicity to surrounding tissues with a second course of radiation limits the radiation dose. A high incidence of late complications, mostly neurological damage and soft tissue fibrosis, was commonly observed after external beam reirradiation. The potential neuroendocrine injury,[38] temporal lobe necrosis,[39] cranial nerve palsies, and other problems such as trismus and deafness can be incapacitating. The use of three-dimensional conformal radiotherapy—and more recently IMRT—has improved the outlook of patients receiving external reirradiation. In one study using three-dimensional conformal radiotherapy for retreatment of NPC, 5-year local control rate was 71%, but the actuarial incidence of major late toxicities was still high. All patients developed at least grade 3 toxicities and nearly half of patients had grade 4 toxicities at 5 years.[40] In one report, following as a second course of radiation, a salvage rate of 32% was achieved; the cumulative incidence of late postreirradiation sequela was 24%, with treatment mortality of 1.8%.[41] External beam reirradiation is employed when other therapeutic options are not applicable.

Brachytherapy

When brachytherapy is used, the radiation dosage is highest at the radiation source and decreases rapidly with increasing distance from the source. This enables a high dose of radiation to be delivered to the residual or recurrent tumor in the nasopharynx, while at the same time reducing the dose to the surrounding tissue. Brachytherapy radiation also delivers radiation at a continuous low dose rate, which gives further radiobiological advantage over fractionated doses of external radiation. Intracavitary brachytherapy has been used traditionally for NPCs.[42] In this method, the radiation source is placed in either a tube or a mold and this device is then inserted into the nasopharynx for therapy. Intracavitary brachytherapy has also been reported with success.[43,44] Clinician experience together with patient selection is the key issue for a favorable outcome. In view of the irregular contour and dimension of the nasopharynx and the location of the persistent or recurrent tumor, it is difficult to position the radiation source accurately in the nasopharynx for tumoricidal effect. To circumvent this problem, radioactive interstitial implants such as gold grains (^{198}Au) have been used to treat small localized residual or recurrent tumor in the nasopharynx. When gold grain implants were applied to treat persistent and recurrent tumors after radiotherapy, the 5-year local tumor control rates were 87 and 63%, respectively, and the corresponding 5-year disease-free survival rates were 68 and 60%, respectively.[45] Gold grain implantation is an effective salvage method for those small tumors localized in the nasopharynx, without bone invasion, and not encroaching onto the eustachian tube cartilage.[46] Studies show that the morbidity was low and there were no other significant sequelae associated with this form of treatment.

Stereotactic Radiosurgery

Stereotactic radiosurgery is a technique in which a target is stereotactically localized and irradiated by multiple convergent beams. This uses a large single dose of radiation. Stereotactic radiosurgery alone was reported to achieve a crude local control rate of 53 to 86% for locally recurrent NPC.[47,48] For recurrent disease confined to nasopharynx or adjacent soft tissues, the reported local control rate at 2 years was 72%.[49] When stereotactic radiosurgery was administered as a boost dose after reirradiation, the 3-year control rate ranged from 52 to 58%.[50,51] The same technique may also be used to deliver multiple fractions of radiation and is termed stereotactic radiotherapy. These results indicate that radiosurgery is an effective salvage treatment for local failures of NPC, although long-term follow-up data are still not available.

Surgery for Residual or Recurrent Tumor

Another salvage option for residual or recurrent tumor localized in the nasopharynx is surgical resection. This is employed when the localized disease cannot be managed adequately by brachytherapy. This could be because the tumor is too large and extends into the paranasopharyngeal space or because its location precludes gold grain implantation (e.g., close to the cartilage of the eustachian tube crura). Surgical resection will obviate the serious long-term consequences of reirradiation.

Endoscopic Resection

Successful resection of small, localized residual or recurrent tumor with endoscopes has recently been reported.[52–54] For this approach to be successful, the location of the tumor in the nasopharynx is most important. This factor determines a successful oncologic resection with rigid instruments. Small tumor located in the posterior wall of the nasopharynx can be removed adequately with endoscope and instruments inserted through the nasal cavity (**Fig. 34.5**). In addition, curved instruments can be introduced into the nasopharynx through the oral cavity behind the soft palate. As a limited portion of the nasopharynx is included in the resection, there is no need for any reconstruction; the wound will heal by secondary intention.

Microwave coagulation therapy has also been used for tumor extirpation, and successful outcomes have been reported with the instrument introduced transnasally.[55] In general with the rigid endoscopic instruments, resection of the deep margins of laterally situated tumors is limited. To help circumvent this problem, the da Vinci robot (Intuitive

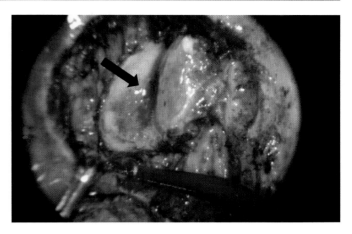

Figure 34.5 Endoscopic resection of a small recurrent nasopharyngeal carcinoma (arrow) at the posterior wall of the nasopharynx. The sucker is shown on the left and the diathermy on the right.

Surgical Inc., Sunnyvale, California) can be employed. With the versatile EndoWrist of the da Vinci robot inserted through a split palate approach, the lateral wall of the nasopharynx and the tumor including the opening of the auditory tympanic tube can be removed en bloc (**Fig. 34.6**).[56]

Nasopharyngectomy

Adequate tumor removal with a negative resection margin is important for a successful salvage surgery.[57] For a more extensive tumor, the nasopharynx has to be exposed widely for an oncologic resection to be performed. This is challenging because the nasopharynx lies in the center of the head; it is not easy to adequately expose pathology in the nasopharynx and its vicinity so that complete tumor extirpation can be performed.

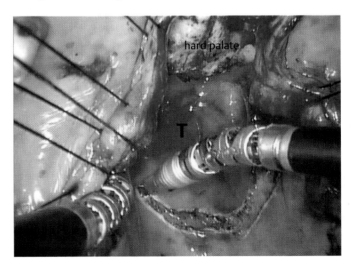

Figure 34.6 Resection of the recurrent nasopharyngeal carcinoma with the da Vinci robot. The tumor (T) was exposed by splitting the soft palate that is slinged with stitches. The EndoWrist with the grasping forceps is shown on the left, whereas the EndoWrist with a diathermy is shown on the right.

In the past, various anterior approaches were used, either the transantral or the transnasal route, but did not provide adequate exposure of the nasopharynx for adequate tumor removal.[58] From the front, even with down fracture of the hard palate as in a Le Fort I[59] or midfacial degloving approach with removal of the medial wall of the maxilla, exposure of the lateral aspect of the nasopharynx is not entirely satisfactory.[60] These approaches were mainly used for the centrally located tumor over the posterior wall of the nasopharynx.

The lateral or infratemporal fossa approach to the nasopharynx has also been described.[61] To reach the nasopharynx with this approach, a mastoidectomy has to be performed and some important structures have to be mobilized. These include the internal carotid artery, the fifth cranial nerve, and the floor of middle cranial fossa. A study on 11 patients who had surgical salvage with this approach reported a 2-year disease-free survival rate of 72%.[62] Although laterally located tumors in the nasopharynx can be removed by this approach, it is difficult to remove the tumor that has crossed the midline, and the associated morbidity of this approach is not negligible.

Approaching the nasopharynx from the inferior aspect, using transpalatal, transmaxillary, and transcervical routes, has been reported as useful.[63] With this approach, it is difficult to carry out dissection of the lateral wall of the nasopharynx under direct vision, especially when the tumor is close to the internal carotid artery. This approach is useful for tumors situated in the central part of the nasopharynx. As long as the internal carotid artery is safeguarded, the associated morbidity of the operation with this approach is low.

The maxillary swing, or anterolateral approach, to the nasopharynx provides adequate exposure of the nasopharynx and the vicinity region.[64]

Following a Weber-Fergusson incision and three osteotomies (anterior wall of the maxilla below the inferior orbital rim, hard palate in the midline maxilla, and separating the pterygoid plates from the maxillary tuberosity), the maxilla is detached from the facial skeleton. It is, however, still attached to the anterior cheek flap and the whole complex is swung laterally as an osteocutaneous flap. The nasopharynx with the recurrent or residual tumor and the paranasopharyngeal space tissue are all widely exposed (**Fig. 34.7**). An oncologic resection can be performed under direct vision (**Fig. 34.8**). The internal carotid artery below the skull base of the skull can be dissected free from the residual or recurrent NPC. After tumor resection, the maxilla is returned and fixed onto the facial skeleton with miniplates. The complications of this procedure are generally minor; some patients develop trismus or a palatal fistula. With modification of surgical techniques, the palatal fistula rate associated with the maxillary swing approach has been markedly reduced,[65] and the quality of life of these patients was satisfactory.[66,67] Reports of 246 patients who underwent salvage nasopharyngectomy with this maxillary swing approach showed a 5-year actuarial local tumor control rate of 74% and a 5-year

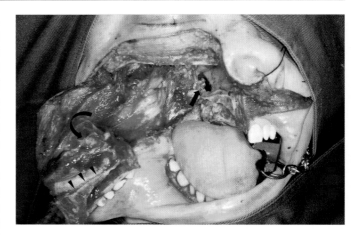

Figure 34.7 The right maxilla is swung to show a recurrent nasopharyngeal carcinoma (arrow) in the nasopharynx. The hard palate (arrowheads) with the teeth and the maxillary antrum (curved arrow) are shown.

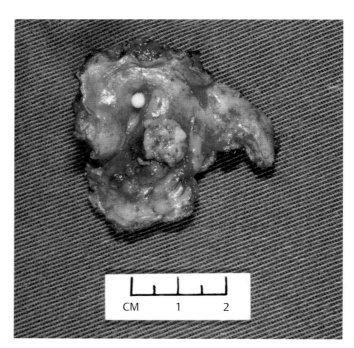

Figure 34.8 Resected nasopharyngeal carcinoma specimen showing the tumor. The yellow tubing marks the right eustachian tube opening.

actuarial survival was 56%.[68] The follow-up period ranged from 6 to 18 years (median 38 months). For more extensive tumor lying close to the internal carotid artery, this vessel would be exposed after tumor removal and might lead to serious complications. Microvascular free tissue transfer, such as a vastus lateralis flap, has been used to cover the exposed vessel to promote healing and prevent vascular complications.[69]

Considering that salvage surgery patients had previous radiotherapy, the mortalities associated with most of these procedures were low. With surgery, as long as the residual or recurrent tumor can be removed adequately, the long-term results have been satisfactory.[70,71–73] The surgical option chosen depends on the location and size of the tumor. When tumor is smaller and localized to easily visualized regions, endoscopic resection, the da Vinci robot, or a combination is applicable.[74] For larger tumors that are still localized to the nasopharynx and the paranasopharyngeal space, surgical resection with an open approach still offers a reasonable chance of cure with limited morbidities.

Conclusion

The treatment of NPC presents a challenge to the clinician. The use of radiation, chemotherapy, and surgery varies with the disease extent and course. Newer regimens using chemotherapy and radiation, as well as surgical techniques spanning open, endoscopic, and robotic methods, hold promise for improving patient outcomes.

References

1. Shao JY, Li YH, Gao HY, et al. Comparison of plasma Epstein-Barr virus (EBV) DNA levels and serum EBV immunoglobulin A/virus capsid antigen antibody titers in patients with nasopharyngeal carcinoma. Cancer 2004;100(6):1162–1170
2. King AD, Ma BB, Yau YY, et al. The impact of 18F-FDG PET/CT on assessment of nasopharyngeal carcinoma at diagnosis. Br J Radiol 2008;81(964):291–298
3. Yen RF, Hung RL, Pan MH, et al. 18-Fluoro-2-deoxyglucose positron emission tomography in detecting residual/recurrent nasopharyngeal carcinomas and comparison with magnetic resonance imaging. Cancer 2003;98(2):283–287
4. Moss WT. Therapeutic Radiology. 2nd ed. St Louis: CV Mosby; 1965
5. Lee AWM, Poon YF, Foo W, et al. Retrospective analysis of 5037 patients with nasopharyngeal carcinoma treated during 1976-1985: overall survival and patterns of failure. Int J Radiat Oncol Biol Phys 1992;23(2):261–270
6. Lee AW, Sze WM, Au JS, et al. Treatment results for nasopharyngeal carcinoma in the modern era: the Hong Kong experience. Int J Radiat Oncol Biol Phys 2005;61(4):1107–1116
7. Lee AW, Sham JS, Poon YF, Ho JH. Treatment of stage I nasopharyngeal carcinoma: analysis of the patterns of relapse and the results of withholding elective neck irradiation. Int J Radiat Oncol Biol Phys 1989;17(6):1183–1190
8. Lee N, Xia P, Quivey JM, et al. Intensity-modulated radiotherapy in the treatment of nasopharyngeal carcinoma: an update of the UCSF experience. Int J Radiat Oncol Biol Phys 2002;53(1):12–22
9. Kam MK, Teo PM, Chau RM, et al. Treatment of nasopharyngeal carcinoma with intensity-modulated radiotherapy: the Hong Kong experience. Int J Radiat Oncol Biol Phys 2004;60(5):1440–1450
10. Kwong DL, Pow EH, Sham JS, et al. Intensity-modulated radiotherapy for early-stage nasopharyngeal carcinoma: a prospective study on disease control and preservation of salivary function. Cancer 2004;101(7):1584–1593
11. Preliminary results of a randomized trial comparing neoadjuvant chemotherapy (cisplatin, epirubicin, bleomycin) plus radiotherapy vs. radiotherapy alone in stage IV(> or = N2, M0) undifferentiated nasopharyngeal carcinoma: a positive effect on progression-free survival. International Nasopharynx Cancer Study Group. VUMCA I trial. Int J Radiat Oncol Biol Phys 1996;35(3):463–469
12. Chua DTT, Sham JST, Choy D, et al; Asian-Oceanian Clinical Oncology Association Nasopharynx Cancer Study Group. Preliminary report of the Asian-Oceanian Clinical Oncology Association randomized trial comparing cisplatin and epirubicin followed by radiotherapy versus radiotherapy alone in the treatment of patients with locoregionally advanced nasopharyngeal carcinoma. Cancer 1998;83(11):2270–2283
13. Ma J, Mai HQ, Hong MH, et al. Results of a prospective randomized trial comparing neoadjuvant chemotherapy plus radiotherapy with radiotherapy alone in patients with locoregionally advanced nasopharyngeal carcinoma. J Clin Oncol 2001;19(5):1350–1357
14. Hareyama M, Sakata K, Shirato H, et al. A prospective, randomized trial comparing neoadjuvant chemotherapy with radiotherapy alone in patients with advanced nasopharyngeal carcinoma. Cancer 2002;94(8):2217–2223
15. Chua DT, Ma J, Sham JS, et al. Long-term survival after cisplatin-based induction chemotherapy and radiotherapy for nasopharyngeal carcinoma: a pooled data analysis of two phase III trials. J Clin Oncol 2005;23(6):1118–1124
16. Rossi A, Molinari R, Boracchi P, et al. Adjuvant chemotherapy with vincristine, cyclophosphamide, and doxorubicin after radiotherapy in local-regional nasopharyngeal cancer: results of a 4-year multicenter randomized study. J Clin Oncol 1988;6(9):1401–1410
17. Chi KH, Chang YC, Guo WY, et al. A phase III study of adjuvant chemotherapy in advanced nasopharyngeal carcinoma patients. Int J Radiat Oncol Biol Phys 2002;52(5):1238–1244
18. Al-Sarraf M, LeBlanc M, Giri PG, et al. Chemoradiotherapy versus radiotherapy in patients with advanced nasopharyngeal cancer: phase III randomized Intergroup study 0099. J Clin Oncol 1998;16(4):1310–1317
19. Lin JC, Jan JS, Hsu CY, Liang WM, Jiang RS, Wang WY. Phase III study of concurrent chemoradiotherapy versus radiotherapy alone for advanced nasopharyngeal carcinoma: positive effect on overall and progression-free survival. J Clin Oncol 2003;21(4):631–637
20. Chan AT, Leung SF, Ngan RK, et al. Overall survival after concurrent cisplatin-radiotherapy compared with radiotherapy alone in locoregionally advanced nasopharyngeal carcinoma. J Natl Cancer Inst 2005;97(7):536–539
21. Wee J, Tan EH, Tai BC, et al. Randomized trial of radiotherapy versus concurrent chemoradiotherapy followed by adjuvant chemotherapy in patients with American Joint Committee on Cancer/International Union against cancer stage III and IV nasopharyngeal cancer of the endemic variety. J Clin Oncol 2005;23(27):6730–6738
22. Kwong DL, Sham JS, Au GK, et al. Concurrent and adjuvant chemotherapy for nasopharyngeal carcinoma: a factorial study. J Clin Oncol 2004;22(13):2643–2653
23. Lee AW, Tung SY, Chua DT, et al. Randomized trial of radiotherapy plus concurrent-adjuvant chemotherapy vs radiotherapy alone for regionally advanced nasopharyngeal carcinoma. J Natl Cancer Inst 2010;102(15):1188–1198
24. Ng WT, Lee MC, Hung WM, et al. Clinical outcomes and patterns of failure after intensity-modulated radiotherapy for nasopharyngeal carcinoma. Int J Radiat Oncol Biol Phys 2011;79(2):420–428
25. Kao CH, Tsai SC, Wang JJ, Ho YJ, Yen RF, Ho ST. Comparing 18-fluoro-2-deoxyglucose positron emission tomography with a combination of technetium 99m tetrofosmin single photon emission computed tomography and computed tomography to detect recurrent or persistent nasopharyngeal carcinomas after radiotherapy. Cancer 2001;92(2):434–439
26. Wei WI, Ho CM, Wong MP, Ng WF, Lau SK, Lam KH. Pathological basis of surgery in the management of postradiotherapy cervical metastasis in nasopharyngeal carcinoma. Arch Otolaryngol Head Neck Surg 1992;118(9):923–929, discussion 930
27. Chua DT, Wei WI, Sham JS, Cheng AC, Au G. Treatment outcome for synchronous locoregional failures of nasopharyngeal carcinoma. Head Neck 2003;25(7):585–594

28. Sham JS, Choy D. Nasopharyngeal carcinoma: treatment of neck node recurrence by radiotherapy. Australas Radiol 1991;35(4):370–373

29. Tu GY, Hu YH, Xu GZ, Ye M. Salvage surgery for nasopharyngeal carcinoma. Arch Otolaryngol Head Neck Surg 1988;114(3):328–329

30. Wei WI, Ho CM, Wong MP, Ng WF, Lau SK, Lam KH. Pathological basis of surgery in the management of postradiotherapy cervical metastasis in nasopharyngeal carcinoma. Arch Otolaryngol Head Neck Surg 1992;118(9):923–929, discussion 930

31. Wei WI, Lam KH, Ho CM, Sham JS, Lau SK. Efficacy of radical neck dissection for the control of cervical metastasis after radiotherapy for nasopharyngeal carcinoma. Am J Surg 1990;160(4):439–442

32. Khafif A, Ferlito A, Takes RP, Thomas Robbins K. Is it necessary to perform radical neck dissection as a salvage procedure for persistent or recurrent neck disease after chemoradiotherapy in patients with nasopharyngeal cancer? Eur Arch Otorhinolaryngol 2010;267(7):997–999

33. Wei WI, Ho WK, Cheng AC, et al. Management of extensive cervical nodal metastasis in nasopharyngeal carcinoma after radiotherapy: a clinicopathological study. Arch Otolaryngol Head Neck Surg 2001;127(12):1457–1462

34. Wang CC. Re-irradiation of recurrent nasopharyngeal carcinoma—treatment techniques and results. Int J Radiat Oncol Biol Phys 1987;13(7):953–956

35. Lee AW, Foo W, Law SC, et al. Reirradiation for recurrent nasopharyngeal carcinoma: factors affecting the therapeutic ratio and ways for improvement. Int J Radiat Oncol Biol Phys 1997;38(1):43–52

36. Oksüz DÇ, Meral G, Uzel Ö, Cağatay P, Turkan S. Reirradiation for locally recurrent nasopharyngeal carcinoma: treatment results and prognostic factors. Int J Radiat Oncol Biol Phys 2004;60(2):388–394

37. Chang JT, See LC, Liao CT, et al. Locally recurrent nasopharyngeal carcinoma. Radiother Oncol 2000;54(2):135–142

38. Lam KSL, Ho JH, Lee AW, et al. Symptomatic hypothalamic-pituitary dysfunction in nasopharyngeal carcinoma patients following radiation therapy: a retrospective study. Int J Radiat Oncol Biol Phys 1987;13(9):1343–1350

39. Lee AW, Ng SH, Ho JH, et al. Clinical diagnosis of late temporal lobe necrosis following radiation therapy for nasopharyngeal carcinoma. Cancer 1988;61(8):1535–1542

40. Zheng XK, Ma J, Chen LH, Xia YF, Shi YS. Dosimetric and clinical results of three-dimensional conformal radiotherapy for locally recurrent nasopharyngeal carcinoma. Radiother Oncol 2005;75(2):197–203

41. Lee AW, Law SC, Foo W, et al. Retrospective analysis of patients with nasopharyngeal carcinoma treated during 1976-1985: survival after local recurrence. Int J Radiat Oncol Biol Phys 1993;26(5):773–782

42. Wang CC, Busse J, Gitterman M. A simple afterloading applicator for intracavitary irradiation of carcinoma of the nasopharynx. Radiology 1975;115(3):737–738

43. Leung TW, Tung SY, Wong VY, et al. High dose rate intracavitary brachytherapy in the treatment of nasopharyngeal carcinoma. Acta Oncol 1996;35(1):43–47

44. Law SC, Lam WK, Ng MF, Au SK, Mak WT, Lau WH. Reirradiation of nasopharyngeal carcinoma with intracavitary mold brachytherapy: an effective means of local salvage. Int J Radiat Oncol Biol Phys 2002;54(4):1095–1113

45. Kwong DL, Wei WI, Cheng AC, et al. Long term results of radioactive gold grain implantation for the treatment of persistent and recurrent nasopharyngeal carcinoma. Cancer 2001;91(6):1105–1113

46. Choy D, Sham JS, Wei WI, Ho CM, Wu PM. Transpalatal insertion of radioactive gold grain for the treatment of persistent and recurrent nasopharyngeal carcinoma. Int J Radiat Oncol Biol Phys 1993;25(3):505–512

47. Cmelak AJ, Cox RS, Adler JR, Fee WE Jr, Goffinet DR. Radiosurgery for skull base malignancies and nasopharyngeal carcinoma. Int J Radiat Oncol Biol Phys 1997;37(5):997–1003

48. Chua DT, Sham JS, Hung KN, Kwong DL, Kwong PW, Leung LH. Stereotactic radiosurgery as a salvage treatment for locally persistent and recurrent nasopharyngeal carcinoma. Head Neck 1999;21(7):620–626

49. Chua DT, Sham JS, Kwong PW, Hung KN, Leung LH. Linear accelerator-based stereotactic radiosurgery for limited, locally persistent, and recurrent nasopharyngeal carcinoma: efficacy and complications. Int J Radiat Oncol Biol Phys 2003;56(1):177–183

50. Chen HJ, Leung SW, Su CY. Linear accelerator based radiosurgery as a salvage treatment for skull base and intracranial invasion of recurrent nasopharyngeal carcinomas. Am J Clin Oncol 2001;24(3):255–258

51. Pai PC, Chuang CC, Wei KC, Tsang NM, Tseng CK, Chang CN. Stereotactic radiosurgery for locally recurrent nasopharyngeal carcinoma. Head Neck 2002;24(8):748–753

52. Wen YH, Wen WP, Chen HX, Li J, Zeng YH, Xu G. Endoscopic nasopharyngectomy for salvage in nasopharyngeal carcinoma: a novel anatomic orientation. Laryngoscope 2010;120(7):1298–1302

53. Chen MK, Lai JC, Chang CC, Liu MT. Minimally invasive endoscopic nasopharyngectomy in the treatment of recurrent T1-2a nasopharyngeal carcinoma. Laryngoscope 2007;117(5):894–896

54. Chen MY, Wen WP, Guo X, et al. Endoscopic nasopharyngectomy for locally recurrent nasopharyngeal carcinoma. Laryngoscope 2009;119(3):516–522

55. Mai HQ, Mo HY, Deng JF, et al. Endoscopic microwave coagulation therapy for early recurrent T1 nasopharyngeal carcinoma. Eur J Cancer 2009;45(7):1107–1110

56. Wei WI, Ho WK. Transoral robotic resection of recurrent nasopharyngeal carcinoma. Laryngoscope 2010;120(10):2011–2014

57. Vlantis AC, Tsang RK, Yu BK, et al. Nasopharyngectomy and surgical margin status: a survival analysis. Arch Otolaryngol Head Neck Surg 2007;133(12):1296–1301

58. Wilson CP. Observations on the surgery of the nasopharynx. Ann Otol Rhinol Laryngol 1957;66(1):5–40

59. Belmont JR. The Le Fort I osteotomy approach for nasopharyngeal and nasal fossa tumors. Arch Otolaryngol Head Neck Surg 1988;114(7):751–754

60. To EW, Teo PM, Ku PK, Pang PC. Nasopharyngectomy for recurrent nasopharyngeal carcinoma: an innovative transnasal approach through a mid-face deglove incision with stereotactic navigation guidance. Br J Oral Maxillofac Surg 2001;39(1):55–62

61. Fisch U. The infratemporal fossa approach for nasopharyngeal tumors. Laryngoscope 1983;93(1):36–44

62. Danesi G, Zanoletti E, Mazzoni A. Salvage surgery for recurrent nasopharyngeal carcinoma. Skull Base 2007;17(3):173–180

63. Morton RP, Liavaag PG, McLean M, Freeman JL. Transcervico-mandibulo-palatal approach for surgical salvage of recurrent nasopharyngeal cancer. Head Neck 1996;18(4):352–358

64. Wei WI, Lam KH, Sham JS. New approach to the nasopharynx: the maxillary swing approach. Head Neck 1991;13(3):200–207

65. Ng RW, Wei WI. Elimination of palatal fistula after the maxillary swing procedure. Head Neck 2005;27(7):608–612

66. Wei WI. Cancer of the nasopharynx: functional surgical salvage. World J Surg 2003;27(7):844–848

67. Ng RW, Wei WI. Quality of life of patients with recurrent nasopharyngeal carcinoma treated with nasopharyngectomy using the maxillary swing approach. Arch Otolaryngol Head Neck Surg 2006;132(3):309–316

68. Wei WI, Chan JY, Ng RW, Ho WK. Surgical salvage of persistent or recurrent nasopharyngeal carcinoma with maxillary swing approach-Critical appraisal after 2 decades. Head Neck 2011; 33(7):969–975

69. Chan JY, Chow VL, Tsang R, Wei WI. Nasopharyngectomy for locally advanced recurrent nasopharyngeal carcinoma: exploring the limits. Head Neck 2012;34(7):923–928

70. Shu CH, Cheng H, Lirng JF, et al. Salvage surgery for recurrent nasopharyngeal carcinoma. Laryngoscope 2000;110(9):1483–1488

71. Wei WI. Nasopharyngeal cancer: current status of management: a New York Head and Neck Society lecture. Arch Otolaryngol Head Neck Surg 2001;127(7):766–769

72. Fee WE Jr, Moir MS, Choi EC, Goffinet D. Nasopharyngectomy for recurrent nasopharyngeal cancer: a 2- to 17-year follow-up. Arch Otolaryngol Head Neck Surg 2002;128(3):280–284

73. Hao SP, Tsang NM, Chang KP, Hsu YS, Chen CK, Fang KH. Nasopharyngectomy for recurrent nasopharyngeal carcinoma: a review of 53 patients and prognostic factors. Acta Otolaryngol 2008;128(4):473–481

74. Yin Tsang RK, Ho WK, Wei WI. Combined transnasal endoscopic and transoral robotic resection of recurrent nasopharyngeal carcinoma. Head Neck 2012;34(8):1190–1193

35 Radiosurgery and Radiotherapy for Benign and Malignant Anterior Skull Base Lesions

Paul B. Romesser, Nataliya Kovalchuk, A. Omer Nawaz, and Minh Tam Truong

Stereotactic radiosurgery (SRS) is the delivery of a single high dose of ionizing radiation to an intracranial target, which is defined by stereotactic image localization. The term stereotactic (derived from Greek "stereo," meaning three dimensional [3D] and "tactos" meaning ordered or arranged) refers to techniques in which targets are precisely localized in three dimensions of space. Stereotactic localization allows for procedures to be performed such as surgery, biopsies, or the delivery of focused radiation. Ideal targets for SRS are small, round, discrete tumors with minimal microscopic spread or discrete functional targets. This allows the maximal target dose to achieve tumor control or functional ablation, while minimizing adjacent normal tissue irradiation.

The term radiosurgery was first coined in 1951 by the neurosurgeon Lars Leksell.[1] He is credited with the development of SRS for the treatment of functional disorders and tumors in the brain. Using the Leksell Gamma Knife (Elekta, Stockholm, Sweden) and linear accelerator (LINAC) radiosurgery units, such as the Radionics X-Knife (Integra Plainsboro, New Jersey), the SRS in the brain uses a rigid head frame externally fixed to the patient's skull by a halo and pins with local anesthesia. The target localizer assembly fitted over the frame is used to determine the target coordinates, when used in conjunction with computed tomography (CT) and/or magnetic resonance imaging (MRI).

In recent years, frameless SRS systems have been developed. These include the CyberKnife radiosurgery system (Accuray, Sunnyvale, California) pioneered by the Stanford neurosurgeon John Adler. Frameless SRS allowed the expansion of radiosurgery principles to extracranial sites without losing the accuracy of the stereotactic approach. Frameless SRS systems have also allowed greater flexibility in terms of radiation delivery using multiple treatments. Stereotactic radiotherapy (SRT) uses the same concept of radiation delivery as SRS. These, however, occur in multiple dose fractions usually using conventional daily dose fractionation schema of 1.8 to 2 Gy per fraction over 5 weeks, or hypofractionated SRT with higher doses delivered in two to five fractions. The decision to use SRS (single fraction) or hypofractionated SRT (2 to 5 fractions), instead of conventionally fractionated SRT is a function of the tumor size, tumor histology, and proximity to adjacent radiosensitive structures. Organs at risk such as the optic chiasm, optic nerves, and brainstem are of particular concern with anterior skull base lesions. The rationale for fractionating radiation treatments is to spare late responding normal tissue from long-term radiation toxicity. Tumors ≤ 3 cm in size are often amenable to single-dose SRS if there is adequate dose fall off to critical normal tissue. Larger tumors or tumors in very close proximity to a critical normal structure are usually amenable to hypofractionated or conventionally fractionated SRT. The overall objective of SRS and SRT is to achieve highly accurate treatment delivery and to maximize the therapeutic ratio of achieving tumor control while minimizing potential treatment-related toxicity to adjacent normal tissue at risk.[2]

SRS uses single fraction treatments ranging from 12 to 24 Gy depending on the disease and location. Fractionated radiosurgery uses hypofractionation over three to five fractions. Fractionated SRT uses conventional daily fractionated doses of 1.8 to 2 Gy delivered to the tumor typically over 5 to 6 weeks of treatment. In the skull base, the gross tumor volume (GTV[3]) is contoured on a high-resolution MRI which display the best set of images to accurately outline the GTV.

Radiation works principally by inducing damage to the deoxyribonucleic acid (DNA) of cells either by direct or indirect damage. Direct damage occurs when a charged particle has sufficient energy to induce damage directly to an atomic structure. About two-thirds of damage to DNA is by indirect action from hydroxyl radicals generated from the radiolysis of water. When cells are irradiated, a single-strand or a double-strand DNA break can occur. Single-strand breaks can usually be repaired (sublethal repair), while double-strand breaks often result in the formation of unstable chromosomes (dicentric chromosomes) and therefore cell death via mitotic catastrophe. The efficacy of radiation and fractionation exploits the differential effect of radiation on tumor cells versus normal tissue. Cancer cells and normal nonmalignant cells are susceptible to radiation damage, but a therapeutic window exists in which radiation selectively damages cells with high mitotic rates. Tumors often have abnormalities in repair of single-stranded DNA breaks; this allows the differential effect between normal tissue repair and tumor cell kill. Cellular response to DNA damage centers on principles of cell cycle kinetics, cell cycle checkpoints (G1/S, intra-S phase, and G2/mitosis), and DNA repair of single-stranded and double-stranded breaks.[4]

Current Radiosurgery Techniques

Gamma Knife Stereotactic Radiosurgery

Current models utilize 192 ^{60}Co sources that converge and focus onto a treatment target at a source to focus distance of approximately 40 cm. While each individual dose from the 192 sources is insignificant, the total convergent dose is therapeutically appropriate with minimal radiation to the surrounding normal tissues. The sources are aligned with the assistance of three collimator systems: the precollimator, the stationary collimator, and the final collimator (on the helmet). An appropriate helmet based on a circular collimator size (4, 8, and 16 mm) is chosen depending on the target size while the Leksell stereotactic frame is fixed to the patient's skull. Heck et al reported the overall, long-term mechanical accuracy, and the precision of the Gamma Knife irradiated volume deviation to be –0.014 ± 0.09 mm, 0.013 ± 0.09 mm, and –0.002 ± 0.06 mm for the x, y, and z coordinates, respectively, with all measured data contained within a 0.2 mm sphere.[5] Since its implementation approximately 30 years ago, over 400,000 patients have received treatment with the Gamma Knife SRS system. The long track record of the Gamma Knife unit coupled with 15-year follow-up clinical data ensures that the Gamma Knife device remains the benchmark and the current gold standard for intracranial radiosurgery.[6–9]

LINAC-Based Stereotactic Radiosurgery with Circular Cone Collimation

A frequently used system for the LINAC-based radiosurgery is the Radionics X-Knife.[10,11] Since most modern LINACs use 6 MV photons, this is the most commonly used energy for LINAC-based radiosurgery. The system uses a series of noncoplanar arcs of circular beams converging at the mechanical isocenter around which the LINAC gantry, collimator, and treatment couch rotate. The physician places a rigid head frame on the patient's skull and inserts four pins to prevent its movement relative to the skull. This frame is then mounted to the couch on the imaging device (CT and/or MRI). Once imaged, the frame is used to define the 3D Cartesian coordinate system for an accurate localization and irradiation of the target. Laser and imaging guidance are used to ensure the patient is positioned on the treatment couch, with the frame docked to the couch, such that the center of the planned treatment beams coincides with the nominal LINAC isocenter. If the head frame slips and the cranial anatomy is no longer at the same coordinates with reference to the head frame, then the process must be restarted. Lutz et al reported average errors of 1.3 ± 0.5 mm for CT imaging and 0.6 ± 0.2 mm for plane film radiograph.[11] Localization errors with MRI were higher than that of CT.[5] However, given better diagnostic abilities with MRI, it remains an integral part of SRS workflow. There have been no clinically significant differences between the Gamma Knife and the X-Knife reported in the literature.[12]

LINAC-Based Stereotactic Radiosurgery with Micro Multileaf Collimators

Another LINAC-based SRS can be used by retrofitting the outside LINAC head with micro multileaf collimators (mMLCs). Traditional multileaf collimators (MLCs) are contained inside the LINAC head and cast a projection of 5 or 10 mm at the LINAC isocenter depending on the make and model of the LINAC. These MLCs are used to shape radiation fields to conform around the GTV. The mMLCs are designed like the standard MLCs, except that the width of their tungsten leaves is considerably smaller providing a typical field width of 1.5 to 6 mm at the LINAC isocenter. This allows the mMLCs to shape the small radiosurgical fields with greater precision and to be used in static 3D SRS treatments, dynamic arc,[13] and intensity-modulated radiation therapy.[14–16] Usually for the LINAC-based SRS with mMLCs, only one isocenter is used for treatment planning.[14,17–19] This design of SRS has considerable appeal because of the availability of multiple treatment techniques and planning options that are not limited by GTV size or geometry but still provide a comparable SRS and SRT option.[20] An alternative approach to the head frame, the infrared optical-guided frameless system has been introduced. It consists of a customized mask and bite block with a rigid array of fiducial markers attached. A ceiling mounted infrared camera detects the array of infrared reflective markers, which in conjunction with the orthogonal kilovoltage images provides the patient setup guidance and intrafractional motion monitoring.[21,22] Wang et al reported that 82% of the patients in their study had setup error of less than 1 mm.[23]

CyberKnife Stereotactic Radiosurgery

The CyberKnife was the first frameless robotic radiosurgery system for intracranial and extracranial tumors.[24,25] A robotic arm with 6 degrees of freedom controls a lightweight 6 MV LINAC. The robotic arm can quickly reposition the LINAC and allows treatment to be delivered from many different angles without the limitations of traditional gantry systems. The CyberKnife system uses a tracking algorithm that computes the offset between live X-ray images and digitally reconstructed radiograph images by identifying and matching landmarks in the images. The landmarks depend on the tracking mode specified by the treatment plan. Different tracking modes include skull tracking, Xsight spine tracking, fiducial tracking, and Xsight lung tracking. Skull and Xsight spine trackings use the fixed relationship between skeletal anatomy and the tumor to identify the tumor throughout the treatment. Fiducial seeds implanted in or around the tumor before the treatment may be used for soft tissue targets, using the fiducial seeds as a reference point for tracking the tumor during treatment. Lung tracking uses a respiratory gating method that tracks the lung volume relative to the soft tissue anatomy to account for patient movement. The CyberKnife system uses repeated planar kilovoltage images throughout the treatment to monitor skeletal landmarks or fiducial markers, and adjusts the robotic arm position accordingly. Typically, 100 to 200 static beams are delivered through fixed collimators for CyberKnife radiosurgery. The "Iris" is a variable aperture collimator recently developed to allow for multiple collimator sizes during a given treatment, without requiring change in collimator attachment during treatment. The reported accuracy of the CyberKnife system is 1.1 ± 0.3 mm.[26] Dosimetric studies have reported excellent tumor dose distribution with the CyberKnife system.[27,28]

Proton Stereotactic Radiosurgery

The first publication theorizing the therapeutic use of protons was published in 1946 by Robert Wilson.[29] Charged particle beam radiosurgery produced by cyclotrons or synchrotrons creates a highly focused dose distribution by virtue of the Bragg peak effect; this deposits radiation over a specified range with minimal exit radiation dose. Hospital-based cyclotrons with high beam energies are able to treat deep-seated tumors, thus making protons a treatment of choice for skull base tumors. Tumors in close proximity to the brain, brainstem, spinal cord, optic chiasm, and cochlea can be treated with protons with sharp dose gradients between tumor and adjacent critical structures and thereby minimizing potential long-term treatment-related morbidity.[30] Another benefit of proton treatment is substantially reduced integral dose (by factor of 2) as compared with photon treatment.[31] This makes proton treatment particularly beneficial for pediatric patients to reduce dose to developing organs and skeletal structures to minimize risk of growth delay. Proton facilities typically use a passive scattering beam delivery method in which the primary proton beam is degraded with scattering foils. A range modulator spreads out the Bragg peak into a clinically useful beam. Additional beam shaping can then be achieved by using patient-specific devices including brass apertures, which are made to shape a specific field to achieve lateral field confirmation and a polymethyl methacrylate range compensator to achieve distal confirmation. Newer techniques include active scanning method in which the proton beam is delivered by a spot or narrow pencil beam and the dose is deposited in layers. With this technique, the beam can also be modulated using intensity-modulated proton beam therapy, in which irregularly shaped tumors can be treated with very high conformity.[32]

Treatment Planning and Dosimetry

Treatment planning relies on reconstruction of axial CT imaging of the patient in the treatment position, commonly referred to as radiation simulation. A virtual patient is created by the treatment planning software by importing the CT scan, and often fusing it with adjunct imaging studies. Most commonly in the skull base, MRI is used to assist target delineation. This allows the physician to delineate both tumor targets and adjacent normal organ structures.[33] The radiation

physicist or dosimetrist programs the software to determine the optimal beam angles, beam weights, and collimation to achieve the dose objectives set by the physician.

The radiation dose distribution can be seen on 2D or 3D reconstructed views from the CT images obtained at the time of radiation simulation. A dose volume histogram (DVH) is generated to determine the percentage of the volume encompassed by the percent of the total dose. The DVH only gives information about the volume of the target as a whole and not necessarily information about the anatomic location of variations in the dose.[34]

Typically in Gamma Knife radiosurgery, the prescription dose is delivered to the 50% isodose line encompassing the target volume (TV), with a central maximum dose being twice that of the prescription dose. In LINAC-based radiosurgery, the prescription dose is often prescribed to higher isodose lines, usually 80%, and hence the maximum dose is less than that delivered by Gamma Knife. Conformity indices (CIs) are used to compare competing plans, evaluate treatment techniques, and assess the risk of potential complications.[27] The CI is defined as the ratio of prescription volume (PV) to TV, and usually ranges from 2.7 for conventional LINAC radiosurgery to 1.8 for mMLC collimator radiosurgery.[35,36] The new conformity index (nCI) used by the University of California, San Francisco, group includes calculating the ratio of the TV within the prescribed isodose surface (TV_{PV}) to the total TV, and dividing the ratio of PV to TV_{PV} by the coverage (to account for the location of the PV with respect to the TV) as devised by Nakamura et al[37] and Paddick.[38] Hence, an ideal plan would have a TV_{PV} = TV = PV, yielding an CI = 1.0 as well as a CI = 1.0. Once the plan is evaluated by these various quantitative and qualitative measures by the physician, the plan is then digitally transferred to the treatment machine.

Consideration of dose to normal tissue in the skull base is important to reduce long-term complications of radiosurgery. In a series of 50 patients treated with SRS for benign skull base tumors, the incidence of optic neuropathy was zero for patients who received a radiation dose of < 10 Gy, 26.7% for patients receiving a dose in the range of 10 to < 15 Gy, and 77.8% for those who received doses of 15 Gy or more ($p < 0.0001$).[39] Previously impaired vision improved in 25.8% and was unchanged in 51.5% of patients. No signs of cranial neuropathy were seen in patients in whom the cranial nerves of the cavernous sinus received doses between 5 and 30 Gy. Tumor control was achieved in 98% of patients. This study demonstrated that structures of the visual pathways (i.e., the optic nerve, chiasm, and tract) exhibit a much higher sensitivity to single-fraction radiation than other cranial nerves. In contrast, the oculomotor and trigeminal nerves were noted to have a higher radiation dose tolerance.[39]

Treatment Execution

For the Gamma Knife system, the stereotactic head frame is attached to the treatment couch at a correct position and docking angle before treatment. During treatment, the couch is moved so that each shot is delivered at the center of the focusing helmet. For conventional LINAC-based radiosurgery, the stereotactic head frame is docked to the treatment couch such that the center of each treatment arc coincides with the nominal LINAC isocenter. For optical-guided frameless LINAC-based radiosurgery, the patient is immobilized with the thermoplastic mask and custom bite block with the infrared reflective markers. During the treatment, both the infrared camera and the kilovoltage images are guiding the robotic couch motion depending on the patient deviation from the baseline position. During CyberKnife treatment, the patient is immobilized with a custom thermoplastic mask for skull base tumors and lies on the robotic couch (before treatment), while the stereo-imaging system tracks the patient in real time and adjusts the robotic couch and robotic arm position (during treatment) accordingly. All radiation machines have a record and verify system to ensure accuracy and to eliminate potential errors of treatment delivery.[34]

Clinical Sites

Radiosurgery is an important treatment modality for the management of skull base tumors, including meningiomas, pituitary adenomas, glomus tumors, and chordomas. Emerging applications of radiosurgery in the treatment of other skull base malignancies include nasopharyngeal cancer and those who have failed previous conventional external beam radiotherapy.

Meningiomas

Meningiomas, which arise from arachnoid cap cells, are benign, slow-growing, well-circumscribed solid tumors.[40] Meningiomas account for 30% of adult intracranial neoplasms with incidence increasing with age, peaking in the 5th or 6th decade, and a 2:1 female predilection.[40] A history of previous radiation exposure has also been reported to increase ones risk. Symptoms at presentation vary widely as they largely reflect tumor location, with common locations including cerebral convexities, falx cerebri, tentorium cerebelli, cerebellopontine angle, sphenoid ridge, and spine. These tumors may undergo malignant transformation, can be locally destructive, and cause adjacent bony erosion or hyperostosis. Meningiomas are graded according to World Health Organization (WHO) grading system, most of which are benign or WHO grade I, but approximately 35% of all meningiomas are atypical (WHO grade II) or malignant (WHO grade III).[41]

Therapeutic options are varied, ranging from observation with serial imaging, surgery, radiosurgery, or fractionated external beam radiotherapy.[41] Determinants of management include the character of the meningioma by imaging (benign versus atypical or malignant), rate of progression on imaging, tumor size, and the presence or absence of surrounding edema. Asymptomatic, small, benign lesions

without any mass effect are often reasonable to follow with observation. Tumors < 3 cm in dimension can be considered for curative SRS. The treatment of choice for symptomatic or progressive benign meningiomas > 3 cm is complete surgical resection. However, meningiomas of the optic nerve sheath[42–44] and skull base tumors located in the petroclival area and cavernous sinus can be primarily treated with radiation therapy, with SRS,[45–55] hypofractionated SRT,[47] or conventionally fractionated SRT[56–59] with excellent functional outcome and local control. Often tumors in these locations are not amenable to surgery without significant morbidity. The decision to use single fraction SRS or fractionated radiation treatment depends on the proximity and potential radiation dose to the adjacent critical organs at risk such as the optic nerves and chiasm. **Fig. 35.1** shows a treatment plan for a left cavernous sinus meningioma.

Outcome data for radiation treatment have been reported in several studies. Flickinger et al from the University of Pittsburgh reported on 219 meningiomas, which underwent Gamma Knife radiosurgery to a median marginal tumor dose of 14 Gy with a median follow-up of 29 months.[60] The actuarial 10-year tumor control rate was 93.2% and the 10-year actuarial rate of developing any postradiosurgical injury was 8.8%. Similarly, an European study evaluated 331 patients with 356 meningiomas treated with Gamma Knife radiosurgery to a median tumor marginal dose of 12.55 Gy. The 5-year actuarial tumor control rate was 97.9%.[61] The overall treatment morbidity was 10.2% with a permanent morbidity rate of 5.7%, and a treatment-specific mortality rate of 0.6%. Tumors > 10 cm^3, peritumoral edema, and meningiomas in the anterior skull base were reported to be at higher risk of posttreatment complications. The University of Maryland identified factors independently associated with treatment outcomes, on multivariate analysis, after Gamma Knife SRS and reported that patients with a GTV > 10 cm^3 were more likely to have tumor recurrence (hazard ratio, 4.58; $p = 0.05$).[62] Additionally, patients who had lower CIs with improved coverage of the dural tail had better control rates on univariate analysis.

Similar outcome data for CyberKnife have been reported. A University of Pittsburgh study reported on the efficacy of CyberKnife in a cohort of 73 patients (60 WHO grade I, 11 WHO grade II, and 2 WHO grade III).[63] The actuarial 1-year local control rate was 95, 71, and 0% for WHO grades I, II, and III, respectively, when treated to a median dose of 17.5 Gy over a median of three fractions. A subjective improvement in existing tumor-related symptoms was noted in 60% of patients. In a series of 199 meningiomas, predominantly of the skull base, the 5-year local actuarial control rate was 93.5% after CyberKnife radiosurgery to a mean dose of 18.5 Gy.[47] Importantly, in 150 patients, the dose was delivered in two to five daily fractions of which 63 patients had lesions that would have been defined as previously untreatable by radiosurgery (volume > 13.5 cm^3 and/or distance < 3 mm from the optic pathway). Clinical symptoms (ocular movement, visual function, exophthalmos, and pain)

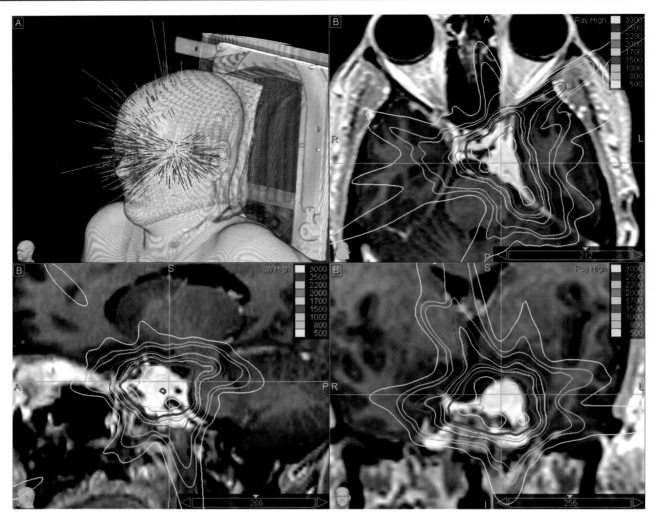

Figure 35.1   A 49-year-old woman with a history of left cavernous sinus meningioma presented with headaches and facial numbness. Single-dose stereotactic radiosurgery would place the cranial nerves in the cavernous sinus at risk for transient or permanent injury. Fractionating the treatment would enable local control of tumor with an improved toxicity profile. Treatment planning was performed using fusion of a dedicated computed tomography and high-resolution T1-weighted magnetic resonance imaging.

worsened in 2.2% of cases, remained unchanged in 82.9%, and improved in 14.9% of cases.

Treatment of tumors close to the optic nerve and/or optic chiasm can be challenging. Stanford University reported on the use of CyberKnife radiosurgery in the treatment of perioptic tumors in 49 patients (27 with meningioma, 19 with pituitary adenoma, 2 with craniopharyngioma, and 1 with mixed germ cell tumor).[64] Patients were treated two to five fractions to a total margin dose of 20.3 Gy (range, 15 to 30 Gy). Patients with optic chiasm involvement (19 out of 49 patients) were treated with five fractions at 5 Gy per fraction. Over a median follow-up of 45 months, radiographic control was reported in 94% of patients and visual fields remained stable or improved in 94% of patient. Furthermore, Stanford University reported on the safety and efficacy of CyberKnife for large (> 15 cm³) cranial base meningiomas with good treatment efficacy without increased cranial nerve toxicity when treated with five fractions at 5 Gy per fraction.[65] These

data have provided evidence suggesting that perichiasmic and cavernous sinus lesions can be effectively and safely treated by CyberKnife radiosurgery over five fractions at 5 Gy per fraction.

Radiation may be indicated as an adjuvant treatment to surgery depending on surgical pathologic findings. With complete surgical resection, meningioma recurrence rates are 7 to 12% at 5 years and 20 to 25% at 10 years.[66,67] While subtotal resection is known to have a higher rate of relapse (39 to 47% at 5 years and 60 to 61% at 10 years), postoperative radiation has been shown to benefit patients who underwent subtotal resections.[68,69] A comparison of patients who received subtotal resection with and without postoperative radiation demonstrated that 60% of the nonirradiated patients had recurrence in contrast to 32% of those who received radiotherapy with a significant difference noted in the median time to recurrence (66 months in the nonirradiated versus 125 months in the irradiated cohort,

$p < 0.05$).[69] These data were further confirmed by Taylor et al, who reported that 15% of patients who received postoperative radiation recurred as compared with 69% who did not ($p = 0.01$).[68] Postoperative radiation is indicated in atypical meningiomas and malignant meningiomas,[70] which are completely resected.[71] Postoperative radiation therapy is usually delivered ranging from 54 to 60 Gy in 30 fractions by conformal external beam radiotherapy for atypical meningiomas, and to 60 Gy in 30 fractions over 6 weeks for malignant meningiomas.

Pituitary Tumors

Pituitary adenomas are identified in nearly 20% of pituitary glands in autopsy studies and represent 10 to 20% of primary adult brain tumors.[72] The large majority of adenomas arise from the anterior lobe, which produces many endocrine hormones (growth hormone [GH], prolactin [PRL], adrenocorticotropic hormone [ACTH], thyroid-stimulating hormone [TSH], follicle-stimulating hormone [FSH], and luteinizing hormone [LH]).[40] Pituitary tumors are usually divided into functional (usually microadenomas, < 1 cm) or nonfunctional (macroadenomas, ≥ 1 cm). Functional adenomas usually present with endocrine dysfunction depending on the hormone. Such syndromes include acromegaly from oversecretion of GH and Cushing disease from ACTH. Approximately 75% of adenomas are functional adenomas, whereas 25% are nonfunctional. Prolactinomas are the most common functional adenomas (30%), followed by somatotropic (25%), and less commonly corticotropic and thyrotrophic.[40]

Macroadenomas are typically nonfunctional. They often present with symptoms related to invasion or compression of adjacent structures (i.e., optic chiasm, optic nerves, and cavernous sinus). Symptoms include headache, cranial nerve deficits secondary to cavernous sinus invasion, and hormonal disturbances. Visual field abnormalities are also seen. Superior temporal deficits, homonymous hemianopsia, and central scotoma may also result. Goals of therapeutic management include control of tumor mass and its effect on normal function, and correcting any endocrine deficiencies. Therefore, treatment can include medical, surgical, and radiation-based plans.

Radiosurgery plays an important role in the management of pituitary adenomas.[73–77] It can be used as an ablative therapy for functional arrest of secretory microadenomas in patients who have failed medical therapy (**Fig. 35.2**).[78,79] For macroadenomas, surgery is used for decompression of pituitary adenomas that invade the optic nerves or chiasm, and radiation is used in the adjuvant setting for residual disease or regrowth after surgery or in nonsurgical candidates.[40] At least 3 to 5 mm of clearance from the optic chiasm is required for single fraction SRS for pituitary adenomas. This allows dose fall off from the tumor and keep the dose of the optic chiasm below 8 Gy in a single fraction. If this cannot be achieved, consideration of fractionated treatment with either hypofractionated radiosurgery (5 Gy × 5 fractions; **Fig. 35.3**) or conventional fractionated SRT over 5 weeks may be used for nonsecretory (nonfunctional) pituitary adenomas.[64]

In a series of 267 patients who were treated for pituitary adenomas using Gamma Knife radiosurgery, there were 131 cases of nonfunctioning and 136 cases of functioning adenomas, in which 71 GH-producing, 33 PRL-producing, and 32 ACTH-producing adenomas were included.[73] Retreatment with Gamma Knife was done in eight cases because of large tumors or uncontrolled hormone secretion. Microadenomas were treated by Gamma Knife radiosurgery alone. Surgical or chemical debulking was necessary before radiosurgery for large tumors with extrasellar extension. Nonfunctioning adenomas had higher control rates than functioning adenomas, despite receiving a lower dose. Cushing disease showed the best response to single fraction SRS because of the small tumor size and high-dose radiation. Acromegaly and prolactinoma were difficult to control. The rate of hormone normalization was also high in Cushing disease but lower in prolactinoma and lowest in acromegaly. High-dose treatment was necessary for functioning adenomas to control tumor growth and oversecretion of hormones. This study demonstrated that careful consideration of radiation dose and volume needed to be tailored according to the type of pituitary adenoma, size, and the secreting functional component present.[73]

Radiosurgery can be used in GH-secreting tumors. In a study of 83 acromegalic patients treated with SRS from 1994 to 2006, 52 women and 31 men with a mean age of 42.6 ± 1.2 years were followed for a median of 69 months (interquartile range, 44 to 107 months).[78] Patients were followed for normalization of age- and sex-adjusted insulin growth factor I (IGF-I) levels together with a basal GH level below 2.5 µg/L without concomitant GH-suppressive drugs. Fifty patients (60.2%) achieved normalization of IGF-I levels and GH levels. The rate of remission was 52.6% at 5 years (95% CI, 40.6 to 64.6). Thirteen patients (15.7%), who were resistant to somatostatin analogs, achieved remission after SRS. Multivariate analysis correlated low basal GH and IGF-I levels with a more favorable outcome. No serious side effects occurred after SRS. The 5-year cumulative risk of new onset hypogonadism, hypothyroidism, or hypoadrenalism was 3.6% (95% CI, 0 to 8.6), 3.3% (95% CI, 0 to 7.7), and 4.9% (95% CI, 0 to 10.4), respectively. A similar study of 149 patients with GH-secreting pituitary adenoma, including 97 males and 52 females, with a mean volume of tumor of 2.36 cm^3 (range, 0.11 to 12.7 cm^3), were treated by Gamma Knife SRS.[80] The mean dose to tumor margin was 20.87 Gy (range, 10 to 30 Gy). The serum GH returned to normal in 74 patients (64.9%) and decreased compared with preradiosurgery levels in 23 patients (18.5%). SRS was found to be safe and effective in the treatment of GH-secreting pituitary adenoma.

Longer follow-up data for radiotherapy and functional outcomes have been reported in a study conducted at the University of Florida; 141 patients with pituitary

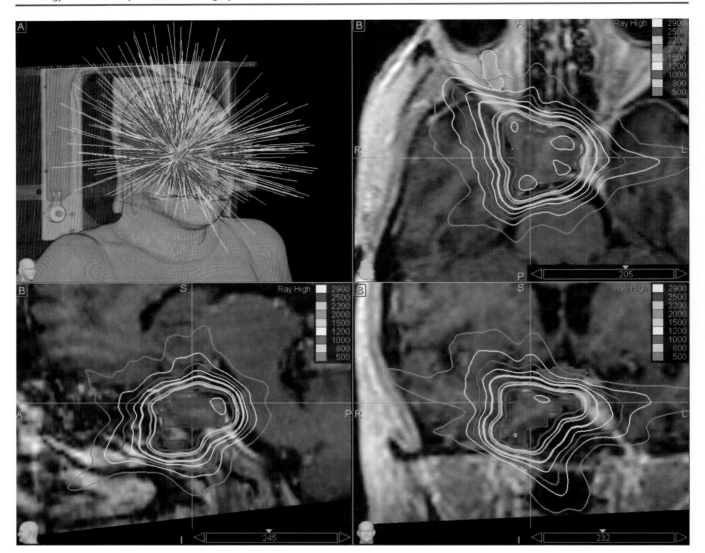

Figure 35.2 A 70-year-old woman with a right cavernous sinus pituitary adenoma presented with headaches and ophthalmoplegia. Brain magnetic resonance imaging (MRI) noted a $2 \times 1.3 \times 1.5$ cm^3 heterogeneously enhancing pituitary lesion within the sella with right lateral extension into the cavernous sinus and toward the right superior and inferior orbital fissures. Endoscopic subtotal resection was performed. Pathology demonstrated a pituitary adenoma with strong staining for synaptophysin, significant staining for adrenocorticotropic hormone, and rare staining for prolactin. Postoperative MRI of the brain showed a $12 \times 15 \times 5$ mm lesion within the lateral right cavernous sinus with extension to the orbital apex, but no optic chiasm involvement. The patient's ophthalmoplegia resolved postoperatively. Postoperatively, the patient underwent CyberKnife stereotactic radiotherapy targeting the right cavernous sinus residual tumor. The lesion was 6 mm away from the optic chiasm. She was treated with a hypofractionated regimen to a total dose of 25 Gy delivered in five fractions. Organs at risk include the optic chiasm (pink) and the right optic nerve (yellow). During each treatment, the patient was temporarily immobilized with a frameless thermoplastic head and neck mask on the robotic couch. Proper alignment was confirmed daily using real-time (intrafractional) kilovolt imaging and skull tracking. Fifteen months after the treatment, the patient is doing well with stable MRI findings, stable vision, and no sequelae from radiation.

adenomas (56% nonfunctional and 44% functional) received radiotherapy, of whom 108 received surgery with adjuvant radiotherapy and 33 received radiotherapy alone.[81] The median total dose was 47.2 Gy (range, 45 to 55 Gy) with a median dose per fraction of 1.8 Gy. At 10 years, tumor control rates were 95 versus 90%, an insignificant difference ($p = 0.58$), for the surgery/adjuvant radiotherapy versus radiotherapy alone, respectively. While only 2% of patients developed worsening visual field defects attributable to radiotherapy, 54.9% of surgery combined with adjuvant

radiotherapy and 22.5% of patients treated with radiotherapy alone developed worsening pituitary hormone deficiencies. Other studies have demonstrated the efficacy and safety of 45 Gy in over 1.8 Gy per fraction prescribed to the 95% isodose line.[82–84]

Long-term outcomes for pituitary adenomas after Gamma Knife radiosurgery have shown good local control rates. In a study done at the University of Virginia, 48 patients with nonfunctioning pituitary adenoma who underwent Gamma Knife radiosurgery had an overall control rate of 83%.[85]

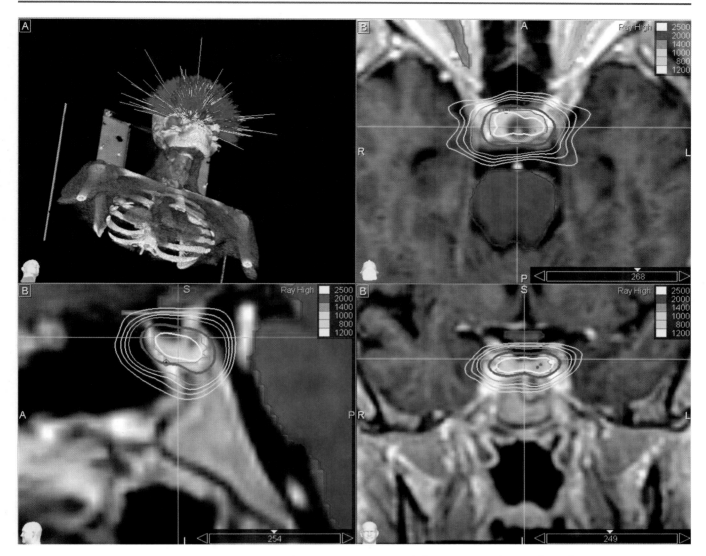

Figure 35.3   Radiosurgery plan for functional pituitary adenoma to 20 Gy in a single fraction. Optic chiasm is limited to 8 Gy.

New hormone deficiencies occurred in 39% of patients, most commonly thyroid and GH-related deficiencies with an occurrence of 20.8 and 16.7%, respectively. The Mayo Clinic published its 15-year experience with Gamma Knife radiosurgery in nonfunctioning pituitary adenomas in a retrospective review of 62 patients treated to a median tumor margin dose of 16 Gy of which 95% were treated postoperatively.[86] Over a median follow-up of 64 months, it was reported that tumor size decreased in 60% of cases and remained unchanged in 37% with 3% local failures and a 32% risk of developing new anterior pituitary deficits at a median of 24 months postradiosurgery.

Similarly, CyberKnife radiosurgery has been explored in the treatment of pituitary adenomas. The Barrow Neurological Institute reported a case series of 20 patients with recurrent or residual pituitary adenomas, 70% nonfunctioning, within 2 mm of the optic chiasm, of which 30% were functional adenomas, treated to 25 Gy over five fractions.[87] About 60% of lesions were unchanged and 40% smaller over a mean

follow-up duration of 29.3 months. Approximately 5% of patients had worsening pituitary hormonal deficiencies and no patients had deterioration of their vision, though one patient had a transient 3-month period of diplopia, which resolved after a short course of dexamethasone. A Stanford series on adjuvant CyberKnife therapy in nine acromegaly patients with residual disease after transsphenoidal resection reported a 44.4% complete hormonal remission rate and a 100% radiographic control rate at a mean follow-up of 25.4 months.[88] Patients were treated to a mean prescribed marginal dose of 21 Gy. The mean biological effective dose was higher in patients who achieved normal IGF-1 levels compared with those with persistent active disease. At least one new pituitary deficiency was observed after CyberKnife treatment in 33% of patients.

The use of proton therapy in the treatment of pituitary adenomas is under active study. Loma Linda University reported on their experience with proton therapy for pituitary adenomas in 47 patients (51% nonfunctioning and 49% functioning), of which 42 had previous resection.[89] Doses specified at the treatment isocenter ranged from 50.4 to 55.9 cobalt-gray equivalent (CGE) with 72.3% of patients receiving a dose of 54.0 CGE to the GTV over 1.8 CGE daily fractions in 85.1% and 2 CGE fractions in 14.9%. Over a median follow-up of 47 months, all tumors had regressed or stabilized and 85.7% had normalized or decreased hormone levels consistent with biochemical control.

Craniopharyngiomas

Craniopharyngioma is a rare benign but locally destructive tumor arising from Rathke pouch at the junction of the infundibular stalk and the pituitary gland in the sellar region.[90] Over 90% of craniopharyngiomas contain a cystic component that can appear calcified on CT imaging. While the majority arise in children predominately in the first or second decade, craniopharyngiomas have a bimodal incidence with a second peak in fifth to seventh decades.[91] Given its sellar location, craniopharyngiomas often present symptomatically with bitemporal hemianopsia or other visual field cuts; neuroendocrine deficits such as diabetes insipidus; growth retardation; and disorders of sexual development, increased intracranial pressure (headaches, vomiting, papilledema), or cognitive (memory loss), and behavior changes.[90]

The primary treatment of choice for craniopharyngiomas is surgery, as patients who undergo gross total resection have local control rates between 50 and 90% as compared with 0 and 40% following subtotal resection.[92] Adherence to surrounding vascular structures is a common cause of incomplete tumor resection.[93] The Children's Memorial Hospital in Chicago examined 25 patients who underwent primary surgery and reported that tumor recurrence following total resection was 32% compared with 100% following subtotal resection.[92] Radiation is a critical modality in patients who undergo subtotal resection, as local control rates increase from approximately 40% in nonirradiated patients to greater than 75% in those who undergo adjuvant radiotherapy.[94,95] A study from the Children's Hospital Boston and Joint Center for Radiation Therapy reported 10-year actuarial freedom from progression rates of 31% in the surgery-only group, 100% in the radiation therapy–only group, and 86% for patients treated with surgery and adjuvant radiotherapy (p = 0.001).[96] Furthermore, they reported that a significantly higher proportion of patients developed diabetes insipidus in the surgery-only group (79%) versus the radiation group (22%).[96]

SRS has been demonstrated to be an effective and safe primary treatment modality for craniopharyngioma. The University of Virginia reported a 3-year progression-free survival rate of 84.8% in 37 consecutive patients treated with Gamma Knife radiosurgery to a median maximum dose of 30 Gy.[97] Similarly, a University of Pittsburgh study of 46 patients with craniopharyngioma who underwent 51 stereotactic radiosurgical procedures to a median

prescribed dose of 13.0 Gy reported a 5-year progression-free survival rate of 91.6%.[93] Importantly, no patients with normal pituitary function developed hypopituitarism after SRS.[93] A meta-analysis of 10 Gamma Knife studies, in which patients were treated to a mean marginal dose of 12.3 Gy, reported tumor control in 75% of cases (90 solid, 80 cystic, and 59% mixed), overall SRS morbidity rate of 4%, and overall SRS mortality rate of 0.5%.[98]

Esthesioneuroblastoma

Esthesioneuroblastoma is a rare malignant neuroectodermal tumor rising from the olfactory rim of the nasal cavity, which is also commonly referred to as olfactory neuroblastoma.[99] As esthesioneuroblastoma has the potential to metastasize, there is a debate into the necessity to address metastatic or micrometastatic disease in the neck, with reported nodal failure rates ranging from 17 to 33%.[100] Given its rarity, there are no widely accepted treatment algorithms, but surgical resection is considered the mainstay of therapy in conjunction with radiation or chemoradiation.[101]

In a meta-analysis of 477 patients with documented follow-up, the University of Milan reported that patients undergoing combined modality treatment had the best overall survival rates as compared with surgery and radiotherapy alone (72.5 versus 62.5 and 53.9%, respectively).[99] Meta-analysis of 26 studies done by Dulguerov et al, reported on 390 patients that survival rates were greatest in patients undergoing surgery plus radiation (65%) as compared with radiotherapy and chemotherapy (51%), surgery alone (48%), surgery plus radiotherapy plus chemotherapy (47%), and radiotherapy alone (37%).[101] This conclusion was further supported by Gruber et al, who reported that despite finding that radical complete resection delivers the highest rates of local tumor control, surgery alone was not sufficient to avoid the occurrence of relapse. After a comprehensive literature review, they estimated a 33% absolute reduction in the local failure rate with the addition of adjuvant radiotherapy (20 versus 53% for surgery alone surgery and adjuvant radiotherapy, respectively).[102] Both Dulguerov et al and Gruber et al concluded that a total radiation dose of > 60 Gy was necessary for adequate tumor control.

The Massachusetts General Hospital and Massachusetts Eye and Ear Infirmary reported their experience in treating 10 esthesioneuroblastoma patients with proton-based radiotherapy.[103] All patients underwent craniofacial resection and adjuvant proton-based radiotherapy, to a median dose of 62.7 Cobalt Gray Equivalents (CGEs) (range, 54 to 70 CGEs), with 40% of patients receiving chemotherapy. Over a median follow-up of 52.8 months, the 5-year disease-free and overall survival rates were 90 and 85.7%, respectively. Importantly no patient suffered severe radiation toxicity, but 70% did suffer mild-to-moderate ocular complications of which the majority spontaneously resolved. As esthesioneuroblastoma can recur many years after treatment, long-term follow-up is necessary.[101]

The role of chemotherapy in the management of esthesioneuroblastoma remains widely debated. At least one study demonstrated a lower cervical nodal failure risk in patients who underwent systemic chemotherapy ($n = 9$), the majority of whom (78%) received etoposide and cisplatin, as compared with those who did not receive systemic chemotherapy ($n = 5$) (0 vs. 60%, respectively; $p = 0.027$).[100] Another retrospective study demonstrated superior outcomes in patients with high-grade, advanced stage esthesioneuroblastomas who underwent adjuvant chemotherapy of which the majority received cisplatin and etoposide. The median time to relapse for patients who received adjuvant chemotherapy was 35 months as compared with 10.5 months for those who did not. While meta-analyses, such as Dulguerov et al, have demonstrated inferior outcomes in patients who underwent adjuvant chemotherapy, even when combined with surgery and radiation therapy, selection bias must be considered, as patients selected to undergo adjuvant chemotherapy typically have aggressive cancers (higher grade) and advanced stage disease. Prospective studies are necessary to identify patients who will benefit from the incorporation of adjuvant chemotherapy.

Chordomas

Chordomas and chondrosarcomas are rare neoplasms of the axial skeleton that are locally destructive, slow-growing, and malignant bone tumors.[40] While 50% of chordomas occur in the sacrococcygeal area, 35% occur in the base of the skull and typically involve the clivus.[40] They commonly present in the fifth or sixth decade with a male predilection (2.5:1).[40] Chondrosarcomas are malignant primary bone tumors that arise in cartilaginous elements and are frequently found within synchondroses in the base of the skull, most commonly in the sphenoid bone. Overall survival is directly related to tumor location, as aggressive behavior and high local recurrence rate are problematic. Surgery is considered the primary treatment of both chordomas and chondrosarcomas. When tumor location, patient comorbid conditions, or other factors make surgical resection an undesirable option, radiation can be utilized as a primary therapy despite the fact that chordomas are considered relatively radiation resistant. Despite often being lumped together in studies, chondrosarcomas typically have good responses to radiotherapy. A European report on 45 patients with chordoma or chondrosarcoma who underwent postoperative stereotactic fractionated radiotherapy to a median dose of 66.6 or 64.9 Gy, respectively, demonstrated the differential response rates for these two tumors.[104] The 2- and 5-year local control rates of chordomas were 82 and 50%, versus 97 and 82% for chondrosarcomas, respectively.[104]

At the Massachusetts General Hospital, a study on the use of protons in the treatment of chordomas of the skull base and cervical spine was reported on 204 patients who underwent combined photon and proton therapy for base of skull or cervical spine chordomas to a median prescribed dose of 70.1 (range, 66.6 to 77.4) cobalt Gy equivalent.[105] Over a median follow-up of 54 months, the rate of failure was 31%. Of those who failed, 95% experienced local recurrence, 3% developed regional lymph node relapse, and 5% developed surgical pathway recurrence. Distant failures occurred in 20% of patients including the lung and bones. Protons allow the safe delivery of high doses of radiation necessary to achieve acceptable local control, as local failure is the predominant type of treatment failure. Given the poor long-term survival in this disease, it is important to acknowledge that a combined multimodality treatment approach is required at the time of initial treatment.

Gamma Knife radiosurgery has been used as an adjuvant treatment after resection for residual tumor volumes of less than 20 mL. Hasegawa et al reported the results of 37 patients with 48 lesions (73% were chordomas, 19% were chondrosarcomas, and 8% were without pathology) treated to a mean marginal dose of 14 Gy (mean maximal dose of 28 Gy) for all lesions. Patients with low-grade chondrosarcomas all achieved long-term control.[106] Actuarial 5-year survival and progression-free survival rates were 80 and 47%, respectively. Substantial differences were noted between the actuarial 5-year progression-free survival rates of chordomas versus chondrosarcomas, 42 versus 80%, respectively.

Conclusion

Radiosurgery is an important treatment modality for the management of skull base tumors, including meningiomas, pituitary adenomas, glomus tumors, and chordomas. SRS is ideal for small, round, discrete tumors with minimal microscopic spread or discrete functional targets. While multiple treatment modalities exist, selective utilization is often based on the disease, anatomical location, size of the primary target, and its proximity to adjacent critical organs. While SRS is often used as a primary definitive therapy, it has also been demonstrated to improve postoperative outcomes. A multidisciplinary approach should be used for each patient to best utilize all the potential treatment options available to ensure the best chance of disease control and functional outcomes.

References

1. Leksell L. The stereotaxic method and radiosurgery of the brain. Acta Chir Scand 1951;102(4):316–319
2. Jagannathan J, Sherman JH, Mehta GU, Chin LS. Radiobiology of brain metastasis: applications in stereotactic radiosurgery. Neurosurg Focus 2007;22(3):E4
3. International Commission on Radiation Units and Measurements. Prescribing, Recording and Reporting Photon Beam Therapy Issue 62. Michigan, MI: International Commission on Radiation Units and Measurements; 1999
4. Hall EJ, Giaccia AJ. Radiobiology for the Radiologist. 7th ed. New York, NY: Lippincott Williams & Wilkins; 2011
5. Heck B, Jess-Hempen A, Kreiner HJ, Schöpgens H, Mack A. Accuracy and stability of positioning in radiosurgery: long-term results of the Gamma Knife system. Med Phys 2007;34(4):1487–1495

6. Chopra R, Kondziolka D, Niranjan A, Lunsford LD, Flickinger JC. Long-term follow-up of acoustic schwannoma radiosurgery with marginal tumor doses of 12 to 13 Gy. Int J Radiat Oncol Biol Phys 2007;68(3):845–851

7. Hasegawa T, McInerney J, Kondziolka D, Lee JY, Flickinger JC, Lunsford LD. Long-term results after stereotactic radiosurgery for patients with cavernous malformations. Neurosurgery 2002;50(6):1190–1197, discussion 1197–1198

8. Jagannathan J, Petit JH, Balsara K, Hudes R, Chin LS. Long-term survival after gamma knife radiosurgery for primary and metastatic brain tumors. Am J Clin Oncol 2004;27(5):441–444

9. Kondziolka D, Martin JJ, Flickinger JC, et al. Long-term survivors after gamma knife radiosurgery for brain metastases. Cancer 2005;104(12):2784–2791

10. Patil AA. Radiosurgery with the linear accelerator. Neurosurgery 1989;25(1):143

11. Lutz W, Winston KR, Maleki N. A system for stereotactic radiosurgery with a linear accelerator. Int J Radiat Oncol Biol Phys 1988;14(2):373–381

12. Debus J, Pirzkall A, Schlegel W, Wannenmacher M. [Stereotactic one-time irradiation (radiosurgery). The methods, indications and results]. Strahlenther Onkol 1999;175(2):47–56

13. Solberg TD, Boedeker KL, Fogg R, Selch MT, DeSalles AA. Dynamic arc radiosurgery field shaping: a comparison with static field conformal and noncoplanar circular arcs. Int J Radiat Oncol Biol Phys 2001;49(5):1481–1491

14. Cardinale RM, Benedict SH, Wu Q, Zwicker RD, Gaballa HE, Mohan R. A comparison of three stereotactic radiotherapy techniques; ARCS vs. noncoplanar fixed fields vs. intensity modulation. Int J Radiat Oncol Biol Phys 1998;42(2):431–436

15. Lee CM, Watson GA, Leavitt DD. Dynamic collimator optimization compared with fixed collimator angle in arc-based stereotactic radiotherapy: a dosimetric analysis. Neurosurg Focus 2005;19(1):E12

16. Shiu A, Parker B, Ye JS, Lii J. An integrated treatment delivery system for CSRS and CSRT and clinical applications. J Appl Clin Med Phys 2003;4(4):261–273

17. Bourland JD, McCollough KP. Static field conformal stereotactic radiosurgery: physical techniques. Int J Radiat Oncol Biol Phys 1994;28(2):471–479

18. Hamilton RJ, Kuchnir FT, Sweeney P, et al. Comparison of static conformal field with multiple noncoplanar arc techniques for stereotactic radiosurgery or stereotactic radiotherapy. Int J Radiat Oncol Biol Phys 1995;33(5):1221–1228

19. Kubo HD, Pappas CT, Wilder RB. A comparison of arc-based and static mini-multileaf collimator-based radiosurgery treatment plans. Radiother Oncol 1997;45(1):89–93

20. Urie MM, Lo YC, Litofsky S, FitzGerald TJ. Miniature multileaf collimator as an alternative to traditional circular collimators for stereotactic radiosurgery and stereotactic radiotherapy. Stereotact Funct Neurosurg 2001;76(1):47–62

21. Lightstone AW, Benedict SH, Bova FJ, Solberg TD, Stern RL; American Association of Physicists in Medicine Radiation Therapy Committee. Intracranial stereotactic positioning systems: Report of the American Association of Physicists in Medicine Radiation Therapy Committee Task Group no. 68. Med Phys 2005;32(7):2380–2398

22. Bova FJ, Meeks SL, Friedman WA, Buatti JM. Optic-guided stereotactic radiotherapy. Med Dosim 1998;23(3):221–228

23. Wang JZ, Rice R, Pawlicki T, et al. Evaluation of patient setup uncertainty of optical guided frameless system for intracranial stereotactic radiosurgery. J Appl Clin Med Phys 2010;11(2):3181

24. Adler JR Jr, Chang SD, Murphy MJ, Doty J, Geis P, Hancock SL. The Cyberknife: a frameless robotic system for radiosurgery. Stereotact Funct Neurosurg 1997;69(1-4, pt 2):124–128

25. Chang SD, Adler JR. Robotics and radiosurgery—the CyberKnife. Stereotact Funct Neurosurg 2001;76(3-4):204–208

26. Chang SD, Main W, Martin DP, Gibbs IC, Heilbrun MP. An analysis of the accuracy of the CyberKnife: a robotic frameless stereotactic radiosurgical system. Neurosurgery 2003;52(1):140–146, discussion 146–147

27. Yu C, Shepard D. Treatment planning for stereotactic radiosurgery with photon beams. Technol Cancer Res Treat 2003;2(2):93–104.

28. Gibbs IC. Frameless image-guided intracranial and extracranial radiosurgery using the Cyberknife robotic system. Cancer Radiother 2006;10(5):283–287

29. Wilson RR. Radiological use of fast protons. Radiology 1946;47(5):487–491

30. Blomquist E, Bjelkengren G, Glimelius B. The potential of proton beam radiation therapy in intracranial and ocular tumours. Acta Oncol 2005;44(8):862–870

31. Lomax A. Intensity modulation methods for proton radiotherapy. Phys Med Biol 1999;44(1):185–205

32. Levin WP, Delaney TF. Charged particle therapy. In: Gunderson LL, Tepper JE, eds. Clinical Radiation Oncology. 3rd ed. Philadelphia, PA: Elsevier Saunders; 2012:361–376

33. Gehring MA, Mackie TR, Kubsad SS, Paliwal BR, Mehta MP, Kinsella TJ. A three-dimensional volume visualization package applied to stereotactic radiosurgery treatment planning. Int J Radiat Oncol Biol Phys 1991;21(2):491–500

34. Khan FM. The Physics of Radiation Therapy. 4th ed. New York, NY: Lippincott Williams & Wilkins; 2009

35. Nedzi LA, Kooy HM, Alexander E III, Svensson GK, Loeffler JS. Dynamic field shaping for stereotactic radiosurgery: a modeling study. Int J Radiat Oncol Biol Phys 1993;25(5):859–869

36. Kubo HD, Wilder RB, Pappas CT. Impact of collimator leaf width on stereotactic radiosurgery and 3D conformal radiotherapy treatment plans. Int J Radiat Oncol Biol Phys 1999;44(4):937–945

37. Nakamura JL, Verhey LJ, Smith V, et al. Dose conformity of gamma knife radiosurgery and risk factors for complications. Int J Radiat Oncol Biol Phys 2001;51(5):1313–1319

38. Paddick I. A simple scoring ratio to index the conformity of radiosurgical treatment plans. Technical note. J Neurosurg 2000;93(Suppl 3):219–222

39. Leber KA, Berglöff J, Pendl G. Dose-response tolerance of the visual pathways and cranial nerves of the cavernous sinus to stereotactic radiosurgery. J Neurosurg 1998;88(1):43–50

40. DeVita VT, Lawrence TS, Rosenberg SA, eds. DeVita, Hellman, and Rosenberg's Cancer: Principles and Practice of Oncology. 9th ed. New York, NY: Lippincott Williams & Wilkins; 2011

41. Sheehan JP, Williams BJ, Yen CP. Stereotactic radiosurgery for WHO grade I meningiomas. J Neurooncol 2010;99(3):407–416

42. Paulsen F, Doerr S, Wilhelm H, Becker G, Bamberg M, Classen J. Fractionated stereotactic radiotherapy in patients with optic nerve sheath meningioma. Int J Radiat Oncol Biol Phys 2012;82(2):773–778

43. Baumert BG, Villà S, Studer G, et al. Early improvements in vision after fractionated stereotactic radiotherapy for primary optic nerve sheath meningioma. Radiother Oncol 2004;72(2):169–174

44. Andrews DW, Faroozan R, Yang BP, et al. Fractionated stereotactic radiotherapy for the treatment of optic nerve sheath meningiomas: preliminary observations of 33 optic nerves in 30 patients with historical comparison to observation with or without prior surgery. Neurosurgery 2002;51(4):890–902, discussion 903–904

45. Zada G, Pagnini PG, Yu C, et al. Long-term outcomes and patterns of tumor progression after gamma knife radiosurgery for benign meningiomas. Neurosurgery 2010;67(2):322–328, discussion 328–329

46. Spiegelmann R, Cohen ZR, Nissim O, Alezra D, Pfeffer R. Cavernous sinus meningiomas: a large LINAC radiosurgery series. J Neurooncol 2010;98(2):195–202

47. Colombo F, Casentini L, Cavedon C, Scalchi P, Cora S, Francescon P. Cyberknife radiosurgery for benign meningiomas: short-term results in 199 patients. Neurosurgery 2009;64(2, Suppl):A7–A13

48. Han JH, Kim DG, Chung HT, et al. Gamma knife radiosurgery for skull base meningiomas: long-term radiologic and clinical outcome. Int J Radiat Oncol Biol Phys 2008;72(5):1324–1332

49. Pollock BE, Stafford SL. Results of stereotactic radiosurgery for patients with imaging defined cavernous sinus meningioma. Int J Radiat Oncol Biol Phys 2005;62(5):1427–1431

50. Lee JY, Niranjan A, McInerney J, Kondziolka D, Flickinger JC, Lunsford LD. Stereotactic radiosurgery providing long-term tumor control of cavernous sinus meningiomas. J Neurosurg 2002;97(1):65–72

51. Nicolato A, Foroni R, Alessandrini F, Maluta S, Bricolo A, Gerosa M. The role of Gamma Knife radiosurgery in the management of cavernous sinus meningiomas. Int J Radiat Oncol Biol Phys 2002;53(4):992–1000

52. Shin M, Kurita H, Sasaki T, et al. Analysis of treatment outcome after stereotactic radiosurgery for cavernous sinus meningiomas. J Neurosurg 2001;95(3):435–439

53. Roche PH, Régis J, Dufour H, et al. Gamma knife radiosurgery in the management of cavernous sinus meningiomas. J Neurosurg 2000;93(Suppl 3):68–73

54. Morita A, Coffey RJ, Foote RL, Schiff D, Gorman D. Risk of injury to cranial nerves after gamma knife radiosurgery for skull base meningiomas: experience in 88 patients. J Neurosurg 1999;90(1):42–49

55. Chang SD, Adler JR Jr, Martin DP. LINAC radiosurgery for cavernous sinus meningiomas. Stereotact Funct Neurosurg 1998;71(1):43–50

56. Metellus P, Batra S, Karkar S, et al. Fractionated conformal radiotherapy in the management of cavernous sinus meningiomas: long-term functional outcome and tumor control at a single institution. Int J Radiat Oncol Biol Phys 2010;78(3):836–843

57. Litré CF, Colin P, Noudel R, et al. Fractionated stereotactic radiotherapy treatment of cavernous sinus meningiomas: a study of 100 cases. Int J Radiat Oncol Biol Phys 2009;74(4):1012–1017

58. Brell M, Villà S, Teixidor P, et al. Fractionated stereotactic radiotherapy in the treatment of exclusive cavernous sinus meningioma: functional outcome, local control, and tolerance. Surg Neurol 2006;65(1):28–33, discussion 33–34

59. Metellus P, Regis J, Muracciole X, et al. Evaluation of fractionated radiotherapy and gamma knife radiosurgery in cavernous sinus meningiomas: treatment strategy. Neurosurgery 2005;57(5): 873–886, discussion 873–886

60. Flickinger JC, Kondziolka D, Maitz AH, Lunsford LD. Gamma knife radiosurgery of imaging-diagnosed intracranial meningioma. Int J Radiat Oncol Biol Phys 2003;56(3):801–806

61. Kollová A, Liscák R, Novotný J Jr, Vladyka V, Simonová G, Janousková L. Gamma Knife surgery for benign meningioma. J Neurosurg 2007;107(2):325–336

62. DiBiase SJ, Kwok Y, Yovino S, et al. Factors predicting local tumor control after gamma knife stereotactic radiosurgery for benign intracranial meningiomas. Int J Radiat Oncol Biol Phys 2004;60(5):1515–1519

63. Bria C, Wegner RE, Clump DA, et al. Fractionated stereotactic radiosurgery for the treatment of meningiomas. J Cancer Res Ther 2011;7(1):52–57

64. Adler JR Jr, Gibbs IC, Puataweepong P, Chang SD. Visual field preservation after multisession cyberknife radiosurgery for perioptic lesions. Neurosurgery 2006;59(2):244–254, discussion 244–254

65. Tuniz F, Soltys SG, Choi CY, et al. Multisession CyberKnife stereotactic radiosurgery of large, benign cranial base tumors:

preliminary study. Neurosurgery 2009;65(5):898–907, discussion 907 discussion

66. Condra KS, Buatti JM, Mendenhall WM, Friedman WA, Marcus RB Jr, Rhoton AL. Benign meningiomas: primary treatment selection affects survival. Int J Radiat Oncol Biol Phys 1997;39(2):427–436

67. Stafford SL, Perry A, Suman VJ, et al. Primarily resected meningiomas: outcome and prognostic factors in 581 Mayo Clinic patients, 1978 through 1988. Mayo Clin Proc 1998;73(10):936–942

68. Taylor BW Jr, Marcus RB Jr, Friedman WA, Ballinger WE Jr, Million RR. The meningioma controversy: postoperative radiation therapy. Int J Radiat Oncol Biol Phys 1988;15(2):299–304

69. Barbaro NM, Gutin PH, Wilson CB, Sheline GE, Boldrey EB, Wara WM. Radiation therapy in the treatment of partially resected meningiomas. Neurosurgery 1987;20(4):525–528

70. Aghi MK, Carter BS, Cosgrove GR, et al. Long-term recurrence rates of atypical meningiomas after gross total resection with or without postoperative adjuvant radiation. Neurosurgery 2009;64(1):56–60, discussion 60

71. Hug EB, Devries A, Thornton AF, et al. Management of atypical and malignant meningiomas: role of high-dose, 3D-conformal radiation therapy. J Neurooncol 2000;48(2):151–160

72. Laws ER, Sheehan JP, Sheehan JM, Jagnathan J, Jane JA Jr, Oskouian R. Stereotactic radiosurgery for pituitary adenomas: a review of the literature. J Neurooncol 2004;69(1-3):257–272

73. Kobayashi T. Long-term results of stereotactic gamma knife radiosurgery for pituitary adenomas. Specific strategies for different types of adenoma. Prog Neurol Surg 2009;22:77–95

74. Tinnel BA, Henderson MA, Witt TC, et al. Endocrine response after gamma knife-based stereotactic radiosurgery for secretory pituitary adenoma. Stereotact Funct Neurosurg 2008;86(5):292–296

75. Becker G, Kocher M, Kortmann RD, et al. Radiation therapy in the multimodal treatment approach of pituitary adenoma. Strahlenther Onkol 2002;178(4):173–186

76. Ikeda H, Jokura H, Yoshimoto T. Transsphenoidal surgery and adjuvant gamma knife treatment for growth hormone-secreting pituitary adenoma. J Neurosurg 2001;95(2):285–291

77. Shin M, Kurita H, Sasaki T, et al. Stereotactic radiosurgery for pituitary adenoma invading the cavernous sinus. J Neurosurg 2000;93(Suppl 3):2–5

78. Losa M, Gioia L, Picozzi P, et al. The role of stereotactic radiotherapy in patients with growth hormone-secreting pituitary adenoma. J Clin Endocrinol Metab 2008;93(7):2546–2552

79. Milker-Zabel S, Zabel A, Huber P, Schlegel W, Wannenmacher M, Debus J. Stereotactic conformal radiotherapy in patients with growth hormone-secreting pituitary adenoma. Int J Radiat Oncol Biol Phys 2004;59(4):1088–1096

80. Wang MH, Liu P, Liu AL, Luo B, Sun SB. [Efficacy of gamma knife radiosurgery in treatment of growth hormone-secreting pituitary adenoma]. Zhonghua Yi Xue Za Zhi 2003;83(23):2045–2048.

81. McCord MW, Buatti JM, Fennell EM, et al. Radiotherapy for pituitary adenoma: long-term outcome and sequelae. Int J Radiat Oncol Biol Phys 1997;39(2):437–444

82. Rush S, Cooper PR. Symptom resolution, tumor control, and side effects following postoperative radiotherapy for pituitary macroadenomas. Int J Radiat Oncol Biol Phys 1997;37(5):1031–1034

83. Rush SC, Newall J. Pituitary adenoma: the efficacy of radiotherapy as the sole treatment. Int J Radiat Oncol Biol Phys 1989;17(1):165–169

84. Rush S, Donahue B, Cooper P, Lee C, Persky M, Newall J. Prolactin reduction after combined therapy for prolactin macroadenomas. Neurosurgery 1991;28(4):502–505

85. Gopalan R, Schlesinger D, Vance ML, Er EL, Sheehan J. Long-term outcomes following Gamma Knife radiosurgery for patients with a nonfunctioning pituitary adenoma. Neurosurgery 2011;69(2): 284–293

86. Pollock BE, Cochran J, Natt N, et al. Gamma knife radiosurgery for patients with nonfunctioning pituitary adenomas: results from a 15-year experience. Int J Radiat Oncol Biol Phys 2008;70(5): 1325–1329

87. Killory BD, Kresl JJ, Wait SD, Ponce FA, Porter R, White WL. Hypofractionated CyberKnife radiosurgery for perichiasmatic pituitary adenomas: early results. Neurosurgery 2009;64(2, Suppl):A19–A25

88. Roberts BK, Ouyang DL, Lad SP, et al. Efficacy and safety of CyberKnife radiosurgery for acromegaly. Pituitary 2007;10(1):19–25

89. Ronson BB, Schulte RW, Han KP, Loredo LN, Slater JM, Slater JD. Fractionated proton beam irradiation of pituitary adenomas. Int J Radiat Oncol Biol Phys 2006;64(2):425–434

90. Matson DD, Crigler JF Jr. Management of craniopharyngioma in childhood. J Neurosurg 1969;30(4):377–390

91. Bunin GR, Surawicz TS, Witman PA, Preston-Martin S, Davis F, Bruner JM. The descriptive epidemiology of craniopharyngioma. J Neurosurg 1998;89(4):547–551

92. Kalapurakal JA, Goldman S, Hsieh YC, Tomita T, Marymont MH. Clinical outcome in children with craniopharyngioma treated with primary surgery and radiotherapy deferred until relapse. Med Pediatr Oncol 2003;40(4):214–218

93. Niranjan A, Kano H, Mathieu D, Kondziolka D, Flickinger JC, Lunsford LD. Radiosurgery for craniopharyngioma. Int J Radiat Oncol Biol Phys 2010;78(1):64–71

94. Rajan B, Ashley S, Gorman C, et al. Craniopharyngioma—a long-term results following limited surgery and radiotherapy. Radiother Oncol 1993;26(1):1–10

95. Stripp DC, Maity A, Janss AJ, et al. Surgery with or without radiation therapy in the management of craniopharyngiomas in children and young adults. Int J Radiat Oncol Biol Phys 2004;58(3):714–720

96. Hetelekidis S, Barnes PD, Tao ML, et al. 20-year experience in childhood craniopharyngioma. Int J Radiat Oncol Biol Phys 1993;27(2):189–195

97. Xu Z, Yen CP, Schlesinger D, Sheehan J. Outcomes of Gamma Knife surgery for craniopharyngiomas. J Neurooncol 2011;104(1):305–313

98. Gopalan R, Dassoulas K, Rainey J, Sherman JH, Sheehan JP. Evaluation of the role of Gamma Knife surgery in the treatment of craniopharyngiomas. Neurosurg Focus 2008;24(5):E5

99. Broich G, Pagliari A, Ottaviani F. Esthesioneuroblastoma: a general review of the cases published since the discovery of the tumour in 1924. Anticancer Res 1997;17(4A):2683–2706

100. Noh OK, Lee SW, Yoon SM, et al. Radiotherapy for esthesioneuroblastoma: is elective nodal irradiation warranted in the multimodality treatment approach? Int J Radiat Oncol Biol Phys 2011;79(2): 443–449

101. Dulguerov P, Allal AS, Calcaterra TC. Esthesioneuroblastoma: a meta-analysis and review. Lancet Oncol 2001;2(11):683–690

102. Gruber G, Laedrach K, Baumert B, Caversaccio M, Raveh J, Greiner R. Esthesioneuroblastoma: irradiation alone and surgery alone are not enough. Int J Radiat Oncol Biol Phys 2002;54(2):486–491

103. Nichols AC, Chan AW, Curry WT, Barker FG, Deschler DG, Lin DT. Esthesioneuroblastoma: the Massachusetts eye and ear infirmary and Massachusetts general hospital experience with craniofacial resection, proton beam radiation, and chemotherapy. Skull Base 2008;18(5):327–337

104. Debus J, Schulz-Ertner D, Schad L, et al. Stereotactic fractionated radiotherapy for chordomas and chondrosarcomas of the skull base. Int J Radiat Oncol Biol Phys 2000;47(3):591–596

105. Fagundes MA, Hug EB, Liebsch NJ, Daly W, Efird J, Munzenrider JE. Radiation therapy for chordomas of the base of skull and cervical spine: patterns of failure and outcome after relapse. Int J Radiat Oncol Biol Phys 1995;33(3):579–584

106. Hasegawa T, Ishii D, Kida Y, Yoshimoto M, Koike J, Iizuka H. Gamma Knife surgery for skull base chordomas and chondrosarcomas. J Neurosurg 2007;107(4):752–757

36 Robotics in Endoscopic Skull Base Surgery

Nicholas C. Sorrel, M. Kupferman, Ehab Y. Hanna, and F. Christopher Holsinger

Surgical Robotics

The coining of the term "robot" is attributed to the Czechoslovakian Joseph Capek who lent it to his brother Karel Capek for use in a play *Rossum's Universal Robots* in 1920. The term was used to describe automated nonhuman laborers and is derived from the Czech word for "forced labor"—*robota*. Since that time the idea of automated machines designed to perform tasks has transformed from fiction to reality. The current definition of robot is as follows: a machine capable of carrying out a complex series of actions automatically, especially one programmable by a computer. Robotic surgery may be further defined as active, semiactive, or passive. Active robotics implies that the robot performs a programmed task independent of a human operator, but semiactive robotics require an operator input at certain set points to carry out an automated action. In passive robotics, the robot functions only at the specific direction of human action. In medicine, the use of robots has evolved dramatically over the past two decades, from machines designed to help precisely hold and guide instruments to advanced physician-controlled telerobotic devices that allow surgeons to perform complex endoscopic surgery from local or remote locations (even across oceans).[1,2]

The da Vinci surgical system (Intuitive Surgical Inc., Sunnyvale, California, United States) is currently the only commercially available surgical robot in the United States. The system consists of the patient-side cart with three or four arms (**Fig. 36.1**). One arm holds the endoscope and other arms hold instruments for surgical manipulation, including cutting, suturing, cautery, clip application, and grasping. Lasers are also often attached to a grasper for laser surgery. The endoscope consists of dual-mounted right and left high-definition telescopes, which project images to the viewing port for the respective eye on the surgical console. This produces a three-dimensional view with pristine clarity and allows for precision dissection in a microscopic environment. The surgical arms are equipped with EndoWrist technology, which provides 7 degrees of freedom and mimics the movement of the human wrist (traditional endoscopic surgery only allows 4 degrees of freedom). The patient-side cart is controlled by a surgeon from a separate console (**Fig. 36.2**). While viewing the field through the three-dimensional projection system the surgeon may articulate the arms and adjust the endoscopic view using the control handles. The computer tracks the surgeon's movements and filters out tremors. In addition, an

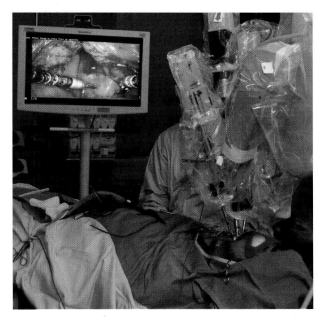

Figure 36.1 The surgical robot seen docked during a transoral robotic surgery.

assistant should be available at the operative table to adjust the instruments, clean the endoscope, and occasionally to provide additional suction and cautery. The leading uses for surgical robotics at this time are in the disciplines of urology, gynecologic surgery, and cardiothoracic surgery, yet there has been a surge of interest in this technology in the field of otolaryngology, which shares similar concerns about limited surgical access in areas of vital structures.[3,4]

Robotics in Otorhinolaryngology

The use of surgical robotics in otorhinolaryngology began with simple automated drill guides used to precisely drill out the stapes footplate.[5] Coinciding advances in technology and interest in minimally invasive surgery fueled the study of the surgeon-operated robot for further indications in the head and neck. Success in studies in porcine, mannequin, and cadaver models led to a variety of applications in live patients for surgery of the upper airway and neck.[2,3,6–9] Although not completely abated, initial concerns about operative time, complications, and cost have been dampened as reports of great outcomes have led to surgical robotics being, in some centers, relatively commonplace for a myriad of otolaryngologic indications.

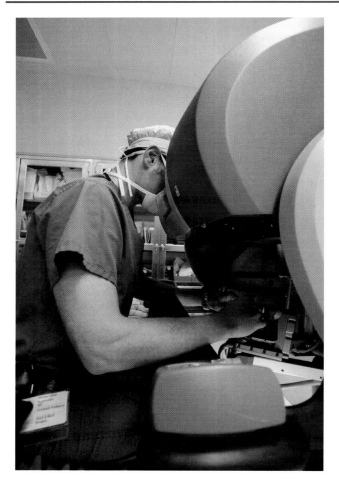

Figure 36.2 The surgeon console for the robot system.

As endoscopic minimally invasive head and neck surgery has evolved around the common natural routes of exposure, the most rapidly advancing discipline has been transoral robotic surgery (TORS) for carcinoma of the upper airway. TORS provides the unique advantage of visualization and precise instrumentation in difficult-to-access areas without large external incisions, and applications now include resections of carcinoma in the oral cavity, oropharynx, supraglottis, glottis, and hypopharynx.[3,10–14] Long-term results are yet to be reported, and TORS has not been compared with other treatment strategies in any randomized controlled trials. However, the mounting literatures on the feasibility, oncologic, and functional outcomes are very encouraging.[3,11–16] The use of the surgical robot for minimally invasive head and neck surgery has also extended beyond the transoral route and includes neck surgery for thyroid gland resection and neck dissection.[2]

One of the least studied but most fertile areas for study and application of surgical robotics in the head and neck is for minimally invasive skull base surgery. The following sections will provide a discussion of the current studied applications of robotics at the skull base, advantages and disadvantages compared with more traditional minimally invasive surgery, and some of the authors' experiences.

Minimally Invasive Skull Base Surgery

The most direct route for endoscopic skull base surgery is via the transnasal route, and endoscopic approaches via this route have been increasingly used for surgical access and treatment of neoplastic and nonneoplastic lesions of the anterior and central skull base.[17] Examples of nonneoplastic conditions include cerebrospinal fluid (CSF) leaks, mucoceles, encephaloceles, cholesterol granulomas, and allergic and invasive fungal sinusitis.[18–26] Endoscopic surgery is also used with increasing frequency for surgical resection of tumors of the sinonasal tract, such as inverted papilloma, angiofibroma, osteomas, and other benign fibro-osseous lesions, and even in selected patients with malignant sinonasal tumors.[27–39] The endoscopic approach has become one of the standard surgical techniques for transsphenoidal access to the sella turcica, and it is considered by many centers the preferred surgical approach for treatment of pituitary adenomas.[40–48] More recently, there has been an emerging trend to expand the use of transnasal endoscopic approaches in the surgical treatment of suprasellar, petroclival, infratemporal, and other intracranial skull base tumors.[49–52]

The main advantage of transnasal endoscopic skull base approaches is to provide more direct access to the anterior and central skull base while avoiding craniofacial incisions and extensive bone removal commonly used in open surgical approaches.[17] Advances in optical clarity of endoscopic telescopes and high-definition video technology have allowed surgeons to have a magnified view of the skull base, which is not possible with the operating microscope. The wider angle of vision and the ability to use angled lenses also increase the range of the endoscopic visual surgical field compared with the "line of sight" visual field gained by surgical loupes or microscopes.[42] Other technological advances that have allowed for the development of this surgical technique include powered instrumentation, improved preoperative imaging quality, and intraoperative image-guidance technologies.

Both neurosurgical and otolaryngological disciplines are now using endoscopic and open with endoscopic-assisted surgery to access lesions from the cribriform plate anteriorly to the craniocervical junction posteriorly, as well as the infratemporal fossa laterally.[53] A full discussion of these approaches to the skull base is located elsewhere in this text. However, for the purpose of this chapter, it is important to reiterate that endoscopic resection of both neoplastic and nonneoplastic lesions of the skull base has been shown to provide equal outcomes in terms of control of the primary lesion with reduced morbidity in carefully selected patients.[27,28,54–56] What follows is a discussion of how some of the inherent technical advantages of surgical robotics may overcome some of the limitations of traditional endoscopic surgery and are leading to this modality defining a role as a viable and useful method for minimally invasive endoscopic skull base surgery.

Technical Advantages and Disadvantages of Surgical Robotics in Skull Base Surgery

One of the major limitations of traditional endoscopic surgery is optical visibility. The two-dimensional visualization provided by single-channel optical systems in current endoscopes lacks three-dimensional vision; thus, depth perception relies more on tactile than on visual cues. Visual depth perception is particularly important when operating on critical intracranial neurovascular structures, especially when working in a deep and limited space. Current endoscopic techniques also have several ergonomic limitations. Bimanual surgery is only feasible if the endoscope is held by an assistant or a mechanical holder. A surgical assistant is preferred because of the constant need to adjust the position (depth and angle) of the endoscope during endoscopic surgery. This not only limits the direct control of the endoscope by the primary surgeon but also requires the assistance of a relatively experienced endoscopic surgeon who can seamlessly follow the primary surgeon in every step of the operation. Also, both surgeons have to work within a confined space that, in some cases, limits ergonomic freedom. In addition, as the surgical field gets deeper, longer instruments are needed; with lack of proper arm support, precision may be limited by fine tremor, especially when using fine instrumentation for delicate dissection of critical neurovascular structures. Finally and perhaps the most significant limitation of current transnasal endoscopic techniques is the inability to suture and provide watertight dural closure or reconstruction of dural defects. Endoscopic repair of dural defects relies on nonvascularized fat, mucosal or allogeneic grafts, or vascularized septal or nasal rotational mucosal flaps.[23,57,58] These reconstructions are then covered with fibrin sealants and supported by either absorbable or nonabsorbable packing. Although these methods may provide an adequate reconstruction of minor dural tears or defects, their ability to provide safe and reliable reconstruction of larger dural defects remains untested.[18,19] Preliminary results suggest that endoscopic repair of larger defects (greater than 2 cm) confers a higher CSF leak rate and complication rate compared with the more standard dural reconstruction using pedicled (axial) flaps, such as the pericranial flap or microvascular free flaps.[53,59] Adequate and reliable dural reconstruction is critical in minimizing the morbidity of skull base resections, particularly in patients who received or will undergo high-dose radiation therapy.

The line of site microscopic approach via transnasal or limited incisions does alleviate some of the optical, ergonomic, and reconstructive limitations. Three-dimensional view with a good optical clarity is possible, but the field of view is limited. Further, bimanual instrumentation is afforded by this approach, which may make suturing of dural defects possible. However, there are limitations in obtaining wide exposure of the surgical site and precision is limited by natural human tremor amplified by the fulcrum of the long instruments required to access the skull base.

A robotic system may overcome optical disadvantages as the dual-channel optical system allows for marriage of the advantages of three-dimensional visualization of microscopic approach and the wider microscopic field of view provided by the endoscopic approach. The robotic system may overcome the ergonomic disadvantages of both endoscopic and microscopic approaches in the following ways. With the da Vinci robotic system, the surgeon controls simultaneously the binocular three-dimensional endoscope and two additional surgical arms. Further, the EndoWrist technology provides movement at the instrument tip with 7 degrees of freedom and 90 degrees of articulation and motion scaling. This allows the surgeon, who sits comfortably at the console with an adjustable arm support, to perform precise tremor-free movement in a deep and confined space, with working angles usually not achievable with nonrobotic instruments. Combined these advantages lead to the feasibility of precise resection and closure of dural defects and may drastically impact the usage and safety of endoscopic surgery of intracranial intradural lesions of the skull base (**Table 36.1**).

Although there are theoretic and, as discussed below, some demonstrated advantages of the robotic approach to the skull base, the modality is not without disadvantages. Concerns have been pointed out about the setup time that can be required with the robotic system and that this may increase the operative time. However, this must be weighed against the generally faster operative time with the robot and depends on experience; further evaluation of this is needed. One major disadvantage of surgical robotics in general is the lack of tactile feedback provided by endoscopic and microscopic surgery. Although there is work being done to provide tactile feedback cues to the surgeon, the current da Vinci system does not allow for this and the surgeon must rely on visual cues. Another disadvantage of the robotic system is that of access. The robotic endoscope is either 8.5 or 12 mm in diameter in contrast with the 2.7 or 4 mm endoscopes used with traditional endoscopic surgery, thus causing difficulty fitting into the nasal cavity. Further,

Table 36.1 Comparative Advantages of Minimally Invasive Approaches to the Skull Base

Advantages	Robotic Approach	Endoscopic Approach	Microscope Approach
Access	++	+++	++
Instrument freedom and precision	+++	+	++
Visibility	+++	+++	++
3-D/depth perception	Yes	No	Yes
Tactile feedback	No	Yes	Yes

3-D, three-dimensional.

pure transnasal access is prohibited by the lack of room to place the robotic arms. The robotic arms not only move at the wrist but translational movement is also provided by the elbows. This poses not only spatial but also some geometric disadvantage to placing all the arms through such a small area as the nasal cavity, as the design of the system requires the two surgical arms to be aligned at a 90-degree angle to one another to avoid physical interference with the camera. Simply put, additional surgical manipulation would be required to access the skull base with the robotic system. Therefore, cadaver models have been developed to evaluate methods of accessing the skull base using the mouth and nose as entry sites without or with limited external incisions.

Techniques

Approach to the Anterior Cranial Fossa

The feasibility of using the surgical robot to access the anterior and central skull base and perform primary dural repair has been described and used and will be discussed here. The following technique was developed by the authors of this chapter in a cadaver model.[60] Entry points for the surgical arms may be obtained through the maxillary sinuses. Sublabial incisions and bilateral anterior maxillary antrostomies are performed, followed by middle meatal antrostomy. Sufficient access can be obtained without compromising the infraorbital nerve. Further posterior septectomy is done to provide a common bilateral surgical field. The robotic endoscope is then placed into the patient's naris and the right and left surgical arms introduced through the respective maxillary sinus. The surgical robot may then be used to carry out anterior and posterior ethmoidectomy with our without resection of the middle or superior turbinates depending on the extent of surgical exposure needed. Sphenoidotomy may also be performed with the surgical robot to expose the planum sphenoidale, sella turcica, and parasellar regions. Finally, access to the anterior cranial fossa is provided by sharp dissection of the anterior skull base and incision of the dura. The dual robotic arms can be used for primary repair of the dura.[60] This approach provides an excellent access to the anterior and central skull base, including the cribriform plate, fovea ethmoidalis, medial orbits, planum sphenoidale, nasopharynx, pterygopalatine fossa, and clivus (**Fig. 36.3**). The most significant advantage of this approach is the ability to perform two-handed, tremor-free endoscopic closure of dural defects. Since the description of this technique in a cadaver model, it has been implemented in live patients with encouraging results.

Approach to the Clivus

The prevalence of pituitary tumors exceeds 15% in the general population, and more than 5000 pituitary surgeries are performed yearly in the United States. Various surgical

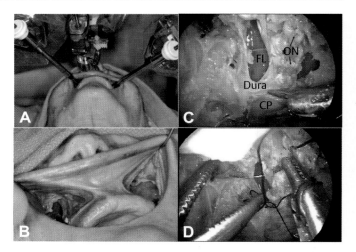

Figure 36.3 (A) Bilateral maxillary antrostomies. (B) Robotic arm and endoscope placement. (C) Surgical exposure revealing the dura, cribriform plate (CP), frontal lobes (FL), and optic nerve (ON). (D) Primary repair of the dura.

approaches to the sella have been described, but the most commonly used approach is the sublabial technique with a microscope-assisted surgical resection. Because of the small surgical field of the pituitary fossa, there has been an evolution toward a transnasal endoscopic approach to take advantage of magnification and angled telescopes.[61,62] The surgical robot may provide this endoscopic advantage as well as maintain the advantage of three-dimensional view and bimanual instrumentation of the microscopic approach. So, an approach that allows endoscopic access for resection of tumors involving the pituitary fossa has been developed.[63]

Similar to the approach to the anterior cranial fossa, access involves creating bilateral maxillary antrostomies. The robot is then docked by introducing three articulated arm ports: the camera through the nostril and the right and left surgical arms through antrotomies. An anterior sphenoidotomy is then performed and the sellar floor is removed to expose the dura of the pituitary fossa. The dura is opened sharply with the robotic scissors to allow for exploration of the pituitary gland. The diaphragma sella is then incised and the pituitary stalk sharply transected. Blunt and sharp dissection is then performed to excise the pituitary gland after the optic chiasm and hypothalamus are exposed. Dissection of the lateral wall of the sphenoid sinus may also be performed with high-speed drills and fine rongeurs to access the cavernous sinus. Using this technique the surgeon obtains access to the central skull base, including the planum sphenoidale, the pituitary gland, cavernous carotid, mammillary bodies, and optic chiasm, and the most significant advantage is the ability of the surgeon to perform precise two-handed endoscopic resection of the anterior pituitary gland.

O'Malley and Weinstein have also reported on the transcervical placement of the robotic instruments in canine and cadaver models. They reported accessing the sphenoid, clivus, sella, and suprasellar anterior fossa successfully by placing a 30-degree robotic endoscope transorally and placing the right and left robotic arms through the neck behind the submandibular gland and into the pharynx.[64]

Approach to the Nasopharynx

Radiation therapy remains the primary treatment for nasopharyngeal carcinoma. However, managing recurrent nasopharyngeal carcinoma has been very difficult because of morbidity associated with open resections or re-irradiation.[65] Endoscopic nasopharyngectomy for recurrent nasopharyngeal carcinoma has been described with good results.[66] Access to the nasopharynx has also been described using the surgical robot via the palatal split. The method was first described in a cadaver by Ozer et al in 2008 and then in a live patient by Wei and Ho in 2010.[67,68] This technique has been performed by the author of this chapter via the following method.

A Dingman retractor may be used to open the oral cavity and view the oropharynx. The soft palate is split under direct visualization using Bovie cautery and each side retracted laterally using sutures suspended to the Dingman. The da Vinci robot is placed at the head of the bed and robotic arms and 0-degree endoscope positioned into the oral cavity. The patient's head may be gently flexed to help eliminate an instrument collision between the camera and the tongue blade of the retractor (**Fig. 36.4**). The nasopharynx soft tissue may then be progressively degloved between the carotid arteries and eustachian tubes laterally and the skull base and prevertebral musculature posteriorly by using the grasper and the spatula cautery (**Fig. 36.5**). The palate is closed in three layers with absorbable suture. The advantage of this technique is that it allows for en bloc excision of nasopharyngeal lesions and may have the distinct advantage of reduced morbidity with similar oncologic outcome

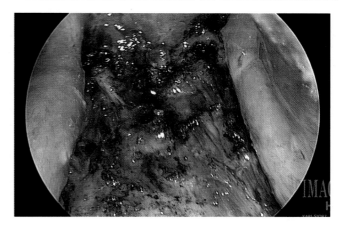

Figure 36.5 Surgical exposure for robotic nasopharyngectomy—view after resection of the lesion.

compared with re-irradiation for recurrent nasopharyngeal carcinoma, although further studies in this regard are needed.

Approach to the Infratemporal Fossa

In 2007, O'Malley and Weinstein reported on preclinical investigation in cadaver and canine models for approaches to the infratemporal fossa and parapharyngeal space.[69] They describe a transoral approach using Crowe-Davis retractor of exposure. Dissection may then be performed through the lateral pharyngeal wall to access the parapharyngeal space. Using a 30-degree endoscope directed superiorly, the surgeon can carefully explore the parapharyngeal space to identify the neurovascular contents—jugular vein, internal carotid, and cranial nerves IX, X, XI, and XII. To gain exposure superiorly and laterally (to the infratemporal fossa) the styloid musculature can be resected and pterygoid muscles partially released. The live canine portion of this experiment confirmed the ability to safely perform the approach by retracting and not injuring the great vessels. O'Malley and colleagues report the feasibility of this approach, but admit limitations that wide resection may not be possible because of lack of effective robotic bone-dissecting instrumentation. They propose this approach best suited for well-circumscribed benign lesions.

In 2010, McCool et al reported on a modification of this technique to access the infratemporal fossa by using a suprahyoid port to place one of the robot's surgical arms through the vallecula and into the surgical field. The other surgical arm and 30-degree endoscope were placed through the mouth. They reported excellent access and surgical control in a cadaver model.[70]

Conclusion

Although a significant body of literature on patients is yet to be reported, the theoretical benefits of robotic approaches to the skull base are apparent. Safe and effective minimally

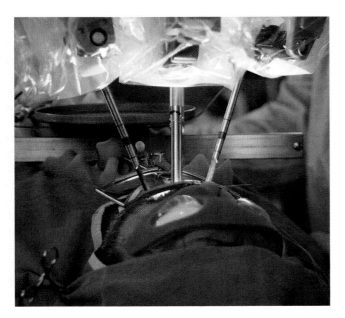

Figure 36.4 Patient positioning for transoral robotic nasopharyngectomy.

invasive robotic approaches have been demonstrated in human, canine, and cadaver models to the anterior skull base, clivus, nasopharynx, and infratemporal fossa. The authors of this chapter are currently considering robotic approach to the skull base as part of the treatment algorithm for selected benign and malignant neoplasms of the skull base and believe that further refinement of robotic instruments and techniques will revolutionize the surgical approach to the skull base.

References

1. Hockstein NG, Gourin CG, et al. A history of robots: from science fiction to surgical robotics. J Robot Surg 2007;1:113–118

2. Parmar A, Grant DG, Loizou P. Robotic surgery in ear nose and throat. Eur Arch Otorhinolaryngol 2010;267(4):625–633

3. Weinstein GS, O'Malley BW Jr, Desai SC, Quon H. Transoral robotic surgery: does the ends justify the means? Curr Opin Otolaryngol Head Neck Surg 2009;17(2):126–131

4. Maan ZN, Gibbins N, Al-Jabri T, D'Souza AR. The use of robotics in otolaryngology-head and neck surgery: a systematic review. Am J Otolaryngol 2012;33(1):137–146

5. Brett PN, Baker DA, Reyes L, Blanshard J. An automatic technique for micro-drilling a stapedotomy in the flexible stapes footplate. Proc Inst Mech Eng H 1995;209(4):255–262

6. Terris DJ, Haus BM, Gourin CG, Lilagan PE. Endo-robotic resection of the submandibular gland in a cadaver model. Head Neck 2005;27(11):946–951

7. Haus BM, Kambham N, Le D, Moll FM, Gourin C, Terris DJ. Surgical robotic applications in otolaryngology. Laryngoscope 2003;113(7):1139–1144

8. Hockstein NG, Nolan JP, O'malley BW Jr, Woo YJ. Robotic microlaryngeal surgery: a technical feasibility study using the daVinci surgical robot and an airway mannequin. Laryngoscope 2005;115(5):780–785

9. Hockstein NG, Nolan JP, O'Malley BW Jr, Woo YJ. Robot-assisted pharyngeal and laryngeal microsurgery: results of robotic cadaver dissections. Laryngoscope 2005;115(6):1003–1008

10. Holsinger FC, Sweeney AD, Jantharapattana K, et al. The emergence of endoscopic head and neck surgery. Curr Oncol Rep 2010;12(3):216–222

11. Weinstein GS, O'Malley BW Jr, Snyder W, Sherman E, Quon H. Transoral robotic surgery: radical tonsillectomy. Arch Otolaryngol Head Neck Surg 2007;133(12):1220–1226

12. Weinstein GS, O'Malley BW Jr, Snyder W, Hockstein NG. Transoral robotic surgery: supraglottic partial laryngectomy. Ann Otol Rhinol Laryngol 2007;116(1):19–23

13. Park YM, Lee WJ, Lee JG, et al. Transoral robotic surgery (TORS) in laryngeal and hypopharyngeal cancer. J Laparoendosc Adv Surg Tech A 2009;19(3):361–368

14. Boudreaux BA, Rosenthal EL, Magnuson JS, et al. Robot-assisted surgery for upper aerodigestive tract neoplasms. Arch Otolaryngol Head Neck Surg 2009;135(4):397–401

15. Moore EJ, Olsen KD, Kasperbauer JL. Transoral robotic surgery for oropharyngeal squamous cell carcinoma: a prospective study of feasibility and functional outcomes. Laryngoscope 2009;119(11):2156–2164

16. Iseli TA, Kulbersh BD, Iseli CE, Carroll WR, Rosenthal EL, Magnuson JS. Functional outcomes after transoral robotic surgery for head and neck cancer. Otolaryngol Head Neck Surg 2009;141(2):166–171

17. Batra PS, Citardi MJ, Worley S, Lee J, Lanza DC. Resection of anterior skull base tumors: comparison of combined traditional and endoscopic techniques. Am J Rhinol 2005;19(5):521–528

18. Basu D, Haughey BH, Hartman JM. Determinants of success in endoscopic cerebrospinal fluid leak repair. Otolaryngol Head Neck Surg 2006;135(5):769–773

19. Locatelli D, Rampa F, Acchiardi I, Bignami M, De Bernardi F, Castelnuovo P. Endoscopic endonasal approaches for repair of cerebrospinal fluid leaks: nine-year experience. Neurosurgery 2006;58(4, Suppl 2):ONS-246–NS-257

20. Castelnuovo P, Dallan I, Pistochini A, Battaglia P, Locatelli D, Bignami M. Endonasal endoscopic repair of Sternberg's canal cerebrospinal fluid leaks. Laryngoscope 2007;117(2):345–349

21. Bolger WE. Management of cerebral vascular structures during endoscopic treatment of encephaloceles: a clinical report. Ann Otol Rhinol Laryngol 2006;115(3):167–170

22. Kanowitz SJ, Bernstein JM. Pediatric meningoencephaloceles and nasal obstruction: a case for endoscopic repair. Int J Pediatr Otorhinolaryngol 2006;70(12):2087–2092

23. Mehta RP, Cueva RA, Brown JD, et al. What's new in skull base medicine and surgery? Skull Base Committee Report. Otolaryngol Head Neck Surg 2006;135(4):620–630

24. Casler JD, Doolittle AM, Mair EA. Endoscopic surgery of the anterior skull base. Laryngoscope 2005;115(1):16–24

25. Chandra RK, Palmer JN. Epidermoids of the paranasal sinuses and beyond: endoscopic management. Am J Rhinol 2006;20(4):441–444

26. Kinsella JB, Rassekh CH, Bradfield JL, et al. Allergic fungal sinusitis with cranial base erosion. Head Neck 1996;18(3):211–217

27. Hanna E, DeMonte F, Ibrahim S, Roberts D, Levine N, Kupferman M. Endoscopic resection of sinonasal cancers with and without craniotomy: oncologic results. Arch Otolaryngol Head Neck Surg 2009;135(12):1219–1224

28. Nicolai P, Battaglia P, Bignami M, et al. Endoscopic surgery for malignant tumors of the sinonasal tract and adjacent skull base: a 10-year experience. Am J Rhinol 2008;22(3):308–316

29. Lund V, Howard DJ, Wei WI. Endoscopic resection of malignant tumors of the nose and sinuses. Am J Rhinol 2007;21(1):89–94

30. Suriano M, De Vincentiis M, Colli A, Benfari G, Mascelli A, Gallo A. Endoscopic treatment of esthesioneuroblastoma: a minimally invasive approach combined with radiation therapy. Otolaryngol Head Neck Surg 2007;136(1):104–107

31. Baradaranfar MH, Dabirmoghaddam P. Endoscopic endonasal surgery for resection of benign sinonasal tumors: experience with 105 patients. Arch Iran Med 2006;9(3):244–249

32. Batra PS, Citardi MJ. Endoscopic management of sinonasal malignancy. Otolaryngol Clin North Am 2006;39(3):619–637, x–xi

33. Buchmann L, Larsen C, Pollack A, Tawfik O, Sykes K, Hoover LA. Endoscopic techniques in resection of anterior skull base/paranasal sinus malignancies. Laryngoscope 2006;116(10):1749–1754

34. Busquets JM, Hwang PH. Endoscopic resection of sinonasal inverted papilloma: a meta-analysis. Otolaryngol Head Neck Surg 2006;134(3):476–482

35. Chen MK. Minimally invasive endoscopic resection of sinonasal malignancies and skull base surgery. Acta Otolaryngol 2006;126(9):981–986

36. Karkos PD, Fyrmpas G, Carrie SC, Swift AC. Endoscopic versus open surgical interventions for inverted nasal papilloma: a systematic review. Clin Otolaryngol 2006;31(6):499–503

37. Lane AP, Bolger WE. Endoscopic management of inverted papilloma. Curr Opin Otolaryngol Head Neck Surg 2006;14(1):14–18

38. Banhiran W, Casiano RR. Endoscopic sinus surgery for benign and malignant nasal and sinus neoplasm. Curr Opin Otolaryngol Head Neck Surg 2005;13(1):50–54

39. Shipchandler TZ, Batra PS, Citardi MJ, Bolger WE, Lanza DC. Outcomes for endoscopic resection of sinonasal squamous cell carcinoma. Laryngoscope 2005;115(11):1983–1987

40. Haruna S, Otori N, Moriyama H, Kamio M. Endoscopic transnasaltransethmosphenoidal approach for pituitary tumors: assessment of technique and postoperative findings of nasal and paranasal cavities. Auris Nasus Larynx 2007;34(1):57–63

41. Anand VK, Schwartz TH, Hiltzik DH, Kacker A. Endoscopic transphenoidal pituitary surgery with real-time intraoperative magnetic resonance imaging. Am J Rhinol 2006;20(4):401–405

42. Frank G, Pasquini E, Farneti G, et al. The endoscopic versus the traditional approach in pituitary surgery. Neuroendocrinology 2006;83(3-4):240–248

43. Kelley RT, Smith JL II, Rodzewicz GM. Transnasal endoscopic surgery of the pituitary: modifications and results over 10 years. Laryngoscope 2006;116(9):1573–1576

44. Frank G, Pasquini E, Doglietto F, et al. The endoscopic extended transsphenoidal approach for craniopharyngiomas. Neurosurgery 2006; 59(1, Suppl 1):ONS75–ONS83, discussion ONS75–ONS83

45. Sethi DS, Leong JL. Endoscopic pituitary surgery. Otolaryngol Clin North Am 2006;39(3):563–583, x x

46. Schwartz TH, Stieg PE, Anand VK. Endoscopic transsphenoidal pituitary surgery with intraoperative magnetic resonance imaging. Neurosurgery 2006;58(1, Suppl):ONS44–ONS51, discussion ONS44–ONS51

47. Kabil MS, Eby JB, Shahinian HK. Fully endoscopic endonasal vs. transseptal transsphenoidal pituitary surgery. Minim Invasive Neurosurg 2005;48(6):348–354

48. Teo C. Application of endoscopy to the surgical management of craniopharyngiomas. Childs Nerv Syst 2005;21(8-9):696–700

49. Kassam A, Snyderman CH, Mintz A, Gardner P, Carrau RL. Expanded endonasal approach: the rostrocaudal axis. Part I. Crista galli to the sella turcica. Neurosurg Focus 2005;19(1):E3

50. Kassam A, Snyderman CH, Mintz A, Gardner P, Carrau RL. Expanded endonasal approach: the rostrocaudal axis. Part II. Posterior clinoids to the foramen magnum. Neurosurg Focus 2005;19(1):E4

51. Kassam AB, Gardner P, Snyderman C, Mintz A, Carrau R. Expanded endonasal approach: fully endoscopic, completely transnasal approach to the middle third of the clivus, petrous bone, middle cranial fossa, and infratemporal fossa. Neurosurg Focus 2005;19(1):E6

52. Solari D, Magro F, Cappabianca P, et al. Anatomical study of the pterygopalatine fossa using an endoscopic endonasal approach: spatial relations and distances between surgical landmarks. J Neurosurg 2007;106(1):157–163

53. Nogueira JF, Stamm A, Vellutini E. Evolution of endoscopic skull base surgery, current concepts, and future perspectives. Otolaryngol Clin North Am 2010;43(3):639–652, x–xi

54. Snyderman CH, Carrau RL, Prevedello DM, Gardner P, Kassam AB. Technologic innovations in neuroendoscopic surgery. Otolaryngol Clin North Am 2009;42(5):883–890, x

55. Cohen MA, Liang J, Cohen IJ, Grady MS, O'Malley BW Jr, Newman JG. Endoscopic resection of advanced anterior skull base lesions: oncologically safe? ORL J Otorhinolaryngol Relat Spec 2009; 71(3):123–128

56. Ong YK, Solares CA, Carrau RL, Snyderman CH. New developments in transnasal endoscopic surgery for malignancies of the sinonasal tract and adjacent skull base. Curr Opin Otolaryngol Head Neck Surg 2010;18(2):107–113

57. Hadad G, Bassagasteguy L, Carrau RL, et al. A novel reconstructive technique after endoscopic expanded endonasal approaches: vascular pedicle nasoseptal flap. Laryngoscope 2006;116(10): 1882–1886

58. Leong JL, Citardi MJ, Batra PS. Reconstruction of skull base defects after minimally invasive endoscopic resection of anterior skull base neoplasms. Am J Rhinol 2006;20(5):476–482

59. Kassam A, Carrau RL, Snyderman CH, Gardner P, Mintz A. Evolution of reconstructive techniques following endoscopic expanded endonasal approaches. Neurosurg Focus 2005;19(1):E8

60. Hanna EY, Holsinger C, DeMonte F, Kupferman M. Robotic endoscopic surgery of the skull base: a novel surgical approach. Arch Otolaryngol Head Neck Surg 2007;133(12):1209–1214

61. Liu JK, Weiss MH, Couldwell WT. Surgical approaches to pituitary tumors. Neurosurg Clin N Am 2003;14(1):93–107

62. Cappabianca P, Cavallo LM, de Divitiis O, Solari D, Esposito F, Colao A. Endoscopic pituitary surgery. Pituitary 2008;11(4):385–390

63. Kupferman M, Demonte F, Holsinger FC, Hanna E. Transantral robotic access to the pituitary gland. Otolaryngol Head Neck Surg 2009;141(3):413–415

64. O'Malley BW Jr, Weinstein GS. Robotic anterior and midline skull base surgery: preclinical investigations. Int J Radiat Oncol Biol Phys 2007;69(2, Suppl)S125–S128

65. Wei WI, Sham JS. Nasopharyngeal carcinoma. Lancet 2005;365(9476):2041–2054

66. Chen MY, Wen WP, Guo X, et al. Endoscopic nasopharyngectomy for locally recurrent nasopharyngeal carcinoma. Laryngoscope 2009;119(3):516–522

67. Ozer E, Waltonen J. Transoral robotic nasopharyngectomy: a novel approach for nasopharyngeal lesions. Laryngoscope 2008;118(9): 1613–1616

68. Wei WI, Ho WK. Transoral robotic resection of recurrent nasopharyngeal carcinoma. Laryngoscope 2010;120(10):2011–2014

69. O'Malley BW Jr, Weinstein GS. Robotic skull base surgery: preclinical investigations to human clinical application. Arch Otolaryngol Head Neck Surg 2007;133(12):1215–1219

70. McCool RR, Warren FM, Wiggins RH III, Hunt JP. Robotic surgery of the infratemporal fossa utilizing novel suprahyoid port. Laryngoscope 2010;120(9):1738–1743

Index